# Drug Interactions
# in Infectious Diseases

# Infectious Disease

SERIES EDITOR: *Vassil St. Georgiev*
*National Institute of Allergy and Infectious Diseases*
*National Institutes of Health*

# Drug Interactions in Infectious Diseases

## Second Edition

*Edited by*

## Stephen C. Piscitelli, PharmD

*Director, Discovery Medicine–Antivirals, GlaxoSmithKline,
Research Triangle Park, NC*

## Keith A. Rodvold, PharmD

*Professor of Pharmacy Practice and Associate Professor of Medicine in Pharmacy,
College of Pharmacy and Medicine, University of Illinois at Chicago, Chicago, IL*

*Foreword by*

## Henry Masur, MD

*Chief, Critical Care Medicine Department,
National Institutes of Health, Bethesda, MD*

HUMANA PRESS ✳ TOTOWA, NEW JERSEY

© 2005 Humana Press Inc.
999 Riverview Drive, Suite 208
Totowa, New Jersey 07512

**www.humanapress.com**

The content and opinions expressed in this book are the sole work of the authors and editors, who have warranted due diligence in the creation and issuance of their work. The publisher, editors, and authors are not responsible for errors or omissions or for any consequences arising from the information or opinions presented in this book and make no warranty, express or implied, with respect to its contents.

Due diligence has been taken by the publishers, editors, and authors of this book to assure the accuracy of the information published and to describe generally accepted practices. The contributors herein have carefully checked to ensure that the drug selections and dosages set forth in this text are accurate and in accord with the standards accepted at the time of publication. Notwithstanding, since new research, changes in government regulations, and knowledge from clinical experience relating to drug therapy and drug reactions constantly occur, the reader is advised to check the product information provided by the manufacturer of each drug for any change in dosages or for additional warnings and contraindications. This is of utmost importance when the recommended drug herein is a new or infrequently used drug. It is the responsibility of the treating physician to determine dosages and treatment strategies for individual patients. Further, it is the responsibility of the health care provider to ascertain the Food and Drug Administration status of each drug or device used in their clinical practice. The publishers, editors, and authors are not responsible for errors or omissions or for any consequences from the application of the information presented in this book and make no warranty, express or implied, with respect to the contents in this publication.

This publication is printed on acid-free paper. ∞

ANSI Z39.48-1984 (American Standards Institute) Permanence of Paper for Printed Library Materials.

Production Editor: Nicole E. Furia

Cover design by Patricia F. Cleary

For additional copies, pricing for bulk purchases, and/or information about other Humana titles, contact Humana at the above address or at any of the following numbers: Tel: 973-256-1699; Fax: 973-256-8341; E-mail: orders@humanapr.com, or visit our Website: http://www.humanapress.com.

**Photocopy Authorization Policy:**

eISBN 1-59259-924-9

Printed in the United States of America. 10 9 8 7 6 5 4 3 2 1

Library of Congress Cataloging-in-Publication Data

Drug interactions in infectious diseases / edited by Stephen C. Piscitelli,
Keith A. Rodvold ; foreword by Henry Masur.-- 2nd ed.
    p. cm. -- (Infectious disease)
  Includes bibliographical references and index.
  ISBN 1-58829-455-2 (alk. paper)
  1. Anti-infective agents--Side effects. 2. Drug interactions. I.
Piscitelli, Stephen C. II. Rodvold, Keith. III. Series: Infectious disease
(Totowa, N.J.)
  RM267.D776 2005
  615'.7045--dc22

                         2005000474

# Foreword

Over the past 25 years, the world's population has witnessed an explosion in knowledge about infectious diseases. The global population is coming to the realization that diseases long recognized to cause substantial suffering, such as malaria, tuberculosis, schistosomiasis, and hepatitis, can be diagnosed and treated, and that transmission can be prevented using tools that are available, and which may be becoming increasingly affordable. The global population is recognizing that few infections are local: the travel of humans, other animals, insects, and food transport pathogens around the world, often with astonishing rapidity. New pathogens are appearing, either newly recognized or newly developing, such as severe acute respiratory syndrome (SARS), avian influenza, metapneumovirus, or hepatitis C, which are causing human morbidity and mortality. Finally, there is growing fear that dangerous pathogens may be intentionally introduced into human populations by deranged individuals or terrorist organizations.

The potential to use drugs or biologic agents to treat and prevent infectious diseases has increased dramatically over the past quarter century as we have learned more about the biology of many of these agents, and as we have developed techniques to discover new agents by high throughput screening programs and by sophisticated drug design and synthesis. The development of more than 20 licensed drugs for therapy of HIV infection within 20 years of discovering the etiologic retrovirus is a prime example of the extraordinary capacity the scientific community has to produce safe and effective agents. New drugs to treat hepatitis C, hepatitis B, influenza, staphylococci, enterococci, plasmodia, flukes, candida, and molds also demonstrate the impressive potential the health care industry has to produce new agents.

For all clinicians, it is clear that the scientific advances in understanding pathogenesis of infectious diseases, and in developing new diagnostic tests, new therapeutic agents, and new preventive strategies have made management of diseases both impressively more successful and yet immensely more complex. It is also clear that noninfectious diseases are being managed more successfully with pharmacologic interventions, such that patients may be on multiple agents to treat related or unrelated processes, and to prevent processes, when they develop an acute or chronic infection that needs to be treated. Patients are not uncommonly on drugs for diabetes, lipid disorders, cardiac dysfunction, or inflammatory disorders. In the United States, more and more individuals have altered their dietary habits substantially to reduce weight or improve some other aspect of their health. These diets, or nonprescription drugs or supplements used in the United States or abroad, can have substantial impact on drug pharmacokinetics.

Though therapy with drugs or biologic agents can be highly effective, many factors influence the efficacy and safety of therapy, including adherence, absorption, metabolism, excretion, and drug interactions. Interactions may occur between or among drugs used specifically for treating the infection, such as interactions between two

*v*

antiretroviral agents or interactions between rifampin and quinolones or macrolides. Such interactions can be used for therapeutic advantage, such as the interaction between ritonavir and other protease inhibitors, or these interactions may be potentially harmful, as the interaction between didanosine and stavudine. Interactions may occur between drugs used to manage the infectious disease, and drugs used to manage unrelated problems, such as the interaction between coumadin or phenytoin and ritonavir. Some of the outcomes can be highly undesirable, such as the interaction between rifampin and oral contraceptives. Lastly, interaction can occur between nutritional substances or nonprescription drugs and antiinfectives, such as the interaction between garlic or St. John's Wort or Echinaceae and protease inhibitors.

The first edition of *Drug Interactions in Infectious Diseases* became an important reference for all health care practitioners, and not only pharmacists, since all needed specific data on how to prescribe multidrug regimens in a manner that maximized efficacy and minimized toxicity. The second edition has been revised and updated. The chapter on mechanisms of drug interactions has been expanded into two chapters to allow increased description of absorption, metabolism, and excretion, and to describe the growing knowledge about transport proteins. A useful chapter on regulatory issues including CYP450 probe studies has also been added.

Stephen Piscitelli, PharmD, and Keith Rodvold, PharmD have been pioneers and leaders in recognizing the importance of drug interactions to patient outcome. They have been leaders in designing pharmacokinetic studies that can answer both conceptual questions and practical problems. Most importantly, however, they have recognized the need for health care professionals to have a well organized, definitive source of information to enhance patient care. Safe and effective care for patients is becoming an increasingly complex task best performed by well-trained health care professionals who know how to access data that is vital to their management strategy. The approach to drug interactions described in *Drug Interactions in Infectious Diseases, Second Edition*, and the factual information presented are an essential part of the resources needed to maximize the likelihood that patients will derive the most benefit from available drugs with the least likelihood of harm.

*Henry Masur, MD*

# Preface

Drug interactions in the field of infectious diseases continue to expand as new drugs are approved, new mechanisms are identified, and recommendations for co-administration of drugs are revised. The editors of *Drug Interactions in Infectious Diseases* are gratified that the first edition was well received and we are enthusiastic about the additions and improvements to this second edition.

Major changes have taken place in our understanding of interaction mechanisms. The literature on P-glycoprotein and other transporters has dramatically increased since the first edition. There is so much new knowledge on transport proteins that an entire chapter has been devoted to this issue. We have also included a chapter outlining the regulatory perspective on interaction studies in drug development since guidances from various countries have been put forth. In addition to these new chapters, our authors have updated their chapters to include new drugs that have become available since the first edition. This is especially true in the field of HIV infection, where several new drugs have been approved over the past three years. Finally, the aspects of this text that make it unique are once again present. The chapter on study design and data analysis is one of the best of its kind. New cases have been added to each chapter and highly acclaimed chapters, such as food interactions and drug–cytokine interactions, are updated and revised.

We feel strongly that *Drug Interactions in Infectious Diseases* has something to offer everyone working in the field of infectious diseases. The practicing clinician, academician, or researcher will all find this book useful. The information contained within here ranges from detailed tables on specific drug–drug interactions to in-depth discussions of mechanisms and research issues.

We would again like to thank our excellent group of authors who have devoted so much time into making this more than just a reference book. Their commitment to this textbook clearly shows. Finally, we could not complete such an undertaking without the support of our families who have encouraged us throughout.

*Stephen C. Piscitelli,* PharmD
*Keith A. Rodvold,* PharmD

# Contents

# Contributors

JARRETT R. AMSDEN, PharmD • *Department of Pharmacy Practice, College of Pharmacy, University of Arkansas for Medical Sciences, Little Rock, AR*

JOSEPH S. BERTINO, JR., PharmD • *Scientific Director, Clinical Pharmacology Studies Unit, Ordway Research Institute, Albany, NY*

LARRY H. DANZIGER, PharmD • *Professor of Pharmacy, College of Pharmacy, University of Illinois at Chicago, Chicago, IL*

GEORGE DRUSANO, MD • *Co-Director, Ordway Research Institute, New York State Department of Health, Albany, NY*

STEVEN C. EBERT, PharmD • *Clinical Professor of Pharmacy, University of Wisconsin; Clinical Specialist, Infectious Diseases, Department of Pharmacy, Meriter Hospital, Madison, WI*

DOUGLAS N. FISH, PharmD • *Associate Professor, Department of Clinical Pharmacy, School of Pharmacy, University of Colorado Health Sciences Center; Clinical Specialist in Infectious Diseases/Critical Care, University of Colorado Hospital, Denver, CO*

KEITH GALLICANO, PhD • *Associate Director, Biopharmaceutics, Watson Laboratories, Inc., Corona, CA*

KEVIN W. GAREY, PharmD • *Assistant Professor, College of Pharmacy, University of Houston, Houston, TX*

DAVID R. P. GUAY, PharmD • *Professor, Institute for the Study of Geriatric Pharmacotherapy, College of Pharmacy, University of Minnesota–Minneapolis, Minneapolis, MN; Clinical Specialist, Partnering Care Senior Services, Division of Geriatrics, HealthPartners, Minneapolis, MN*

PAUL O. GUBBINS, PharmD • *Professor, Department of Pharmacy Practice, College of Pharmacy, University of Arkansas for Medical Sciences, Little Rock, AR*

CURTIS E. HAAS, PharmD • *Assistant Professor, School of Pharmacy and Pharmaceutical Sciences, State University of New York at Buffalo, Buffalo, NY*

KELLY A. HARRIS, PharmD • *Clinical Research Scientist, Upsher-Smith Laboratories Inc., Maple Grove, MN*

ANGELA D. M. KASHUBA, PharmD • *Associate Professor, School of Pharmacy, University of North Carolina at Chapel Hill, Chapel Hill, NC*

HENRY MASUR, MD • *Chief, Critical Care Medicine Department, Clinical Center, National Institutes of Health, Bethesda, MD*

SCOTT A. MCCONNELL, PharmD • *Assistant Professor, Department of Pharmacy Practice, College of Pharmacy, University of Arkansas for Medical Sciences, Little Rock, AR*

ROCSANNA NAMDAR, PharmD • *Assistant Professor of Pharmacy, University of New Mexico Health Sciences Center, College of Pharmacy, Albuquerque, NM*

JAMIE L. NELSEN, PharmD • *Research Fellow, School of Pharmacy and Pharmaceutical Sciences, State University of New York at Buffalo, Buffalo, NY*

MELINDA M. NEUHAUSER, PharmD • *Clinical Pharmacy Specialist, Infectious Diseases, Clinical Center Pharmacy Department, National Institutes of Health, Bethesda, MD*

DAVID E. NIX, PharmD • *Associate Professor, Department of Pharmacy Practice and Science, The University of Arizona College of Pharmacy; Clinical Pharmacist, Infectious Diseases, University Medical Center, Tucson, AZ*

CHARLES A. PELOQUIN, PharmD • *Director, Infectious Disease Pharmacokinetics Laboratory, National Jewish Medical and Research Center; Professor of Pharmacy and Medicine, University of Colorado, Denver, CO*

SCOTT R. PENZAK, PharmD • *Coordinator, Clinical Pharmacokinetics Research Laboratory, Warren G. Magnuson Clinical Center, Pharmacy Department, National Institutes of Health, Bethesda, MD*

STEPHEN C. PISCITELLI, PharmD • *Director, Discovery Medicine - Antivirals, GlaxoSmithKline, Research Triangle Park, NC*

KELLIE SCHOOLAR REYNOLDS, PharmD • *Clinical Pharmacology Team Leader, Office of Clinical Pharmacology and Biopharmaceutics, Center for Drug Evaluation and Research, United States Food and Drug Administration, Rockville, MD*

KEITH A. RODVOLD, PharmD • *Professor of Pharmacy Practice and Associate Professor of Medicine in Pharmacy, College of Pharmacy and Medicine, University of Illinois at Chicago, Chicago, IL*

KIMBERLY A. STRUBLE, PharmD • *Senior Clinical Analyst, Division of Antiviral Drug Products, Center for Drug Evaluation and Research, United States Food and Drug Administration, Rockville, MD*

GREGORY M. SUSLA, PharmD • *Pharmacy Manager, VHA Inc., Frederick, MD*

ALICE TSENG, PharmD, FCSHP • *Assistant Professor, Faculty of Pharmacy, University of Toronto; HIV Clinical Pharmacist, Immunodeficiency Clinic, Toronto General Hospital, Toronto, Ontario, Canada*

# Introduction to Drug Interactions

## Keith Gallicano and George Drusano

## INTRODUCTION

Human immunodeficiency virus (HIV), more than any other disease, is responsible for the renewed interest in drug interactions by physicians, pharmacists, nurses, scientists, and regulatory agencies. The importance of managing drug interactions in infectious diseases moved to the forefront as more drugs spanning the different classes of infectious disease agents became available to treat HIV and prevent or treat opportunistic infections and HIV-related malignancies. This has led to recognition of the potential for and impact of drug interactions in other infectious diseases and with a variety of anti-infective drug classes. Recent reviews *(1–4)*, including those in this volume, and the development of computerized drug interaction databases *(5)* further attest to the revived interest and importance of drug interactions in the different therapeutic areas of infectious diseases.

Numerous workshops and symposia devoted specifically to drug interactions have emerged since 1995. Pharmaceutical manufacturers are conducting more pharmacokinetic drug interaction studies earlier rather than during late Phase II and Phase III of clinical drug development or during postmarket surveillance. Many of these studies are rationally designed from in vitro studies that use specific human cell lines, tissues, or tissue components. Regulatory authorities in Canada (Therapeutic Products Programme) *(6)*, the United States (Food and Drug Administration) *(7,8)*, and Europe (The European Agency for the Evaluation of Medicinal Products) *(9)* have produced guidance for conducting in vitro and clinical drug interaction studies. These guides emphasize the importance of appropriate study design and data analysis techniques, which are highlighted in Chapter 15 of this volume. Further regulatory perspective is presented in Chapter 4. Drug product labels and monographs now frequently include detailed information on drug interactions. This widespread interest in drug interactions has resulted in more scientific and clinical data available to the consumer and prescriber. Consequently, the management of drug interactions has become more challenging.

Drug interactions represent one of eight categories of drug-related problems that have been identified as events or circumstances of drug therapy that may interfere with optimal clinical outcome *(10)*. Identification, resolution, and prevention of drug-related prob-

From: *Infectious Disease: Drug Interactions in Infectious Diseases, Second Edition*
Edited by: S. C. Piscitelli and K. A. Rodvold © Humana Press Inc., Totowa, NJ

**Table 1**
**Drug-Related Factors Affecting Drug Interactions**

- Narrow therapeutic range
- Low bioavailability
- Drug formulation (presence of interacting excipients)
- Drug stereochemical and physiochemical properties
- Drug potency
- Steep dose–response curve
- Duration of therapy (acute vs chronic administration)
- Drug dosage (a higher dose yields a more significant interaction)
- Drug concentration in blood and tissue
- Timing and sequence of administration of interacting drugs
  (staggered vs simultaneous administration)
- Route of administration
- Baseline blood concentration of interacting drug and its therapeutic index
- Extent of drug metabolism (fraction of systemic clearance from metabolism)
- Rate of drug metabolism (hepatic extraction ratio and hepatic clearance)
- Degree of protein binding of interacting drugs
- Volume of distribution of affected drug

**Table 2**
**Patient-Related Factors Affecting Drug Interactions**

- Body weight, composition, and size
- Quantity and activity of specific drug-metabolizing enzymes
  (genetic polymorphism)
- Inherent inter- and intraindividual variability in pharmacokinetics
  and pharmacological response
- Age
- Gender
- Race
- Tobacco use
- Alcohol use (acute or chronic)
- Diet
- Underlying disease states and their severity (acute, chronic, unstable)
- Malfunction and disease of organs of drug elimination (e.g., liver, kidney)
- Polypharmacy (particularly with enzyme inhibitors or inducers)

lems are important determinants for patient management and are the responsibility of those providing pharmaceutical care. The continued development of new, high-potency drugs increases the potential for drug interactions. However, the incidence of clinically important interactions remains difficult to quantify because both drug-related (Table 1) and patient-related (Table 2) factors influence the likelihood of a clinically relevant interaction occurring. Consideration must also be given to the level of documentation of the interaction, the frequency of use of the coadministered agents, and the mechanism and time-course of the interaction.

A drug interaction occurs when the pharmacokinetics or pharmacodynamics of a drug in the body are altered by the presence of one or more interacting substances. The most commonly encountered or perceived interactions are those between two drugs. However, multiple drug interactions are possible with the polypharmaceutical drug regimens often encountered in the prophylaxis and treatment of infectious diseases. Other than drug–drug interactions, drugs may interact with food *(11)*; drink *(12)*; nutrients (e.g., vitamins, minerals); alternative medicines (herbal products, homeopathic remedies) *(13,14)*; drug formulations (e.g., excipients) *(15)*; cytokines; or environmental chemical agents (e.g., cigarette smoke) *(16)*. Drug–food and drug–cytokine interactions are discussed in Chapters 12 and 13, respectively. Various disease states may also alter the magnitude and duration of interaction.

The term *drug interaction* is sometimes used to describe in vitro and ex vivo interactions that occur outside the body. These pharmaceutical or physicochemical interactions result from the physical incompatibility of drugs (e.g., admixtures in intravenous lines), from contact with pharmaceutical packaging or devices, or in loss of drug during laboratory analysis (e.g., binding to storage containers). This volume focuses on drug interactions that occur within the body.

## PHARMACOKINETIC DRUG INTERACTIONS

Pharmacokinetic interactions alter the absorption, transport, distribution, metabolism, or excretion of a drug. Corresponding or independent changes in pharmacological response or therapeutic outcome may or may not occur *(6,12,17,18)*. The rate and extent of absorption can be affected by physicochemical factors such as complexation and nonspecific adsorption of the drug and by physiological factors such as gastrointestinal motility, gastrointestinal pH, presence of gastrointestinal disease, gastric emptying time, intestinal blood flow, intestinal metabolism, and inhibition/induction of transport proteins (e.g., P-glycoprotein). In infectious diseases, changes in extent are more clinically important than changes in rate of absorption. As safety and effectiveness are concerns in pharmacokinetic interaction studies, the use of *exposure* rather than *rate and extent of absorption* concepts is encouraged, because the term exposure expresses more clinical relevance and focuses on the shape of the drug concentration–time profile *(19)*.

Altered distribution in drug interactions is explained mainly by displacement of drug from plasma proteins or receptor-binding sites. The most common binding proteins are the high-affinity, low-capacity protein $\alpha_1$-acid glycoprotein and the low-affinity, high-capacity protein albumin. Protein-binding displacement interactions after oral and intravenous dosing of low hepatically and nonhepatically extracted drugs are generally clinically unimportant because unbound drug concentrations at steady state in plasma do not change or are only transiently changed by displacement *(20–22)*. Average unbound plasma concentrations at steady state of high hepatically extracted drugs administered orally are also not expected to be affected by displacement, provided that changes in bioavailability and unbound clearance are proportional. Moreover, drugs that are bound to both $\alpha_1$-acid glycoprotein and albumin may show no overall change in fraction of unbound drug in plasma because displacement from $\alpha_1$-acid glycoprotein can be buffered by binding to albumin (e.g., saquinavir; *[23]*). Protein-displacement interactions may cause adverse events if the displaced drug is highly bound (>95%) to plasma proteins at therapeutic concentrations and has a small volume of distribution and a narrow therapeutic range.

Most clinically relevant interactions result from changes in drug elimination caused by inhibition or induction of metabolic enzymes present in the liver and extrahepatic tissues *(17,24)*. These processes can cause changes in intrinsic clearance of elimination pathways, which result in alterations in unbound plasma concentrations at steady state for orally administered drugs. The clinical consequences of inhibition or induction can be difficult to predict when active or toxic metabolites are present. Inhibition results in accumulation of the parent drug, whereas induction decreases concentrations of the parent drug. However, concentrations of active metabolites can increase or decrease depending on whether their formation and elimination are directly or indirectly affected by inhibition or induction and thus influence whether a metabolite predisposes patients to drug toxicity or lack of drug effectiveness. Furthermore, metabolites may persist longer than parent drug in plasma after an inhibitor is discontinued. The extent of pharmacokinetic consequences depends on the contribution to overall drug elimination and the relative importance of the affected pathways. Pharmacokinetic mechanisms are discussed in further detail in Chapters 2 and 3.

The outcome of a pharmacokinetic drug interaction may be no measurable pharmacological or toxicological effects or enhancement or diminution of these effects. Harm may result from interactions that cause elevated drug exposure, leading to an increase in adverse effects or reduced drug exposure, leading to a decrease in the desired effect or the development of drug-resistant organisms. However, benefit may be obtained from interactions that increase drug exposure, improve therapeutic outcome, and minimize side effects. The use of ritonavir to enhance blood concentrations of other protease inhibitors in antiretroviral treatment of HIV is an example of a beneficial pharmacokinetic interaction that provides enhanced viral suppression *(4)*.

## PHARMACODYNAMIC DRUG INTERACTIONS

Pharmacodynamic interactions are an alteration in the pharmacological response of a drug. They may be caused by direct competition at certain sites of action or by indirectly involving altered physiological mechanisms but do not always modify a drug's concentration in tissue fluids. Different terminology is used to describe outcomes depending on whether two drugs are active or inactive *(25)*. If the response from the combination is greater than predicted, then the outcome is termed *synergism* (both drugs active), *potentiation* (one drug active), or *coalism* (neither drug active). If the response is equal to that predicted, then the outcome is termed *additivity/independence* (both drugs active) or *inertism* (one or both drugs inactive). *Antagonism* refers to a less-than-predicted response if one or both drugs are active. Idiosyncratic interactions produce effects that are not expected based on the known effects of either agent when given alone.

Pharmacodynamic interactions can be beneficial in that an improved therapeutic response may occur or be detrimental in that toxicity may be heightened. Also, therapeutic activity and toxic effects may occur simultaneously in opposite directions, resulting in a balance between positive and negative responses. Beneficial pharmacodynamic drug interactions abound in infectious disease therapy because of the many of drug combinations used to treat infections. An example of such an interaction is the effective synergistic combination of ampicillin and gentamicin or streptomycin in the treatment of enterococcal endocarditis *(26)*.

## PHARMACOEPIDEMIOLOGY

The reports of overall frequency of drug–drug interactions vary widely in the literature *(27)*. Incidence rates reported in the 1970s and 1980s ranged between 2.2 and 70.3% for ambulatory, hospitalized, or nursing-home patients *(28–34)*. Overall, the incidence of potentially harmful drug interactions is generally low, but certain populations, such as the elderly, extensive or poor metabolizers, those with hepatic or renal dysfunction, and those who are likely to take multiple medications, particularly for off-label use, are more at risk. Data collected over 1995–1997 suggest that potential interactions are as high as 75% in the population with HIV, with an actual 25% incidence of clinically significant interactions *(35)*.

Some studies have attempted to quantify the incidence of symptoms resulting from these potential interactions. A range of 0 to 1% has been reported in hospitalized patients (36), but the incidence is likely increasing *(35)*. Although the number of potential interactions may be high and the number of clinically significant interactions in many reports appears low, there are still data that indicate drug interactions can lead to harmful consequences *(37–40)*. An inability to quantify the actual incidence accurately should not minimize the importance of this drug-related problem.

The variance in incidence in the early literature can be attributed to a number of factors *(27–29,41)*. Study methodologies differed with respect to design (retrospective or prospective), population studied, interactions/categories that were assessed, definitions of clinical significance, denominators used to calculate incidence, and methods used to determine the incidence of the significant interactions *(36)*. Underreporting of drug interactions also likely occurred.

Literature reports of drug interactions began in the 1970s, when there were fewer drugs on the market. Knowledge of mechanisms of interactions, particularly in drug metabolism, has since grown, leading to recognition of more potential interactions. Improvements in analytical methods to measure drug levels in biological fluids has led to more refined and robust techniques with better selectivity, sensitivity, and efficiency for characterizing drug interactions. This has led to inclusion of pharmacokinetics (e.g., therapeutic drug monitoring) with clinical decision making for a number of agents. The means to evaluate drug interactions, either mechanistically or clinically, are now readily accessible to the clinician.

## PHARMACOECONOMICS

The literature suggests that up to 2.8% of hospitalizations result from drug interactions *(36)*. An association also has been found between the risk of hospitalization and interactions of various medications, including anti-infective agents, thus supporting the premise that drug interactions compromise health and incur costs *(42)*. Individual case reports can demonstrate the measurable financial impact of drug interactions. However, quality of life and cost to the patient and society are less apparent but equally or more important *(43)*. Although data are scarce regarding cost increases secondary to drug interactions, the impact of such events remains a concern *(44)*.

## CLINICAL VS STATISTICAL SIGNIFICANCE

The term *clinical significance* describes the degree to which a drug interaction changes the underlying disease or the condition of the patient *(45)*. The magnitude of the change in effects may be statistically significant but not clinically relevant. A measurable effect such as a change in blood drug concentrations or laboratory parameters must be interpreted regarding whether the effect produces a change in clinical outcome. An interaction is considered clinically relevant when the therapeutic activity or toxicity of a drug is changed to such an extent that a dosage adjustment of the medication or medical intervention may be required *(9)*. Next, the desired outcome must be assessed in relation to benefit and risk before changes in management are made.

An important statistical and clinical consideration is the evaluation of changes in both "mean" and individual pharmacokinetic and pharmacodynamic variables. Drug interaction reports may conclude that a mean change is statistically and clinically insignificant, but certain individuals may be affected by the drug interaction. Evaluation of individual changes in study participants is therefore important to determine if a particular subset of individuals responds differently to the treatment. Conversely, some individuals are not affected by drug interactions even though significant mean changes may occur.

The aim of many interaction studies is to demonstrate that there is no clinically relevant interaction. The currently accepted bioequivalence approach (i.e., the inclusion of the 90% confidence limits for the ratio/difference of the means or medians within some prespecified equivalence range) seems appropriate *(46)*. The equivalence interval represents the range of clinically acceptable variation in mean or median pharmacokinetic changes and is the only link between clinical and blood concentration significance. For agents with wide therapeutic windows, an equivalence range of ±20% or higher appears reasonable, depending on the drug. However, a smaller equivalence range may be required for agents with a narrow therapeutic window. A detailed presentation on biostatistical concepts in drug interaction studies is provided in Chapter 15.

## CLINICAL SIGNIFICANCE GRADING

The clinical significance grading of a detrimental drug interaction can be difficult. The level of documentation must be assessed to determine the degree of confidence that the interaction exists. The predictability of drug interactions from documentation can be divided into five levels: established (well documented), probable, suspected, possible, or unlikely. The data may be from in vitro studies, animal studies, anecdotal case reports, or randomized controlled trials in the target population or healthy volunteers.

The severity of the interaction must also be graded and can be classified into three levels: minor, moderate, or major. An interaction of minor severity is one that may occur but is not considered significant as potential harm to the patient is likely slight. An example is the minor decrease in ciprofloxacin absorption with antacids when doses are taken more than 2 hours apart *(47)*. An interaction of moderate severity is one for which potential harm to the patient may be possible, and some type of intervention/monitoring is often warranted. An example of a moderate interaction is the combination of vancomycin and gentamicin, for which monitoring for nephrotoxicity is important *(48)*. An interaction of major severity is one that has a high probability of harm to the patient, including outcomes that are life threatening. An example is the development of arrhythmias caused by the coadministration of erythromycin and terfenadine *(49)*.

The *Drug Interaction Facts* classification scheme combines the three severity levels and five documentation levels into 15 interaction categories, with five levels of clinical significance assigned to those 15 categories *(50)*. A scale of the clinical significance of drug–drug interactions that reflects the professional judgments of practicing pharmacists has been proposed by Roberts et al. *(45)*.

## EVALUATION OF DRUG INTERACTION LITERATURE

Each report of a drug interaction must be assessed for a variety of criteria *(17)*. Management decisions should be in response to clinically important outcomes resulting from coadministration of drugs. Consideration must be given to the time-course of the interaction (or lack thereof if a negative report is under assessment) to be sure that the occurrence of the most prominent effect is captured. The timing and order of administration of drugs must be evaluated in drug interaction reports because the sequence of administration can determine if an interaction will manifest. Interactions that affect drug absorption can often be mitigated by staggering the dosages and giving the object drug (i.e., drug with the effect that is altered) first. Examples are drug–food (Chapter 12) and quinolone–antacid (Chapter 8) interactions. Dose also affects interactions. A smaller-than-usual dose reduces the chance of observing an interaction, whereas a larger-than-usual dose increases the possibility of detecting an interaction.

Drug interactions reported for one member of a drug class may not reflect those of other members of that class *(51)*. Drugs within a class usually have different pharmacokinetic properties, which lead to differing interaction patterns for individual drugs. Studies in healthy volunteers instead of diseased subjects must be viewed with caution. Patients may be at higher risk of adverse outcomes associated with a predisposition to drug interactions because of their disease. Also, study populations may be too restrictive and not representative of the target population. As mentioned in the Clinical vs Statistical Significance section, another consideration is the reporting of mean pharmacokinetic changes that do not reflect the range of observed changes in certain individuals.

## CLINICAL MANAGEMENT

After assessing the level of documentation in the literature and the significance grading of the interaction, consideration must be given to the onset and offset of the event, the mechanism, the change in outcome, management suggestions, and any discussion in the available literature concerning the interaction. When a patient has been identified to be at risk of experiencing a clinically relevant drug interaction, steps must be taken to prevent or minimize this potential event *(17)*. If possible, the combination should be avoided or one or more of the agents stopped. The medication(s) may be replaced by noninteracting medication(s) that are therapeutically equivalent, doses may be staggered, dose strength or interval may be modified, or the route of administration may be changed.

An important consideration is not to overreact to potential interactions. Actions such as discontinuation of an important agent in the management of the patient, an unnecessary increase or decrease in dose, needless increased visits for monitoring, or extraneous orders for drug concentration measurements or laboratory work are not desirable. A five-class categorization system for management has been recommended and is presented in Table 3 *(52)*.

**Table 3**
**Classification Scheme for Management of Drug Interactions**

| | |
|---|---|
| Class 1 | Avoid administration of the drug combination. The risk of adverse patient outcome precludes the concomitant administration of the drugs. |
| Class 2 | Combination should be avoided unless it is determined that the benefit of coadministration of the drugs outweighs the risk to the patient. The use of an alternative to one of the interacting drugs is recommended when appropriate. Patients should be monitored carefully if the drugs are coadministered. |
| Class 3 | Several potential management options are available: use of an alternative agent, change in drug regimen (dose, interval) or route of administration to minimize the interaction, or monitor patient if drugs are coadministered. |
| Class 4 | Potential for harm is low and no specific action is required other than to be aware of the possibility of the drug interaction. |
| Class 5 | Available evidence suggests no interaction. |

## CURRENT TRENDS: PREDICTION OF IN VIVO INTERACTIONS FROM IN VITRO DATA

Although human studies provide the most definitive data on the likelihood and magnitude of a drug interaction, there are important limitations to performing such studies. There is always potential risk to the subject, even if it is small or unlikely. Regulatory requirements for control and monitoring of these studies are becoming increasingly costly and time consuming. Consequently, the number and spectrum of studies that can be performed are limited. A search for alternatives has led to the use of human liver components (e.g., microsomes, hepatocytes) or other tissues to represent or predict the interaction in vivo *(53)*. Chapters 2 and 3 provide an overview of in vitro methods to predict drug interactions.

There are now human liver banks that have microsomes and purified or recombinant human cytochrome P450 enzymes available for extensive in vitro study of metabolic pathways of new drugs *(54)*. During early development of a new drug, these in vitro systems can predict if the drug will display variations in clearance from genetic polymorphism, and if the drug will be susceptible to clinically significant interactions. They also allow the determination of mechanisms of previously observed, unexplained interactions. Moreover, multiple drug interactions are easier to investigate in vitro than in vivo. Some concerns of in vitro/in vivo scaling include differences in the concentrations used in vitro compared to those obtained in vivo at the metabolizing enzyme *(53,54)*, the isolation of the enzyme when studied in vitro, and the lack of specific markers available for in vivo studies to confirm in vitro findings *(54)*. Nevertheless, in vitro screens offer a useful early warning system for the rational selection of in vivo studies provided there is careful analysis of all pharmacokinetic information available.

## CONCLUSION

With the increasing appreciation of known and potentially important drug interactions covering the broad spectrum of infectious diseases, the need for clarification of the clinical importance of these interactions has become imperative. An awareness of the role of pharmacokinetics, pharmacodynamics, and factors that alter these processes and insight into differentiating clinical and statistically significant effects are important variables in the clinician's process of decision making.

This volume is intended to provide an in-depth review of drug interactions related to a number of topics in infectious diseases. An emphasis on the clinical approach with specific examples and cases will guide the reader in developing skills for identifying drug interactions and problem drugs as well as strategies for circumventing of drug interactions.

## REFERENCES

1. Piscitelli SC, Gallicano KD. Interactions among drugs for HIV and opportunistic infections. N Engl J Med 2001;344:984–996.
2. Albengres E, Le Louet H, Tillement JP. Systemic antifungal agents: drug interactions of clinical significance. Drug Safety 1998;18:83–97.
3. Von Rosenstiel N-A, Adam D. Macrolide antibiotics: drug interactions of clinical significance. Drug Safety 1995;13:105–122.
4. Malaty LI, Kuper JJ. Drug interactions of HIV protease inhibitors. Drug Safety 1999;20: 147–169.
5. Foisy MM, Tseng A. Development of an interactive computer-assisted program to manage medication therapy in HIV-infected patients. Drug Inf J 1998;32:649–656.
6. Therapeutic Products Programme Guidance Document. Drug–drug interactions: studies in vitro and in vivo (September 21, 2000). Therapeutics Products Directorate, Health Canada.
7. Center for Drug Evaluation and Research, Center for Biologics Evaluation and Research. Guidance for Industry in vivo drug metabolism/drug interaction studies—study design, data analysis, and recommendations for dosing and labeling (November 1999). US Department of Health and Human Services, Food and Drug Administration.
8. Center for Drug Evaluation and Research, Center for Biologics Evaluation and Research. Guidance for Industry drug metabolism/drug interaction studies in the development process: studies in vitro (April 1997). US Department of Health and Human Services, Food and Drug Administration.
9. Committee for Proprietary Medicinal Products (CPMP). Note for Guidance on the investigation of drug interactions (December 1997). The European Agency for the Evaluation of Medicinal Products Human Medicines Evaluation Unit.
10. Hepler CD, Strand LM. Opportunities and responsibilities in pharmaceutical care. Am J Hosp Pharm 1990;47:533–543.
11. Gauthier I, Malone M. Drug–food interactions in hospitalized patients. Drug Safety 1998; 18:383–393.
12. Fuhr U. Drug interactions with grapefruit juice: extent, probable mechanism and clinical relevance. Drug Safety 1998;18:251–272.
13. D'Arcy PF. Adverse reactions and interactions with herbal medicines. Adverse Drug React Toxicol Rev 1991;10:189–208.
14. D'Arcy PF. Adverse reactions and interactions. Part 2. Adverse Drug React Toxicol Rev 1993;12:147–162.
15. Sahai J, Gallicano K, Oliveras L, Khaliq S, Hawley-Foss N, Garber, G. Cations in didanosine tablet reduce ciprofloxacin bioavailability. Clin Pharmacol Ther 1993;53:292–297.
16. Schein JR. Cigarette smoking and clinically significant drug interactions. Ann Pharmacother 1995;29:1139–1148.
17. Hansten P. Drug interactions. In: Applied Therapeutics: The Clinical Use of Drugs. Vancouver, WA: Applied Therapeutics, 1995, pp. 2–10.

18. Gibaldi M. Drug interactions: part II. Ann Pharmacother 1992;26:829–834.

19. Tozer TN, Bois FY, Hauck WW, Chen M-L, Williams RL. Absorption rate vs exposure: which is more useful for bioequivalence testing? Pharm Res 1996;13:453–456.

20. Rolan PE. Plasma protein binding displacement interactions—why are they still regarded as clinically important? Br J Clin Pharmacol 1994;37:125–128.

21. MacKichan JJ. Protein binding drug displacement interactions fact or fiction? Clin Pharmacokinet 1989;16:65–73.

22. Benet LZ, Hoener B-A. Changes in plasma protein binding have little clinical relevance. Clin Pharmacol Ther 2002;71:115–121.

23. Halifax KL, Lindup WE, Barry MG, Wiltshire HR, Back DJ. Binding of the HIV protease inhibitor saquinavir to human plasma proteins. Br J Clin Pharmacol 1998;46:291P.

24. Michalets EL. Update: clinically significant cytochrome P-450 drug interactions. Pharmacotherapy 1998;18:84–112.

25. Greco WR, Bravo G, Parsons JC. The search for synergy: a critical review from a response surface perspective. Pharmacol Rev 1995;47:331–385.

26. Murillo J, Standiford HC, Holley HP, Tatem BA, Caplan ES. Prophylaxis against enterococcal endocarditis: comparison of the aminoglycoside component of parenteral antimicrobial regimens. Antimicrob Agents Chemother 1980;18:448–453.

27. Jankel CA, Speedie SM. Detecting drug interactions: a review of the literature. DICP, Ann Pharmacother 1990;24:982–988.

28. Gosney M, Tallis R. Prescription of contraindicated and interacting drugs in elderly patients admitted to hospital. Lancet 1984;1:564–567.

29. Shinn AF, Shrewsbury RP, Anderson KW. Development of a computerized drug interaction database (MEDICOM) for use in a patient specific environment. Drug Inf J 1983;17:205–210.

30. Jinks MJ, Hansten PD, Hirschman JL. Drug interaction exposures in an ambulatory Medicaid population. Am J Hosp Pharm 1979;36:923–927.

31. Mitchell GW, Stanaszek WF, Nichols NB. Documenting drug–drug Interactions in ambulatory patients. Am J Hosp Pharm 1979;36:653–657.

32. Cooper JW, Wellins I, Fish KH, Loomis ME. Frequency of potential drug–drug interactions. J Am Pharm Assoc 1975;15:24–31.

33. Durrence CW III, DiPiro JT, May JR, Nesbit RR, Sisley JF, Cooper JW. Potential drug interactions in surgical patients. Am J Hosp Pharm 1985;42:1553–1556.

34. Puckett WH, Visconti JA. An epidemiologic study of the clinical significance of drug–drug interactions in a private community hospital. Am J Hosp Pharm 1971;28:247–253.

35. Foisy MM, Gough K, Quan CM, Harris K, Ibanez D, Phillips A. Hospitalizations due to adverse drug reactions and interactions pre- and post-HAART [abstract B215]. Can J Infect Dis 1999;10(suppl B):24B.

36. Jankel CA, Fitterman LK. Epidemiology of drug-drug interactions as a cause of hospital admissions. Drug Safety 1993;9:51–59.

37. Honig PK, Wortham DC, Amani K, Conner D, Mullin JC, Cantilena LR. Terfenadine–ketoconazole interaction: pharmacokinetic and electrocardiographic consequences. JAMA 1993;269:1513–1518.

38. Henry JA, Hill IR. Fatal interaction between ritonavir and MDMA. Lancet 1998;352:1751–1752.

39. Lees RS, Lees AM. Rhabdomyolysis from the coadministration of lovastatin and the antifungal agent itraconazole. N Engl J Med 1995;333:664–665.

40. Pollak PT, Sketris IS, MacKenzie SL, Hewlett TJ. Delirium probably induced by clarithromycin in a patient receiving fluoxetine. Ann Pharmacother 1995;29:486–488.

41. Kwan TC, Wahba WW, Wildeman RA. Drug interactions: a retrospective study of its epidemiology, clinical significance and influence upon hospitalization. Can J Hosp Pharm 1979;32:12–16.

42. Hamilton RA, Briceland LL, Andritz MH. Frequency of hospitalization after exposure to known drug–drug interactions in a Medicaid population. Pharmacother 1998;18:1112–1120.
43. Kennedy DT, Hayney MS, Lake KD. Azathioprine and allopurinol: the price of an avoidable drug interaction. Ann Pharmacother 1996;30:951–954.
44. Nightingale CH, Quintiliani R. Cost of oral antibiotic therapy. Pharmacother 1997;17:302–307.
45. Roberts JS, Watrous ML, Schulz RM, Mauch RP, Nightengale BS. Quantifying the clinical significance of drug–drug interactions: scaling pharmacists' perceptions of a common interaction classification scheme. Ann Pharmacother 1996;30:926–934.
46. Steinijans VW, Hartmanns M, Huber R, Radtke HW. Lack of pharmacokinetic interaction as an equivalence problem. Int J Clin Pharmacol Ther Toxicol 1991;29:323–328.
47. Nix DE, Watson WA, Lener ME, et al. Effects of aluminum and magnesium antacids and ranitidine on the absorption of ciprofloxacin. Clin Pharmacol Ther 1989;46:700–705.
48. Rybak MJ Albrecht LM, Boike SC, Chandrasekar PH. Nephrotoxicity of vancomycin, alone and with an aminoglycoside. J Antimicrob Chemother 1990;25:679–687.
49. Honig PK, Woosley RL, Zamani K, Conner DP, Cantilena LR Jr. Changes in the pharmacokinetics and electrocardiographic pharmacodynamics of terfenadine with concomitant administration of erythromycin. Clin Pharmacol Ther 1992;52:231–238.
50. Tatro DS, ed. Drug interaction facts. Facts and comparisons. St. Louis, MO: Wolters Kluwer, 1998.
51. Rapp RP. Pharmacokinetics and pharmacodynamics of intravenous and oral azithromycin: enhanced tissue activity and minimal drug interactions. Ann Pharmacother 1998;32:785–793.
52. Hansten PD, Horn JR, eds. Hansten and Horn's Drug Interactions Analysis and Management. Vancouver, WA: Applied Therapeutics, 1999.
53. Von Moltke LL, Greenblatt DJ, Schmider J, Wright CE, Harmatz JS, Shader RI. In vitro approaches to predicting drug interactions in vivo. Biochem Pharmacol 1998;55:113–122.
54. Touw DJ. Clinical implications of genetic polymorphisms and drug interactions mediated by cytochrome P450 enzymes. Drug Metab Drug Interact 1997;14:55–82.

# 2

# Mechanisms of Drug Interactions I

*Absorption, Metabolism, and Excretion*

## Angela D. M. Kashuba and Joseph S. Bertino, Jr.

## INTRODUCTION

Each year, 150 million outpatient prescriptions for antibiotics are dispensed in the United States *(1)*. In institutional settings, 25 to 35% of hospitalized patients receive antibiotic treatment for active infections or to prevent infections *(2)*. Given that antibiotics represent global sales of approx $20 billion of a $370 billion pharmaceutical market, one can assume that many patients who are prescribed antibiotics are also receiving other agents *(3)*. Therefore, the potential for drug interactions is significant.

It is difficult to assess the overall clinical importance of many drug interactions. Often, drug interaction reports are based on anecdotal or case reports, and their mechanisms are not clearly defined. In addition, determining clinical significance requires an assessment of the severity of potential harm. This makes an unequivocal determination of "clinically significant" difficult.

Drug interactions can be pharmacokinetic or pharmacodynamic. Pharmacokinetic interactions result from alterations in a drug's absorption, distribution, metabolism, or excretion characteristics. Pharmacodynamic interactions are a result of the influence of combined treatment at a site of biological activity and yield altered pharmacological actions at standard plasma concentrations. Although drug interactions occur through a variety of mechanisms, the effects are the same: the potentiation or antagonism of the effects of drugs.

The mechanisms by which changes in absorption, distribution, and excretion occur have been understood for decades. However, only recently has technology allowed for a more thorough understanding of drug-metabolizing isoforms and influences thereon. Much information has been published regarding drug interactions involving the cytochrome P450 (CYP) enzyme system *(4–8)*. This is an important focus of this chapter because the majority of currently available anti-infectives are metabolized by, or influence the activity of, the CYP enzyme system. This chapter provides a detailed review of the mechanisms by which clinically significant pharmacokinetic drug interactions occur.

From: *Infectious Disease: Drug Interactions in Infectious Diseases, Second Edition*
Edited by: S. C. Piscitelli and K. A. Rodvold © Humana Press Inc., Totowa, NJ

**Table 1**
**Potential Mechanisms of Drug Interactions**
**Involving Absorption and Distribution**

Absorption
- Altered gastric pH
- Chelation of compounds
- Adsorption of compounds
- Altered gastric emptying
- Altered intestinal motility
- Altered intestinal blood flow
- Altered active and passive intestinal transport
- Altered intestinal cytochrome P450 isozyme activity
- Altered intestinal P-glycoprotein activity

Distribution
- Altered protein binding

## DRUG INTERACTIONS AFFECTING ABSORPTION

Mechanisms of absorption include passive diffusion, convective transport, active transport, facilitated transport, ion-pair transport, and endocytosis *(9)*. Certain drug combinations can affect the rate or extent of absorption of anti-infectives by interfering with one or more of these mechanisms *(10)*. Generally, a change in the extent of a medication's absorption of greater than 20% may be considered clinically significant *(11)*. The most common mechanisms of drug interactions affecting absorption are discussed in Table 1.

### Changes in pH

The rate of drug absorption by passive diffusion is limited by the solubility, or dissolution, of a compound in gastric fluid. Basic drugs are more soluble in acidic fluids, and acidic drugs are more soluble in basic fluids. Therefore, compounds that create an environment with a specific pH may decrease the solubility of compounds needing an opposing pH for absorption. However, drug solubility does not completely ensure absorption because only un-ionized molecules are absorbed. Although acidic drugs are soluble in basic fluids, basic environments can also decrease the proportion of solubilized acidic molecules that are in an un-ionized state. Therefore, weak acids ($pK_a = 3–8$) may have limited absorption in an alkaline environment, and weak bases ($pK_a = 5–11$) have limited absorption in an acidic environment.

These interactions can be clinically significant. For example, because the nucleoside analog didanosine is acid labile and requires a neutral-to-basic pH to be absorbed, all didanosine formulations are buffered. However, medications known to require an acidic environment for dissolution, such as ketoconazole, itraconazole, and dapsone, have demonstrated significantly decreased absorption when given concomitantly *(12–15)*.

Antacids, histamine receptor antagonists, and proton pump inhibitors all raise gastric pH to varying degrees. Antacids transiently (0.5–2 hours) raise gastric pH by 1–2 units *(16)*, $H_2$-antagonists dose-dependently maintain gastric pH above 5.0 for many hours, and proton pump inhibitors dose-dependently raise gastric pH above 5.0 for up to 19 hours *(17)*. The concomitant administration of these compounds leads to significant alterations in the extent of absorption of basic compounds such as certain azole antifungals and β-lactam antibiotics *(11,18–23)*. However, because of large interindividual variability in the extent of altered gastric pH, significant interactions may not occur in all patients.

## Chelation and Adsorption

Drugs may form insoluble complexes by chelation in the gastrointestinal tract. Chelation involves the formation of a ring structure between a metal ion (e.g., aluminum, magnesium, iron, and to a lesser degree calcium) and an organic molecule (e.g., anti-infective medication), which results in an insoluble compound that is unable to permeate the intestinal mucosa because of the lack of drug dissolution.

A number of examples of the influence on anti-infective exposure by this mechanism exist in the literature, involving primarily the quinolone antibiotics in combination with magnesium- and aluminum-containing antacids, sucralfate, ferrous sulfate, or certain buffers. These di- and trivalent cations complex with the 4-oxo and 3-carboxyl groups of the quinolones, resulting in clinically significant decreases in the quinolone area under the concentration–time curve (AUC) by 30 to 50% *(24–27)*. Cations present in enteral feeding formulations do not appear to interfere significantly with the absorption of these compounds *(28,29)*. A second well-documented, clinically significant example of this type of interaction involves the complexation of tetracycline and iron. By this mechanism, tetracycline antibiotic AUCs are decreased by up to 80% *(30–32)*.

Adsorption is the process of ion binding or hydrogen binding and may occur between anti-infectives such as penicillin G, cephalexin, sulfamethoxazole, or tetracycline and adsorbents such as cholestyramine. Because this process can significantly decrease antibiotic exposure *(33,34)*, the concomitant administration of adsorbents and antibiotics should be avoided.

## Changes in Gastric Emptying and Intestinal Motility

The presence or absence of food can affect the absorption of anti-infectives by a variety of mechanisms *(35)*. High-fat meals can significantly increase the extent of absorption of fat-soluble compounds such as griseofulvin, cefpodoxime, and cefuroxime axetil. Prolonged stomach retention can cause excessive degradation of acid-labile compounds such as penicillin and erythromycin *(10)*.

Because the primary location of drug absorption is the small intestine, changes in gastric emptying and gastrointestinal motility may have significant effects on drug exposure. Rapid gastrointestinal transit effected by prokinetic agents such as cisapride, metoclopramide, and domperidone may decrease the extent of absorption of poorly soluble drugs or drugs that are absorbed in a limited area of the intestine *(36)*. However, clinically significant effects on anti-infectives have not been documented.

## Effects of Intestinal Blood Flow

Intestinal blood flow can be modulated by vasoactive agents and theoretically can affect the absorption of lipophilic compounds. However, there is no evidence to date that this results in clinically significant drug interactions *(37)*.

## Changes in Active and Passive Transport

A rapidly expanding field of research is that of intestinal transcellular transport. Multiple intestinal transporters located on the brush-border and basolateral membrane of the enterocyte have been identified *(38–40)*. The potential for competitive inhibition of these transporters with quinolone antibiotics has been documented *(41)*. This contributes an additional mechanism by which anti-infective drug interactions may occur.

The Caco-2 cell model is a human colonic cell line sharing similarities with enterocytes and is used as a model for oral absorption *(42)*. Investigations using this cell line have demonstrated that certain compounds can modulate the tight junctions of the intestinal epithelia and alter paracellular drug absorption *(43,44)*. Future research that focuses on understanding the functional characteristics of enterocyte transporters and tight-junction modulators will provide information regarding which compounds may participate in these interactions and to what extent. Mechanisms related to transporters are described in Chapter 3.

## Changes in Presystemic Clearance

Knowledge of first-pass drug elimination and systemic availability of many anti-infectives in humans has increased tremendously in the last decade. The drug-metabolizing CYP 3A4 and 3A5 (CYP3A4/5) are expressed at high concentrations in the intestine and contribute to drug inactivation. P-Glycoprotein is expressed at the lumenal surface of the intestinal epithelium and serves to extrude unchanged drug from the enterocyte into the lumen. Both CYP3A4/5 and P-glycoprotein share a significant overlap in substrate specificity *(45–47)*, although there is no correlation between affinities *(48)*. Determining the relative contributions of intestinal P-glycoprotein and CYP3A4/ 5 activity to drug bioavailability and interactions is an active area of investigation. Potential drug interactions involving these mechanisms are discussed in detail next.

## Cytochrome P450 Isozymes

Gastrointestinal CYP isozymes, responsible for Phase I oxidative metabolism (for a more detailed discussion of CYP isoforms, *see* Phase I Drug Metabolism section), are most highly concentrated in the proximal two-thirds of the small intestine *(49)*. Two intestinal CYP isoforms, CYP3A4 and CYP3A5 (CYP3A4/5), account for approx 70% of total intestinal P450 protein and are a major determinant of the systemic bioavailability of orally administered drugs *(50–53)*.

For example, the benzodiazepine midazolam is a specific CYP3A4/5 substrate with no affinity for P-glycoprotein. An investigation of oral and intravenous midazolam plasma clearance in 20 healthy young volunteers *(54)* revealed an incomplete correlation between the two measures ($r = 0.70$). The large variability in midazolam oral clearance not accounted for by hepatic metabolism most likely represents the contribution of intestinal CYP3A4/5. Therefore, it appears that at least 30–40% of the clearance of many CYP3A compounds may be significantly influenced by CYP3A4/5 located in enterocytes. Because the activity of intestinal CYP3A4/5 can also be influenced by a variety of environmental factors *(53,55,56)*, the potential for drug interactions to occur during drug absorption is great.

Some of the most significant effects of drug interactions occurring at the intestinal isozyme level involve the potential suicide inhibition of CYP3A4/5 with grapefruit juice *(57,58)*. Generally, this interaction results in a minimum threefold increase in the extent of absorption and toxicity of the concomitantly administered agent *(59)*, but can also result in decreased efficacy of prodrugs needing CYP3A for conversion to active moieties. The concern of this interaction is strictly limited to orally administered agents because the active components of grapefruit juice are either inactivated in the gut or are present in such minute quantities in the portal circulation that no effect on hepatic metabolism occurs *(60–62)*.

Clinical data available for anti-infective–grapefruit juice interactions include the protease inhibitor saquinavir *(63)*, the antifungal agent itraconazole *(64)*, and the macrolide clarithromycin *(65)*. Whereas saquinavir AUC increases twofold with a single 400-mL dose of commercially available grapefruit juice, itraconazole and clarithromycin AUCs do not change significantly. The absence of an effect of grapefruit juice on the oral clearance of these last two compounds suggests that their first-pass metabolism does not rely significantly on intestinal CYP3A4/5 *(45)*.

Anti-infectives can also inhibit intestinal CYP isozyme activity *(55,56,66)*. For example, the protease inhibitor ritonavir is a potent inhibitor of CYP3A4 activity. This characteristic can be clinically useful, as demonstrated by the increased bioavailability of the protease inhibitors saquinavir *(67)* and lopinavir *(68)* when given in combination with small doses of ritonavir.

Other CYP isozymes present in enterocytes may also influence drug absorption. Environmental factors may influence their activity as well, and drug–environment interactions may result in significantly altered absorption *(69)*. However, further research is needed to better characterize these influences before specific interactions can be predicted.

## Effects of P-Glycoprotein

P-Glycoprotein is a multidrug-resistance gene product found in a variety of human tissues, including the gastrointestinal epithelium *(70)*. This efflux pump is expressed at the lumenal surface of the intestinal epithelium and opposes the absorption of unchanged drug by transporting lipophilic compounds out of enterocytes back into the gastrointestinal lumen. P-Glycoprotein has demonstrated up to 10-fold variability in activity between subjects *(71)* and has a significant role in oral drug absorption. Decreased bioavailability occurs because intact drug molecules are pumped back into the gastrointestinal tract lumen and exposed multiple times to enterocyte metabolism.

P-Glycoprotein has broad substrate specificity, and inhibiting or inducing the activity of this protein can lead to significant alterations in drug exposure *(72)*. However, because many drugs have affinities for both P-glycoprotein and CYP3A4/5 *(45,46)*, it is difficult to determine by which specific mechanism drug interactions occur. For some compounds, inhibition of both P-glycoprotein function and CYP3A4/5 activity may be required to produce clinically significant interactions.

Many anti-infectives have binding affinity for P-glycoprotein. These include erythromycin, clarithromycin *(73)*, ketoconazole, sparfloxacin *(74)*, the nucleoside analog adefovir *(75)*, and the human immunodeficiency virus (HIV)-1 protease inhibitors *(76–78)*. Because drugs that have affinity for P-glycoprotein are not necessarily removed from the enterocyte by this efflux pump *(79)*, anti-infectives may participate in, but are not necessarily influenced by, drug interactions involving P-glycoprotein. This concept was illustrated by an in vitro investigation of ketoconazole and erythromycin *(80)*. Both drugs demonstrated significant affinity for P-glycoprotein. However, in combination with verapamil (a classic P-glycoprotein inhibitor), significantly decreased P-glycoprotein-mediated efflux occurred only with erythromycin. Therefore, although ketoconazole exhibits binding affinity for P-glycoprotein, it can be concluded that P-glycoprotein does not contribute significantly to the process of first-pass metabolism of ketoconazole.

In vitro data revealed that grapefruit juice, in addition to inactivating enterocyte CYP3A isozymes, may also increase P-glycoprotein activity *(81)*. The clinical implications of this have yet to be determined. P-Glycoprotein is further discussed in Chapter 3.

## DRUG INTERACTIONS AFFECTING DISTRIBUTION

### Protein Binding and Displacement

Drug interactions affecting distribution are those that alter protein binding. Generally, the importance of drug displacement interactions has been overestimated, with the extrapolation of data from in vitro investigations without consideration for subsequent physiological phenomena. The lack of well-designed studies has prevented precise quantification of the influence of protein binding on anti-infective therapeutic efficacy in vivo. However, redistribution and excretion of drugs generally occurs quickly after displacement, and the effects of any transient rise in unbound concentration of the object drug are rarely clinically important *(82)*.

Albumin constitutes the main protein fraction (~5%) in blood plasma. As albumin contains both basic and acidic groups, it can bind basic and acidic drugs. Acidic drugs (i.e., penicillins, sulfonamides, doxycycline, and clindamycin; *83*) are strongly bound to albumin at a small number of binding sites, and basic drugs (i.e., erythromycin) are weakly bound to albumin at a larger number of sites. Basic drugs may also preferentially bind to $\alpha$-1-acid glycoprotein *(84)*.

Depending on relative plasma concentrations and protein-binding affinities, one drug may displace another with clinically significant results. This interaction is much more likely to occur with drugs that are at least 80 to 90% bound to plasma proteins, with small changes in protein binding leading to large relative changes in free drug concentration. Drugs that are poorly bound to plasma proteins may also be displaced, but the relative increase in free drug concentration is generally of less consequence. When a protein displacement interaction occurs, the increased free drug in plasma quickly distributes throughout the body and will localize in tissues if the volume of distribution is large. An increase in unbound drug concentrations at metabolism and elimination sites will also lead to increased rates of elimination. Therefore, many clinically significant drug interactions that have been attributed to protein binding have often involved a second, unrecognized mechanism of interaction *(85)*.

Generally, interactions between basic drugs and albumin are not clinically significant. In subjects with normal concentrations of albumin and anti-infective concentrations of less than 100 µg/mL, the degree of protein binding will be relatively constant. At higher anti-infective concentrations, available binding sites may theoretically become saturated and the extent of binding subsequently decreased *(83)*. Clinically significant displacement interactions for $\alpha$-1-acid glycoprotein have not been described. This is most likely caused by the large volume of distribution of these drugs, with plasma containing a very small proportion of the total amount of drug in the body.

**Table 2**
**Potential Mechanisms of Drug**
**Interactions Involving Metabolism**

Phase I (nonsynthetic)
- Genetic polymorphisms
- Inhibition of activity
- Suppression of activity
- Induction of activity

Phase II (synthetic)
- Genetic polymorphisms
- Inhibition of activity
- Induction of activity

In summary, drug interactions involving albumin-binding displacement may potentially be clinically significant if the compound is greater than 80% protein bound, has a high hepatic extraction ratio, a narrow therapeutic index, and a small volume of distribution. Although temporary increase in drug concentrations may be clinically significant with such drugs as warfarin and phenytoin, mean steady-state free drug concentrations will remain unaltered *(86)*.

## DRUG INTERACTIONS AFFECTING DRUG METABOLISM

The principal site of drug metabolism is the liver. Metabolism generally converts lipophilic compounds into ionized metabolites for renal elimination. Drug-metabolizing activity can be classified according to nonsynthetic (Phase I) and synthetic (Phase II) reactions. Phase I reactions include oxidation, reduction, and hydrolysis and occur in the membrane of hepatocyte endoplasmic reticula. Phase II reactions result in conjugation (i.e., glucuronidation, sulfation) and occur in the cytosol of the hepatocyte.

### Phase I Drug Metabolism

The majority of oxidative reactions are catalyzed by a superfamily of mixed-function mono-oxygenases called the CYP enzyme system. Although CYP isozymes are located in numerous tissues throughout the body, the liver is the largest source of CYP protein *(50)*. Many significant pharmacokinetic drug interactions involve the hepatic CYP isozymes *(87–91)* (Table 2).

Nomenclature for this superfamily is based on amino acid sequence homology and groups enzymes and genes into families and subfamilies *(92)*. To designate the CYP enzymes, the CYP prefix is used. All isozymes having at least 40% amino acid sequence homology are members of an enzyme family, as designated by an Arabic number (e.g., CYP3). All isozymes that have at least 55% amino acid sequence homology are members of an enzyme subfamily, as designated by a capital letter (e.g., CYP3A). An Arabic number is used to represent an individual enzyme (e.g., CYP3A4). Italicized nomenclature represents the gene coding for a specific enzyme (e.g., *CYP3A4*).

To date, at least 14 human families, 22 human subfamilies, and 36 human CYP enzymes have been identified *(93)*. However, the CYP1, 2, and 3 families account for 70% of the total hepatic P450 content *(94,95)*. Approximately 95% of all therapeutic

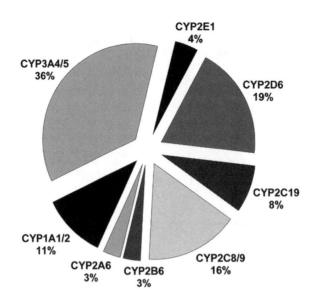

**Fig. 1.** Proportion of drugs metabolized by P450 isozymes.

drug oxidation can be accounted for by the activities of CYP1A2, CYP2C8/9, CYP2C19, CYP2D6, CYP2E1, and CYP3A4/5 (Fig. 1). Drug interactions involving these isozymes result from enzyme inhibition or induction, although genetic polymorphism can attenuate these interactions *(96)*.

*Genetic Polymorphisms*

Polymorphisms are generated by nonrandom genetic mutations that occur in at least 1% of a population and give rise to distinct subgroups within that population that differ in their ability to metabolize xenobiotics. Clinically significant polymorphisms have been documented for CYP2D6, CYP2C9, and CYP2C19 *(97)*. Extensive or rapid metabolizers (generally the largest proportion of a population) have heterozygous or homozygous dominant alleles, poor metabolizers possess variant homozygous autosomal recessive alleles, and ultraextensive metabolizers exhibit gene amplification of autosomal dominant alleles.

Poor-metabolizer phenotypes can be at high risk for toxicity from drugs that require CYP inactivation and at high risk for therapeutic inefficacy from prodrugs that need CYP activation *(98)*. However, they are at low risk for drug interactions that involve enzyme inhibition or induction because their activity is preemptively compromised and cannot be induced.

In addition, because of the large variability (e.g., 40-fold or greater) in enzyme activity documented in extensive metabolizers *(99)*, drug interactions may not manifest in all subjects with this phenotype. Inhibition of drug-metabolizing enzymes may result in more significant effects in those with high initial enzyme activity, and induction of drug-metabolizing enzymes may result in more significant effects in those individuals with low initial enzyme activity.

## Mechanisms of Inhibition

Enzyme inhibition can result in sudden catastrophic drug interactions. Several mechanisms of inhibition exist, and many drugs can interact by multiple mechanisms *(100,101)*. Reversible inhibition is most common. Reversible inhibition occurs when compounds quickly form weak bonds with CYP isozymes without permanently disabling them. This can occur both competitively (competition for the same binding site between inhibitor and substrate) and noncompetitively (inhibitor binds at a site on the enzyme distinct from the substrate).

The magnitude of this type of inhibition depends both on the affinity of substrate and inhibitor for the enzyme and on the concentration of the inhibitor at the enzyme site *(48)*. Affinity is represented by an inhibitor constant $K_i$, which is the concentration of inhibitor required to decrease the maximal rate of the reaction to half of the uninhibited value. For example, potent reversible CYP3A inhibitors generally have $K_i$ values below 1 $\mu M$ (e.g., ketoconazole, itraconazole, ritonavir, and indinavir), although drugs with $K_i$ values in the low micromolar range can also demonstrate competitive inhibition (e.g., erythromycin and nelfinavir). Compounds with $K_i$'s greater than 100 $\mu M$ for the CYP3A subfamily tend not to produce clinically significant inhibition *(52)*.

CYP inhibition can also occur as a result of a slowly reversible reaction. When an inhibitor binds to a CYP isozyme and undergoes oxidation to a nitrosoalkane species, it can form a slowly reversible complex with the reduced heme in the CYP isozyme *(52)*. This interaction has been documented between the macrolide antibiotics and CYP3A *(102)* and explains why clinically significant interactions (i.e., erythromycin and terfenadine) can occur with compounds that have modest $K_i$ values *(88,103)*.

It is postulated that irreversible, mechanism-based inhibition (or suicide inhibition) occurs with the CYP-mediated formation of a reactive metabolite. This metabolite can covalently and irreversibly bind to the catalytic site residue and permanently inactivate the enzyme for subsequent reactions. The extent of the clinical importance of this reaction depends on the total amount of CYP isozyme present, the total amount of inhibitor to which the isozyme is exposed, and the rate of new isozyme synthesis *(104)*.

## Mechanisms of Suppression

As early as the 1960s, inflammation and infection were demonstrated to decrease Phase I metabolism of drugs and toxins in animals, thereby modulating pharmacological and toxicological effects *(105,106)*. One of the earliest reports of infection altering human drug-metabolizing enzyme activity occurred a decade later, with quinidine concentrations consistently elevated in subjects experimentally infected with *Plasmodium falciparum* malaria *(107)*. Since that time, numerous reports have described alterations in drug metabolism with viral and bacterial infections *(108–114)*, in addition to complex events such as surgery and bone marrow transplantation *(115,116)*.

The effects of inflammation and infection on CYP activity are ascribed to stimulation of the cellular immune response *(117)*. Although many different mediators may be involved, there has been particular focus on the major proinflammatory cytokines interleukin (IL)-1, IL-6, and tumor necrosis factor (TNF)-α. Generally, IL-1, IL-6, and TNF-α demonstrate a suppressive effect on CYP isozymes by decreasing messenger ribonucleic acid (mRNA) up to 80%. However, correlations among mRNA, enzyme protein content, and enzyme activity are incomplete both within and between investigations *(118–125)*. To date, the majority of investigations examining cytokine-induced effects on drug-metabolizing isozyme activities have been performed in the rodent model. Very few of these investigations have been repeated in human hepatocytes. Although rodents are an inexpensive and readily available model, qualitative and quantitative interspecies differences in regulation and activity of drug-metabolizing enzymes *(126–128)* as well as response to cytokines do not allow the effects of inflammation on isozyme activities, or the underlying mechanisms, to be easily extrapolated to humans *(129–132)*.

A small number of clinical investigations have documented decreased drug-metabolizing enzyme activity during the administration of therapeutic interferons and interleukins. These studies demonstrated variable and conflicting results with respect to the magnitude of drug–cytokine interactions *(114,133–139)*. With the increasing use of cytokines as therapeutic agents for a variety of disease states, further investigation is required to elucidate the mechanisms of drug–cytokine interactions to optimize anti-infective therapeutic regimens. Drug–cytokine interactions are described in detail in Chapter 13.

*Mechanisms of Induction*

An increase in CYP activity through induction is less of an immediate concern than inhibition because induction occurs gradually rather than rapidly and generally leads to compromised therapeutic goals rather than profound toxicity. Because the time-course of enzyme induction is determined by the half-life of the substrate as well as the rate of isozyme turnover, it is often difficult to predict this time-course specifically. Clinically significant induction results from a more than 50-fold increase in the number of enzyme molecules. This generally occurs through an increase in P450 synthesis by either receptor-mediated transcriptional activation or mRNA stabilization. However, protein stabilization leading to decreased rates of P450 degradation has also been noted.

Induction of the CYP1 family by cigarette smoke, charcoal-broiled foods, indoles (found in broccoli, cauliflower, cabbage, brussels sprouts, kale, watercress), and omeprazole occurs primarily by substrate binding to the Ah-receptor (dioxin receptor). This complex subsequently binds with a receptor nuclear translocator, enters the hepatocyte nucleus, and binds with regulatory deoxyribonucleic acid (DNA) sequences to enhance gene transcription and stabilize mRNA *(140,141)*.

The CYP2 family is induced by a variety of structurally diverse compounds. Although the mechanism of CYP2 gene induction is not well understood and a specific receptor has not been identified, transcriptional CYP2C gene activation and mRNA stabilization were demonstrated to occur with the azole antifungal agents ketoconazole, clotrimazole, and miconazole *(141)*.

A transcriptional mechanism for CYP3 induction has been identified *(142)*. Investigators have established that a human orphan nuclear receptor, termed the pregnane X receptor (PXR), binds to a response element in the *CYP3A4* promoter region. PXR is activated by a range of drugs known to induce CYP3A4 expression (i.e., rifampicin, clotrimazole, etc.). PXR is expressed most abundantly in the liver but is also present in the small intestine and colon. CYP3A can also be induced by posttranscriptional message stabilization and protein stabilization with the following anti-infectives: macrolides, imidazole antifungal agents, and rifampin. The specific mechanisms for this are currently unknown but most likely involve interaction with a cyclic adenosine 5′-monophosphate-dependent phosphorylation process involved in protein denaturation.

## Phase II Drug Metabolism

The term *Phase II metabolism* was developed originally to represent synthetic reactions occurring after Phase I processes. It is now known that many xenobiotics do not require Phase I metabolism before undergoing conjugation reactions. The group of Phase II isozymes consists of uridine 5'-diphosphate (UDP)-glucuronosyltransferases, sulfotransferases, acetyltransferases, glutathione-S-transferase, and methyltransferases. Many of these families of enzymes are still growing in complexity, and drug interactions involving these isozymes are under investigation.

### Genetic Polymorphism

Many of the Phase II enzymes exhibit polymorphism *(143–146)*. Although these polymorphisms have been implicated in selected anti-infective-associated adverse drug reactions (e.g., dapsone, isoniazid, sulfonamides; *146–148*), influences of these polymorphisms on anti-infective drug interactions have not been documented.

### Inhibition

Phase II drug-metabolizing enzymes do not currently appear to play as prominent a role in clinical drug interactions with anti-infectives as the CYP enzyme system. This may be because of the large capacity of the conjugation system, in which only profound disturbances result in clinically significant alterations in drug pharmacokinetics *(149)*.

UDP-glucuronosyltransferase represents the most common conjugation reaction in drug metabolism. Many drugs have been characterized as competitive inhibitors of UDP-glucuronosyltransferases *(150)*, but the roles of these interactions in practical drug metabolism issues are unexplored.

### Induction

Far less is known about the potential for induction of Phase II enzymes than the CYP enzyme system. The UDP-glucuronosyltransferases can be induced, but the clinical significance of this is not fully understood *(151)*. However, the increased clearance of zidovudine that has been documented with the coadministration of rifampin suggests that induction of these enzymes may be clinically significant *(152)*. Glutathione-S-transferase is also known to be inducible, although these activities rarely exceed two- to threefold times baseline and are not involved in anti-infective metabolism *(153)*.

## DRUG INTERACTIONS AFFECTING EXCRETION

Renal elimination of drugs involves glomerular filtration, tubular secretion, and tubular reabsorption. Five mechanisms of drug–drug interactions can occur at the site of renal elimination *(154)*. The most common mechanisms are discussed next (Table 3).

### Glomerular Filtration

Rates of glomerular filtration can be affected by changes in renal blood flow, cardiac output, and extent of protein binding *(155)*. With highly protein-bound drugs (e.g., >80%), a significant increase in the unbound fraction can lead to an increase in glomerular filtration and subsequent increased drug elimination *(156)*. Conversely, with transporter saturation and renal elimination at maximal, elimination rates may decrease significantly with increased free drug.

**Table 3**
**Potential Mechanisms of Drug**
**Interactions Involving Excretion**

- Glomerular filtration
- Tubular secretion
- Tubular reabsorption

## Tubular Secretion

The most common renal drug interactions occur at the transport site of tubular secretion. Sharing the same proximal tubular active transport system, many organic anionic and cationic drugs and metabolites compete with each other for secretion. A classic example of this interaction, used long ago intentionally for therapeutic benefit, is the combination of probenecid and penicillin to increase antibiotic serum concentrations *(157)*. Examples of other anti-infectives that may exhibit interactions by this mechanism include the sulfonamides, penicillins, and zidovudine *(158–160)*.

P-Glycoprotein has been identified in the apical membrane of the proximal tubule and can transport a large variety of drugs into the lumen. A number of experimental drug interaction investigations have implicated the inhibition of renal p-glycoprotein to an increase in plasma drug concentrations. Quinolones *(161)*, macrolides *(73)*, and azole antifungals *(162)* demonstrate affinity for renal P-glycoprotein and can potentially contribute to significant drug interactions. Although renal nucleoside transporters have been shown to mediate the secretion and reabsorption of purine and pyrimidine nucleoside analog drugs, their role in clinically significant drug interactions is unknown *(163,164)*.

## Tubular Reabsorption

Reabsorption of drugs from the tubular lumen involves both passive diffusion and active transport processes. Only nonionized compounds are passively reabsorbed from the renal tubule, and thus manipulating urinary pH can alter the reabsorption of weak organic acids and bases. Renal clearance of weak organic bases ($pK_a = 7–10$) is increased with urine acidification (i.e., by salicylates and ascorbic acid) and decreased with urine alkalinization (i.e., by antacids, calcium carbonate, thiazide diuretics, and sodium bicarbonate). Likewise, renal elimination of weak organic acids ($pK_a = 3–7$; nitrofurantoin, sulfonamides, aminoglycosides, and vancomycin) is increased with urine alkalinization and decreased with urine acidification. Generally, these interactions are not clinically significant because few drugs can have altered urinary excretion to a large enough extent to affect plasma half-life. The role of active transport reabsorption in anti-infective drug interactions is currently unknown *(165)*.

## SIGNIFICANCE OF DRUG INTERACTIONS

Many drug interactions are primarily assessed in vitro (*see* the Preclinical Methods for Predicting Drug Interactions section). However, absolute in vitro/in vivo correlations are infrequent. Even with clinical trials, not all statistically significant drug interactions are clinically significant. In particular, drugs with wide therapeutic indices that demonstrate a less than 20% change in pharmacokinetic parameters when combined with a second agent will most likely be of little, if any, clinical significance.

The greatest risk of documented clinically significant pharmacokinetic drug interactions involving anti-infective-induced altered protein binding, drug-metabolizing enzyme inhibition, and altered renal elimination is the combination of anti-infectives with anticoagulants, antidepressants, and cardiovascular agents *(90)*. The most clinically significant anti-infective drug interactions involving enzyme induction are subtherapeutic concentrations resulting from the combination of rifampin with warfarin *(166)*, cyclosporine *(167)*, and oral contraceptives *(168,169)*. Conversely, the reduction of $C_{max}$ or AUC of anti-infectives by other drugs or environmental influences can result in a much greater chance of therapy failure and possibly an increase in the development of resistance.

Not all pharmacokinetic drug interactions involving anti-infectives are detrimental, however. Ketoconazole has been used for a number of years to inhibit the metabolism of oral cyclosporine by approx 80%, thereby reducing the cost of therapy as well as the rates of rejection and infection *(170,171)*. As mentioned in the section Cytochrome P450 Isozymes, the administration of ritonavir to enhance the oral absorption of saquinavir is a well-known component of potent antiretroviral combination regimens *(172)*.

Beneficial and detrimental pharmacodynamic antimicrobial drug interactions also exist. The use of lower concentrations of two synergistic antibacterials to reduce the toxicity of each but to have the same pharmacological effect has been advocated *(173)*, although the clinical data supporting superior efficacy is weak. Synergistic combinations of antimicrobials may produce better results in the treatment of *Pseudomonas aeruginosa* and *Enterococcus* species *(174,175)*. Clinical data are also lacking for detrimental effects of potentially antagonistic combinations of antimicrobials (e.g., a bacteriostatic drug combined with a bactericidal agent) *(176)*. However, these combinations are best avoided unless clinically warranted for the treatment of multiple pathogens.

## PRECLINICAL METHODS FOR PREDICTING DRUG INTERACTIONS

Although understanding and anticipating pharmacokinetic drug interactions are important components of rational therapeutics, there is a limit to the number and scope of clinical studies that can reasonably be performed. The development of human in vitro models allows information to be obtained without the expense and potential risks involved in conducting human trials. However, scaling of in vitro data to the clinical situation is not always accurate, and the results of these methods may not be definitive. A primary focus of preclinical screening methods for assessing drug–drug interactions is the identification of isozymes responsible for the metabolism of these compounds and the relative contribution of an inhibited pathway to a compound's overall elimination.

Modern technology has allowed in vitro screening techniques to become widely available, and the bulk of these data are currently included in package inserts. However, extrapolating in vitro results to an in vivo situation is often complicated. Preclinical screening of promising compounds frequently uses nonhuman mammalian species, although interspecies differences in expression and regulation of transporters and enzymes are well documented *(177,178)*. Supratherapeutic, as opposed to clinically relevant, concentrations of inhibitors and substrates may be utilized. In addition, experimental conditions such as enzyme protein concentration and buffers can critically affect specific results

**Table 4**
**Preclinical Methods for Predicting Drug Interactions**

| | |
|---|---|
| • Purified P450 isozymes | • Immortalized cell lines |
| • Recombinant P450 isozymes | • Liver slices |
| • Human microsomes | • Hepatocyte cultures |

and confound in vitro/in vivo correlations *(179)*. To account for variability in individual enzyme expression, positive controls for inhibition and induction should always be used (e.g., troleandomycin or ketoconazole for CYP3A inhibition, quinidine for CYP2D6 inhibition, and rifampin for CYP3A induction).

The following briefly summarizes the strengths and weaknesses of currently available in vitro human methodologies for assessing CYP drug interactions and predicting their clinical significance (Table 4).

### Purified P450 Isozymes

In an attempt to identify specific isozymes responsible for the metabolism of compounds, human CYP enzymes have been isolated and purified from hepatic tissue *(180)*. However, only small amounts of protein can be isolated at any one time, and specific isozymes from certain subfamilies often cannot be separated (i.e., CYP2C9 vs CYP2C19 vs CYP2C10). To ensure correct interpretation of the results obtained from this method, it is most critical to examine the isozyme purification methods and quality control procedures. This method has been primarily superceded by the use of recombinant human CYP isozymes.

### Recombinant Human P450 Isozymes

Complementary DNA (cDNA) expression has been used to produce recombinant human CYP isozymes in yeast, insects, bacteria, and mammalian cells *(181,182)*. An advantage of this system is the ability to identify specific isozymes of a subfamily that are responsible for the metabolism of a compound and to confirm suspected isozyme-selective inhibitors *(183)*. However, this remains an artificial system, and discrepancies can exist between results obtained by cDNA methods and other in vitro systems. Generally, data obtained from cDNA systems should be confirmed by at least one other in vitro system *(184,185)*.

### Microsomes

Microsomes isolated from human hepatocytes have become the "gold standard" of in vitro experimentation for drug interactions. Microsomes are isolated membranes of hepatocyte endoplasmic reticula and contain the CYPs in proportion to their in vivo representation. This is an important consideration because most often multiple isozymes are responsible for drug metabolism. Given the large interindividual variability in CYP expression, using microsomes from a single individual may produce distorted results. To circumvent this, pooling microsomes from multiple sources to obtain an average representation of activity is advocated. Human microsomes are widely available at relatively low cost, but they can only be used to determine direct inhibition of metabolism. Investigations of drug–drug interactions involving induction or suppression of CYP isozymes require intact cellular machinery.

### Immortalized Cell Lines

An ideal in vitro model for studying drug–drug interactions involving induction, inhibition, and suppression would be a validated, immortalized, readily available cell line, the results from which could be extrapolated directly to the clinical environment. However, no such model currently exists. All available immortalized human cell lines do not maintain a full complement of CYP enzyme activities or maintain other potentially important physiological processes. One commonly used immortalized cell line is derived from a human hepatoma (HepG2 cells). This model has been investigated for CYP1A1 induction but does not significantly express other CYPs *(186,187)*.

### Liver Slices

Human liver slices have been used with moderate success in determining the hepatic metabolism of certain compounds. Liver slices are relatively easy to prepare, and they maintain the hepatic ultrastructure. However, up to half of constitutive (baseline) CYP activity is lost within the first 24 hours after isolation, and all constitutive CYP activity is lost by 96 hours *(188)*. This makes investigations of induction and suppression of drug-metabolizing enzyme activity difficult. In addition, a distribution equilibrium is not achieved between all hepatocytes within the slice and the incubation media, resulting in decreased rates of metabolism compared to a hepatocyte monolayer culture system *(189)*.

### Human Hepatocyte Cultures

Human hepatocyte monolayer culture systems are ideal for studying drug interactions because they maintain both Phase I and II activity and form and maintain physiological processes such as biliary canaliculi and transporters *(190)*. Determining drug interactions in this system often allows for the closest prediction of potential drug interactions *(191)*. Although this system does not mimic the pharmacokinetic alterations in drug concentrations seen clinically, it does allow quantitation of "best" and "worst" scenarios that may be extrapolated to the clinical setting. Induction, suppression, and inhibition interactions can all be performed with this model *(192,193)*. Although maintaining constitutive levels of CYP activity has been challenging, currently available enriched media and improved culture conditions allow for maintenance of control activity for at least 72–96 hours after isolation. Challenges encountered with this system are primarily in obtaining fresh hepatic tissue for digestion and the specialized technique of perfusion for isolation of the hepatocytes. In addition, with the wide variability in enzyme activity seen clinically, investigations in a limited number of hepatocyte preparations will not be able to reflect definitively the occurrence of drug interactions in an entire population but only suggest the potential for interactions to occur.

## OVERVIEW OF CLINICAL METHODS
## FOR PREDICTING DRUG INTERACTIONS

The primary cause of clinically significant drug interactions is the involvement of drug-metabolizing enzymes. Because great variability exists in drug-metabolizing enzyme activity among subjects, and drug interactions may not achieve clinical significance in all patients, interactions may be better clinically predicted by the knowledge of individual patient isozyme activities. However, there is currently a need for the development of reliable, accurate, and noninvasive methods to monitor drug-metabolizing enzyme expression in humans to guide drug dosage, reduce toxicity, and predict potential drug interactions.

Genotyping involves identification of variant genes causing poor- or ultraextensive metabolizer activity or phenotype. Genotyping has been demonstrated to predict the clinical outcome of drug interactions involving both Phase I and II metabolism *(194,195)*. However, drug-metabolizing enzyme activity can be exquisitely sensitive to environmental and physiological influences. Therefore, genotyping allows for the determination of an individual's genetic predisposition to a specific enzyme activity but may not reflect true phenotype at any one point in time.

An analytical technique that allows the characterization of specific in vivo drug-metabolizing enzyme activity is the process of phenotyping: using the ratios of parent drug and drug metabolites in blood or urine as a surrogate marker of isozyme activity. Specific methods have been developed to phenotype CYP1A2, CYP2C9, CYP2C19, CYP2D6, CYP2E1, CYP3A, glutathione-*S*-transferase, glucuronyl-transferase, and *N*-acetyltransferase activities *(196)*. Phenotyping offers the primary advantage of quantitating time-sensitive enzyme activity and accounts for combined genetic, environmental, and endogenous influences on drug-metabolizing enzyme activity. However, a number of currently available phenotyping methods are invasive and impractical, and analytical methods are not readily available. With a simplification of phenotyping methods and an increase in the availability of analytical procedures, it may be possible to use these methods to determine correlations between enzyme activity and the risk of significant drug interactions in individual patients.

## IN VITRO/IN VIVO SCALING OF DRUG INTERACTIONS

The process of using in vitro models to predict in vivo drug interactions is still in its infancy, and extensive validation of this approach is needed. In vitro models predictive of in vivo drug interactions will be essential for rapid, cost-effective screening of pharmaceutical compounds and are important for reducing risks to patient safety. Currently, these models are constructed from a combination of laboratory and theoretical components. Ideally, in a valid model, the in vivo decrease in clearance caused by coadministration of an inhibitor would be specifically predicted by the decrease in reaction velocity (e.g., formation rate of a metabolite) for the same compound in vitro when the inhibitor is present in the same concentration.

However, presently available models contain a number of weaknesses and assumptions that make scaling of in vitro data to the clinical situation complicated and not always accurate. Poor predictions occur with compounds that have flow-dependent hepatic clearance, with mechanism-based inhibition, and with compounds that concurrently induce and inhibit enzyme activity. In addition, inhibitor and substrate plasma concentrations are not always proportional to the inhibitor and substrate concentrations to which the enzyme is exposed. In vitro and cell culture models demonstrate extensive partitioning of lipophilic compounds into cells, with uptake not restricted by plasma protein binding. As an example, the mean in vivo liver:plasma partition ratios for benzodiazepine derivatives range from 6.4 to 17.4, making predictions of these concentrations at the site of enzyme activity very difficult *(197,198)*. Some examples of in vitro scaling with azole antifungal agents can be found in a commentary by von Moltke et al. *(198)*.

To establish the feasibility of in vitro-to-in vivo scaling, most currently reported predictions of inhibitory drug interactions are retrospective. Presently available methods allow a general assessment of what may occur (i.e., an unlikely interaction vs a probable interaction; *199,200*). However, to be most useful, in vitro data should not only indicate the possibility of an interaction but also predict its magnitude and clinical importance. Until such a time, the clinical study remains the ultimate means by which a drug interaction and its importance can be assessed.

## CASE STUDY 1

O.N., a 40-year-old white male with hypercholesterolemia, has had appropriate low-density lipoprotein levels by taking 40 mg pravastatin daily along with a controlled diet. His normal dietary routine includes a breakfast of cereal, low-fat milk, decaffeinated coffee, and orange juice each morning; salad for lunch; a sensible dinner; and an evening snack of grapefruit juice and graham crackers. With the turning of the year, O.N.'s health maintenance organization sends a letter stating that pravastatin will no longer be covered by his prescription plan; however, atorvastatin and simvastatin will be covered. O.N.'s physician switches him to 20 mg daily of simvastatin.

Following 1 week of therapy with simvastatin, O.N. is feeling weak and sore. Two days later, his urine turns red, and he goes to the emergency department of the local hospital. He is admitted with acute renal failure.

This case illustrates a drug–food interaction between simvastatin and grapefruit juice. Grapefruit juice contains furanocoumarin deratives *(201)*. These compounds have been shown to inhibit CYP3A isoforms (but have no significant effect on other CYP isoforms). This is a combination of reversible and irreversible inhibition and generally occurs only at the level of the small intestine with little hepatic effect. Simvastatin is a substrate of CYP3A. Generally, bioavailability of simvastatin is low (~5%); however, administration with grapefruit juice can increase the exposure of simvastatin up to 20-fold. Because individuals vary in the amount of CYP3A in their gut, it is impossible to predict who will get a significant inhibitory effect from drugs and food that inhibits this enzyme.

Increased exposure to simvastatin resulted in rhabomyolysis, with resulting renal failure most likely because of high simvastatin exposures with this drug–food interaction.

## CASE STUDY 2

ClarkiePharma, a drug development firm, contracts with a Japanese research organization to investigate the potential for drug interactions for their new antifungal compound. This compound is primarily metabolized by CYP2C19, with an average drug clearance in Caucasian males of 120 mL/minute. The researchers perform a study in 16 Japanese males, finding a baseline drug clearance of 50 mL/minute. With the addition of ketoconazole, clearance drops to approx 38 mL/

minute, and tests of bioequivalence do not reveal a drug interaction. When the drug is put into Phase II studies in humans (Caucasians and African Americans) with fungal infections, addition of ketoconazole results in a substantial increase in the investigational drug exposure and significant toxicity.

This case shows the importance of examining a metabolic drug interaction in an appropriate population. Asians have up to 20% incidence of poor metabolism (presence of two null alleles for CYP2C19) and a substantial incidence of penetrance of one null allele for CYP2C19, making them intermediate metabolizers of CYP2C19 substrates. The use of this Asian population underestimated the extent of this drug interaction.

## CONCLUSIONS AND FUTURE DIRECTIONS

It is difficult to assess the true incidence and clinical significance of drug interactions. Understanding the mechanisms underlying drug interactions is important for the prediction and avoidance of drug toxicity when initiating combination therapy. Although multiple in vitro methods are currently in use to assess drug interactions, not all have allowed the prediction of clinically significant events *(202,203)*. As drug interactions most commonly result from influences on drug-metabolizing enzymes, future research defining the origins of enzyme activity variability and characterizing individual patient activity will certainly improve our ability to predict these interactions and improve drug therapy.

## REFERENCES

1. Levy SB. The challenge of antibiotic resistance. Sci Am 1998;278:46–53.
2. US Congress, Office of Technology Assessment. Impacts of Antibiotic Resistant Bacteria. OTA-H 629, September 1995. Washington, DC: US Government Printing Office.
3. IMS America Web-site. Available at: http://www.imshealth.com/frameset/frameset global. htm. Accessed December 2004.
4. Tanaka E. Clinically important pharmacokinetic drug–drug interactions: role of cytochrome P450 enzymes. J Clin Pharm Ther 1998;23:403–416.
5. Lin JH, Lu AY. Inhibition and induction of cytochrome P450 and the clinical implications. Clin Pharmacokinet 1998;35:361–390.
6. Greenblatt DJ, von Moltke LL, Harmatz JS, et al. Drug interactions with newer antidepressants: role of human cytochromes P450. J Clin Psychiatry 1998;59(suppl 15):19–27.
7. Shannon M. Drug–drug interactions and the cytochrome P450 system: an update. Pediatr Emerg Care 1997;13:350–353.
8. Guengerich FP. Role of cytochrome P450 enzymes in drug-drug interactions. Adv Pharmacol 1997;43:7–35.
9. Ritschel WA, ed. Handbook of Basic Pharmacokinetics. 4th Ed. Hamilton, IL: Drug Intelligence.
10. Welling PG. Interactions affecting drug absorption. Clin Pharmacokinet 1984;9:404–434.
11. Gugler R, Allgayer H. Effects of antacids on the clinical pharmacokinetics of drugs; an update. Clin Pharmacokinet 1990;18:210–219.
12. Lee BL, Safrin S. Interactions and toxicities of drugs used in patients with AIDS. Clin Infect Dis 1992;14:773–779.
13. Horowitz HW, Jorde UP, Wormser GP. Drug interactions in use of dapsone for *Pneumocystis carinii* prophylaxis. Lancet 1992;339:747.
14. Moreno F, Hardin TC, Rinaldi MG, et al. Itraconazole-didanosine excipient interaction. JAMA 1993;269:1508.

15. Metroka CE, McMechan MF, Andrada R, et al. Failure of prophylaxis with dapsone in patients taking dideoxyinosine. N Engl J Med 1991;325:737.

16. Fisher RS, Sher DJ, Donahue D, et al. Regional differences in gastric acidity and antacid distribution: is a single pH electrode sufficient? Am J Gastroenterol 1997;92:263–270.

17. Burget DW, Chiverton SG, Hunt RH. Is there an optimal degree of acid suppression for healing duodenal ulcers? Gastroenterology 1990;99:345–351.

18. Kanda Y, Kami M, Matsuyama T, et al. Plasma concentration of itraconazole in patients receiving chemotherapy for hematological malignancies: the effect of famotidine on the absorption of itraconazole. Hematol Oncol 1998;16:33–37.

19. Jaruratanasirikul S, Sriwiriyajan S. Effect of omeprazole on the pharmacokinetics of itraconazole. Eur J Clin Pharmacol 1998;54:159–161.

20. Chin TW, Loeb M, Fong IW. Effects of an acidic beverage (Coca-Cola) on absorption of ketoconazole. Antimicrob Agents Chemother 1995;39:1671–1675.

21. Hansten PD. Drug interactions with antisecretory agents. Aliment Pharmacol Ther 1991;5(suppl 1):121–128.

22. Somogyi A, Muirhead M. Pharmacokinetic interactions of cimetidine 1987. Clin Pharmacokinet 1987;12:321–366.

23. Sadowski DC. Drug interactions with antacids. Mechanisms and clinical significance. Drug Safety 1994;11:395–407.

24. Knupp CA, Barbhaiya RH. A multiple-dose pharmacokinetic interaction study between didanosine (Videx) and ciprofloxacin (Cipro) in male subjects seropositive for HIV but asymptomatic. Biopharmaceut Drug Disp 1997;18:65–77.

25. Polk RE. Drug–drug interactions with ciprofloxacin and other fluoroquinolones. Am J Med 1989;87:76S–81S.

26. Sahai J, Gallicano K, Oliveras L, et al. Cations in the didanosine tablet reduce ciprofloxacin bioavailability. Clin Pharmacol Ther 1993;53:292–297.

27. Lomaestro BM, Bailie GR. Quinolone-cation interactions: a review. DICP 1991;25:1249–1258.

28. Yuk JH, Nightingale CH, Sweeney KR, et al. Relative bioavailability in healthy volunteers of ciprofloxacin administered through nasogastric tube with or without enteral feeding. Antimicrob Agents Chemother 1989;33:1118–1120.

29. Yuk JH, Nightingale CH, Quintiliani R, et al. Absorption of ciprofloxacin administered through a nasogastric or a nasoduodenal tube in volunteers and patients receiving enteral nutrition. Diagn Microbiol Infect Dis 1990;13:99–102.

30. Neuvonen PJ, Gothon G, Hackman R, et al. Interference of iron with the absorption of tetracyclines in man. Br Med J 1970;4:532–534.

31. Leyden JJ. Absorption of minocycline hydrochloride and tetracycline hydrochloride. Effect of food, milk, and iron. J Am Acad Dermatol 1985;12(2 Pt 1):308–312.

32. Campbell NR, Hasinoff BB. Iron supplements: a common cause of drug interactions. Br J Clin Pharmacol 1991;31:251–255.

33. Questran product monograph. Cholestyramine for oral suspension. September 1993. Bristol-Myers-Squibb.

34. Parsons RL, Paddock GM. Absorption of two antibacterial drugs, cephalexin and cotrimoxazole, in malabsorption syndromes. J Antimicrob Chemother 1975;1(suppl):59–67.

35. Fraga Fuentes MD, Garcia Diaz B, de Juana Velasco P, et al. Influence of foods on the absorption of antimicrobial agents. Nutricion Hospitalaria 1997;12:277–288.

36. Tonini M. Recent advances in the pharmacology of gastrointestinal prokinetics. Pharmacol Res 1996;33:217–226.

37. Kedderis GL. Pharmacokinetics of drug interactions. Adv Pharmacol 1997;43:189–203.

38. Tsuji A, Tamai I. Carrier-mediated intestinal transport of drugs. Pharm Res 1996;13:963–977.

39. Zhang L, Brett CM, Giacomini KM. Role of organic cation transporters in drug absorption and elimination. Annu Rev Pharmacol Toxicol 1998;38:431–460.

40. Saitoh H, Fujisaki H, Aungst BJ, et al. Restricted intestinal absorption of some β-lactam antibiotics by an energy-dependent efflux system in rat intestine. Pharm Res 1997;14: 645–649.

41. Rabbaa L, Dautrey S, Colas-Linhart N, et al. Absorption of ofloxacin isomers in the rat small intestine. Antimicrob Agents Chemother 1997;41:2274–2277.

42. Yee S. In vitro permeability across Caco-2 cells (colonic) can predict in vivo (small intestinal) absorption in man—fact or myth. Pharm Res 1997;14:763–766.

43. Delie F, Rubas W. A human colonic cell line sharing similarities with enterocytes as a model to examine oral absorption: advantages and limitations of the Caco-2 model. Crit Rev Ther Drug Carrier Syst 1997;14:221–286.

44. Lu AY. Drug-metabolism research challenges in the new millennium: individual variability in drug therapy and drug safety. Drug Metab Dispos 1998;26:1217–1222.

45. Hall SD, Thummel KE, Watkins PB, et al. Molecular and physical mechanisms of first-pass extraction. Drug Metab Dispos 1999;27:161–166.

46. Wacher VJ, Wu C-Y, Benet LZ. Overlapping substrate specificities and tissue distribution of cytochrome P450 3A and P-glycoprotein: implications for drug delivery and activity in cancer chemotherapy. Mol Carcinog 1995;13:129–134.

47. Schuetz EG, Beck WT, Schuetz JD. Modulation and substrates of P-glycoprotein and cytochrome P4503A coordinately up-regulate these proteins in human colon carcinoma cells. Mol Pharmacol 1996;49:311–318.

48. Bertz RJ, Granneman GR. Use of in vitro and in vivo data to estimate the likelihood of metabolic pharmacokinetic interactions. Clin Pharmacokinet 1997;32:210–258.

49. Bonkovsky HL, Hauri HP, Marti U, et al. Cytochrome P450 of small intestinal epithelial cells. Gastroenterology 1985;88:458–467.

50. Krishna DR, Klotz U. Extrahepatic metabolism of drugs in humans. Clin Pharmacokinet 1994;26:144–160.

51. Paine MF, Khalighi M, Fisher JM, et al. Characterization of interintestinal and intraintestinal variations in human CYP3A-dependent metabolism. J Pharmacol Exp Ther 1997;283:1552–1562.

52. Thummel KE, Wilkinson GR. In vitro and in vivo drug interactions involving human CYP3A. Ann Rev Pharmacol Tox 1998;38:389–430.

53. Kolars JC, Schmiedlin-Ren P, Schuetz JD, et al. Identification of rifampin-inducible P450IIIA4 (CYP3A4) in human small bowel enterocytes. J Clin Invest 1992;90:1871–1878.

54. Thummel KE, O'Shea D, Paine MF, et al. Oral first-pass elimination of midazolam involves both gastrointestinal and hepatic CYP3A-mediated metabolism. Clin Pharmacol Ther 1996;59:491–502.

55. Gibbs MA, Thummel KE, Shen DD, et al. Inhibition of cytochrome P-450 3A (CYP3A) in human intestinal and liver microsomes: comparison of $K_i$ values and impact of CYP3A5 expression. Drug Metab Dispos 1999;27:180–187.

56. Gorski JC, Jones DR, Haehner-Daniels BD, et al. The contribution of intestinal and hepatic CYP3A to the interaction between midazolam and clarithromycin. Clin Pharmacol Ther 1998;64:133–143.

57. Lown KS, Bailey DG, Fontana RJ, et al. Grapefruit juice increases felodipine oral availability in humans by decreasing intestinal CYP3A protein expression. J Clin Invest 1997;99:2245–2253.

58. Schmiedlin-Ren P, Edwards DJ, Fitzsimmons ME, et al. Mechanisms of enhanced oral availability of CYP3A4 substrates by grapefruit constituents: decreased enterocyte CYP3A4 concentration and mechanism-based inactivation by furanocoumarins. Drug Metab Dispos 1997;25:1228–1233.

59. Ameer B, Weintraub RA. Drug interactions with grapefruit juice. Clin Pharmacokinet 1997;33:103–121.

60. Kupferschmidt HH, Ha HR, Ziegler WH, et al. Interaction between grapefruit juice and midazolam in humans. Clin Pharmacol Ther 1995;58:20–28.

61. Lundahl J, Regardh CG, Edgar B, et al. Effects of grapefruit juice ingestion—pharmaco-kinetics and haemodynamics of intravenously and orally administered felodipine in healthy men. Eur J Clin Pharmacol 1997;52:139–145.

62. Rashid TJ, Martin U, Clarke H, et al. Factors affecting the absolute bioavailability of nifedipine. Br J Clin Pharmacol 1995;40:51–58.

63. Kupferschmidt HH, Fattinger KE, Ha HR, et al. Grapefruit juice enhances the bioavail-ability of the HIV protease inhibitor saquinavir in man. Br J Clin Pharmacol 1998;45: 355–359.

64. Kawakami M, Suzuki K, Ishizuka T, et al. Effect of grapefruit juice on pharmacokinetics of itraconazole in healthy subjects. Int J Clin Pharmacol Ther 1998;36:306–308.

65. Cheng KL, Nafziger AN, Peloquin CA, et al. Effect of grapefruit juice on clarithromycin pharmacokinetics. Antimicrob Agents Chemother 1998;42:927–929.

66. Tsunoda SM, Velez RL, Greenblatt DJ. Ketoconazole inhibition of intestinal and hepatic cytochrome P450 3A4 (CYP3A4) activity using midazolam as an in vivo probe. Clin Phar-macol Ther 1999;65:172.

67. Hsu A, Granneman GR, Cao G, et al. Pharmacokinetic interactions between two human immunodeficiency virus protease inhibitors, ritonavir and saquinavir. Clin Pharmacol Ther 1998;63:453–464.

68. Sham HL, Kempf DJ, Molla A, et al. ABT-378, a highly potent inhibitor of the human immunodeficiency virus protease. Antimicrob Agents Chemother 1998;42:3218–3224.

69. Paine MF, Schmiedlin-Ren P, Watkins PB. Cytochrome P-450 1A1 expression in human small bowel: interindividual variation and inhibition by ketoconazole. Drug Metab Dispos 1999;27:360–364.

70. Stein WD. Kinetics of the multidrug transporter (P-glycoprotein) and its reversal. Physiol Rev 1997;77:545–590.

71. Lown KS, Fontana RJ, Schmiedlin-Ren P, et al. Interindividual variation in intestinal mdr1:lack of short term diet effects. Gastroenterology 1995;108:A737.

72. Willie RT, Lown KS, Huszezo UR, et al. Short term effect of medications on CYP3A and P-glycoprotein expression in human intestinal mucosa. Gastroenterology 1997;112 (suppl):A419.

73. Wakasugi H, Yano I, Ito T, et al. Effect of clarithromycin on renal excretion of digoxin: interaction with P-glycoprotein. Clin Pharmacol Ther 1998;64:123–128.

74. Cormet-Boyaka E, Huneau JF, Mordrelle A, et al. Secretion of sparfloxacin from the human intestinal Caco-2 cell line is altered by P-glycoprotein inhibitors. Antimicrob Agents Chemother 1998;42:2607–2611.

75. Annaert P, Van Gelder J, Naesens L, et al. Carrier mechanisms involved in the transepithelial transport of bis(POM)-PMEA and its metabolites across Caco-2 monolay-ers. Pharm Res 1998;15:1168–1173.

76. Alsenz J, Steffen H, Alex R. Active apical secretory efflux of the HIV protease inhibitors saquinavir and ritonavir in Caco-2 cell monolayers. Pharm Res 1998;15:423–428.

77. Srinivas RV, Middlemas D, Flynn P, et al. Human immunodeficiency virus protease inhibi-tors serve as substrates for multidrug transporter proteins MDR1 and MRP1 but retain anti-viral efficacy in cell lines expressing these transporters. Antimicrob Agents Chemother 1998;42:3157–3162.

78. Kim AE, Dintaman JM, Waddell DS, et al. Saquinavir, an HIV protease inhibitor, is transported by P-glycoprotein. J Pharmacol Exp Ther 1998;286:1439–1445.

79. Salphati L, Benet LZ. Effects of ketoconazole on digoxin absorption and disposition in rat. Pharmacology 1998;56:308–313.

80. Takano M, Hasegawa R, Fukuda T, Yumoto R, Nagai J, Murakami T. Interaction with P-glycoprotein and transport of erythromycin, midazolam and ketoconazole in Caco-2 cells. Eur J Pharmacol 1998;358:289–294.

81. Soldner A, Christians U, Susanto M, et al. Grapefruit juice activates P-glycoprotein-mediated drug transport. Pharm Res 1999;16:478–485.

82. Sansom LN, Evans AM. What is the true clinical significance of plasma protein binding displacement interactions? Drug Safety 1995;12:227–233.

83. Craig WA, Welling PG. Protein binding of antimicrobials: clinical pharmacokinetics and therapeutic implications. Clin Pharmacokinet 1977;2:252.

84. McElnay JC, D'Arcy PF. Protein binding displacement interactions and their clinical importance. Drugs 1983;25:495–513.

85. Rowland M. Plasma protein binding and therapeutic drug monitoring. Ther Drug Monit 1980;2:29–37.

86. Rolan PR. Plasma protein binding displacement interactions—why are they still regarded as clinically important? Br J Clin Pharmacol 1994;37:125–128.

87. Monahan BP, Ferguson CL, Killeavy ES, et al. Torsades des pointes occurring in association with terfenadine use. JAMA 1990;264:2788–2790.

88. Honig PK, Woosley RL, Zamani K, et al. Changes in the pharmacokinetics and electro-cardiographic pharmacodynamics of terfenadine with concomitant administration of erythromycin. Clin Pharmacol Ther 1992;52:231–238.

89. Pohjola-Sintonen S, Viitasalo M, Toivonen L, et al. Itraconazole prevents terfenadine metabolism and increases risk of torsades de pointes ventricular tachycardia. Eur J Clin Pharmacol 1993;45:191–193.

90. Honig PK, Wortham DC, Zamani K, et al. Terfenadine-ketoconazole interaction, pharmacokinetic and electrocardiographic consequences. JAMA 1993;269:1513–1518.

91. Michalets EL. Update: clinically significant cytochrome P-450 drug interactions. Pharmacotherapy 1998;18:84–112.

92. Nelson DR, Koymans L, Kamataki T, et al. P450 superfamily: update on new sequences, gene mapping, accession numbers and nomenclature. Pharmacogenetics 1996;6:1–42.

93. Degtyarenko KN, Fábián P. Directory of P450-Containing Systems. Available at: http://www.icgeb.trieste.it/p450/P450Nom_Full.html#Animalia. (December 2004)

94. Wrighton SA, Stevens JC. The human hepatic cytochromes P450 involved in drug metabolism. Crit Rev Tox 1992;22:1–21.

95. Smith G, Stubbins MJ, Harries LW, et al. Molecular genetics of the human cytochrome P450 monooxygenase superfamily. Xenobiotica 1998;28:1129–1165.

96. Pelkonen O, Maenpaa J, Taavitsainen P, et al. Inhibition and induction of human cytochrome P450 (CYP) enzymes. Xenobiotica 1998;28:1203–1253.

97. Daly AK, Fairbrother KS, Smart J. Recent advances in understanding the molecular basis of polymorphisms in genes encoding cytochrome P450 enzymes. Toxicol Lett 1998;102–103:143–147.

98. Kroemer HK, Eichelbaum M. "It's the genes, stupid." Molecular bases and clinical consequences of genetic cytochrome P450 2D6 polymorphism. Life Sci 1995;56:2285–2298.

99. Rendic S, Di Carlo FJ. Human cytochrome P450 enzymes: a status report summarizing their reactions, substrates, inducers, and inhibitors. Drug Metab Rev 1997;29:413–580.

100. Vanden Bossche H, Koymans L, Moereels H. P450 inhibitors of use in medical treatment: focus on mechanisms of action. Pharmacol Ther 1995;67:79–100.

101. Murray M. Drug-mediated inactivation of cytochrome P450. Clin Exp Pharmacol Physiol 1997;24:465–470.

102. Babany G, Larrey D, Pessayre D. Macrolide antibiotics as inducers and inhibitors of cytochrome P-450 in experimental animals and man. In: Gibson GG, ed. Progress in Drug Metabolism. London, UK: Taylor and Francis, 1988, pp. 61–98.

103. Ludden TM. Pharmacokinetic interactions of the macrolide antibiotics. Clin Pharmacokinet 1985;10:63–79.
104. Gray MR, Tam YK. Pharmacokinetics of drugs that inactivate metabolic enzymes. J Pharmaceut Sci 1991;80:121–127.
105. Wooles WR, Borzelleca JF. Prolongation of barbiturate sleeping time in mice by stimulation of the reticuloendothelial system (RES). J Reticuloendothel Soc 1966;3:41–47.
106. Leeson GA, Biedenbach SA, Chan KY, et al. Decrease in the activity of the drug-metabolizing enzymes of rat liver following the administration of tilorone hydrochloride. Drug Metab Dispos 1976;4:232–238.
107. Trenholme GM, Williams RL, Rieckmann KH, et al. Quinine disposition during malaria and during induced fever. Clin Pharmacol Ther 1976;19:459–467.
108. Chang KC, Bell TD, Lauer BA, et al. Altered theophylline pharmacokinetics during acute respiratory viral illness. Lancet 1978;1:1132,1133.
109. Kraemer MJ, Furukawa CT, Koup JR, et al. Altered theophylline clearance during an influenza B outbreak. Pediatrics 1982;69:476–480.
110. Renton KW, Mannering GJ. Depression of the hepatic cytochrome P-450 mono-oxygenase system by administered tilorone (2,7-bis(2-(diethylamino)ethoxy)fluoren-9-one dihydrochloride). Drug Metab Dispos 1976;4:223–231.
111. Sonne J, Dossing M, Loft S, et al. Antipyrine clearance in pneumonia. Clin Pharmacol Ther 1985;37:701–704.
112. Shedlofsky SI, Israel BC, McClain CJ, et al. Endotoxin administration to humans inhibits hepatic cytochrome P450-mediated drug metabolism. J Clin Invest 1994;94:2209–2214.
113. Shelly MP, Mendel L, Park GR. Failure of critically ill patients to metabolize midazolam. Anaesthesia 1987;42:619–626.
114. Brockmeyer NH, Barthel B, Mertins L, et al. Changes of antipyrine pharmacokinetics during influenza and after administration of interferon-α and -β. Int J Clin Pharmacol Ther 1998;36:309–311.
115. Gidal BE, Reiss WG, Liao JS, et al. Changes in interleukin-6 concentrations following epilepsy surgery: potential influence on carbamazepine pharmacokinetics. Ann Pharmacother 1996;30:545,546.
116. Chen YL, Le Vraux V, Leneveu A, et al. Acute-phase response, interleukin-6, and alteration of cyclosporine pharmacokinetics. Clin Pharmacol Ther 1994;55:649–660.
117. Morgan ET. Regulation of cytochromes P450 during inflammation and infection. Drug Metab Rev 1997;29:1129–1188.
118. Sewer MB, Morgan ET. Nitric oxide-independent suppression of P450 2C11 expression by interleukin-1β and endotoxin in primary rat hepatocytes. Biochem Pharmacol 1997;54:729–737.
119. Tinel M, Robin MA, Doostzadeh J, et al. The interleukin-2 receptor down-regulates the expression of cytochrome P450 in cultured rat hepatocytes. Gastroenterology 1995;109:1589–1599.
120. Chen J, Nikolova-Karakashian M, Merrill AH Jr, et al. Regulation of cytochrome P450 2C11 (CYP2C11) gene expression by interleukin-1, sphingomyelin hydrolysis, and ceramides in rat hepatocytes. J Biol Chem 1995;270:25,233–25,238.
121. Morgan ET, Thomas KB, Swanson R, et al. Selective suppression of cytochrome P-450 gene expression by interleukins 1 and 6 in rat liver. Biochim Biophys Acta 1994;1219:475–483.
122. Wright K, Morgan ET. Regulation of cytochrome P450IIC12 expression by interleukin-1 α, interleukin-6, and dexamethasone. Mol Pharmacol 1991;39:468–474.
123. Abdel-Razzak Z, Corcos L, Fautrel A, et al. Interleukin-1 β antagonizes phenobarbital induction of several major cytochromes P450 in adult rat hepatocytes in primary culture. FEBS Lett 1995;366:159–164.

124. Fukuda Y, Ishida N, Noguchi T, et al. Interleukin-6 down regulates the expression of transcripts encoding cytochrome P450 IA1, IA2 and IIIA3 in human hepatoma cells. Biochem Biophys Res Commun 1992;184:960–965.
125. Barker CW, Fagan JB, Pasco DS. Interleukin-1 β suppresses the induction of P4501A1 and P4501A2 mRNAs in isolated hepatocytes. J Biol Chem 1992;267:8050–8055.
126. Berthou F, Ratanasavanh D, Alix D, et al. Caffeine and theophylline metabolism in newborn and adult human hepatocytes; comparison with adult rat hepatocytes. Biochem Pharmacol 1988;37:3691–3700.
127. Veronese ME, McManus ME, Laupattarakasem P, et al. Tolbutamide hydroxylation by human, rabbit and rat liver microsomes and by purified forms of cytochrome P-450. Drug Metab Dispos 1990;18:356–361.
128. Parkinson A. An overview of current cytochrome P450 technology for assessing the safety and efficacy of new materials. Toxicol Pathol 1996;24:48–57.
129. Kurokohchi K, Matsuo Y, Yoneyama H, et al. Interleukin 2 induction of cytochrome P450-linked monooxygenase systems of rat liver microsomes. Biochem Pharmacol 1993; 45:585–592.
130. Cantoni L, Carelli M, Ghezzi P, et al. Mechanisms of interleukin-2-induced depression of hepatic cytochrome P-450 in mice. Eur J Pharmacol 1995;292:257–263.
131. Ansher SS, Puri RK, Thompson WC, et al. The effects of interleukin 2 and α-interferon administration on hepatic drug metabolism in mice. Cancer Res 1992;52:262–266.
132. Craig PI, Williams SJ, Cantrill E, et al. Rat but not human interferons suppress hepatic oxidative drug metabolism in rats. Gastroenterology 1989;97:999–1004.
133. Pageaux GP, le Bricquir Y, Berthou F, et al. Effects of interferon-α on cytochrome P-450 isoforms 1A2 and 3A activities in patients with chronic hepatitis C. Eur J Gastroenterol Hepatol 1998;10:491–495.
134. Okuno H, Kitao Y, Takasu M, et al. Depression of drug metabolizing activity in the human liver by interferon-α. Eur J Clin Pharmacol 1990;39:365–367.
135. Okuno H, Takasu M, Kano H, et al. Depression of drug-metabolizing activity in the human liver by interferon-β. Hepatology 1993;17:65–69.
136. Williams SJ, Farrell GC. Inhibition of antipyrine metabolism by interferon. Br J Clin Pharmacol 1986;22:610–612.
137. Israel BC, Blouin RA, McIntyre W, et al. Effects of interferon-α monotherapy on hepatic drug metabolism in cancer patients. Br J Clin Pharmacol 1993;36:229–235.
138. Piscitelli SC, Vogel S, Figg WD, et al. Alteration in indinavir clearance during interleukin-2 infusions in patients infected with the human immunodeficiency virus. Pharmacotherapy 1998;18:1212–1216.
139. Elkahwaji J, Robin MA, Berson A, et al. Decrease in hepatic cytochrome P450 after interleukin-2 immunotherapy. Biochem Pharmacol 1999;57:951–954.
140. Kleman MI, Overvik E, Poellinger L, et al. Induction of cytochrome P4501A isozymes by heterocyclic amines and other food-derived compounds. Princess Takamatsu Symp 1995;23:163–171.
141. Dogra SC, Whitelaw ML, May BK. Transcriptional activation of cytochrome P450 genes by different classes of chemical inducers. Clin Exp Pharmacol Physiol 1998;25:1–9.
142. Lehmann JM, McKee DD, Watson MA, et al. The human orphan nuclear receptor PXR is activated by compounds that regulate CYP3A4 gene expression and cause drug interactions. J Clin Invest 1998;102:1016–1023.
143. Patel M, Tang BK, Kalow W. Variability of acetaminophen metabolism in Caucasians and Orientals. Pharmacogenetics 1992;2:38–45.
144. Weinshilboum R. Sulfotransferase pharmacogenetics. Pharmacol Ther 1990;45:93–107.
145. Weinshilboum R. Methyltransferase pharmacogenetics. Pharmacol Ther 1989;43:77–90.
146. Evans DA. N-Acetyltransferase. Pharmacol Ther 1989;42:157–234.

147. Lennard MS. Genetically determined adverse drug reactions involving metabolism. Drug Safety 1993;9:60–77.
148. Spielberg SP. N-Acetyltransferases: pharmacogenetics and clinical consequences of polymorphic drug metabolism. J Pharmacokinet Biopharm 1996;24:509–519.
149. Park BK, Kitteringham NR. Assessment of enzyme induction and enzyme inhibition in humans: toxicological implications. Xenobiotica 1990;20:1171–1185.
150. Burchell B, McGurk K, Brierly CH, et al. UDP-glucuronosyltransferases. In: Guengerich FP, ed. Biotransformation, Vol. 3, Comprehensive Toxicology. Oxford, UK: Elsevier Science, 1997, pp. 401–435 .
151. Abid A, Sabolovic N, Batt AM, et al. Induction of UDP-glucuronosyltransferases and cytochromes P450 in human hepatocytes. Cell Pharmacol 1994;1:257–262.
152. Burger DM, Meenhorst PL, ten Napel CHH, et al. Pharmacokinetic variability of zidovudine in HIV-infected individuals: subgroup analysis and drug interactions. AIDS 1994;8:1683–1689.
153. Hayes JD, McLeod R, Pulford DJ, et al. Regulation and activity of glutathione S-transferases. ISSX Proc 1996;10:12–18
154. Bonate PL, Reith K, Weir S. Drug interactions at the renal level: implications for drug development. Clin Pharmacokinet 1998;34:375–404.
155. van Ginneken CA, Russel FG. Saturable pharmacokinetics in the renal excretion of drugs. Clin Pharmacokinet 1989;16:38–54.
156. Kirby WMM, DeMaine JB, Serrill WS. Pharmacokinetics of the cephalosporins in healthy volunteer and uremic patients. Postgrad Med J 1971;47:41–46.
157. Kampmann J, Molholm-Hansen J, Siersbaeck-Nielsen K, et al. Effect of some drugs on penicillin half-life in blood. Clin Pharmacol Ther 1972;13:516–519.
158. Prescott LF. Clinically important drug interactions. Drugs 1973;5:161–186.
159. Chatton JY, Munafo A, Chave JP, et al. Trimethoprim, alone or in combination with sulphamethoxazole, decreases the renal excretion of zidovudine and its glucuronide. Br J Clin Pharmacol 1992;34:551–554.
160. Fletcher CV, Henry WK, Noormohamed SE, et al. The effect of cimetidine and ranitidine administration with zidovudine. Pharmacotherapy 1995;15:701–708.
161. Ito T, Yano I, Tanaka K, et al. Transport of quinolone antibacterial drugs by human P-glycoprotein expressed in a kidney epithelial cell line, LLC-PK1. J Pharmacol Exp Ther 1997;282:955–960.
162. Kaukonen KM, Olkkola KT, Neuvonen PJ. Itraconazole increases plasma concentrations of quinidine. Clin Pharmacol Ther 1997;62:510–517.
163. Bendayan R, Georgis W, Rafi-Tari S. Interaction of 3′-azido-3′-deoxythymidine with the organic base transporter in a cultured renal epithelium. Pharmacotherapy 1995;15:338–344.
164. Sweeney KR, Hsyu PH, Statkevich P, et al. Renal disposition and drug interaction screening of (–)-2′-deoxy-3′-thiacytidine (3TC) in the isolated perfused rat kidney. Pharm Res 1995;12:1958–1963.
165. Bendayan R. Renal drug transport: a review. Pharmacotherapy 1996;16:971–985.
166. O'Reilly RA. Interaction of sodium warfarin and rifampin. Studies in man. Ann Intern Med 1974;81:337–340.
167. Modry DL, Stinson EB, Oyer PE, et al. Acute rejection and massive cyclosporine requirements in heart transplant recipients treated with rifampin. Transplantation 1985;39:313–314.
168. Barditch-Crovo P, Trapnell CB, Ette E, et al. The effects of rifampin and rifabutin on the pharmacokinetics and pharmacodynamics of a combination oral contraceptive. Clin Pharmacol Ther 1999;65:428–438.
169. LeBel M, Masson E, Guilbert E, et al. Effects of rifabutin and rifampicin on the pharmacokinetics of ethinylestradiol and norethindrone. J Clin Pharmacol 1998;38:1042–1050.

170. Keogh A, Spratt P, McCosker C, et al. Ketoconazole to reduce the need for cyclosporine after cardiac transplantation. N Engl J Med 1995;333:628–633.

171. Jones TE. The use of other drugs to allow a lower dosage of cyclosporine to be used. Therapeutic and pharmacoeconomic considerations. Clin Pharmacokinet 1997;32:357–367.

172. Kempf DJ, Marsh KC, Kumar G, et al. Pharmacokinetic enhancement of inhibitors of the human immunodeficiency virus protease by coadministration with ritonavir. Antimicrob Agents Chemother 1997;41:654–660.

173. Caranasos GJ, Stewart RB, Cluff LE. Clinically desirable drug interactions. Ann Rev Pharmacol Toxicol 1985;25:67–95.

174. Pizzo PA. Management of fever in patients with cancer and treatment-induced. N Engl J Med 1993;328:1323–1332.

175. Eliopoulos GM. The 10 most commonly asked questions about resistant enterococcal infections. Infect Dis Clin Pract 1994;13:125–129.

176. Lepper MC, Dowling HF. Treatment of pneumococcal meningitis with penicillin compared with penicillin plus aureomycin. Arch Intern Med 1951;88:489–494.

177. Rice JM, Diwan BA, Ward JM, et al. Phenobarbital and related compounds: approaches to interspecies extrapolation. Prog Clin Biol Res 1992;374:231–249.

178. Strolin Benedetti M, Dostert P. Induction and autoinduction properties of rifamycin derivatives: a review of animal and human studies. Environ Health Perspect 1994;102 (suppl 9):101–105.

179. Maenpaa J, Hall SD, Ring BJ, et al. Human cytochrome P450 3A (CYP3A) mediated midazolam metabolism: the effect of assay conditions and regioselective stimulation by α-naphthoflavone, terfenadine and testosterone. Pharmacogenetics 1998;8:137–155.

180. Guengerich FP. Characterization of human microsomal cytochrome P-450 enzymes. Annu Rev Pharmacol Toxicol 1989;29:241–264.

181. Rodrigues AD. Integrated cytochrome P450 reaction phenotyping: attempting to bridge the gap between cDNA-expressed cytochromes P450 and native human liver microsomes. Biochem Pharmacol 1999;57:465–480.

182. Gonzalez FJ, Korzekwa KR. Cytochromes P450 expression systems. Annu Rev Pharmacol Toxicol 1995;35:369–390.

183. Zhang Z, Fasco MJ, Huang Z, et al. Human cytochromes P4501A1 and P4501A2: R-warfarin metabolism as a probe. Drug Metab Dispos 1995;23:1339–1346.

184. Fischer V, Vogels B, Maurer G, et al. The antipsychotic clozapine is metabolized by the polymorphic human microsomal and recombinant cytochrome P450 2D6. J Pharmacol Exp Ther 1992;260:1355–1360.

185. Dahl ML, Llerena A, Bondesson U, et al. Disposition of clozapine in man: lack of association with debrisoquine and S-mephenytoin hydroxylation polymorphisms. Br J Clin Pharmacol 1994;37:71–74.

186. Lipp HP, Schrenk D, Wiesmuller T, et al. Assessment of biological activities of mixtures of polychlorinated dibenzo-*p*-dioxins (PCDDs) and their constituents in human HepG2 cells. Arch Toxicol 1992;66:220–223.

187. Krusekopf S, Kleeberg U, Hildebrandt AG, et al. Effects of benzimidazole derivatives on cytochrome P450 1A1 expression in a human hepatoma cell line. Xenobiotica 1997; 27:1–9.

188. VandenBranden M, Wrighton SA, Ekins S, et al. Alterations of the catalytic activities of drug-metabolizing enzymes in cultures of human liver slices. Drug Metab Dispos 1998; 26:1063–1068.

189. Dogterom P. Development of a simple incubation system for metabolism studies with precision-cut liver slides. Drug Metab Dispos 1993;21:699–704.

190. Borchardt RT, Wilson G, Smith P, eds. Model Systems for Biopharmaceutical Assessment of Drug Absorption and Metabolism. New York, NY: Plenum, 1996.

191. LeCluyse EL, Madan A, Hamilton G, Carroll K, DeHaan R, Parkinson A. Expression and regulation of cytochrome P450 enzymes in primary cultures of human hepatocytes. J Biochem Mol Toxicol 2000;14:177–188.

192. Strom SC, Pisarov LA, Korko K, et al. Use of human hepatocytes to study P450 gene induction. Meth Enzymol 1996;272:388–401.

193. Li AP, Maurel P, Gomez-Lechon MJ, et al. Preclinical evaluation of drug–drug interaction potential: present status of the application of primary human hepatocytes in the evaluation of cytochrome P450 induction. Chemico-Bio Interact 1997;107:5–16.

194. Buchert E, Woosley RL. Clinical implications of variable antiarrhythmic drug metabolism. Pharmacogenetics 1992;2:2–11.

195. Lewis LD, Benin A, Szumlanski CL, et al. Olsalazine and 6-mercaptopurine-related bone marrow suppression: a possible drug–drug interaction. Clin Pharmacol Ther 1997;62: 464–475.

196. Brockmoller J, Roots I. Assessment of liver metabolic function. Clinical implications. Clin Pharmacokinet 1994;27:216–248.

197. Scavone JM, Friedman H, Greenblatt DJ, et al. Effect of age, body composition, and lipid solubility on benzodiazepine tissue distribution in rats. Arzeneimittelforschung 1987;37: 2–6.

198. von Moltke LL, Greenblatt DJ, Schmider J, et al. In vitro approaches to predicting drug interactions in vivo. Biochem Pharmacol 1998;55:113–122.

199. Greenblatt DJ, von Moltke LL, Harmatz JS, et al. Inhibition of triazolam clearance by macrolide antimicrobial agents: in vitro correlates and dynamic consequences. Clin Pharmacol Ther 1998;64:278–285.

200. Thummel KE, Wilkinson GR. In vitro and in vivo drug interactions involving human CYP3A. Annu Rev Pharmacol Toxicol 1998;38:398–430.

201. Greenblatt, DJ, Patki KC, von Moltke LL, Shader RI. Drug interactions with grapefruit juice: an update. J Clin Psychopharmacol 2001;21:357–359.

202. Posicor. Voluntary Market Withdrawal. Nutley, NJ: Roche Laboratories, June 8, 1998.

203. Food and Drug Administration. FDA Talk Paper Seldane and Generic Terfenadine Withdrawn From Market. Rockville, MD: US Department of Health and Human Services, Public Health Service, February 27, 1998.

# 3

# Mechanisms of Drug Interactions II

*Transport Proteins*

**Scott R. Penzak**

## INTRODUCTION

Drug interactions continue to be an important consideration for patients receiving antimicrobial chemotherapy. The clinical significance of drug interactions in patients receiving anti-infectives has been spotlighted by numerous reports of drug interactions among patients taking antiretroviral therapy *(1)*. As a result, considerable progress has been made in describing the mechanisms by which drug interactions occur; this has led to increased ability to recognize and manage clinically significant drug interactions. Although much of the success in managing drug interactions can be attributed to increased knowledge of cytochrome P450 (CYP)-mediated drug metabolism, drug transport mechanisms are increasingly recognized as a means by which clinically relevant drug interactions occur among anti-infective agents *(2)*.

Modulation of drug transport mechanisms is a long-recognized phenomenon by which one drug may alter the pharmacokinetics of another. For years, clinicians have appreciated probenecid's ability to inhibit the renal secretion and increase the systemic exposure of β-lactam antibiotics *(3)*. Probenecid is also used in combination with the nucleotide analog cidofovir to prevent nephrotoxicity *(4)*. Despite probenecid's lengthy history as an adjunct in antibiotic treatment, its role as a renal transport protein inhibitor, which is examined in this chapter, has been characterized only recently *(5)*.

Considerable advancement has occurred in the molecular characterization of transport proteins *(6)*. This knowledge has led to improved understanding of the role of transport proteins in the disposition of medications—including antimicrobial agents—throughout various organs and cell types, including the intestine, liver, brain, kidney, testes, placenta, and lymphocyte subsets, including $CD4^+$, $CD8^+$, and CD56 natural killer (NK) cells *(7)*. A variety of transport proteins are involved in drug distribution throughout these sites; these include the product of the multidrug resistance 1 (MDR1) gene P-glycoprotein (P-gp), multidrug resistance-related proteins (MRPs) 1–9, human organic anion transporting polypeptides (OATPs), organic anion transporters (OATs), and organic cation transporters (OCTs) *(6,8)*. When any of these transport proteins are

From: *Infectious Disease: Drug Interactions in Infectious Diseases, Second Edition*
Edited by: S. C. Piscitelli and K. A. Rodvold © Humana Press Inc., Totowa, NJ

modulated (i.e., inhibited or induced) by xenobiotics, the absorption, distribution, metabolism, and excretion of coadministered medications may be affected. As such, drug transport proteins represent an important mechanism by which one drug may alter the disposition and pharmacological effects of another.

Despite the progress that has been made in characterizing drug transport mechanisms, drug interactions because of alterations in drug transport are complex and frequently difficult to predict; reasons for this include

1. Transport proteins are present in a variety of organs and cells throughout the human body, so determining the anatomic site of a particular drug interaction and which transport system is involved is inherently difficult.
2. The expression of many transport proteins is under genetic control, resulting in different transporter phenotypes with altered susceptibility to drug interactions.
3. Many transporters are expressed differently among mammalian species, sometimes making it hard to extrapolate animal data to humans.
4. Different cell lines variably express certain transport proteins, and drug concentrations used in cellular systems are not always clinically relevant.
5. Some transporters (i.e., P-gp) contain multiple drug-binding sites, which can result in a drug having disparate effects on the pharmacokinetics of coadministered drugs (i.e., drug interactions may be substrate dependent).
6. Most transport systems alter drug distribution into various sanctuary sites, such as the central nervous system (CNS); therefore, drug interaction studies that only assess plasma concentrations do not fully characterize the transport-mediated influence of one drug on another.
7. In human studies, it is often difficult to distinguish between the effects of drug transport and drug metabolism regarding the mechanism by which a particular drug interaction occurs.

This chapter reviews the most common drug transport proteins, their anatomic and cellular location, and their documented or potential role in drug interactions involving anti-infective medications. Data from humans, animals, and in vitro cellular systems are discussed to highlight specific transport mechanisms by which clinically significant drug interactions occur. Individual transport proteins are considered for their documented or putative involvement in drug interactions involving antimicrobial agents.

## P-GLYCOPROTEIN

P-gp is the first known and best studied of the adenosine-triphosphate (ATP)-binding cassette (ABC) proteins, which also include MRPs 1–8 *(8,9)*. P-gp-mediated drug extrusion was initially identified as a mechanism by which chemically diverse anticancer agents were ejected from tumor cells, resulting in multidrug resistance *(10)*. In addition to tumor cells, P-gp is also located on the canalicular surface of hepatocytes, the apical surface of renal tubular epithelial cells, the apical surface of intestinal and placental epithelial cells, and the luminal surface of capillary endothelial cells at the blood-brain barrier (BBB) *(2,6,9)*. P-gp is also localized on a number of lymphocyte subsets, including CD4[+], CD8[+], CD19[+], and CD56 NK cells *(7)*. Because of its presence in multiple anatomic locations, P-gp may influence the absorption, distribution, metabolism, and excretion of drugs that are P-gp substrates. As such, modulation of P-gp activity by one drug may affect the pharmacokinetics of another, resulting in a transport-mediated drug–drug interaction.

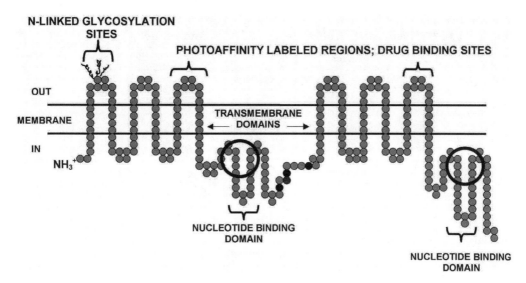

**Fig. 1.** Schematic representation of P-glycoprotein. Large open and small closed circles denote ATP-binding sites and phosphorylation sites, respectively.

P-gp is encoded by the MDR1 gene and is a 150- to 170-kDa membrane protein composed of two symmetrical homologous cassettes (Fig. 1) *(11)*. Each cassette contains six transmembrane domains separated by a flexible linker polypeptide loop, each containing an ATP-binding motif *(11,12)*. The two cassettes of P-gp interact in a cooperative manner to function as a single transporting unit, and ATP hydrolysis supplies the energy for the extrusion process *(2,11,12)*. Numerous substrate binding sites have been identified throughout the transmembrane domains of P-gp *(13)*; these sites differentially interact with P-gp substrates and inhibitors. Therefore, the tendency of a drug to inhibit or induce P-gp may depend on the P-gp substrate with which it is coadministered *(14)*. To illustrate, colchicine and quercetin were both found to stimulate transport of the P-gp substrate rhodamime-123; conversely, these drugs were found to inhibit the transport of the P-gp substrate Hoechst 33342 *(13)*. These results, along with those from others, suggest the need to test more than one P-gp substrate when screening for drug interactions *(13,14)*; these data also advise cautious interpretation of studies that report a drug as a P-gp inhibitor or inducer (exclusively) when the drug has only been studied in combination with a single substrate.

Partly because of the presence of multiple binding sites, P-gp is nondiscriminatory in the compounds that it transports. P-gp recognizes and transports drugs, drug metabolites, drug conjugates, and endogenous compounds with a wide variety of chemical structures and weight *(8)*. Clinically relevant P-gp substrates, inhibitors, and inducers are listed in Table 1 *(7,15–22)*. Although P-gp transports a variety of chemically diverse compounds, in general molecules that are uncharged or weakly basic are transported most efficiently *(8)*.

Partitioning of the cellular lipid membrane is the first step of the interaction between a drug and P-gp-binding sites. Because all P-gp substrates are amphipathic, they can adequately diffuse across biological membranes *(2,6,8,9)*. Thus, in the absence of active

**Table 1**
**Summary of P-Glycoprotein Substrates, Inhibitors, and Inducers**

| Drug class | Substrates | Inhibitors | Inducers |
|---|---|---|---|
| Antivirals | Amprenavir<br>Indinavir<br>Nelfinavir<br>Ritonavir<br>Saquinavir | Amprenavir<br>Nelfinavir<br>Ritonavir<br>Saquinavir<br>Indinavir | Ritonavir<br>Saquinavir<br>Indinavir |
| CNS agents<br>(antidepressants,<br>antipsychotics,<br>and anticonvulsants) | Amitriptyline<br>Nortriptyline<br>Chlorpromazine<br>Phenytoin | | St. John's wort |
| Anticancer agents and<br>immunosuppressants | Numerous [a] | Cyclosporine<br>Sirolimus<br>Tacrolimus<br>Tamoxifen<br>Vinblastine | |
| Antibiotics | Erythromycin<br>Clarithromycin<br>Ciprofloxacin<br>Norfloxacin<br>Cefoperazone<br>Trimethoprim<br>Levofloxacin<br>Grepafloxacin | Erythromycin<br>Clarithromycin<br>Troleandomycin | Erythromycin<br>Rifampin |
| Antifungals | Itraconazole | Itraconazole<br>Ketoconazole | Clotrimazole |
| Anti-infectives<br>(miscellaneous) | Ivermectin<br>Quinine | | |
| Antihistamines | Fexofenadine | Astemizole<br>Terfenadine | |
| Antidiarrheals | Loperamide | | |
| Antihyperlipidemics | Atorvastatin<br>Pravastatin | Lovastatin<br>Simvastatin | |
| Cardiac agents | Losarten<br>Digoxin<br>Quinidine<br>Talinolol<br>Verapamil<br>Lidocaine<br>Propranolol | Amiodarone<br>Bepredil<br>Diltiazem<br>Dipyridamole<br>Felodipine<br>Nicardipine<br>Quinidine<br>Verapamil | Amiodarone<br>Diltiazem<br>Nicardipine<br>Nifedipine<br>Verapamil |
| Steroids, hormones<br>and analogues | Dexamethasone<br>Methylprednisolone<br>Estradiol | Cortisol<br>Progesterone | Bromocriptine<br>Dexamethasone |

**Table 1 *(Continued)***
**Summary of P-Glycoprotein Substrates, Inhibitors, and Inducers**

| Drug class | Substrates | Inhibitors | Inducers [c] |
|---|---|---|---|
| Gastrointestinal agents | Domperidone<br>Cimetidine<br>Ondansetron<br>Ranitidine<br>Omeprazole<br>Lansoprozole<br>Pantoprazole | | |
| Narcotic analgesics | Methadone<br>Fentanyl<br>Morphine | | Morphine |
| Miscellaneous | Colchicine<br>Rhodamine 123<br>Imatinab mesylate | Disulfiram<br>Valspodar (Psc 833)[b]<br>Gf 120918[b]<br>Ly 335979[b]<br>Imatinab mesylate<br>Grapefruit juice<br>  constituents:<br>  furanocoumarins<br>  and flavonoids | Colchicine<br>Probenecid<br>Yohimbine<br>Grapefruit juice<br>  constituents:<br>  furanocoumarins<br>  and flavonoids |

*Source*: From refs. *7,15–22.*

[a] The following anticancer agents have been identified as P-gp substrates: cyclosporine, chlorambucil, cisplatin, cytarabine, daunorubicin, doxorubicin, docetaxel, etoposide, vinblastine methotrexate, hydroxyurea, fluorouracil, mitoxantrone, paclitaxel, tacrolimus, tamoxifen, topotecan, and vincristine.

[b] Second-generation P-gp inhibitors.

[c] The following anticancer agents have been identified as P-gp inducers: chlorambucil, cyclosporine, cisplatin, daunorubicin, doxorubicine, etoposide, fluorouracil, hydroxyurea, methotrexate, mitoxantrone, sirolimus, tacrolimus, tamoxifen, vinblastine, and vincristine.

transport mechanisms (e.g., P-gp-mediated efflux) P-gp substrates cross cellular membranes and penetrate into tissues and cellular compartments. Back-transport (extrusion or efflux) by P-gp only affects drug distribution if the rate of active (back) transport for that drug is considerable compared to the rate of passive diffusion inward *(2,9)*. If this is not the case, the efflux transport system will be saturated by the inward diffusion of drug. This phenomenon explains why P-gp does not alter the disposition of all drugs that are P-gp substrates *(2,9)*; it also explains why P-gp inhibition by a drug does not necessarily alter the disposition of coadministered P-gp substrates. This is discussed in further detail in the consideration of intestinal P-gp. Interactions known or strongly suspected to occur secondary to P-gp modulation at a specific anatomic site will are also discussed under individual organ/cellular systems.

Significant interpatient variability exists in P-gp expression in the human intestine and possibly other organs *(6,23,24)*. Genetic polymorphisms in the MDR1 gene have been recognized as a variable that may contribute to interindividual heterogeneity in drug disposition, therapeutic response, and predisposition to drug interactions *(25,26)*.

Indeed, messenger ribonucleic acid (mRNA) and protein levels of P-gp vary approx 8-to 10-fold between individuals *(6,23,24)*. Data suggest a possible role for MDR1 genotype in contributing to drug–drug interactions.

Kurata et al. reported that the absolute bioavailability of the P-gp substrate digoxin was increased to a greater extent by the P-gp inhibitor clarithromycin in individuals with the G/G2677C/C3435 (wild-type) genotype compared to individuals with the T/T2677T/T3435 (mutant) genotype *(27)*. The CC/GG, CT/GT,A, and TT/TT haplotypes at positions 3435/2677 have been associated with high, intermediate, and low levels of P-gp expression, respectively (although conflicting data have been reported) *(28)*. The most plausible reason for differences in the extent of the digoxin–clarithromycin interaction among different MDR1 genotypes is that individuals with the GG/CC haplotype harbored higher levels of intestinal P-gp compared to TT/TT individuals; thus, when P-gp was inhibited by clarithromycin, there was a comparatively greater increase in digoxin availability in CC/GG vs TT/TT individuals *(27)*. Similarly, in a healthy volunteer study, increases in digoxin exposure were greater in CC/GG subjects vs TT/TT subjects taking liquid-filled digoxin capsules with and without the putative P-gp inhibitor ritonavir *(29)*; however, because of the small number of subjects studied, results did not reach statistical significance in either study.

Although further investigation is needed, these preliminary results suggest that certain individuals may be genetically predisposed to P-gp-mediated drug–drug interactions with P-gp-inhibiting antibiotics such as clarithromycin and erythromycin; this may also prove true for other anti-infective medications purported to inhibit P-gp (i.e., human immunodeficiency virus [HIV] protease inhibitors). A comprehensive review of MDR1 pharmacogenetics has been published *(30)*.

## Principles of P-gp Inhibition

Most of the P-gp-mediated drug interactions discussed in this chapter arise from inhibition or induction of the protein at one or more organs or cell types in the body. Commonly sited inhibitors of P-gp are listed in Table 1 *(7,15–21)*. Competitive inhibition of P-gp-mediated transport occurs when two substrates act on the same binding site, to which only one of the substrates can bind at any one time. Noncompetitive inhibition may also occur; in this case, two substrates simultaneously bind to P-gp at the same time at different, functionally independent sites. P-gp inhibition can also occur when a drug prevents ATP hydrolysis, thereby disengaging P-gp and reducing the transport of a coadministered medication *(2)*. Drugs can inhibit P-gp function through one or more of these mechanisms; and as these mechanisms would suggest, P-gp inhibition by a particular drug is often dependent on the drug with which it is coadministered (i.e., P-gp inhibition is substrate dependent) *(13,14)*. Interestingly, many P-gp inhibitors are also inhibitors of CYP3A4; examples include erythromycin, itraconazole, cyclosporine, diltiazem, and HIV protease inhibitors *(7,15)*. Because of the complex nature of P-gp inhibition and substrate overlap with CYP3A4, it is difficult to qualitatively and quantitatively predict drug–drug interactions via this mechanism *(2)*.

## Principles of P-gp Induction

A number of medications have been shown to induce P-gp in a variety of animal and human cell lines *(7,15–21,31–36)*. These studies confirmed that there are species differences in P-gp inducibility, possibly because of sequence differences in the ligand-binding domain of pregnane X receptor (PXR) among animal species *(2)*. Preclinical studies have also reported that P-gp induction appears to depend on the animal model, tissue type, and drug dose and length of exposure employed *(34,35)*.

Similar to P-gp inhibition, there is considerable overlap between CYP3A4 and P-gp inducers; examples include phenobarbital, phenytoin, dexamethasone, rifampin, and St. John's wort *(7,15)*. This overlap in CYP3A4 and P-gp inducers has been hypothesized to result from the fact that CYP3A4 and MDR1 are coordinated through similar mechanisms, which includes PXR activation *(37)*. Activation of PXR is purported to result in increased P-gp expression (induction). Data that showed that PXR is activated by the P-gp inducers rifampin and paclitaxel support this concept *(38,39)*. For a more detailed review of the mechanism of PXR-mediated induction of P-gp, refer to a review by Lin and Yamazaki *(2)*. Similar to P-gp inhibition, P-gp induction is a complex process that is qualitatively and quantitatively difficult to predict.

## P-gp and Drug Absorption

P-gp is present in high levels on the villus tip of the apical membrane of enterocytes, where it is involved in the efflux of substrates from inside cells back into the intestinal lumen *(2,7–9)*. The highest concentrations of P-gp are present on the apical surface of superficial columnar cells in the jejunum and colon *(40)*. P-gp is unevenly distributed throughout the gastrointestinal tract. The content of mRNA expression from P-gp was found to increase progressively from the stomach to the jejunum to the colon *(41,42)*. This uneven distribution of P-gp influenced cyclosporine area under the concentration–time curve (AUC) in 10 healthy volunteers who were given the drug at different parts of the gastrointestinal tract, including the stomach, jejunum, and colon *(42)*. Consistent with P-gp mRNA levels, cyclosporine AUC was highest in the stomach and lowest in the jejunum *(2)*. Presumably, uneven distribution of intestinal P-gp can influence drug absorption and predisposition to P-gp-mediated drug interactions among antimicrobial agents, particularly in critically ill patients receiving multiple medications through intestinal feeding tubes. To date however, no clinical studies have clearly described this phenomenon.

Numerous preclinical studies using in vitro cellular systems and *mdr1* knockout mice (mice lacking *mdr1* that subsequently do not express P-gp) have documented the involvement of P-gp in drug disposition, including absorption *(43–49)*. A general finding in all of these studies was that absence or blockade of intestinal P-gp results in reduced efflux and increased bioavailability of P-gp substrates; as a result, enhanced toxicity or improved clinical efficacy may theoretically occur. This has been noted with HIV protease inhibitors *(45)*. Conversely, induction of intestinal P-gp would be expected to reduce the oral availability of P-gp substrates, which in the case of HIV protease inhibitors may result in suboptimal plasma concentrations, accumulation of HIV resistance mutations, and clinical failure. Specific interactions involving anti-infective agents that are caused by P-gp inhibition and induction are addressed in this section.

With the identification of HIV protease inhibitors as P-gp substrates came the belief that intestinal P-gp (at least partially) accounts for the low and variable oral bioavailability of these drugs, and that inhibition of intestinal P-gp by coadministered drugs—often protease inhibitors themselves—may improve drug absorption *(2,9)*.

However, this assumption has drawn criticism *(2,9)*. Indeed, it is a common mistaken belief that the extent of oral absorption of a drug is always significantly limited by intestinal P-gp if that drug is a P-gp substrate *(45,50)*. Many drugs that are well-described substrates for P-gp exhibit reasonably good bioavailability; this is caused by saturation of intestinal P-gp at clinically relevant doses. Examples of P-gp substrates with good oral availability include digoxin liquid-filled capsules, vinblastine, etoposide, verapamil, ritonavir, and indinavir *(9)*.

Illustrating the concept directly above, indinavir, when administered as a single protease inhibitor, is given as an 800-mg dose. At this high dose, indinavir concentrations in the intestinal lumen are substantial (in the millimolar concentration range); these concentrations are much higher than the indinavir affinity constant $K_m$ for P-gp, which is 140 µM *(51)*. Therefore, at clinically relevant doses, it is likely that intestinal P-gp is saturated by indinavir, in which case the cellular influx of drug is much greater than the P-gp-mediated efflux. This presumably explains why indinavir exhibits reasonably good oral bioavailability (>60%) in patients with HIV infection despite its designation as a P-gp substrate *(52)*. Extrapolating from these data, one would not expect a coadministered medication to appreciably increase indinavir oral bioavailability through inhibition of intestinal P-gp. However, it must be remembered that indinavir concentrations in other areas of the body (brain, liver, and kidney) may be at or below the indinavir $K_m$ for P-gp transport; as such, P-gp may still influence cellular or organ distribution of the drug, in which case drug interactions at these anatomic locations secondary to P-gp inhibition or induction may still occur with indinavir.

Ritonavir is another HIV protease inhibitor that is a P-gp substrate with good oral bioavailability (>60%) *(53)*. Like indinavir, ritonavir is also given at a high (>50 mg) oral dose of 600 mg. Thus, the administration of high doses of P-gp substrates tends to reduce the impact of intestinal P-gp-mediated efflux on their absorption, particularly when one considers that $K_m$ values for P-gp transport for most drugs is low (4–213 µmol/L), thus allowing for saturation of intestinal P-gp at clinically relevant doses *(2)*.

Nevertheless, exceptions exist in that some drugs given at high doses are still influenced by the effects of intestinal P-gp. Typically, such drugs are poorly water soluble, dissolve slowly, and are large in size (>800 Da) *(2)*. Well-described examples of such drugs include cyclosporine and paclitaxel *(2,9)*. The HIV protease inhibitor saquinavir—particularly the hard-gel capsule formulation—may also represent a P-gp substrate with oral bioavailability (4% when given as a single 600-mg dose) *(54)* that is negatively impacted by P-gp. Saquinavir is a large lipophilic molecule (free base molecular weight = 670.86) that is slowly absorbed (time to maximal concentration $[T_{max}]$ = 3–5 hours) *(54,55)*. As such, saquinavir concentrations below its $K_m$ value for P-gp transport may be expected in the intestine. In further support of this concept, saquinavir exposure is significantly increased by the putative intestinal P-gp inhibitors ritonavir and grapefruit juice (by 20- to 50-fold with ritonavir and 60% with grapefruit juice) *(56–59)*. However, because saquinavir is both a P-gp and CYP3A4 substrate, ritonavir inhibits intestinal as well as hepatic CYP3A4, and grapefruit juice inhibits intestinal CYP3A4, it is difficult to appreciate the contribution of intestinal P-gp inhibition with these agents on saquinavir exposure.

In addition to inhibition, induction of intestinal P-gp may be involved in clinically significant drug interactions *(2)*. The influence of the P-gp inducer rifampin on digoxin pharmacokinetics was described in 8 healthy volunteers receiving both oral and intravenous digoxin doses *(27)*. Of note, digoxin is a P-gp substrate that is not appreciably metabolized in humans *(60)*. Digoxin pharmacokinetic parameter values were derived before and after rifampin administration at 600 mg daily for 10 days *(61)*. Rifampin coadministration resulted in decreases of 31 and 52% in digoxin AUC and $C_{max}$, respectively, when digoxin was given orally. When given intravenously, digoxin pharmacokinetics were not appreciably altered by rifampin. Moreover, duodenal biopsies revealed that P-gp content increased 3.5-fold with rifampin administration, which correlated inversely with the digoxin AUC after oral dosing. These data provide strong evidence that the interaction between rifampin and orally administered digoxin occurs at the intestinal level secondary to P-gp induction. In a similar study in eight healthy volunteers, the influence of rifampin on talinolol disposition and duodenal P-gp expression was described *(62)*. Talinolol, like digoxin, is a P-gp substrate that is not appreciably metabolized in humans *(63)*. Oral administration of 600 mg rifampin daily for 9 days reduced the steady-state AUC of orally administered talinolol by 35% ($p < 0.05$). Treatment with rifampin also resulted in a statistically significant increase in duodenal P-gp content (4.2-fold above baseline).

Like digoxin and talinolol, cyclosporine is also a P-gp substrate; however, contrary to digoxin, cyclosporine is also metabolized by CYP3A4 in the liver and to a lesser extent in the intestine *(2)*. The influence of rifampin (600 mg per day for 11 days) was assessed in healthy volunteers on both orally and intravenously administered cyclosporine *(64)*. Rifampin increased the clearance of cyclosporine from 5 mL/min/kg to 7 mL/min/kg and decreased its bioavailability from 27 to 10%. Presumably, induction of intestinal P-gp was at least partially responsible for the observed interaction between the drugs. However, because cyclosporine is a substrate for both CYP3A4 and P-gp and rifampin induces both of these proteins, the influence of rifampin on cyclosporine disposition is most likely caused by coinduction of both P-gp and CYP3A4. Further, the respective roles of intestinal vs hepatic induction of P-gp and CYP3A4 are difficult to define regarding the mechanism of this interaction.

In general, the influence of intestinal P-gp inhibition as a mechanism for clinically significant drug interactions tends to be overstated. Drug interactions caused by P-gp inhibition at the intestinal level are more likely to be quantitatively important for those antimicrobial agents given as small oral doses or with slow dissolution or membrane diffusion rates *(9)*. Conversely, drug interactions caused by induction of intestinal P-gp are supported by data from several investigations using different P-gp substrates *(61,62,64)*.

Because many drugs are both P-gp and CYP3A4 substrates, it is frequently difficult to differentiate between P-gp and CYP3A4 modulation when attempting to elucidate the mechanism behind specific P-gp-mediated interactions. In fact, many such interactions are appreciated by clinicians under the auspices of CYP inhibition. For example, the large increases in plasma saquinavir concentrations that occur when the drug is coadministered with ritonavir are well known; presumably, P-gp inhibition by ritonavir contributes to this interaction to some degree. However, the mechanism of the ritonavir–saquinavir interaction is typically cited as CYP3A4 inhibition. An important group of drugs that may be underrecognized by clinicians as susceptible to drug interactions are P-gp substrates that are not appreciably metabolized by CYP enzymes. The interaction between ritonavir and digoxin is an example of such an interaction *(29)*. As such, clinicians should remain diligent in keeping up-to-date in identifying medications that are not CYP substrates (i.e., digoxin and colchicine) yet are still susceptible to potentially clinically significant interactions secondary to P-gp modulation.

### P-gp and Drug Metabolism and Biliary Excretion

P-gp appears to play an important role in drug metabolism for two primary reasons. First, there is significant overlap in substrate recognition between P-gp and CYP3A4 *(2,7, 9)*; second, both of these proteins are co-localized in the intestine, liver, and kidney *(2,7,9)*. The influence of P-gp on drug metabolism is related to its intracellular relationship to CYP3A4. In the liver, P-gp is located at the canalicular (basolateral) membrane of hepatocytes facing the bile duct lumen (i.e., at the exit site of the cell) *(9)*. Drugs, drug metabolites, and drug conjugates do not come into contact with P-gp in the liver until after they have been taken up into the hepatocyte (via passive diffusion or active transport) and undergone intracellular distribution and metabolism *(2,9)*. After excretion into the bile, only a small fraction of the drug (or metabolite or conjugate) is typically reabsorbed. Therefore, it is necessary to consider hepatic uptake processes, hepatic metabolism, and biliary excretion by other drug transport systems (i.e., MRPs) when attempting to assess the influence of P-gp on hepatic drug excretion *(2,9)*. As might be imagined, this is a daunting process that frequently requires use of various animal and cellular models.

Based on the localization of P-gp in hepatocytes, only drugs that are not significantly metabolized in the liver yet undergo appreciable biliary excretion via P-gp will be susceptible to drug interactions secondary to modulation of hepatic P-gp; digoxin and fexofenadine are examples of such medications. In humans, approx 20–25% of an oral digoxin dose is excreted unchanged in the bile *(65)*. Numerous antibacterial and antifungal medications increase serum concentrations of digoxin. These include the P-gp inhibitors erythromycin, clarithromycin, itraconazole, and ketoconazole *(66)*.

Although inhibition of P-gp-mediated digoxin transport in the liver (and intestine) likely contributes to these interactions, most data suggest that the interactions occur primarily at the level of the kidney *(2,9)*. Conversely, ritonavir was found to increase digoxin exposure by 22 and 86% in separate healthy volunteer studies, one of which did not show an effect on renal digoxin clearance *(29,67)*. Because digoxin (more than 90% bioavailable) liquid-filled capsules were used in this investigation, the most plausible mechanism for this interaction was inhibition of P-gp-mediated digoxin transport in the liver. Similarly, ritonavir was found to inhibit fexofenadine transport in an in vitro cell culture model with an $IC_{50}$ value of 5.4 $\mu M$ (3.9 $\mu$g/mL), which is well within the range of ritonavir plasma concentrations achieved with low-dose regimens (100–200 mg twice daily) *(68)*; in humans, one would expect this interaction to occur primarily at the hepatic level considering that 80% of a fexofenadine dose is recovered in the feces, presumably because of significant biliary excretion, although this assumption has been challenged *(2)*. Of note, unlike digoxin, increases or decreases in fexofenadine exposure secondary to P-gp modulation are not expected to result in clinically relevant toxicity; however, fexofenadine (like digoxin) serves as a useful probe to detect P-gp inhibition or induction with a variety of anti-infective agents.

In addition to ritonavir, other anti-infective agents have also been reported to alter fexofenadine disposition, presumably because of their effects on P-gp-mediated fexofenadine transport in the liver *(69,70)*. In healthy volunteers, a 6-day course of 600 mg rifampin daily reduced the AUC and $C_{max}$ of fexofenadine two- and threefold, respectively, when fexofenadine was administered as single 60-mg doses before and after rifampin dosing *(69)*. Conversely, the P-gp inhibitor ketoconazole did not alter fexofenadine transport in the small intestines of eight healthy volunteers undergoing a jejunal perfusion study *(71)*. Another healthy volunteer jejunal perfusion investigation showed that the P-gp inhibitor verapamil, like ketoconazole, also failed to alter intestinal fexofenadine transport *(72)*.

Collectively, these data establish fexofenadine as an effective probe drug for P-gp transport in the liver. Moreover, results from these investigations suggest that certain anti-infectives have the potential to interact with coadministered medications by influencing their P-gp-mediated hepatic transport. Future studies involving fexofenadine in combination with antimicrobial agents should yield important information regarding the potential of certain anti-infectives to interact with other medications via modulation of hepatic P-gp. However, it bears emphasizing that the characteristics of a drug most likely to be affected by P-gp modulation would be one that is a P-gp substrate, not appreciably metabolized in the liver, and significantly excreted into the bile. Because few drugs meet these criteria in full, hepatic P-gp modulation does not appear to be a major mechanism for P-gp-mediated drug interactions, although exceptions will most certainly exist.

Contrary to P-gp's localization in hepatocytes, P-gp is located on the apical surface of epithelial cells of intestines (i.e., at the entrance site of the cell). As such, P-gp "sees" a drug before it undergoes intracellular distribution and metabolism *(2,9)*. Intestinal P-gp extrudes drugs from enterocytes back into the intestinal lumen, and the drug is then typically reabsorbed. This repetitive process of efflux and reasbsorption increases the intracellular contact time between drug molecules and drug-metabolizing enzymes, such as intestinal CYP3A4. Several studies in animal and cell culture models have shown that the intestinal metabolism of indinavir was increased when it was subjected to repetitive P-gp-mediated efflux *(73,74)*.

However, it is important not to overstate the potential clinical significance of these data given that the influence of intestinal P-gp on presystemic drug metabolism is less important when high drug doses (>50 mg) are administered orally *(2,9)*. Indeed, the intestinal extraction ratio of indinavir increased from 5 to 25% when an oral dose of indinavir was decreased from 10 to 0.1 mg/kg in rats *(75)*. These data highlight the importance of P-gp saturation and cellular localization when considering potential P-gp and CYP-mediated drug interactions in the liver and intestines. In general, unless intestinal P-gp is markedly upregulated by a P-gp inducer (i.e., rifampin) or the concurrently administered P-gp substrate is given as a low dose and is poorly and slowly absorbed, intestinal P-gp-mediated efflux will not produce major alterations in the intestinal metabolism and absorption of coadministered P-gp substrates in most cases.

### P-gp and Renal Excretion of Drugs

P-gp is localized on the apical (exit site) brush border membrane of renal proximal tubular cells—the major site of renal secretion—facing the lumen of the renal tubule *(2,9)*. As in the liver, renal P-gp does not see drugs, drug metabolites, or drug conjugates until intracellular trafficking has been completed, at which point compounds are excreted into the urine by P-gp *(2,9)*. Drugs that are secreted unchanged in the urine are most likely to be affected by P-gp inhibition in the kidney, in which case drug efflux into renal tubules would be compromised, renal clearance reduced, and plasma concentrations increased.

Increased drug exposure secondary to inhibition of renal P-gp may lead to the development of unexpected toxicities or improved clinical efficacy. A preclinical study noted that the antibiotics dicloxacillin and trimethoprim are P-gp substrates with transport that is inhibited by the P-gp inhibitors, including cyclosporine, ketoconazole, and vinblastine *(76)*. The authors of this study proposed that P-gp may be responsible for the increase in renal clearance of these, and possibly other, antibiotics in patients with cystic fibrosis *(76)*. If this proves true in humans, drugs targeted to inhibit renal P-gp may reduce the renal clearance of certain antibiotics in such patients. It has also been hypothesized that modulation of tubular secretion may affect intracellular drug accumulation and potentiate the nephrotoxic potential of certain antibiotics, such as cephalosporins and vancomycin *(77)*; this concept is expanded in the discussion of MRPs.

A variety of anti-infective agents has been noted to inhibit P-gp in the kidney. Clarithromycin was found to increase the $AUC_{0-24}$ of digoxin 1.7-fold in 12 healthy volunteers; a 68% increase in the nonglomerular renal clearance of digoxin was also observed (from $34 \pm 39$ mL/minute to $57 \pm 41$ mL/minute; $p = 0.03$) *(78)*. In another study in healthy volunteers, itraconazole coadministration resulted in a significant reduction in the renal clearance of digoxin *(79)*. Similar to the liver, when considering the potential for P-gp-mediated drug interactions in the kidney, other transporter systems must be considered, particularly because they may be upregulated in the presence of P-gp inhibition or downregulation. In general, P-gp-mediated inhibition in the kidney should be considered a potentially clinically relevant mechanism by which renally eliminated P-gp substrates interact with inhibitors. Clinicians must keep this mechanism in mind as P-gp substrates and inhibitors are increasingly identified, particularly because these types of drug interactions are unlikely to be routinely cited in tertiary literature sources and package inserts. Practitioners must frequently extrapolate information on drug transport processes from a variety of primary sources, including data from animal and cell culture experiments, to anticipate potential interactions.

### P-gp and Drug Distribution Into the Central Nervous System

The BBB, which consists of closely joined endothelial cells in brain capillary blood vessels, prevents the passive diffusion of many drugs into the CNS *(2,6,9,80)*. Large, hydrophilic, and highly protein-bound molecules are frequently impeded from crossing the BBB; in comparison, lipophilic molecules traverse the BBB more efficiently *(2,6–9)*. However, not all lipophilic drugs sufficiently penetrate the BBB because of their extrusion from the CNS by P-gp and other transport systems.

P-gp is highly expressed on the apical surface of brain capillary epithelial cells *(81,82)*. Because of P-gp's efficiency in preventing xenobiotics from permeating the CNS, the brain is far more sensitive, compared to other organs, to modulation in P-gp activity *(2,6,9)*. As such, P-gp inhibition at the BBB has the potential to enhance the efficacy or potentiate the toxicity of anti-infective medications.

Successful treatment of certain infections, such as acquired immunodeficiency syndrome (AIDS) dementia complex and other HIV-related neurological disorders, and bacterial, fungal, or viral meningitis require adequate CNS penetration of anti-infective medications. In patients with HIV infection, the CNS can act as a sanctuary site for HIV, thereby protecting the virus from antiretroviral therapy *(83)*. Pharmacological seques-tration of HIV in the CNS occurs partly because of P-gp mediated efflux of antiretroviral medications—HIV protease inhibitors in particular—from the brain. A series of elegant animal studies have shown that the HIV protease inhibitors saquinavir, indinavir, nelfinavir, and amprenavir are all extruded from the CNS by P-gp, and that it is possible to partially reverse that extrusion by coadministering a P-gp inhibitor *(45,48,84)*.

In addition to their role as P-gp substrates, HIV protease inhibitors have been stud-ied for their ability to modulate P-gp at the BBB and alter the CNS penetration of coadministered medications. Kravcik et al. reported cerebrospinal fluid (CSF) concen-trations and CSF:plasma ratios of saquinavir and ritonavir in 11 HIV-infected treat-ment responders (HIV RNA <20 copies/mL for >6 months) receiving these drugs in combination for over 12 months. Saquinavir could only be detected in the CSF of 2 of 11 patients (at 0.1 and 0.2% of concentrations in plasma), suggesting that ritonavir-mediated P-gp inhibition at the BBB was not sufficient to appreciably enhance the CNS penetration of saquinavir in this group of patients *(85)*. Consistent with these findings, separate investigations reported that ritonavir failed to enhance the penetra-tion of coadministered HIV protease inhibitors into the CNS of mice *(84,86)*. Simi-larly, the P-gp inhibitors erythromycin and verapamil also failed to significantly inhibit P-gp at the BBB in clinical investigations *(6)*. On the other hand, the P-gp inhibitor ketoconazole increased the unbound CSF:plasma ratio of ritonavir by 181% (95% confi-dence interval 47–437%) in HIV-infected patients *(87)*. These generally negative results may be partly caused by the relatively low concentrations of many drugs at the BBB after oral administration *(6)*. Furthermore, the large molecular weight (>500 Da) and high protein-binding characteristics of the protease inhibitors (98%) also contribute to poor CNS penetration by these drugs.

In contrast to these data, P-gp inhibitors of greater potency that are not currently avail-able have indeed proven highly effective at inhibiting P-gp at the BBB and enhancing the CNS penetration of coadministered P-gp substrates *(48,84,88,89)*. However, until such medications are approved for use in humans and found to be safe and effective for their intended purpose of enhancing CSF concentrations of a coadministered medication, the therapeutic usefulness of targeted P-gp inhibition at the BBB with currently available medications is questionable.

Although numerous studies have assessed P-gp inhibition at the BBB, few have examined the effects of P-gp induction at the BBB. In principle, P-gp induction at the BBB could increase the efficiency with which P-gp extrudes drugs from the CNS. This could lead to suboptimal antimicrobial concentrations in the brains of patients with CNS infections. However, in animal studies the P-gp-inducing agents rifampin, phenytoin, and phenobarbital all proved ineffective in reducing the CNS penetration of coadministered compounds *(90,91)*. Although human data are necessary to con-firm these study results, these data offer reassurance given the frequent use of seizure prophylaxis as well as rifampin therapy in patients with serious CNS infections, such as meningitis. To date, there are no data to suggest that patients receiving such medi-cations are prone to P-gp induction at the BBB, which could theoretically lead to reduced CNS penetration of concurrent medications, particularly anti-infectives.

It is unclear why P-gp at the BBB does not appear to be readily inducible. One possibility is that high basal levels of P-gp in the brain prevent potential inducers (e.g., cyclosporine, rifampin, phenobarbital, phenytoin, etc.) from achieving intracellular concentrations necessary to induce P-gp *(2)*. In addition, it is possible that variability exists among tissues regarding their ability to respond to P-gp inducers *(2)*. Further study is clearly necessary to explore these hypotheses.

## *P-gp and Drug Distribution Across the Placenta*

P-gp is thought to play a protective role in reducing fetal exposure to xenobiotics *(92,93)*. P-gp is highly expressed in human placental trophoblasts, in which it is present on the apical membrane facing the maternal blood compartment *(94)*. The level of P-gp expression in the placenta appears to change throughout the course of pregnancy; however, the direction and magnitude of this change has yet to be fully described *(95)*. The potential benefits of placental P-gp in protecting the human fetus from harmful toxins or medications is evident; however; in certain clinical situations, such as pregnancy in the setting of HIV infection, it may be beneficial to increase the placental transfer of drugs.

Several trials in humans suggested that the nucleoside reverse transcriptase inhibitors zidovudine, lamivudine, and didanosine penetrate the placental barrier reasonably well *(96,97)*. One likely reason that these agents readily transverse the placental barrier is the fact that none are well-described substrates for P-gp. Similarly, the nonnucleoside reverse transcriptase inhibitor nevirapine is also not a P-gp substrate; this is consistent with its excellent transplacental ratio of 0.8 (newborn:mother blood concentration) *(98)* and its documented clinical efficacy in reducing vertical transmission of HIV *(99)*.

In contrast, the HIV protease inhibitors have been noted to exhibit poor penetration across the placental barrier in several clinical and preclinical studies *(100–102)*. Among 10 maternal–cord blood sample pairs, Marzolini et al. reported median umbilical cord blood concentrations at delivery for nelfinavir, ritonavir, saquinavir, and lopinavir that were <250, <250, <100, and <250 ng/mL, respectively *(100)*. Of note, maternal plasma drug concentrations collected at the same time as cord blood samples were within expected ranges. An ex vivo placental transfusion study reported the mean fetal transfer rate of saquinavir was 1.8% *(102)*. A similar study with ritonavir revealed that the drug did not accumulate in placental tissue *(101)*.

One of the major reasons HIV protease inhibitors do not readily traverse the placental barrier is most likely because of their extrusion by P-gp. Other factors, such as high plasma protein binding (>98%) and large molecular weight, may also contribute. Interestingly, there are no data on the placental transfer of indinavir, which is the only HIV protease inhibitor that is not highly bound to plasma proteins; data on the fetal penetration of indinavir would offer a means of speculating on the relative contributions of plasma protein binding and P-gp efflux to poor placental penetration with these drugs.

Despite a growing body of preclinical data that suggests the possibility of fetal toxicity when a P-gp substrate is coadministered with a P-gp inhibitor during pregnancy, the clinical importance of this phenomenon is unclear. Moreover, at least one study suggested that the well-known P-gp inhibitors quinidine and verapamil do not inhibit digoxin transport in human placental cells, possibly suggesting that the placenta, like the brain, may be unique in its ability to respond to P-gp modulation *(103)*. Whether targeted P-gp inhibition in the placenta can be used to enhance fetal penetration of certain drugs, such as HIV protease inhibitors, is unknown; in theory, this could result in increased antiretroviral activity in the fetus, potentially leading to reduced vertical transmission of HIV. Of interest, there are no studies to date describing P-gp induction in the placenta.

Genetic variation in MDR1 expression has been described for placental P-gp, which may result in interindividual differences in drug penetration across the placental barrier *(2,9)*. Whether genetic variability in placental P-gp can predispose certain individuals to drug interactions mediated through P-gp inhibition is unknown. To date, however, there are insufficient data to suggest a clinical role for targeted P-gp inhibition in the placenta, although future studies may eventually alter this interpretation.

### P-gp and Drug Distribution Into the Genital Tract

Similar to the CNS, the testes represent a sanctuary site for antimicrobial chemotherapy *(104)*; this is primarily because of the blood–testes barrier, which like the BBB, consists of continuous cell layers containing the efflux proteins P-gp and MRP1 *(82)*. In the testes, P-gp is expressed at the luminal side of endothelial cells as well as the myoid-cell layer surrounding the seminiferous tubule *(104)*. After a drug passively diffuses from the blood to the testicular interstitium, it can then be extruded via efflux pumps such as P-gp *(104)*. Agents that have been reported to be transported and excreted by P-gp at the testes level include carcinogens, xenobiotics, hormones, carcinogens, and HIV-1 protease inhibitors *(104–109)*.

Median genital-tract-to-blood-plasma ratios for lopinavir, nelfinavir, ritonavir, and saquinavir range between <0.04 and 0.070 *(109)*. These ratios for amprenavir and indinavir were reported to be between 0.20 and 1.4–1.9 *(109)*. Indinavir's superior penetration across the blood–testes barrier likely results from its comparatively lower plasma protein binding, which in addition to transport systems, can also affect drug penetration into the genital tract. Inadequate penetration of HIV protease inhibitors into the genital tract may compromise the usefulness of these agents in the setting of postexposure prophylaxis *(109)*. In addition, low protease inhibitor concentrations in the genital tract may fail to suppress local viral replication, leading to the development of resistant viral variants and perhaps increased transmissibility of the virus through sexual contact *(109)*.

Targeted inhibition of P-gp at the testes level may improve penetration of the HIV protease inhibitors into the genital tract, resulting in clinical benefit. Van Praag et al. measured indinavir trough concentrations in 13 HIV-infected patients receiving zidovudine or stavudine plus lamivudine, abacavir, and nevirapine at standard clinical doses; they also received 1000 mg indinavir three times daily (increased from the standard dose of 800 mg three times daily to account for induction of indinavir metabolism by nevirapine) *(110)*. When investigators observed inadequate indinavir trough plasma concentrations with this regimen, indinavir was switched to the combination of 800 mg indinavir plus 100 mg ritonavir twice daily. Addition of ritonavir increased the median indinavir trough plasma concentration from 65 to 336 ng/mL (5.2-fold; $p = 0.002$). Seminal indinavir concentrations, measured in 6 patients before and after the addition of ritonavir, increased 8.2-fold (95% confidence interval 5.2–11.6). Higher indinavir plasma trough concentrations alone did not sufficiently account for the observed increases in indinavir concentrations in semen after the addition of ritonavir. Ritonavir-mediated inhibition of P-gp in the testes may have contributed to the observed drug interaction *(110)*.

These results were supported in concept by at least one preclinical study in which [$^{14}$C]nelfinavir testes:plasma ratios increased two- to fivefold after coadministration with the P-gp inhibitor LY-335979. Although such data are preliminary, they suggest that ritonavir-boosted protease inhibitor regimens may offer the advantage of increased genital tract penetration by the coadministered protease inhibitor; in theory, this could result in improved virological efficacy against HIV in the genital tract and reduced potential to transmit HIV through sexual contact. Clearly, definitive studies are necessary to confirm or refute such speculation.

## P-gp and Drug Distribution Into Lymphocytes

Several ABC proteins, including P-gp, are detectable and functionally active on subclasses of lymphocytes *(111,112)*. Studies have suggested that the highest levels of P-gp are expressed on NK CD8$^+$ and CD4$^+$ cells *(7)*. P-gp expression is variable on human monocytes and granulocytes *(7)*. P-gp functions at the lymphocyte level to extrude drugs, thereby limiting their intracellular accumulation. Intracellular drug concentrations are an important consideration when treating certain infectious diseases, such as HIV infection. Indeed, the HIV virus replicates and is primarily contained within CD4$^+$ cells and CD34$^+$ progenitor cells *(111,112)*.

Similar to the brain and testes, it is possible that human CD4$^+$ cells may represent a sanctuary for replicating virus. Some studies have reported that inhibition of viral replication is impeded in cells that express P-gp *(113)*; other investigations, however, have found conflicting results *(114,115)*. Assuming that P-gp does play a significant role in reducing penetration of HIV protease inhibitors into cells, then blocking P-gp via coadministration of a P-gp inhibitor would represent an attractive option for improving antiretroviral activity. Another consideration when assessing the cellular role of P-gp is the fact that P-gp expression itself on CD4$^+$ cells has been reported to reduce the infectivity and replicative capacity of HIV, although the clinical importance of this phenomenon remains a topic of debate *(116,117)*.

A study examined the relationship between P-gp expression on peripheral blood mononuclear cells (PBMCs) isolated from HIV-infected patients and intracellular accumulation of ritonavir and saquinavir *(118)*. Ritonavir accumulation was significantly higher in patients with lower P-gp expression (< median for all specimens) compared to patients with higher expression (*p* = 0.014). Saquinavir accumulation in PBMCs was not related to P-gp expression in this study *(118)*. Additional experiments conducted in in vitro cell lines offered additional evidence that P-gp can significantly reduce the rate of uptake and lower steady-state intracellular concentrations of HIV protease inhibitors, including ritonavir, indinavir, saquinavir, and nelfinavir *(119)*.

Several studies have shown that HIV protease inhibitors themselves, with the possible exception of indinavir, are inhibitors of P-gp on peripheral blood lymphocytes *(114)*. In one study, P-gp inhibition occurred in the following order: ritonavir > saquinavir > nelfinavir > indinavir *(120)*. In a separate investigation, nelfinavir was found to effectively inhibit P-gp on CD4$^+$ as well as CD8$^+$ cells from both HIV-negative and HIV-positive donors *(121)*. Furthermore, reduced P-gp activity was observed in 59% of HIV-positive patients (27 of 46 individuals) receiving nelfinavir.

Chaillou et al. examined plasma and intracellular (PBMC) peak and trough drug concentrations in 49 HIV-infected patients receiving a variety of protease inhibitor-containing antiretroviral regimens *(122)*. Mean ratios of intracellular:plasma concentrations for the different regimens were reported, along with MDR1 expression and HIV RNA. Patients who overexpressed MDR1 had significantly lower intracellular protease inhibitor concentrations compared to those with normal P-gp expression ($p = 0.042$). In addition, patients treated with low-dose ritonavir as a pharmacoenhancing agent (100 mg twice daily), who had detectable intracellular ritonavir concentrations, did not express MDR1. Last, patients with HIV RNA below 40 copies/mL had significantly higher intracellular concentrations of ritonavir ($p = 0.029$). These data suggest that P-gp effectively limits intracellular protease inhibitor penetration, and that ritonavir can reverse this process, thereby increasing intracellular drug accumulation. Whether this is a significant mechanism by which ritonavir contributes to the antiviral activity of combination drug regimens is unclear but is certainly plausible. Further study is necessary to determine whether other, more potent P-gp inhibitors will be clinically useful in enhancing intracellular accumulation of HIV protease inhibitors and improving their virological efficacy.

Conversely, although P-gp inhibition enhances intracellular penetration of substrates, induction is expected to produce the opposite effect. Perhaps because of substantial intra- and interpatient variability in lymphocyte P-gp expression, studies have reported conflicting results regarding the induction potential of lymphocyte P-gp by certain drugs *(123–126)*. Indeed, HIV protease inhibitors, generally regarded as P-gp inhibitors to varying degrees, have also been reported to have no effect and to induce P-gp activity in some preclinical studies *(124,127–129)*. Similarly, rifampin has been reported to induce, and to have no affect on, P-gp expression on lymphocytes *(125,126)*. In theory, induction of P-gp on lymphocytes may lead to reduced intracellular penetration of coadministered P-gp substrates (e.g., protease inhibitors) and reduced virological efficacy with long-term drug administration. The clinical relevance of this observation is unclear. However, based on the clinical data reported by Chaillou et al., inhibition of lymphocyte P-gp by ritonavir would appear to be clinically relevant *(122)*; whether long-term administration of ritonavir or other protease inhibitors is associated with P-gp induction and reduced intracellular drug accumulation over time is unknown. Longitudinal studies in HIV-infected patients that assessed plasma and intracellular drug concentrations and their relationship to virological suppression are necessary to answer this question; currently, however, data are insufficient to be of particular clinical use.

In addition to HIV protease inhibitors, other anti-infectives, such as macrolide antibiotics, also accumulate intracellularly *(130–132)*. Intracellular concentrations of azithromycin, erythromycin, and telithromycin were markedly increased when these drugs were coadministered with the P-gp inhibitors verapamil, cyclosporine, and GF 120918 in an in vitro investigation *(132)*. In a separate study, human KB and G-185 cells, which overexpress P-gp, were shown to reduce intracellular macrolide accumulation and antimicrobial activity vs intracellular forms of *Listeria monocytogenes (133)*. The potential for targeted P-gp inhibition to influence the intracellular pharmacokinetics and pharmacodynamics of macrolides and other anti-infectives is largely unknown and requires further evaluation. Thus, no specific conclusions that have an impact on macrolide dosing and administration to patients can yet be drawn from these preclinical investigations.

## MULTIDRUG RESISTANCE (-ASSOCIATED) PROTEINS

As mentioned in the P-glycoprotein section, MRPs *(1–9)* are contained within the superfamily of mammalian ABC transporters *(8)*. In general, the MRP homologues are functionally analogous to P-gp, although their structures and amino acid sequences differ *(8)*. As a group, the MRPs transport numerous medications and share many substrates with P-gp *(108)*. In general, MRPs are widely distributed in nearly all human tissues *(134–136)*. The overwhelming majority of published information on MRP transporters deals with their role in conferring multidrug resistance to anticancer agents. Next, MRPs are considered individually in relation to their role as potential mediators of drug interactions among anti-infectives. A list of MRP substrates, inhibitors, and inducers is presented in Table 2 *(6,8,137–154)*.

### Multidrug Resistance (-Associated) Protein 1

MRP1, like P-gp, was first identified for its ability to confer multidrug resistance against numerous anticancer medications secondary to cellular efflux *(155,156)*. MRP1 functions primarily as a (co-)transporter of amphipathic organic ions; it can transport hydrophobic drugs that are complexed to oxidized glutathione, sulfate, or glucuronic acid *(136,167–159)*. MRP1 is localized on the basolateral membrane (tissue side) of epithelial cells and is located in various tissues, including the intestine, liver, choroid plexus in the brain, lung, PBMCs, CD4+ cells, kidney, testes, and oropharnyx *(6,8,104,136,160)*.

Most preclinical investigations have identified the HIV protease inhibitors as MRP1 substrates. Using various in vitro cellular system models, ritonavir, indinavir, nelfinavir, and saquinavir were found to undergo transport by MRP1 *(119,161–163)*. Of note, MRP-1 did not affect the intracellular accumulation of amprenavir in two different cell lines, suggesting that—unlike the other protease inhibitors—amprenavir is not transported by MRP1 *(163)*. In contrast to the above findings, one investigation using a canine kidney cell model found that saquinavir, indinavir, and ritonavir were not transported by MRP1 *(137)*. The reasons for these disparate results are not clear but are hypothesized to arise in part from differences in transporter protein expression among various cell lines and differences in experimental conditions *(164)*.

To address the potential clinical relevance of the protease inhibitors as MRP1 substrates, the relationship between MRP1 and P-gp expression on lymphocytes and intracellular accumulation of ritonavir and saquinavir was examined in HIV-infected patients *(118)* Patients with low MRP1 expression (less than the median) had increased intracellular accumulation of ritonavir and saquinavir compared to patients with high MRP1 expression (above the median) ($p = 0.035$). Moreover, when MRP1 and P-gp expression were combined, there was a statistically significant relationship between transporter expression and ritonavir and saquinavir intracellular accumulation ($p = 0.035$).

To test whether MRP1 and P-gp compromise the anti-HIV activity of the protease inhibitors, Srinivas and colleagues assessed the intracellular accumulation of saquinavir, ritonavir, and nelfinavir in addition to their capacity to inhibit HIV replication in T-lymphocytes *(115)*. Results from this study showed that HIV replication was effectively inhibited by all protease inhibitors, even in cells that overexpressed MRP1

**Table 2**
**Reported Substrates, Inhibitors, and Inducers for Multidrug-Resistance Proteins**

| Drug class | Characteristics of transported molecules | Substrates | Inhibitors | Inducers |
|---|---|---|---|---|
| MRP1 | Amphipathic organic ions; can transport glutathione, sulfate, and glucuronide conjugates | Indinavir<br>Nelfinavir<br>Ritonavir<br>Saquinavir | Ritonavir<br>Probenecid<br>MK 571 | Ritonavir<br>Sulindac<br>Rifampin |
| MRP2 | Amphipathic ions | Probenecid<br>Saquinavir<br>Ritonavir<br>Indinavir<br>Vinblastine<br>Sulfinpyrazone<br>Methotrexate<br>Adefovir<br>Cidofovir<br>Tenofovir (possibly) | Probenecid<br>Adefovir<br>Cidofovir<br>Furosemide<br>Ritonavir | Probenecid<br>Indomethacin<br>Furosemide<br>Sulfinpyrazone<br>Penicillin G<br>Rifampin<br>Phenobarbital |
| MRP3 | Organic anions (broad specificity) | Methotrexate<br>Various bile salts<br>Etoposide<br>Teniposide<br>Vincristine | Probenecid<br>Indomethacin<br>Furosemide<br>Sulrinpyrazone<br>Benzbromarone | Rifampin |
| MRP4 | Nucleotide and nucleoside analogs and metabolites | Adefovir (PMEA)<br>Zidovudine<br>Lamivudine<br>Stavudine<br>Didanosine<br>Abacavir<br>Cidofovir<br>Various anticancer agents | Dipyridamole<br>MK 571<br>Sildenafil<br>Nonsteroidal anti-inflam-matory drugs<br>Probenecid<br>Sulfinpyrazone | |
| MRP5 | Nucleotide and nucleoside analogs and metabolites | Adefovir (PMEA)<br>Lamivudine | Probenecid<br>Sulfinpyrazone<br>MK 571<br>Dipyridamole<br>Sildenafil | |
| MRP8 | Cyclic nucleosides | Zalcitabine<br>Anticancer fluoropyrimidines | | |

*Source*: From refs. *6,8,46,137–154*.

or P-gp *(115)*. It is unclear whether these results can be extrapolated to the clinical setting or if targeted inhibition of MRP1 could improve intracellular penetration of HIV protease inhibitors and improve their antiviral activity. The potential usefulness of targeted MRP1 inhibition is suggested by preclinical studies in which intracellular accumulation of protease inhibitors was increased secondary to MRP1 inhibition by probenecid and MK 571 *(162,163)*. Preliminary data suggest that protease inhibitors themselves may inhibit MRP1 *(165)*.

Although their status as MRP1 modulators is in question, most data are in agreement that HIV protease inhibitors are substrates for MRP1; accordingly, their penetration into sanctuary sites, including CD4$^+$ cells, may be compromised by MRP1 efflux. As such, further investigation is necessary to define the role of MRP1 alone and in combination with other transporters, such as P-gp, in reducing antiretroviral activity. This information will help delineate the potential role of targeted MRP1 inhibition and determine whether protease inhibitors or other drugs (e.g., probenecid) have a clinical role in enhancing the intracellular accumulation of coadministered anti-infectives. In all likelihood, the most efficient means of targeted transporter inhibition on immune cells will involve the simultaneous inhibition of multiple transport proteins, including MRP1, P-gp, and perhaps others. Whether such strategies will ultimately prove useful in optimizing antiretroviral activity remains to be seen. Currently, no firm recommendations can be made regarding targeted MRP1 or P-gp inhibition for these purposes. It will also be necessary to determine whether ritonavir or other drugs such as nonsteroidal anti-inflammatory drugs (NSAIDs) or rifampin significantly induce MRP1 activity to the extent that they reduce intracellular drug accumulation and compromise therapeutic efficacy *(166,167)*.

## Multidrug Resistance (-Associated) Protein 2

Similar to MRP1 and P-gp, MRP2 is noteworthy for its ability to confer resistance to multiple anticancer agents. Located on the apical side of cells, MRP2 functions as an efflux pump for amphipathic anions; it is involved in the transport of endogenous compounds such as bilirubin and bilirubin conjugates as well as numerous anionic drugs and drug conjugates *(6,168)*. MRP2 is expressed primarily in liver canaliculi, in which it excretes compounds into bile; it is expressed to a lesser degree in the kidney, intestine, placenta, and brain *(168)*. Despite minimal expression in the kidney, data suggest that MRP2 plays a significant role in the renal excretion of some drugs *(169)*.

Inhibition of MRP2 was suggested as a contributing mechanism to the development of Fanconi syndrome in an HIV-infected patient receiving once-daily antiretroviral therapy with 250 mg didanosine, 300 mg lamivudine, 300 mg tenofovir, and 800/200 mg lopinavir-ritonavir *(169)*. Two weeks prior to hospital admission, a single steady-state tenofovir plasma concentration was obtained 10 hours postdose and found to be 0.444 mg/L, which was approximately four times higher than expected. The authors hypothesized that inhibition of MRP2 by low-dose ritonavir may have increased proximal tubular concentrations of tenofovir by decreasing its apical efflux; this in turn may have led to tenofovir-mediated nephrotoxicity. This hypothesis is consistent with data from a pharmacokinetic study in healthy volunteers that showed that the lopinavir-ritonavir combination increased tenofovir exposure by 34%, although this did not lead to increased toxicity among 291 HIV-infected patients *(170,171)*.

Nonetheless, some clinicians are currently suggesting that lopinavir-ritonavir be avoided in patients receiving tenofovir and vice-versa *(169)*. However, such a strong recommendation is not adequately supported by currently available data. Nevertheless, drug regimens containing low-dose ritonavir in combination with tenofovir should be used cautiously, with close monitoring of serum creatinine, serum urea nitrogen, phosphorous, and other electrolytes. Certainly, clinicians may wish to avoid concurrent use of ritonavir and tenofovir in patients with underlying renal dysfunction as these patients may be particularly predisposed to tenofovir-induced renal dysfunction. If this combination cannot be avoided in a patient with compromised renal function, clinicians should take particular care to ensure that tenofovir dosing is appropriately reduced in accordance with manufacturer recommendations *(172)*.

In addition to tenofovir, the nucleoside phosphonates adefovir and cidofovir are both moderate inhibitors as well as substrates of MRP2 *(151)*. Adefovir and cidofovir are antiviral compounds that undergo renal tubular secretion and can cause nephrotoxicity, particularly at higher doses *(151,173–175)*. Nephrotoxicity with these agents occurs as a result of their accumulation in proximal renal tubules via OAT1-mediated cellular uptake (i.e., cellular entry) *(151,174)*. As such, the nephrotoxic effects of the nucleoside phosphonates can be tempered through OAT1 inhibition by probenecid, which is discussed in this section. In addition to OAT1, however, MRP2 modulation may also contribute to adefovir and cidofovir nephrotoxicity *(151)*. MRP2 is postulated to mediate the efflux of adefovir and cidofovir (and possibly tenofovir) from proximal tubule cells (i.e., cellular exit) *(151)*. Competitive inhibition of MRP2 in renal cells may result in reduced efflux and increased intracellular accumulation and nephrotoxicity with these drugs. Conversely, MRP2 induction could potentially reduce accumulation of adefovir and cidofovir in tubular cells, thereby producing a nephroprotective effect.

Medications that may interact with the nucleoside phosphonates via MRP2 inhibition or induction are listed in Table 2 *(6,8,137–154)*. Although none of the agents listed are absolutely contraindicated with adefovir, cidofovir, and tenofovir, they should be used cautiously in patients receiving these medications. Other medications that may affect the intracellular accumulation and nephrotoxic potential of these agents—via competition at MRP2 or other transporter sites—include acyclovir, valacyclovir, ganciclovir, and valganciclovir *(170)*; however, there are currently insufficient data to recommend avoiding these medications in combination with nucleoside phosphonates. Nonetheless, clinicians should keep these potential interactions in mind if they observe renal toxicity in patients receiving these drugs in combination.

Probenecid, which has been identified as both an MRP2 inhibitor and inducer in separate studies, was found to enhance the MRP2-mediated transport of saquinavir, ritonavir, and indinavir in in vitro experiments *(137)*. Another uricoscuric agent, sulfinpyrazone, also enhanced saquinavir transport via MRP2 in the same study *(137)*. In a related investigation, the same investigators noted that probenecid reduced saquinavir exposure in rats, although the probenecid dose used in this study (100 mg/ kg) was two orders of magnitude higher than doses used in humans *(176)*.

Because of the increasing number of drugs identified as substrates, inhibitors, or inducers of MRP2, the potential for clinically significant drug interactions involving this transporter is high, even though specific combinations of potentially interacting drugs have not been evaluated *per se* in most cases. As such, combinations of MRP2 inhibitors, inducers, and substrates must be systematically evaluated in humans to better define drug interactions among these agents. For the time being, it should be kept in mind that a number of clinically significant drug interactions may occur secondary to MRP2 modulation, and clinicians should become familiar with medications that interact with this transporter (Table 2).

## Multidrug Resistance (-Associated) Proteins 3, 4, 5, and 8

Among the MRPs, MRP3 possesses the highest degree of structural similarity to MRP1 (58%) (168,177,178). As such, there is overlap in substrate selectivity among MRP3, MRP1, and MRP2 with respect to transport of glutathione and glucuronide conjugates (168). Of note, the ability of MRP3 to confer multidrug resistance to anti-cancer agents is diminished compared to MRP1 and MRP2 (168); this may be because of MRP3's lower affinity for amphipathic anions and glutathione (168). MRP3 is typi-cally expressed at low levels at the basolateral membranes of hepatocytes and bile duct cells; it is also expressed in the pancreas, kidney, adrenal gland, and gallbladder (168). Although several medications have been noted to inhibit and induce MRP3 (Table 2), clinically significant drug interactions caused by MRP3 modulation have not been described. Of note, saquinavir, ritonavir, and indinavir did not undergo transport by MRP3 in a cellular system (137). Clearly, additional information is necessary before the role of MRP3 in drug interactions can be defined and this information applied clini-cally.

MRP4 differs from MRPs 1–3 in that it lacks the N-terminal domain of five pur-ported transmembrane segments within MRPs 1–3 (8). This structural difference likely accounts for differences in substrate selectivity with MRP4. MRP4 is expressed in many tissues, including the lung, kidney, gallbladder, tonsil, bladder, prostate, skeletal muscle, pancreas, spleen, thymus, testes, ovary, and small intestine (179,180). There is discordant information regarding the localization of MRP4 (i.e., apical vs basolateral membrane) and its tissue distribution. MRP4 is noteworthy for its ability to confer resistance to certain nucleotide and nucleoside analog antiviral agents (168).

Schuetz et al. reported that overexpression and amplification of MRP4 in T lym-phoid cells correlated with ATP-dependent efflux of PMEA [9-(2-phosphonylmetho-xyethyl)adenine; adefovir] and azidothymidine (AZT; zidovudine) monophosphate from cells (181). Moreover, MRP4 overexpression significantly reduced the antiviral efficacy of PMEA, zidovudine, lamivudine, stavudine, and didanosine in this cellular model (181). These results are suggestive of an MRP4 phenotype that is associated with enhanced efflux of nucleoside analog monophosphates and reduced accumulation of active nucleoside analog triphosphates (182). In a related investigation, dipyridamole reversed MRP4-mediated drug efflux and potentiated the antiviral activity of nucleo-side analog triphosphates in MRP4-overexpressing cells (182). In a separate preclini-cal investigation, MRP4 transport confirmed low-level resistance to PMEA but not to zidovudine or lamivudine (8,183). Additional nucleoside and nucleotide analogs that undergo transport by MRP4 include abacavir, cidofovir, and a host of anticancer medi-cations (154). Of note, HIV protease inhibitors do not appear to be substrates for MRP4 (137). Dipyridamole, MK571, sildenafil, and NSAIDs have all been reported to effec-tively inhibit MRP4-mediated transport (153,154,182); probenecid and sulfinpyrazone are weaker inhibitors. To date, potent inducers of MRP4 activity have not been identi-fied.

High levels of MRP4 on cells that are targets for HIV infection could lead to reduced virological efficacy of nucleoside analogs secondary to reduced intracellular accumu-lation of these agents (184). Further, reduced antiviral drug accumulation in cells and tissues may result in the formation of a protective sanctuary site for the virus (184). Whether targeted MRP4 inhibition can enhance the cellular and tissue penetration of nucleoside and nucleotide analog reverse transcriptase inhibitors and improve their antiviral activity are currently unclear. Further, the clinical consequences of MRP4 induction on the antiviral activity of nucleoside and nucleotide analogs is unknown; additional study is necessary to examine these relationships and determine the role of MRP4 in the pharmacological treatment of HIV infection.

MRP5 is an organic anion transporter localized to the basal membrane of cells *(185)*; it is expressed in many tissues, including the brain, skeletal muscle, and erythrocyte membranes *(179,186,187)*. Similar to MRP4, MRP5 lacks the initial transmembrane domain; however, its amino acid sequence is only 36% homologous with MRP4 *(184)*. Also like MRP4, MRP5 appears to be a nucleotide analogue pump. MRP5 was noted to extrude PMEA in several preclinical investigations *(185,187)*. Increased expression of an MRP5 homologue (ABCC11) was noted to transport lamivudine in a human T lymphoblastoid cell line *(188)*. Inhibitors of MRP5 include probenecid, sulfinpyrazone, MK571, dipyridamole, and sildenafil (Table 2); it is unclear at this time which drugs induce this transporter. A greater number of MRP5 (and MRP4) substrates, inhibitors, and inducers will likely be described as further information on this new group of transporters is collected. Likewise, the role of MRP5 in anti-infective pharmacotherapy has yet to be defined, as do drug interactions involving this transporter.

MRP8 is a newly identified MRP, gaining classification in 2001 *(189–191)*. MRP8 resembles MRP4 and MRP5 in that it lacks a third (N-terminal) membrane-spanning domain. Sequence comparisons revealed that MRP8 is most similar to MRP5, leading to speculation that MRP8 may also be involved in the transport of cyclic nucleosides *(189,191)*. Although the functional properties and localization of MRP8 in cells and tissues is currently under characterization, initial studies suggested that MRP8 is expressed on macrophages and dendritic cells *(192,193)*. MRP8 is also expressed in moderate levels in breast cancer cells and normal breast and testicular tissue *(189)*; it is expressed at very low levels in the liver, brain, and placenta *(189)*. In a cell culture model, MRP8 was found to transport the nucleoside reverse transcriptase inhibitor zalcitabine and anticancer fluoropyrimidines; it did not appear to transport zidovudine or lamivudine *(194)*. The role of MRP8 in anti-infective therapy, including implications for drug interactions, remains to be defined.

## ORGANIC ANION AND CATION TRANSPORTERS

### *Organic Anion Transporting Polypeptides*

Human OATPs represent a group of membrane carriers that transports a wide spectrum of amphipathic substrates *(195)*. At the end of 2002, there were nine human OATPs identified *(195)*. It should be noted that species differences exist in OATP such that human OATP is not orthologous to rat (Oatp) or mouse (oatp) organic anion transporting polypeptide. The human transporters, which are the focus here, are designated by all capital letters. Some OATPs are exclusively expressed in liver (i.e., OATP-C and OATP-8); however, most OATPS are expressed in various other tissues, including the BBB, choroid plexus, lung, heart, intestine, kidney, placenta, and testes *(196)*. Collectively, OATPs transport a variety of diverse compounds. OATP-C, however, only transports acidic agents, including pravastatin, bilirubin, benzylpenicillin, and 17β-estradiol glucuronide. Similarly, OATP-8 only transports acidic compounds as well.

However, other members of the OATP family have been shown to transport basic zwitterionic and neutral compounds such as rocuronium, fexofenadine, and digoxin *(5,6,197–205)*. As such, the designation of these transporters as organic *anion* transporting polypeptides is misleading in that certain OATPs are capable of transporting compounds that are not acidic *(6)*.

Unlike P-gp and the MRPs, which efflux xenobiotics out of cells, OATPs generally function as uptake transporters that facilitate the influx of compounds *(6)*. The OATP family appears to play a major role in hepatobiliary drug excretion as it is located on the basolateral (sinusoidal) membrane of hepatocytes and mediates drug uptake *(6)*. In addition to the liver, OATPs are active in numerous other cells and tissues throughout the body; however, their precise roles are still being defined. To date, few substrates and modulators of OATPs have been identified (Table 3) *(5,6,197–205)*. The P-gp substrates fexofenadine and digoxin, however, are two medications that are clearly transported by OATPs *(198–206)*.

In a preclinical investigation, ritonavir (10 $\mu M$) was found to produce 76% inhibition of OATP (subtype not reported)-mediated fexofenadine transport *(198)*. These data are consistent with clinical reports showing that ritonavir increases plasma concentrations of the OATP substrate digoxin *(29,67)*. However, because both digoxin and fexofenadine are also P-gp substrates, it is not possible to know the precise mechanism of these interactions. What can be delineated is that clinically significant OATP inhibition in the intestine by ritonavir was unlikely to have occurred; this is because gut OATP inhibition would have resulted in reduced digoxin uptake by enterocytes and decreased absorption (i.e., OATP inhibition in the intestine produces the opposite effect of P-gp inhibition in the intestine). Conversely, ritonavir-mediated OATP inhibition in the liver may have contributed to increased digoxin concentrations via reduced digoxin uptake at the hepatocyte. Unlike what occurs at the intestinal level, OATP and P-gp inhibition in the liver both lead to increased substrate plasma concentrations, albeit by different mechanisms. Digoxin renal clearance was unchanged by ritonavir in one of the studies and decreased by 35% in the other; thus, it is unclear whether ritonavir-mediated OATP inhibition in the kidney was responsible for decreasing digoxin uptake into renal tubules and elevating its concentrations in plasma *(29,67)*. OATP inhibition may also be involved in other drug interactions between digoxin and anti-infectives such as itraconazole, ketoconazole, clarithromycin, and erythromycin.

Additional drugs that have been shown to inhibit transport by OATP(s) in in vitro cellular systems include saquinavir, nelfinavir, lovastatin, quinidine, and ketoconazole *(198)*. In addition, orange juice, apple juice, and grapefruit juice have all been shown to reduce fexofenadine exposure by approx 70% in healthy volunteers; the mechanism of this interaction is presumed to be because of inhibition of OATP(s) in the intestine by components of the various fruit juices *(207)*. Of note, the HMGCo-A reductase inhibitor pravastatin is a substrate for OATP-C. Interestingly, pravastatin's AUC is approximately halved by nelfinavir, efavirenz, and the combination of saquinavir-ritonavir *(208,209)*. It is unclear whether OATP-C modulation by these antiretrovirals contributes to the observed interaction, but this possibility should be considered in future studies. At present, what is clear is that higher doses of pravastatin (>40 mg) may be necessary for adequate antihyperlipidemic activity in HIV-infected patients receiving these antiretroviral medications.

**Table 3**
**Reported Substrates, Inhibitors, and Inducers of Organic Anion Transporting Polypeptides (OATPs), Organic Cation Transporters (OCTs), and Organic Anion Transporters (OATs)**

| Drug class | Characteristics of transported molecules | Substrates | Inhibitors |
|---|---|---|---|
| OATPs | Acidic, basic, and zwitterionic compounds; depends on OATP subtype | | Ritonavir [a]<br>Saquinavir [a]<br>Nelfinavir [a]<br>Lovastatin [a]<br>Quinidine [a]<br>Ketoconazole [a] |
| • OATP-C | Acidic compounds | Pravastatin<br>Bilirubin<br>Benzylpenicillin<br>17-β-Estradiol glucuronide<br>Rifampin | |
| • OATP-A, OATP-B, Oatp1, Oatp2 | Basic, zwitterionic, and neutral compounds | UK 191005<br>Rocuronium<br>N-Methylquinidine<br>Fexofenadine<br>Digoxin | Orange juice (OATP-A)<br>Grapefruit juice (OATP-A) |
| OCT | Small organic cations | Choline<br>N-Methylnicotinamide | Clonidine<br>Quinidine<br>Quinine<br>Verapamil<br>HIV protease inhibitors |

*Continued on next page*

**Table 3 (Continued)**

| Drug class | Characteristics of transported molecules | Substrates | Inhibitors |
|---|---|---|---|
| OAT | Organic anions (all subtypes) | | |
| • OAT1 | | NSAIDs | Probenecid |
| | | Various anticancer drugs | Betamipron |
| | | Cimetidine | |
| | | Ranitidine | |
| | | Angiotensin-converting enzyme inhibitors | |
| | | β-Lactam antibiotics | |
| | | Adefovir | |
| | | Cidofovir | |
| • OAT2 | | Zidovudine | |
| | | Tetracycline | |
| | | Cephalosporin antibiotics | |
| | | Salicylate | |
| • OAT3 | | NSAIDs | |
| | | Various anticancer drugs | |
| | | Cimetidine | |
| | | Ranitidine | |
| | | Angiotensin-converting enzyme inhibitors | |
| | | β-Lactam antibiotics | |
| • OAT4 | | Cimetidine | |
| | | Methotrexate | |
| | | Cidofovir | |
| | | Adefovir | |
| | | Acyclovir | |
| | | Ganciclovir | |
| | | Zidovudine | |
| | | β-Lactam antibiotics | |

*Source*: From refs. *5,6,197–205*.
[a]The study that identified these drugs as OATP inhibitors did not specify a subtype.

66

In addition to pravastatin, OATP-C also appears to transport rifampin *(201)*. In an in vitro cellular system, Tirona et al. showed that OATP-C expression was associated with increased intracellular retention of rifampin; they also observed an increase in rifampin-mediated PXR activation *(201)*. PXR activation by rifampin is involved in the process of enzymatic induction. Therefore, modulation of OATP-C activity may ultimately influence the P-gp and CYP induction potential of rifampin and perhaps other drugs *(201)*. Further delineation of this relationship may help explain a variety of drug interactions with rifampin and perhaps similar medications.

Because of the increasing number of drugs noted to be transported by OATPs and the fact that OATPs are present at a variety of anatomic sites, their potential for involvement in clinically significant drug interactions is high. Future studies will shed light on which compounds are likely to be involved; this knowledge may eventually prove useful in the optimal management of anti-infective medications.

### Organic Cation Transporters

OCT proteins are expressed on the basolateral membrane of epithelial cells in the liver, kidney, and intestine *(6)*. Human OCT-1 is primarily expressed in both the liver and kidney; OCT2 is predominantly located in the kidney *(210,211)*. OCT proteins typically transport small organic cations, yet can be inhibited by basic drugs such as clonidine, quinine, quinidine, verapamil, and HIV protease inhibitors *(6)*. Because of the relatively limited number of compounds transported by OCT, its role in hepatobiliary drug excretion and potential for involvement in drug interactions are considered limited and not of current clinical consequence.

### Organic Anion Transporters

OAT proteins are similar in amino acid sequence to OCT proteins, and they are expressed in the liver, kidney, and brain. OAT2 is expressed on the basolateral side of the proximal tubule and is involved in the renal transport of zidovudine, tetracycline, cephalosporins, and salicylate (Table 3) *(5,6,197–205)*. OAT1 and OAT3 are also localized on the basolateral membrane of the proximal tubule; these proteins transport NSAIDs, antitumor drugs, histamine $H_2$ receptor antagonists, prostaglandins, angiotensin-converting enzyme inhibitors, diuretics, and β-lactam antibiotics. OAT4 is located on the apical side of the proximal tubule and mediates the uptake as well as the efflux of compounds such as cilastatin and estrone sulfate *(212)*. As a group, a primary function of OAT proteins is the active renal secretion of cimetidine, methotrexate, cidofovir, adefovir, acyclovir, ganciclovir, β-lactam antibiotics, and zidovudine *(6,203–205)*.

OAT1 is a key uptake transporter for adefovir and cidofovir (and perhaps tenofovir), both of which have been associated with clinically significant nephrotoxicity in humans *(151)*. Preclinical experiments have shown that both cidofovir and adefovir are taken up by OAT1, and that this process contributes to increased cytotoxicity with both agents. The cytotoxicity of both drugs was sharply reduced, however, in the presence of the OAT1 inhibitors probenecid and betamipron. These data support probenecid-mediated OAT1 inhibition as the mechanism responsible for probenecid's ability to limit the nephrotoxic effects of cidofovir. Other drugs, not yet identified, that inhibit OAT1 might also be expected to abrogate the nephrotoxic effects of cidofovir. Along these lines, it can be speculated that OAT1 enhancement could foster the uptake efficiency of cidofovir and adefovir into renal tubule cells, possibly increasing the nephrotoxic potential of both agents. Further study is necessary to determine which drugs are capable of stimulating OAT1 function. As discussed, intracellular accumulation of adefovir and cidofovir in renal tubule cells is also impacted by MRP2 activity, which is responsible for removing these drugs from cells.

Similar to the interaction between OAT1 and nucleotide analogs, OAT2 was found to mediate the transport of a variety of cephalosporins *(202)*. A preclinical study using proximal tubule cells provided evidence that cephaloridine-induced nephrotoxicity is most likely mediated by OAT proteins *(202)*. Interestingly, in this investigation probenecid was not always able to reverse cellular toxicity with cephaloridine, suggesting that probenecid does not indiscriminantly inhibit all OAT subtypes. Accordingly, probenecid may not be nephroprotective for all OAT substrates. Clearly, modulation of OAT proteins is expected to affect the renal elimination of cephalosporins; further investigation is necessary to identify which drugs may be involved. Fortunately, cephalosporin antibiotics are infrequently associated with nephrotoxicity, and many of these medications currently exhibit an acceptable pharmacokinetic profile, thus suggesting that identification of new OAT inhibitors is not likely to dramatically alter the current manner in which β-lactam antibiotics are administered.

In addition to their influence on renal elimination, OAT proteins also appear to be involved in mediating the distribution of a variety of substrates into and out of the CNS. Probenecid has long been known to increase zidovudine plasma concentrations by inhibiting its metabolism through glucuronosyl transferase enzymes; however, probenecid also decreases zidovudine clearance from CSF and prolongs its half-life in the brain *(213)*. Similar effects occur with the combination of probenecid and β-lactam antibiotics *(214)*. These data suggest that brain uptake and elimination of OAT substrates may be affected by drugs that modulate specific OAT proteins. Despite the effectiveness of probenecid in increasing the CNS exposure of certain β-lactam antibiotics, presumably secondary to altered drug transport, it is infrequently used clinically for this purpose; this may be because probenecid may not markedly improve antibiotic penetration into CSF early in the course of CNS infection when inflammation is present and antibiotic penetration occurs *(215)*.

In summary, OAT proteins transport a variety of anti-infective medications, including antivirals and β-lactam antibiotics. Modulation of OATs in the kidney and brain may result in clinically significant alterations in the distribution and elimination of OAT substrates. Future studies will shed light on specific OAT-mediated interactions that should be avoided or possibly exploited to optimize antimicrobial pharmacotherapy.

## SUMMARY

Drug transport proteins are becoming increasingly appreciated for their role in clinically significant drug interactions in patients receiving antimicrobial chemotherapy. Because of their presence in various human organs and cell types, they have the potential to influence drug absorption, distribution, metabolism, and elimination when their function is pharmacologically altered. Differentiating between drug transport and drug metabolism is inherently difficult in vivo when attempting to characterize the mechanism of a specific drug–drug interaction; therefore, most of the research that has been completed in this field involves the use of cellular systems and animal models. To date, there are few, but an ever-increasing number of, studies in humans that suggest that modulation of drug transport can contribute to clinically significant drug interactions. As more clinical data become available in this rapidly developing field, it is important for clinicians to develop a thorough understanding of drug transport systems, including which drugs are substrates and modulators of the most common drug transport proteins.

## CASE STUDY 1

R.K. is a 48-year-old African American male who presents to his physician complaining of severe pain in his right big toe. His medical history is significant for chronic renal insufficiency (2.4 mg/dL baseline serum creatinine) secondary to long-standing hypertension. He also has onychomycosis of his left thumb nail and is currently on day 4 of a second weak-long treatment pulse with 200 mg itraconazole twice daily. His other medications include 40 mg lisinopril once daily and 25 mg hydrochlorothiazide once daily. He takes no additional prescription, over-the-counter, or herbal medications. R.K. explains that the pain in his toe awoke him at 3 AM the previous night, and he has been in "excruciating" pain ever since.

On physical exam, R.K.'s toe appears red, swollen, tender, and warm to the touch. His blood pressure is 145/85, and he has a low grade fever (38°C); other vital signs are unremarkable. Blood is drawn for liver function tests, a mineral and electrolyte panel, serum urea nitrogen, serum creatinine, uric acid, and glucose; results are pending. A 24-hour urine collection is scheduled to determine urine uric acid and creatinine. In the mean time, R.K.'s physician diagnoses him with acute gouty arthritis and prescribes him 0.5 mg colchicine with instructions to take 2 tablets initially followed by 1–2 tablets every 1–2 hours until the pain in his toe improves, gastrointestinal side effects become intolerable, or a total of 10 mg has been administered.

That day, R.K. experienced resolution of his symptoms after ingesting a total of 8 mg colchicine. He experienced moderate diarrhea and cramping during this time. Over the next 2 days, R.K.'s toe pain returned intermittently, and he ingested a total of 6 mg colchicine during this time (total dose = 14 mg over 3 days). The following morning, R.K. developed severe abdominal cramping, diarrhea, myalgia, and lower extremity parasthesias. His wife took R.K. to their local emergency room, where he was found to be confused, agitated, and unable to ambulate. His temperature was 39.1°C, blood pressure was 180/88, and heart rate was 90 beats/ minute. An acute laboratory panel revealed significant elevations in AST, ALT, GGT, and LDH. He was also found to be pancytopenic. CPK was 2,752 U/L, and serum creatinine was 2.9 mg/dL. R.K. was admitted to the hospital.

### DISCUSSION

This case illustrates a drug–drug interaction between colchicine and itraconazole. Colchicine is a P-gp substrate with a main route of elimination that is secretion into the bile; only 10–20% of a colchicine dose is excreted renally. In a study in human liver microsomes, CYP3A4 was noted to catalyze colchicine demethylation; however, this does not appear to be a major elimination pathway for the drug. Colchicine is an antigout/antimitotic agent that can cause multiple organ dysfunction in cases of excess drug exposure; this has been observed in cases of colchicine overdose and in patients receiving colchicine in combination with certain P-gp inhibitors, including macrolide antibiotics and cyclosporine. Itraconazole is an azole antifungal that has been found to inhibit P-gp transport activity in a number of preclinical investigations. Itraconazole also increases the systemic exposure and decreases the renal clearance of the P-gp substrate digoxin. Digoxin is a P-gp substrate that is not significantly metabolized in humans. The presumed mechanism of this interaction is inhibition of P-gp-mediated digoxin transport in renal tubules by itraconazole. Therefore, the most likely mechanism for the interaction in R.K. is itraconazole-mediated inhibition of hepatic and/or renal secretion of colchicine via P-gp; this likely resulted in increased plasma (and perhaps cellular) colchicine concentrations, resulting in toxicity.

### IDENTIFICATION/MONITORING

This interaction may have been identified *a priori* by an alert pharmacist or physician, especially because drug interactions between colchicine and P-gp inhibitors appear to occur more frequently in patients with underlying renal dysfunction. Moreover, the patient should have been instructed that a 3-day colchicine-free interval should follow each oral course of therapy. As such, R.K. was at risk for experiencing toxicity caused by drug interactions with colchicine. Typically, one might expect a longer duration of colchicine and itraconazole coadministration before observing such severe colchicine toxicity; however, organ dysfunction caused by excessive colchicine exposure has been described after short periods of administration ($\leq 3$ days). In fact, death caused by colchicine intoxication has occurred with as little as 7 mg.

### CASE STUDY 2

T.H. is a 53-year-old white female who was recently diagnosed with pulmonary tuberculosis following a 4-week history of cough, fevers, and night sweats. She was initiated on a regimen of 600 mg rifampin daily, 300 mg isoniazid daily, 1500 mg pyrazinamide daily, and 800 mg ethambutol daily. In addition to her recent tuberculosis diagnosis, T.H.'s medical history is positive for chronic atrial fibrillation and seasonal allergic rhinitis. Her other medications include 100 mg pyridoxine daily, 0.25 mg digoxin daily (1.8 ng/mL steady-state serum digoxin concentration), and 180 mg fexofenadine daily as needed.

Within 2 weeks, T.H.'s sputum became negative for acid-fast bacilli. However, she presented to her physician on day 15 of anti-TB therapy complaining of chest pain, dizziness, and palpitations. Moreover, on visual examination, T.H. was suffering from severe rhinorrhea, watery eyes, and sneezing. Her heart rate was 180 beats/minute and a stat electrocardiogram showed atrial fibrillation. A digoxin level was drawn postelectrocardiogram and found to be < 0.5 ng/mL.

### DISCUSSION

This case illustrates drug–drug interactions between rifampin and digoxin and between rifampin and fexofenadine. Both digoxin, a cardiac glycoside, and fexofenadine, a nonsedating antihistamine, are P-gp substrates that are minimally metabolized in humans. Rifampin has been shown to induce P-gp activity in a variety of clinical and preclinical studies, including pharmacokinetic studies in healthy volunteers, which document rifampin's ability to increase the clearance of digoxin and fexofenadine, respectively. The reduction in digoxin and fexofenadine exposure in this case resulted in inadequate pharmacological response to both drugs (i.e., atrial fibrillation and uncontrolled allergic rhinitis). In addition to P-gp, both digoxin and fexofenadine are substrates for the human OATP. Therefore, it is possible that rifampin may also modulate OATP activity, resulting in enhanced elimination of fexofenadine and digoxin; however, to date this has not been clearly proven.

### IDENTIFICATION/MONITORING

This interaction could reasonably have been predicted ahead of time. However, alternate therapeutic choices for T.H. are limited. Alternatives to digoxin for chronic heart rate control would commonly include verapamil, diltiazem, or β-blockers such as metoprolol, propranolol, and atenolol. With the possible exception of atenolol, plasma concentrations of all of these agents would likely be decreased by rifampin secondary to CYP ± P-gp induction. Atenolol is not metabolized by CYP enzymes and does not appear to be a P-gp substrate; however, there is at least one anecdotal report of reduced atenolol activity when it was coadministered with rifampin. Another therapeutic intervention involves replacing rifampin with rifabutin. Rifabutin is less prone to enzyme induction compared to rifampin and may also be less inclined to induce P-gp activity. Still, digoxin concentrations would need to be monitored closely in this setting. Moreover, if in response to the interaction with digoxin rifampin is discontinued in favor of rifabutin, one might expect a gradual increase in digoxin exposure over the ensuing weeks as P-gp activity normalizes in the absence of rifampin. Vigilant monitoring of digoxin serum concentrations and dosage adjustment as necessary are warranted in this situation.

## REFERENCES

1. Piscitelli SC, Gallicano KD. Interactions among drugs for HIV and opportunistic infections. N Engl J Med. 2001;344:984–996.
2. Lin JH, Yamazaki M. Role of P-glycoprotein in pharmacokinetics: clinical implications. Clin Pharmacokinet. 2003;42:59–98.
3. Karney WW, Turck M, Holmes KK. Comparative therapeutic and pharmacological evaluation of amoxicillin and ampicillin plus probenecid for the treatment of gonorrhea. Antimicrob Agents Chemother 1974;5:114–118.
4. Lea AP, Bryson HM. Cidofovir. Drugs 1996;52:225–230.
5. Ho ES, Lin DC, Mendel DB, Cihlar T. Cytotoxicity of antiviral nucleotides adefovir and cidofovir is induced by the expression of human renal organic anion transporter 1. J Am Soc Nephrol 2000;11:383–393.
6. Ayrton A, Morgan P. Role of transport proteins in drug absorption, distribution and excretion. Xenobiotica 2001;31:469–497.
7. Matheny CJ, Lamb MW, Brouwer KR, Pollack GM. Pharmacokinetic and pharmacodynamic implications of P-glycoprotein modulation. Pharmacotherapy 2001;21:778–796.
8. Schinkel AH, Jonker JW. Mammalian drug efflux transporters of the ATP binding cassette (ABC) family: an overview. Adv Drug Deliv Rev 2003;55:3–29.

9. Lin JH. Drug–drug interaction mediated by inhibition and induction of P-glycoprotein. Adv Drug Deliv Rev 2003;55:53–81.

10. Sharma R, Awasthi YC, Yang Y, Sharma A, Singhal SS, Awasthi S. Energy dependent transport of xenobiotics and its relevance to multidrug resistance. Curr Cancer Drug Targets. 2003;3:89–107.

11. Sauna ZE, Smith MM, Muller M, Kerr KM, Ambudkar SV. The mechanism of action of multidrug-resistance-linked P-glycoprotein. J Bioenerg Biomembr 2001;33:481–491.

12. Gottesman MM, Pastan I. Biochemistry of multidrug resistance mediated by the multidrug transporter P-glycoprotein. Annu Rev Biochem 1993;62:385–427.

13. Shapiro AB, Ling V. Positively cooperative sites for drug transport by P-glycoprotein with distinct drug specificities. Eur J Biochem 1997;250:130–137.

14. Yasuda K, Lan LB, Sanglard D, Furuya K, Schuetz JD, Schuetz EG. Interaction of cytochrome P450 3A inhibitors with P-glycoprotein. J Pharmacol Exp Ther. 2002;303:323–332.

15. Patel J, Mitra AK. Strategies to overcome simultaneous P-glycoprotein mediated efflux and CYP3A4 mediated metabolism of drugs. Pharmacogenomics 2001;2:401–415.

16. Bogman K, Peyer AK, Torok M, Kusters E, Drewe J. HMG-CoA reductase inhibitors and P-glycoprotein modulation. Br J Pharmacol 2001;132:1183–1192.

17. Chen C, Liu X, Smith BJ. Utility of MDR1-gene deficient mice in assessing the impact of P-glycoprotein on pharmacokinetics and pharmacodynamics in drug discovery and development. Curr Drug Metab 2003;4:272–291.

18. Barecki-Roach M, Wang EJ, Johnson WW. Many P-glycoprotein substrates do not inhibit the transport process across cell membranes. Xenobiotica 2003;33:131–140.

19. Hamada A, Miyano H, Watanabe H, Saito H. Interaction of imatinib mesilate with human P-glycoprotein. J Pharmacol Exp Ther 2003;307:824–828.

20. Pauli-Magnus C, Rekersbrink S, Klotz U, Fromm MF. Interaction of omeprazole, lansoprazole, and pantoprazole with P-glycoprotein. Naunyn Schmiedebergs Arch Pharmacol 2001;364:551–557.

21. Tian R, Koyabu N, Takanaga H, Matsuo H, Ohtani H, Sawada Y. Effects of grapefruit juice and orange juice on the intestinal efflux of P-glycoprotein substrates. Pharm Res 2002;19:802–809.

22. Soldner A, Christians U, Susanto M, Wacher VJ, Silverman JA, Benet LZ. Grapefruit juice activates P-glycoprotein-mediated drug transport. Pharm Res 1999;16:478–485.

23. Lown KS, Fontana RJ, Schmiedlin-Ren P, Turgeon DK, Watkins PB. Interindividual variation in intestinal *mdr1* expression: lack of short-term dietary effects. Gastroenterology 1995;108:A737.

24. Lown KS, Mayo RR, Leichtman AB, et al. Role of intestinal P-glycoprotein (*mdr1*) in interpatient variation in the oral availability of cyclosporine. Clin Pharmacol Ther 1997; 62:248–260.

25. Fromm MF. The influence of MDR1 polymorphisms on P-glycoprotein expression and function in humans. Adv Drug Del Rev 2002;54:1295–1310.

26. Fellay J, Marzolini C, Meaden ER, et al. Response to antiretroviral treatment in HIV-1 infected individuals with allelic variants of the multidrug resistance transporter 1: a pharmacogenetics study. Lancet 2002;359:30–36.

27. Kurata Y, Ieiri I, Kimura M, et al. Role of human MDR1 gene polymorphism in bioavailability and interaction of digoxin, a substrate of P-glycoprotein. Clin Pharmacol Ther 2002;72:209–219.

28. Kim RB, Leake BF, Choo EF, et al. Identification of functionally variant MDR1 alleles among European Americans and African Americans. Clin Pharmacol Ther 2001;70: 189–199.

29. Penzak SR, Shen J, Alfaro RM, Remaley A, Falloon J. Ritonavir decreases the non-renal clearance of digoxin in healthy volunteers with known MDR1 genotypes. Ther Drug Monit 2004;26:322–330.

30. Fromm MF. The influence of MDR1 polymorphisms on P-glycoprotein expression and function in humans. Adv Drug Del Rev 2002;54:1295–1310.
31. Lin JH, Lu AYH. Inhibition and induction of cytochrome P450 and the clinical implications. Clin Pharmacokinet 1998;35:361–390.
32. Chin KV, Chauhan SS, Pastan I, et al. Regulation of mdr RNA levels in response to cytotoxic drugs in rodent cells. Cell Growth Differ 1990;1:361–365.
33. LeCluyse EL. Pregnane X receptor: molecular basis for species differences in CYP3A induction by xenobiotics. Chem Biol Interact 2001;134:283–289.
34. Fardel O, Lecureur V, Guillouzo A. Regulation by dexamethasone of P-glycoprotein expression in cultured rat hepatocytes. FEBS Lett 1993;327:189–193.
35. Liu J, Brunner LJ. Chronic cyclosporine administration induces renal P-glycoprotein in rats. Eur J Pharmacol 2001;418:127–132.
36. Jette L, Beaulieu E, Leclerc J-M, et al. Cyclosporine A treatment induces overexpression of P-glycoprotein in the kidney and other tissues. Am J Physiol 1996;270:F756–F765.
37. Wacher VJ, Wu C-Y, Benet LZ. Overlapping substrate specificities and tissue distribution of cytochrome P450 3A and P-glycoprotein: implications for drug delivery and activity in cancer chemotherapy. Mol Carcinog 1995;13:129–134.
38. Synold TW, Dussault I, Forman BM. The orphan nuclear receptor SXR coordinately regulates drug metabolism and efflux. Nat Med 2001;7:584–590.
39. Geik A, Eichelbaum M, Burk O. Nuclear receptor response elements mediate induction of intestinal MDR1 by rifampin. J Biol Chem 2001;276:14,581–14,587.
40. Thiebaut F, Tsuruo T, Hamada H, Gottesman MM, Pastan I, Willingham MC. Cellular localization of the multidrug resistance gene product in normal human tissues. Proc Natl Acad Sci U S A 1987;84:7735–7738.
41. Fojo A, Ueda K, Slamon DJ, Poplack DG, Gottesman MM, Pastan I. Expression of a multidrug resistance gene in human tumors and tissues. Proc Natl Acad Sci USA 1987; 84:265–269.
42. Fricker G, Drewe J, Huwyler J, Gutmann H, Beglinger C. Relevance of P-glycoprotein for the enteral absorption of cyclosporine A: in vitro–in vivo correlation. Br J Clin Pharmacol 1996;118:1841–1847.
43. Hunter J, Jepson MA, Tsuruo T, Simmons NL, Hirst BH. Functional expression of P-glycoprotein in apical membranes of human intestinal Caco-2 cell layers: kinetics of vinblastine secretion and interaction with modulators. J Biol Chem 1993;268:14,991–14,997.
44. Hunter J, Hirst BH, Simmons NL. Drug absorption limited by P-glycoprotein-mediated secretory drug transport in human intestinal epithelial Caco-2 cells. Pharm Res 1993;10: 743–749.
45. Kim RB, Fromm MF, Wandel C, et al. The drug transporter P-glycoprotein limits oral absorption and brain entry of HIV-1 protease inhibitors. J Clin Invest 1998;101:289–294.
46. Gutmann H, Fricker G, Drewe J, Toeroek M, Miller DS. Interactions of HIV protease inhibitors with ATP-dependent drug export proteins. Mol Pharmacol 1999;56:383–389.
47. Drewe J, Gutmann H, Fricker G, Torok M, Beglinger C, Huwyler J. HIV protease inhibitor ritonavir: a more potent inhibitor of P-glycoprotein than the cyclosporine analogue SDZ PSC 833. Biochem Pharmacol 1999;57:1147–1152.
48. Choo EF, Leake B, Wandel C, et al. Pharmacological inhibition of P-glycoprotein transport enhances the distribution of HIV-1 protease inhibitors into brain and testes. Drug Metab Dispos 2000;28:655–660.
49. Alsenz J, Steffen H, Alex R. Active apical secretory efflux of HIV protease inhibitors saquinavir and ritonavir in Caco-2 cells. Pharm Res 1998;15:423–428.
50. Lee CGL, Gottesman MM. HIV protease inhibitors and the MDR1 multidrug transporter. J Clin Invest 1998;101:287–288.

51. Hochman JH, Chiba H, Nishime J, Yamazaki M, Lin JH. Influence of P-glycoprotein on the transport and metabolism of indinavir in Caco-2 cells expressing cytochrome P450 3A4. J Pharmacol Exp Ther 2000;292:310–318.

52. Lin JH. Role of pharmacokinetics in the discovery and development of indinavir. Adv Drug Deliv Rev 1999;39:33–49.

53. Lin JH. Human immunodeficiency virus protease inhibitors: from drug design to clinical studies. Adv Drug Deliv Rev 1997;27:215–233.

54. Invirase [package insert]. Nutley, NJ: Roche Laboratories, 2002.

55. Plosker GL, Scott LJ. Saquinavir: a review of its use in boosted regimens for treating HIV infection. Drugs 2003;63:1299–1324.

56. Kempf DJ, Marsh KC, Kumar G, et al. Pharmacokinetic enhancement of inhibitors of the human immunodeficiency virus protease by coadministration with ritonavir. Antimicrob Agents Chemother 1997;41:654–660.

57. Hsu A, Granneman GR, Cao G, et al. Pharmacokinetic interactions between two human immunodeficiency virus protease inhibitors, ritonavir and saquinavir. Clin Pharmacol Ther 1998;63:453–464.

58. Merry C, Barry MG, Mulcahy F, et al. Saquinavir pharmacokinetics alone and in combination with ritonavir in HIV-infected patients. AIDS 1997;11:F29–F33.

59. Kupferschmidt HH, Fattinger KE, Ha HR, Follath F, Krahenbuhl S. Grapefruit juice enhances the bioavailability of the HIV protease inhibitor saquinavir in man. Br J Clin Pharmacol 1998;45:355–359.

60. Hinderling PH, Hartmann D. Pharmacokinetics of digoxin and main metabolites/derivatives in healthy humans. Ther Drug Monit 1991;13:381–401.

61. Greiner B, Eichelbaum M, Fritz P, et al. The role of intestinal P-glycoprotein in the interaction of digoxin and rifampin. J Clin Invest 1999;104:147–153.

62. Westphal K, Weinbrenner A, Zschiesche M, et al. Induction of P-glycoprotein by rifampin increases intestinal secretion of talinolol in human beings: a new type of drug/drug interaction. Clin Pharmacol Ther 2000;68:345–355.

63. Gramatte T, Oertel R, Terhaag B, Kirch W. Direct demonstration of small intestinal secretion and site-dependent absorption of the β-blocker talinolol in humans. Clin Pharmacol Ther 1996;59:541–549.

64. Hebert MF, Roberts JP, Prueksaritanont T, et al. Bioavailability of cyclosporine with concomitant rifampin administration is markedly less than predicted by hepatic enzyme induction. Clin Pharmacol Ther 1992;52:453–457.

65. Mayer U, Wagenaar E, Beijnen JH, et. al Substantial excretion of digoxin via the intestinal mucosa and prevention of long-term digoxin accumulation in the brain by the mdr 1a P-glycoprotein. Br J Pharmacol 1996;119:1038–1044.

66. Koren G, Woodland C, Ito S. Toxic digoxin-drug interactions: the major role of renal P-glycoprotein. Vet Hum Toxicol 1998;40:45–46.

67. Ding R, Tayrouz Y, Riedel KD, et al. Substantial pharmacokinetic interaction between digoxin and ritonavir in healthy volunteers. Clin Pharmacol Ther 2004;76:73–84.

68. Perloff MD, von Moltke LL, Greenblatt DJ. Fexofenadine transport in Caco-2 cells: inhibition with verapamil and ritonavir. J Clin Pharmacol 2002;42:1269–1274.

69. Hamman MA, Bruce MA, Haehner-Daniels BD, et al. The effect of rifampin administration on the disposition of fexofenadine. Clin Pharmacol Ther 2001;69:114–121.

70. Milne RW, Larsen LA, Jorgensen KL, Bastlund J, Stretch GR, Evans AM. Hepatic disposition of fexofenadine: influence of the transport inhibitors erythromycin and dibromosulphothalein. Pharm Res 2000;17:1511–1515.

71. Tannergren C, Knutson T, Knutson L, Lennernas H. The effects of ketoconazole on the in vivo intestinal permeability of fexofenadine using a regional perfusion technique. Br J Clin Pharmacol 2002;55:182–190.

72. Tannergren C, Petri N, Knutson L, Hedeland M, Bondesson U, Lennernas H. Multiple transport mechanisms involved in the intestinal absorption and first-pass extraction of fexofenadine. Clin Pharmacol Ther 2003;74:423–436.

73. Lin JH, Chiba M, Chen I-W, et al. Effect of dexamethasone on the intestinal first-pass metabolism of indinavir in rats: evidence of cytochrome P-450 and P-glycoprotein induction. Drug Metab Dispos 1999;27:1187–1193.

74. Hochman JH, Chiba M, Yamazaki C, Tang JH, Lin JH. P-glycoprotein-mediated efflux of indinavir metabolites in Caco-2 cells expressing cytochrome P450 3A4. J Pharmacol Exp Ther 2001;298:323–330.

75. Lin JH, Chiba M, Baillie TA. Is the role of the small intestine in first-pas metabolism overemphasized? Pharmacol Rev 1999;51:135–157.

76. Susanto M, Benet LZ. Can the enhanced renal clearance of antibiotics in cystic fibrosis patients be explained by P-glycoprotein transport? Pharm Res 2002;19:457–462.

77. Fanos V, Cataldi L. Renal transport of antibiotics and nephrotoxicity: a review. J Chemother 2001;13:461–472.

78. Rengelshausen J, Goggelmann C, Burhenne J, et al. Contribution of increased oral bioavailability and reduced nonglomerular renal clearance of digoxin to the digoxin-clarithromycin interaction. Br J Clin Pharmacol 2003;56:32–38.

79. Jalava KM, Partanan J, Neuvonen PJ. Itraconazole decreases renal clearance of digoxin. Ther Drug Monit 1997;19:609–613.

80. Pardridge WM. Transport of protein-bound hormones into tissue in vivo. Endocr Rev 1981; 2:103–123.

81. Thiebault F, Tsuruo T, Hamada H, Gottesman MM, Pastan I, Willingham MC. Immuno-histochemical localization in normal tissues of different epitopes in the multidrug transport protein P170: evidence for localization in brain capillaries and crossreactivity of one antibody with a muscle protein. J Histochem Cytochem 1989;37:159–164.

82. Cordon-Cardo C, O'Brien JP, Casals D, et al. Multidrug resistance gene (P-glycoprotein) is expressed by endothelial cells at blood–brain barrier sites. Proc Natl Acad Sci USA 1989;86:695–698.

83. Sawchuck RJ, Yang Z. Investigation of distribution, transport and uptake of anti-HIV drugs to the central nervous system. Adv Drug Del Rev 1999;39:5–31.

84. Polli JW, Jarrett JL, Studenberg SD, et al. Role of P-glycoprotein on the CNS of amprenavir (141W94) an HIV protease inhibitor. Pharm Res 1999;16:1206–1212.

85. Kravcik S, Gallicano K, Roth V, et al. Cerebrospinal fluid HIV RNA and drug levels with combination ritonavir and saquinavir. J Clin Invest 1999;104:147–153.

86. Huisman M, Smit JW, Wiltshire HR, Hoetelmans RMW, Beijnen JH, Schinkel AH. P-Glycoprotein limits oral availability, brain, and fetal penetration of saquinavir even with high doses of ritonavir. Mol Pharmacol 2001;59:806–813.

87. Khaliq Y, Gallicano K, Venance S, Kravcik S, Cameron DW. Effect of ketoconazole on ritonavir and saquinavir concentrations in plasma and cerebrospinal fluid from patients infected with human immunodeficiency virus. Clin Pharmacol Ther 2000;68:637–646.

88. Mayer U, Wagenaar E, Dorobek B, Beijnen JH, Borst P, Schinkel AH. Full blockade of intestinal P-glycoprotein and extensive inhibition of blood-brain barrier P-glycoprotein by oral treatment of mice with PSC833. J Clin Invest 1997;100:2430–2436.

89. Hendrikse NH, Schinkel AH, de Vries EGE, et al. Complete in vivo reversal of P-glyco-protein pump function in the blood-brain barrier visualized with positron emission tomography. Br J Pharmacol 1998;124:1413–1418.

90. Zong J, Pollack GM. Modulation of P-glycoprotein transport activity in the mouse blood–brain barrier by rifampin. J Pharmacol Exp Ther 2003;306:556–562.

91. Seegers U, Poyschka H, Loscher W. Lack of effects of prolonged treatment with phe-nobarbital or phenytoin on the expression of P-glycoprotein in various rat brain regions. Eur J Clin Pharmacol 2002;451:149–155.

92. Smit JW, Huisman MT, van Tellingen O, et al. Absence of pharmacological blocking of placental P-glycoprotein profoundly increases fetal drug exposure. J Clin Invest 1999; 104:1441–1447.

93. Lankas GR, Wise LD, Cartwright ME, Pippert T, Umbenhauer DR. Placenta P-glycoprotein deficiency enhances susceptibility to chemically induced birth defects in mice. Reprod Toxicol 1998;12:457–463.

94. Nakamura Y, Ikeda S, Furukawa T, et al. Function of P-glycoprotein expressed in placenta and mole. Biochem Biophys Res Commun 1997;235:849–853.

95. Young AM, Allen CE, Audus KL. Effluc transporters of the human placenta. Adv Drug Del Rev 2003;55:125–132.

96. Moodley J, Moodley D, Pillay K, et al. Pharmacokinetics and antiretroviral activity of lamivudine alone or when coadministered with zidovudine in human immunodeficiency virus type 1-infected pregnant women and their offspring. J Infect Dis 1998;178: 1327–1333.

97. Wang Y, Livingston E, Patil S, et al. Pharmacokinetics of didanosine in antepartum and postpartum immunodeficiency virus-infected pregnant women and their neonates: an AIDS Clinical Trials Group Study. J Infect Dis 1999;180:1536–1541.

98. Musoke P. Guay LA, Bagenda D, et al. A phase I/II study of the safety and pharmacokinetics of nevirapine in HIV-1-infected pregnant Ugandan women and their neonates (HIV/NET 006). AIDS 1999;13:479–486.

99. Guay LA, Musoke P, Fleming T, et al. Intrapartum and neonatal single-dose nevirapine compared with zidovudine for prevention of mother-to-child transmission of HIV-1 in Kampala, Uganda: HIVNET 012 randomised trial. Lancet 1999;354:795–802.

100. Marzolini C, Rudin C, Decosterd LA, et al. Transplacental passage of protease inhibitors at delivery. AIDS 2002;16:889–893.

101. Casey BM, Bawdon RE. Placental transfer of ritonavir with zidovudine in the ex-vivo placental perfusion model. Am J Obstet Gynecol 1998;178:758–761.

102. Forrestier F, de Renty P, Peytavin G, Dohin E, Farinotti R, Mandelbrot L. Maternal-fetal transfer of saquinavir studied in the ex-vivo placental perfusion model. Am J Obstet Gynecol 2001;185:178–181.

103. Holcberg G, Sapir O, Tsadkin M, et al. Lack of interaction of digoxin and P-glycoprotein inhibitors, quindine and verapamil in human placenta in vitro. Eur J Obstet Reprod Biol 2003;109:133–137.

104. Bart J, van der Graff WT, Hollema H, et al. An oncological view of the blood–testes barrier. Lancet Oncol 2002;3:357–363.

105. Lum BL, Fisher NA, Brophy NA, et al. Clinical trials of modulation of multidrug resistance. Pharmacokinetic and pharmacodynamic considerations. Cancer 1993;72:3502–3514.

106. van der Valk P, van Kalken H, Ketelaars H, et al. Distribution of multi-drug resistance-associated P-glycoprotein in normal and neoplastic human tissues: analysis with three monoclonal antibodies recognizing different epitopes of the P-glycoprotein molecule. Ann Oncol 1990;1:56–64.

107. Thorgeirsson SS, Silverman JA, Gant TW, Marino PA. Multidrug resistance gene family and chemical carcinogens. Pharmacol Ther 1991;49:283–292.

108. Bart J, Groen HJN, Hendrikse NH, et al. The blood–brain barrier and oncology: new insights into function and modulation. Cancer Treat Rev 2000;26:449–462.

109. Reddy YS, Kashuba A, Gerber J, Miller V, on behalf of the roundtable participants. Importance of antiretroviral drug concentrations in sanctuary sites and viral reservoirs. AIDS Res Hum Retroviruses 2003;19:167–176.

110. van Praag RM, Weverling GJ, Portegies P, et al. Enhanced penetration of indinavir in cerebrospinal fluid and semen after the addition of low-dose ritonavir. AIDS 2000;14: 1187–1194.

111. Huisman MT, Smit JW, Schinkel AH. Significance of P-glycoprotein for the pharmacology and clinical use of HIV protease inhibitors. AIDS 2000;14:237–242.

112. Prechtl S, Roellinghoff M, Scheper R, Cole SP, Deeley RG, Lohoff M. The multidrug resistance protein 1: a functionally important activation marker for murine Th1 cells. J Immunol 2000;164:754–761.

113. Lee CG, Gottesman MM, Cardarelli CO, et al. HIV-1 protease inhibitors are substrates for the MDR1 multidrug transporter. Biochemistry 1998;37:3594–3601.

114. Washington CB, Duran GE, Man MC, Sikic BI, Blaschke TF. Interaction of anti-HIV protease inhibitors with the multidrug transporter P-glycoprotein (P-gp) in human cultured cells. J Acquir Immune Defic Syndr Hum Retrovirol 1998;19:203–209.

115. Srinivas RV, Middlemas D, Flynn P, Fridland A. Human immunodeficiency virus protease inhibitors serve as substrates for multidrug transporter proteins MDR1 and MRP1 but retain antiviral efficacy in cell lines expressing these transporters. Antimicrob Agents Chemother 1998;42:3157–3162.

116. Speck RR, Xiao-Fang Yu, Hildreth J, Flexner C. Differential effects of P-glycoprotein and multidrug resistance protein-1 on productive human immunodeficiency virus infection. J Infect Dis 2002;186:332–340.

117. Lee CG, Ramachandra M, Jeang KT, Martin MA, Pastan I, Gottesman MM. Effect of ABC transporters on HIV-1 infection: inhibition of virus production by the MDR1 transporter. FASEB J 2000;14:516–522.

118. Meaden ER, Hoggard PG, Newton P, et al. P-Glycoprotein and MRP1 expression and reduced ritonavir and saquinavir accumulation in HIV-infected individuals. J Antimicrob Chemother 2002;50:583–588.

119. Jones K, Bray PG, Khoo SH, et al. P-Glycoprotein and transporter MRP1 reduce HIV protease inhibitor uptake in CD4 cells: potential for accelerated viral drug resistance? AIDS 2001;15:1353–1358.

120. Lucia MB, Rutella S, Leone G, Vella S, Cauda R. HIV-protease inhibitors contribute to P-glycoprotein efflux function defect in peripheral blood lymphocytes from HIV-positive patients receiving HAART. J Acquir Immun Defic Syndr 2001;27:321–330.

121. Donahue JP, Dowdy D, Ratnam K, et al. Effects of nelfinavir and its M8 metabolite on lymphocyte P-glycoprotein activity during antiretroviral therapy. Clin Pharmacol Ther 2003;73:78–86.

122. Chaillou S, Durant J, Garraffo R, et al. Intracellular concentration of protease inhibitors in HIV-1-infected patients: correlation with MDR-1 gene expression and low dose ritonavir. HIV Clin Trials 2002;3:493–501.

123. Dupuis ML, Flego M, Molinari A, Cianfriglia M. Saquinavir induces stable and functional expression of the multidrug transporter P-glycoprotein in human CD4 T-lymphoblastoid CEMrev cells. HIV Med 2003;4:338–345.

124. Ford J, Meaden ER, Hoggard PG, et al. Effect of protease inhibitor-containing regimens on lymphocyte multidrug resistance transporter expression. J Antimicrob Chemother 2003;52:354–358.

125. Asghar A, Gorski C, Haehner-Daniels B, Hall SD. Induction of multidrug resistance-1 and cytochrome P450 mRNAs in human mononuclear cells by rifampin. Drug Metab Dispos 2002;30:20–26.

126. Becquemont L, Camus M, Eschwege V, et al. Lymphocyte P-glycoprotein expression and activity before and after rifampicin in man. Fundam Clin Pharmacol 2000;14:519–525.

127. Perloff M, van Moltke L, Fahey J, Daily J, Greenblatt D. Induction of P-glycoprotein expression by HIV protease inhibitors in cell culture. AIDS 2000;14;1287–1289.

128. Perloff MD, von Moltke LL, Marchand JE, Greenblatt DJ. Ritonavir induces P-glycoprotein expression, multidrug resistance-associated protein (MRP1) expression, and drug transporter-mediated activity in a human intestinal cell line. J Pharm Sci 2001;90: 1829–1837.

129. Dupuis ML, Tombesi M, Sabatini M, Cianfriglia M. Differential effect of HIV-1 protease inhibitors on P-glycoprotein function in multidrug-resistant variants of the human CD4+ lymphoblastoid CEM cell line. Chemotherapy 2003;49:8–16.

130. Carlier MB, Zenebergh A, Tulkens M. Cellular uptake and subcellular localization of azithromycin in phagocytic cells. Int J Tissue React 1987;16:211-29.

131. Mor NJ, Vanderkolk, Heifets L. Accumulation of clarithromycin in macrophages infected with *Mycobacterium avium*. Pharmacotherapy 1994;14:100–104.

132. Seral C, Michot J-M, Chanteux H, Mingeot-Leclerq M-P, Tulkens PM, Van Bambeke F. Influence of P-glycoprotein inhibitors on accumulation of macrolides in J774 murine macrophages. Antimicrob Agents Chemother 2003;47:1047–1051.

133. Nichterlein T, Kretschmar M, Schadt A, et al. Reduced intracellular activity of antibiotics against Listeria monocytogenes in multidrug resistant cells. Int J Antimicrob Agents 1998;10:119–125.

134. Sugawara I, Kataoka Y, Morishita Y, et al. Tissue distribution of P-glycoprotein encoded by a multidrug-resistant gene as revealed by a monoclonal antibody MRK16. Cancer Res 1988;48:1926–1929.

135. Huai-Yun H, Secrest DT, Mark KS, et al. Expression of multidrug resistance-associated protein (MRP) in brain microvessel endothelial cells. Biochem Biophys Res Commun 1998;243:816–820.

136. Evers R, Zaman GJ, van Deemter L, et al. Basolateral localization and export activity of the human multidrug resistance-associated protein in polarized pig kidney cells. J Clin Invest 1996;97:1211–1218.

137. Huisman MT, Smit JW, Crommentuyn KML, et al. Mulridrug resistance protein 2 (MRP2) transports HIV protease inhibitors, and transport can be enhanced by other drugs. AIDS 2002;16:2295–2301.

138. Sasabe H, Tsuji H, Sugiyama Y. Carrier-mediated mechanism for the biliary excretion of the quinolone antibiotic grepafloxacin and its glucuronide in rats. J Pharmacol Exp Ther 1998;284:1033–1039.

139. Yamazaki M, Akiyama S, Ninuma K, Nishigaki R, Sugiyama Y. Biliary excretion of pravastatin in rats: contribution of the excretion pathways mediated by the canalicular multispecific organic anion transporter. Drug Metab Dispos 1997;26:1123–1129.

140. Sathirakul K, Susuki H, Yamada T, Hanano M, Sugiyama Y. Multiple transport systems for organic anions across the bile canalicular membrane. J Pharmacol Exp Ther 1994;268: 65–73.

141. Hoojberg JH, Broxterman HJ, Kool M, et al. Antifolate resistance mediated by the multidrug resistance proteins MRP1 and MRP2. Cancer Res 1999;59:2532–2535.

142. Bodo A, Bakos E, Szeri F, Varadi A, Sarkadi B. Differential modulation of the human liver conjugate transporters MRP2 and MRP3 by bile acids and organic anions. J Biol Chem 2003;278:23,529–23,537.

143. Bakos E, Evers R, Sinko E, Varadi A, Borst P, Sarkadi B. Interactions of the human multidrug resistance proteins MRP1 and MRP2 with organic anions. Mol Pharmacol 2000;57:760–768.

144. Chen C, Scott D, Hanson E, et al. Impact of Mrp2 on the biliary excretion and intestinal absorption of furosemide, probenecid, and methotrexate using Eisai hyperbilirubinemic rats. Pharm Res 2003;20:31–37.

145. Assaraf YG, Rothem L, Hoojberg JH, et al. Loss of multidrug resistance protein 1 expression and folate efflux activity results in a highly concentrative folate transport in human leukemia cells. J Biol Chem 2003;278:6680–6686.

146. Schrenk D, Baus PR, Ermel N, Klein C, Vorderstemann B, Kauffmann HM. Up-regulation of transporters of the MRP family by drugs and toxins. Toxicol Lett 2001;120: 51–57.

147. Evers R, de Haas M, Sparidans R et al. Vinblastine and sulfinpyrazone export by the multidrug resistance protein MRP2 is associated with glutathione export. Br J Cancer 2000;83:375-83.

148. Potschka H, Fedrowitz M, Loscher W. Multidrug resistance protein MRP2 contributes to blood-brain barrier function and restricts antiepileptic drug activity. J Pharmacol Exp Ther 2003;306:124-31.

149. Horikawa M, Kato Y, Sugiyama Y. Reduced gastrointestinal toxicity following inhibition of the biliary excretion of ironotecan and its metabolites by probenecid in rats. Pharm Res 2002;19:1345-53.

150. Naruhashi K, Tamai I, Inoue N et al. Involvement of multidrug resistance-associated protein 2 in intestinal secretion of grepafloxacin in rats. Antimicrob Agents Chemother 2002;46:344-9.

151. Miller DS. Nucleoside phosphonate interactions with multiple organic anion transporters in renal proximal tubule. J Pharmacol Exp Ther 2001;299:567-74.

152. van Aubel RA, Smeets PH, Peters JG, Bindels RJ, Russel FG. The MRP4/ABCC4 gene encodes a novel apical organic anion transporter in human kidney proximal tubules: putative efflux pump for urinary cAMP and cGMP. J Am Nephrol 2002;13:595–603.

153. Reid G, Wielinga P, Zelcer N, et al. The human multidrug resistance protein MRP4 functions as a prostaglandin efflux transporter and is inhibited by nonsteroidal anti-inflammatory drugs. Proc Natl Acad Sci USA 2003;100:9244–9249.

154. Reid G, Wielinga P, Zelcer N, et al. Characterization of the transport of nucleoside analog drugs by the human multidrug resistance proteins MRP4 and MRP5. Mol Pharmacol 2003;63:1094–1103.

155. Cole SPC, Bhardway G, Gerlach JH, et al. Overexpression of a transporter gene in a multidrug-resistant human lung cancer cell line. Science 1992;258:1650–1654.

156. Cole SPC, Sparks KE, Fraser DW, et al. Pharmacological characterization of multidrug resistant MRP-transfected human tumor cells. Cancer Res 1994;54:5902–5910.

157. Leier I, Jedlitschky G, Buchholz U, Cole SPC, Deeley RG, Keppler D. The MRP gene encodes an ATP-dependent export pump for leukotriene C4 and structurally related conjugates. 1994;269:27,807–27,810.

158. Muller M, Meijer C, Zaman GJR, et al. Overexpression of the gene encoding the multidrug resistance-associated protein results in increased ATP-dependent glutathione S-conjugate transport. Proc Natl Acad Sci USA 1994;91:13,033–13,037.

159. Loe DW, Almquist KC, Cole SPC, Deeley RG. ATP-dependent 17β-estradiol and 17-(β-D-glucuronide) transport by multidrug resistance protein (MRP). J Biol Chem 1996; 271:9683–9689.

160. Wijnholds J, Scheffer GL, van der Valk M, et al. Multidrug resistance protein 1 protects the oropharyngeal mucosal layer and the testicular tubules against drug-induced damage. J Exp Med 1998;188:797–808.

161. Jones K, Hoggard PG, Sales SD, Khoo S, Davey R, Back DJ. Differences in the intracellular accumulation of HIV protease inhibitors in vitro and the effect of active transport. AIDS 2001;15:675–681.

162. Williams GC, Liu A, Knip G, Sinko PJ. Direct evidence that saquinavir is transported by the multidrug resistance-associated protein (MRP1) and canalicular multispecific organic anion transporter (MRP2). Antimicrob Agents Chemother 2002;46:3456–3462.

163. van der Sandt IC, Vos CM, Nabulsi L, et al. Assessment of active transport of HIV protease inhibitors in various cell lines and the in vitro blood-brain barrier. AIDS 2001;15: 483–491.

164. Owen A, Hartkoorn RC, Khoo S, Back D. Expression of P-glycoprotein, multidrug-resistance proteins 1 and 2 in CEM, CEM$_{VBL}$, CEM$_{E1000}$, MDCKII$_{MRP1}$, and MDCKII$_{MRP2}$ cell lines. AIDS 2003;17:2276–2278.

165. Olson DP, Scadden DT, D'Aquila RT, De Pasquale MP. The protease inhibitors ritonavir inhibits the functional activity of the multidrug resistance related-protein 1 (MRP-1). AIDS 2002;16:1743–1747.

166. Tatebe S, Sinicrope FA, Kuo MT. Induction of multidrug resistance proteins MRP1 and MRP3 and γ-glutamylcysteine synthetase gene expression by nonsteroidal anti-inflammatory drugs in human colon cancer cells. Biochem Bipphys Res Commun 2002;290: 1427–1433.

167. Lucia MB, Rutella S, Golotta C, Leone G, Cauda R. Differential induction of P-glycoprotein and MRP by rifamycins in T lymphocytes from HIV-1/tuberculosis co-infected patients. AIDS 2002;16:1563–1565.

168. Kruh GD, Belinsky MG. The MRP family of drug efflux pumps. Oncogene 2003;22: 7537–7552.

169. Rollot F, Nazal E-M, Chauvelot-Moachon L, et al. Tenofovir-related Fanconi syndrome wi th nephrogeneic diabetes insipidus in a patient with acquired immunodeficiency syndrome: the role of lopinavir-ritonavir-didanosine. Clin Infect Dis 2003;37:e174–e176.

170. Viread [package insert]. Foster City, CA: Gilead Sciences, 2004.

171. Kearney BP, Mittan A, Sayre J, et al. Pharmacokinetic drug interaction and long term safety profile of tenofovir DF and lopinavir/ritonavir. Programs and Abstracts of the 41st Interscience Conference of Antimicrobial Agents and Chemotherapy, Chicago, IL, September 14–17, 2003, Abstract A-1617.

172. Panel on Clinical Practices for Treatment of HIV Infection. Guidelines for the Use of Antiretroviral Agents in HIV-1-Infected Adults and Adolescents, March 23, 2004. Available at Website: http://Aidsinfo.nih.gov. Accessed August 2, 2004.

173. Lalezari JP, Stagg RJ, Kupperman BD, et al. Intravenous cidofovir for peripheral cytomegalovirus retinitis in patients with AIDS: a randomized controlled trial. Ann Intern Med 1997;126:257–263.

174. Kahn J, Lagakos S, Wulfsohn M, et al. Efficacy and safety of adefovir dipivoxil with antiretroviral therapy: a randomized controlled trial. JAMA 1999;I:2305–I2312.

175. Cundy KC, Petty BG, Flaherty J, et al. Clinical pharmacokinetics of cidofovir in human immunodeficiency virus-infected patients. Antimicrob Agents Chemother 1995;39:1247–1252.

176. Huisman M, Crommentuyn K, Rosing H, Beijnen J, Schinkel A. Co-administration of multidrug resistance protein 2 (mrp2)-stimulators dramatically reduces saquinavir oral availability. Fourth International Workshop on Clinical Pharmacology of HIV Therapy, Cannes, France, March 27–29, 2003. Abstract 2.3.

177. Hirohashi T, Suzuki H, Sugiyama Y. Characterization of the transport properties of cloned rat multidrug resistance-associated protein 3 (MRP3). J Biol Chem 1999;274:15,181–15,185.

178. Zeng H, Bain LJ, Belinsky MG, Kruh GD. Expression of multidrug resistance protein-3 (multispecific organic anion transporter-D) in human embryonic kidney 293 cells confers resistance to anticancer agents. Cancer Res 1999;59:5964–5967.

179. Kool M, de Haas GL, Scheffer RJ, et al. Analysis of expression of cMOAT (MRP2), MRP3, MRP4, and MRP5, homologs of the multidrug resistance-associated resistance protein (MRP1), in human cancer cell lines. Cancer Res 1997;57:3537–3547.

180. Lee K, Belinsky MG, Bell DW, Testa JR, Kruh GD. Isolation of MOAT-B, a widely expressed multidrug resistance-associated protein/canalicular multispecific organic anion transporter-related transporter. Cancer Res 1998;58:2741–2747.

181. Schuetz JD, Connelly MC, Sun D, et al. MRP4: A previously unidentified factor in resistance to nucleoside-based antiviral drugs. Nat Med 1999;5:1048–1051.

182. Fridland A. Effect of multidrug-resistance associated protein 4 on antiviral nucleotide analogs. Eighth Conference on Retroviruses and Opportunistic Infections, Chicago, IL, February 5–8, 2001. Abstract S2.

183. Lee K, Klein-Szanto AJP, Kruh GD. Analysis of the MRP4 drug resistance profile in transfected NIH3T3 cells. J Natl Cancer Inst 2000;92:1934–1940.

184. Adachi M, Reid G, Schuetz JD. Therapeutic and biological importance of getting nucleotides out of cells: a case for the ABC transporters MRP4 and 5. Adv Drug Del Rev 2002; 54:1333–1342.

185. Wijnholds J, Mol CAAM, van Deemter L, de Haas M, et al. Multidrug resistance protein 5 is a multispecific organic anion transporter able to transport nucleotide analogs. Proc Natl Acad Sci USA 2000;97:7476–7481.

186. McAleer MA, Breen MA, White NL, Matthews N. pABC11 (also known as MOAT-C and MRP5) a member of the ABC family of proteins, has anion transporter activity but does not confer multidrug resistance when overexpressed in human embryonic kidney 293 cells. J Biol Chem 1999;274:23,541–23,548.

187. Jedlitschky G, Burchell B, Keppler D. The multidrug resistance protein 5 functions as an ATP-dependent export pump for cyclic nucleotides. J Biol Chem 2000;275:30,069–30,074.

188. Turriziani O, Schuetz JD, Focher F, et al. Impaired 2′,3′-dideoxy-3′-thiacytidine accumulation in T-lymphoblastoid cells as a mechanism of acquired resistance independent of multidrug resistant protein 4 with a possible role for ATP-binding cassette C11. Biochem J 2002;368:325–332.

189. Bera T, Lee K, Salvatore G, Lee B, Pastan IH. MRP8, a new member of ABC transport superfamily, identified by EST database mining and gene prediction program is highly expressed in breast cancer. Mol Med 2001;7:509–516.

190. Tammur J, Prades C, Arnould I, et al. Two new genes from the human ATP-binding cassette transporter superfamily, ABCC11 and ABCC12, tandemly duplicated on chromosome 16q12. Gene 2001;273:89–96.

191. Yabuuchi H, Shimizu H, Takayanagi S, Ishikawa T. Multiple splicing variants of two new human ATP-binding cassette transporters, ABCC11 and ABCC12. Biochem Biophys Res Commun 2001;288:933–939.

192. Kumar A, Steinkasserer A, Berchtold S. Interleuken-10 influences the expression of MRP8 and MRP14 in human dendritic cells. Int Arch Allergy Immunol 2003;132: 40–47.

193. Frosch M, Vogl T, Waldherr R, Sorg C, Sunderkotter C, Roth J. Expression of MRP8 and MRP14 by macrophages is a marker for severe forms of glomerulonephritis [serial online]. J Leukoc Biol November 3, 2003.

194. Gou Y, Kotova E, Chen Z-S, et al. MRP8, ATP-binding cassette C11 (ABCC11), is a cyclic nucleotide efflux pump and a resistance factor for fluoropyrimidines 2′,3′-dideoxycytidine and 9′-(2′-phosphonylmethoxyethyl)adenine. J Biol Chem 2003;278: 29,509–29,514.

195. Hagenbuch B, Meier PJ. The superfamily of organic anion transporting polypeptides. Biochim Biophys Acta 2003;1609:1–18.

196. Tamai I, Nezu J, Uchino H, et al. Molecular identification and characterization of novel members of the human organic anion transporter (OATP) family. Biochem Biophys Res Commun 2000;273:251–260.

197. Eckhardt U, Stuber W, Dickneite G, Reers M, Petzinger E. First pass elimination of a peptidomimetic thrombin inhibitor is due to carrier-mediated uptake by the liver. Biochem Pharmacol 1996;52:65–96.

198. Cvetkovic M. Leake B, Fromm MF, Eilkinson GR, Kim RB. OATP and P-glycoprotein transporters mediate the cellular uptake and excretion of fexofenadine. Drug Metab Dispos 1999;27:866–871.

199. Morgan P, Beaumont K, Fenner K, Leake B, Kim RB. Identification of OATP-mediated uptake of a series of lipophilic bases. Paper presented at the Ninth North American ISSX Meeting, Nashville, TN, October 25–29, 1999.

200. Van Montfoort JE, Hegenbuch B, Fattinger KE, et al. Polyspecific organic anion transporting polypeptides mediates hepatic uptake of amphipathic type II organic cations. J Pharmacol Exp Ther 1999;291:147–152.

201. Tirona RG, Leake BF, Wolkoff AW, Kim RB. Human organic anion transporting polypeptide-C (SLC21A6) is a major determinant of rifampin-mediated pregnane X receptor activation. J Pharmacol Exp Ther 2003;304:223–228.

202. Khamdang S, Takeda M, Babu E, et al. Interaction of human and rat organic anion transporter 2 with various cephalosporin antibiotics. Eur J Pharmacol 2003;465:1–7.

203. Cundy KC. Clinical pharmacokinetics of the antiviral nucleotide analogues cidofovir and adefovir. Clin Pharmacokinet 1999;36:127–143.

204. Inui K, Masuda S, Saito H. Cellular and molecular aspects of drug transport in the kidney. Kidney Int 2000;58:944–958.

205. Takeda M, Khamdang S, Narikawa S, et al. Human organic anion transporters and human organic cation transporters mediate renal antiviral transport. J Pharmacol Exp Ther 2002; 300:918–924.

206. Kullak-Ublick GA. Regulation of organic anion and drug transporters of the sinusoidal membrane. J Hepatol 1999;31:563–573.

207. Dresser GK, Bailey DG, Leake BF, et al. Fruit juices inhibit organic anion transporting polypeptide-mediated drug uptake to decrease the oral availability of fexofenadine. Clin Pharmacol Ther 2002;71:11–20.

208. Fichtenbaum CJ, Gerber JG, Rosenkranz SL, et al. Pharmacokinetic interactions between protease inhibitors and statins in HIV seronegative volunteers: ACTG Study A5047. AIDS 2002;16:569–577.

209. Gerber JG, Rosenkranz S, Fichtenbaum CJ, et al. The effect of efavirenz (EFV) and nelfinavir (NFV) on the pharmacokinetics of pravastatin. Drug interaction studies presented at the Second IAS Conference on HIV Pathogenesis and Treatment, Paris, France, July 2003. Abstract 870.

210. Koepsell H. Organic cation transporters in intestine, kidney, liver, and brain. Ann Rev Physiol 1998;60:243–266.

211. Zhang Y, Brett CM, Giacomini KM. Role of organic cation transporters in drug absorption and elimination. Annu Rev Pharmacol Toxicol 1998;38:431–460.

212. Enomoto A, Takeda M, Shimoda M, et al. Interaction of human organic anion transporters 2 and 4 with organic anion transport inhibitors. J Pharmacol Exp Ther 2002;301: 797–802.

213. Wong SL, van Belle K, Sawchuck RJ. Distributional transport kinetics of zidovudine between plasma and brain extracellular fluid/cerebrospinal fluid in the rabbit: investigation of the inhibitory effect of probenecid utilizing microdialysis. J Pharmacol Exp Ther 1993;264:899–909.

214. Suzuki H, Sawada Y, Sugiyama Y, Iga T, Hanano M. Facilitated transport of benzylpenicillin through the blood–brain barrier in rats. J Pharmacobiodyn 1989;12:182–185.

215. Craft JC, Feldman WE, Neldon JD. Clinicopharmacological evaluation of amoxicillin and probenecid against bacterial meningitis. Antimicrob Agents Chemother 1979;16: 346–352.

# 4

# Drug Interactions

*Regulatory Perspective**

## Kellie Schoolar Reynolds

## INTRODUCTION

Regulatory review scientists have been interested in the impact of drug interactions on the safety and efficacy of drugs for many years; however, a number of regulatory actions highlight the importance of the issue. The withdrawals of terfenadine, astemizole, and cisapride were related, in part, to safety concerns when drug interactions with cytochrome P450 (CYP) 3A inhibitors led to higher plasma drug concentrations. Mibefradil is a CYP3A inhibitor that was withdrawn because of drug interactions that led to markedly increased concentrations of CYP3A substrates. In 2002, a Food and Drug Administration (FDA) advisory committee recommended against approval of pleconaril for the treatment of the common cold partly because of the potential for drug interactions *(1)*. Pleconaril is a CYP3A inducer, and its administration may decrease plasma concentrations of CYP3A substrates, including some contraceptive steroids *(2)*. We can reflect on these examples when we consider the appropriate timing of drug interaction evaluations and the appropriate methods to communicate the risk of drug interactions.

Two FDA guidances specifically addressed the evaluation of metabolism-based drug interactions. The April 1997 FDA *Guidance for Industry Drug Metabolism/Drug Interaction Studies in the Drug Development Process: Studies In Vitro (3)* describes in vitro techniques for evaluating the potential for metabolism-based drug interactions, the correlation of in vitro and in vivo findings, the timing of the in vitro studies, and labeling that may result from in vitro studies. The November 1999 *FDA Guidance for Industry In Vivo Drug Metabolism/Drug Interaction Studies—Study Design, Data Analysis and Recommendations for Dosing and Labeling (4)* provides recommendations on study design, study population, choice of interacting drug, dose selection, statistical considerations, and labeling that may result from in vivo studies. Although the guidances addressed metabolism-based drug interactions, many of the principles outlined in the in vivo guidance also apply to drug interactions caused by other mechanisms.

*The views presented in this chapter do not necessarily reflect those of the FDA.

From: *Infectious Disease: Drug Interactions in Infectious Diseases, Second Edition*
Edited by: S. C. Piscitelli and K. A. Rodvold © Humana Press Inc., Totowa, NJ

Because of significant concern within the drug industry and regulatory authorities, the issue of drug interactions was discussed at numerous conferences. A report is available from a conference held in Basel, Switzerland, in 2000; the aim of the conference was to arrive at a consensus on the conduct of in vitro and in vivo studies of metabolic and transporter-based drug interactions *(5)*. Based on discussions at the conference, it was evident that guidance documents developed by the European Agency for the Evaluation of Medical Products, the US FDA, and the Ministry of Health, Labor, and Welfare in Japan provide similar recommendations regarding approaches to address metabolism-based drug interactions. Also, the Pharmaceutical Research and Manufacturers of America (PhRMA) Drug Metabolism and Clinical Pharmacology Technical Working Groups prepared a position paper that describes the industry position on the evaluation of drug interactions *(6)*. The intent of the position paper was to define the best practices for in vitro and in vivo pharmacokinetic drug interaction studies during drug development.

There are numerous similarities across the various guidance documents and position papers that address drug interactions. This chapter does not elaborate on most of the scientific issues discussed in the guidance documents and position papers because other chapters address those issues. Instead, this chapter focuses on the regulatory issues that surround the evaluation of drug interactions. The issues discussed in this chapter apply to most drug classes; however, the discussion of clinical implications and the actual examples apply to drugs that are administered to patients with infectious diseases.

The specific objectives of a drug interaction program are to determine whether there are any interactions with an NME (new molecular entity) that necessitate a dose adjustment, a warning, or a contraindication. Although the potential for drug interactions should be considered for all NMEs, in vivo drug interaction studies are not necessary for all NMEs. One should consider the potential for drug interactions within the context of a drug's pharmacokinetic properties, intended clinical use, and known safety and efficacy.

This chapter provides an overview of regulatory considerations when evaluating the potential for an NME to interact with other drugs. The topics covered include

- Timing of drug interaction evaluations during drug development
- Regulatory considerations for in vitro drug metabolism studies
- When in vivo drug interaction studies are necessary
- In vivo study design issues
- In vivo drug interaction cocktail studies
- Interpretation of in vivo study results
- Current thoughts on drug interactions related to drug transporters
- Case study
- Labeling issues
- Considerations for interactions with pharmacokinetically enhanced protease inhibitors
- Other considerations

## TIMING OF DRUG INTERACTION EVALUATIONS DURING DRUG DEVELOPMENT

The effect of an NME on the pharmacokinetics of other drugs and the effects of other drugs on the pharmacokinetics of an NME should be determined early in drug development so the clinical implications can be assessed adequately in clinical studies.

Because suboptimal concentrations of anti-infective and antiviral drugs can lead to treatment failure and drug resistance, it is helpful to have some knowledge of the potential for drug interactions before these drugs are administered to patients. If drug interaction information is not available when studies in patients begin, it is important to restrict the use of concomitant medications. The restriction of concomitant medications may be acceptable in studies of the treatment of some bacterial infections, such as otitis media. However, it is impossible to administer long-term monotherapy for the treatment of human immunodeficiency virus (HIV) or tuberculosis. As a general rule, the evaluation of the potential for drug interactions should be adequate to allow the safe conduct of each phase of development. Thus, if a proposed treatment for HIV can be administered as monotherapy to a group of HIV-infected patients for 10 days, drug interaction information is not needed prior to the conduct of a 10-day monotherapy study. However, investigators need drug interaction information prior to administering a drug as part of combination therapy to HIV-infected patients.

## REGULATORY CONSIDERATIONS
## FOR IN VITRO DRUG METABOLISM STUDIES

In vitro drug metabolism studies can play a powerful role in the assessment of drug interactions, acting as a screening tool. Goals of in vitro drug metabolism studies are to identify the major metabolic pathways that affect the NME and its metabolites, including the specific enzymes involved, and to determine the effects of the NME on drug-metabolizing enzymes. When these goals are met, it is possible to prioritize the conduct of in vivo drug interaction studies. For example, if in vitro drug metabolism studies indicate that an NME is not metabolized by CYP3A, it is not necessary to determine the effect of in vivo CYP3A inhibitors or inducers on the NME. Likewise, if in vitro drug metabolism studies indicate an NME is not a CYP3A inhibitor or inducer, it is not necessary to determine the in vivo effect of the drug on CYP3A substrates. The PhRMA position paper acknowledges the importance of in vitro studies that provide negative findings, because these in vitro studies may provide the only information regarding the lack of an interaction with a specific enzyme. As such, it is essential that data in support of these negative findings be obtained using methods supported by the most up-to-date scientific data, and the methodology should be well documented for submission to regulatory authorities *(6)*. Important considerations for all in vitro drug metabolism studies are the model system, probe drugs (substrates, inhibitors), drug concentrations, tissue handling, and study conditions.

A full in vitro drug metabolism program can provide a large amount of information regarding the potential for drug interactions with an NME. Studies conducted to determine which enzymes metabolize a drug include general experiments that identify the types of metabolites formed, followed by more specific experiments that identify enzymes that metabolize the drug. If the available data indicate that CYP enzymes contribute to 25% or more of a drug's clearance, studies to identify drug metabolizing CYP enzymes in vitro are recommended. It is appropriate to begin the evaluation with the more common CYP enzymes (CYP3A4, CYP2D6, CYP1A2, CYP2C19, CYP2C9) *(6)*. However, if the more common CYP enzymes do not account for all CYP-mediated metabolism, it may be helpful to evaluate less-common enzymes, such as CYP2B6 or CYP2C8.

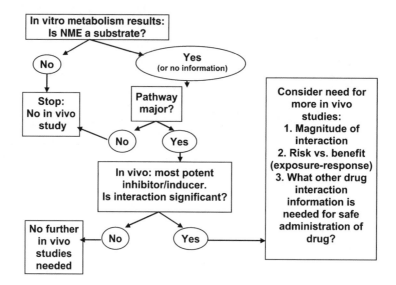

**Fig. 1.** Decision tree for NME as a substrate.

It is important to evaluate the potential for an NME to inhibit and induce CYP-mediated drug metabolism, even if the drug is not metabolized by the enzyme. Most drug interaction programs include an in vitro evaluation of the potential to inhibit the more common CYP enzymes. In vitro evaluations of the potential for CYP induction are becoming more common. The studies must use human materials to provide reliable information about the potential for interactions in humans.

## WHEN IN VIVO DRUG INTERACTION STUDIES ARE NECESSARY

### The Effect of Other Drugs on the NME

In vitro drug metabolism and in vivo pharmacokinetic information help determine whether formal in vivo drug interaction studies are needed. The first consideration is the contribution of renal and metabolic pathways to in vivo clearance. If metabolism does not contribute to clearance, there is usually no need to conduct metabolism-based drug interaction studies. As indicated in Fig. 1, if a particular enzyme contributes significantly to elimination, in vivo studies with inhibitors and inducers of that enzyme are recommended. An efficient approach is first to evaluate the effects of a potent inhibitor and a potent inducer; examples are ketoconazole and rifampin, respectively, if the NME is a CYP3A substrate. If the potent inhibitor and inducer do not have a significant effect on the drug, no further studies are needed for that enzyme. Figure 1 indicates factors to consider if the potent inducer or inhibitor has a significant effect on the drug.

### NME as a Potential Inhibitor

As indicated in Fig. 2, if in vitro evidence does not rule out the possibility that a drug is a metabolic inhibitor, in vivo interaction studies should be conducted. Significant enzyme inhibition should occur when the concentration of the inhibitor present at the

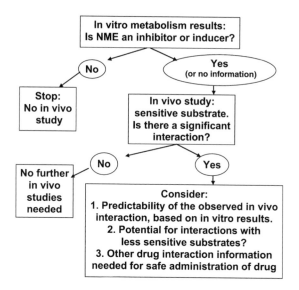

**Fig. 2.** Decision tree for an NME as an inhibitor or inducer.

**Table 1**
**Factors That Affect [I] and $K_i$**

| Factors that affect [I] | Factors that affect $K_i$ |
|---|---|
| 1. Uncertainty regarding the concentration that best represents the concentration at the enzyme binding site (unbound plasma concentration, total plasma concentration, hepatic cytosol concentration) | 1. Substrate specificity (mainly a problem with CYP3A; degree of inhibition of one substrate may not predict degree of inhibition of another substrate for the same enzyme) |
| 2. Uncertainty regarding the impact of first-pass exposure (hepatic and intestinal) | 2. Binding to components of the in vitro incubation system |
| | 3. Substrate and inhibitor depletion during the in vitro experiment |

active site is similar to or greater than $K_i$ (dissociation constant of the enzyme–inhibitor complex; defines the affinity of the inhibitor for the enzyme). If the NME is an inhibitor in vitro and its $K_i$ is equal to or less than in vivo NME concentrations, in vivo inhibition is likely. In theory, the magnitude of the interaction (percentage increase in area under the concentration–time curve [AUC]) can be expressed quantitatively as the following equation:

$$R = 1 + [I]/K_i$$

where $R$ is the percentage increase in AUC, and [I] is the concentration of the inhibitor (NME) present at the active site of the enzyme *(5)*. Many investigators use the ratio of $[I]/K_i$ to predict the likelihood of an in vivo interaction. However, there are a number of limitations for the use of $[I]/K_i$ as a predictor of in vivo inhibition. The limitations are caused by factors that affect interpretation of [I] and $K_i$, as outlined in Table 1 *(5)*.

The second two factors that affect $K_i$ emphasize the importance of good in vitro study design and conduct. Both lists reiterate the fact that the $[I]/K_i$ ratio is not exact enough to predict the degree of inhibition in vivo.

With the listed limitations in mind, $[I]/K_i$ can be used as a screening tool to determine whether an in vivo interaction study is needed. The current recommended approach is quite conservative. When calculating $[I]/K_i$, $[I]$ represents the mean steady-state $C_{max}$ value for total drug (bound plus unbound) following administration of the highest proposed clinical dose. The PhRMA position paper states that if the ratio is below 0.1, the likelihood of an interaction is remote, and an in vivo metabolism-based drug interaction study is not needed for the enzyme (6). Although there is a great deal of debate regarding the appropriate cutoff value, the 0.1 value proposed by PhRMA is reasonable.

If in vitro studies indicate the NME may inhibit an enzyme, the best approach is to conduct an in vivo interaction study with a sensitive substrate for the enzyme, such as midazolam (5) or buspirone (7) for CYP3A. It is acceptable to use any sensitive substrate for the enzyme evaluated if the potential increase in concentrations because of inhibition will not lead to safety concerns. If there is no interaction with a sensitive substrate, no further inhibition studies are needed for that enzyme. However, if coadministration of the NME results in an increase in plasma concentrations of a sensitive substrate, further studies with less-sensitive substrates may be needed.

To prioritize in vivo drug interaction studies, it is reasonable to consider the potential for in vivo inhibition in rank order across the different CYP enzymes. For example, consider an NME with the following in vivo and in vitro characteristics:

In vivo $C_{max} = 0.2\ \mu M$ (use as $[I]$)
CYP3A: $K_i = 0.33\ \mu M$; $[I]/K_i = 0.6$
CYP2D6: $K_i = 1.0\ \mu M$; $[I]/K_i = 0.2$
CYP2C9: $K_i = 2.0\ \mu M$; $[I]/K_i = 0.1$

It is acceptable to conduct the in vivo studies in ascending order of $[I]/K_i$. If the NME interacts with a sensitive CYP3A substrate and increases its AUC, a study with a CYP2D6 substrate is needed. If there is no interaction with the CYP2D6 substrate, there is no need to conduct an in vivo inhibition study with a CYP2C9 substrate. The above scenario is altered if metabolites also inhibit CYP enzymes. In such a case, the rank order needs to consider the effects of the NME and metabolites on other drugs.

The progression listed above applies to reversible inhibition. If an NME demonstrates nonreversible, metabolism-based inhibition of enzymes, in vivo studies are warranted with those enzymes.

## NME as Potential Inducer

Enzyme induction can lead to lack of efficacy, which is an important safety issue for patients taking anti-infective and antiviral agents. There is less experience with interpretation of in vitro induction studies compared to inhibition studies. The most appropriate in vitro end point is the percentage of the positive control induction level (8). As mentioned in the PhRMA position paper, induction of at least 40% of the positive control induction level indicates a positive inductive response (6). If there are no in vitro data or if in vitro data indicate an NME may be an enzyme inducer, in vivo interaction studies should be conducted. It is important that the potential for induction of CYP3A, CYP1A2, CYP2C19, and CYP2C9 be addressed for most drugs.

# IN VIVO STUDY DESIGN ISSUES
## General Design Issues

In vivo drug interaction studies are designed to compare substrate concentrations with and without the interacting drug. The appropriate study design varies depending on the specific objective of the study and the characteristics of the drugs *(4)*. The inhibiting/inducing drug and the substrates should be dosed so that the exposure is relevant to their clinical use. A randomized crossover design is often preferred because the interaction can be evaluated in each individual subject and the design controls for sequence effect. However, a parallel design is acceptable for drugs with long elimination half-lives to decrease the chance of carryover from one treatment to the next. A one-sequence cross-over study is acceptable when both drugs are administered chronically. The choice of single- or multiple-dose administration for each drug is based on the clinical use of the drug and the ability to extrapolate to the clinically relevant situation.

## Selection of Study Population

Drug interaction studies are often conducted in healthy volunteers because there are fewer confounding factors that may alter pharmacokinetics. In some cases, safety concerns may preclude the use of healthy volunteers. If the study enrolls healthy volunteers, it is important to consider whether there are factors that may impede extrapolation to the relevant patient population. For some antibiotics, the relevant patient population is quite similar to healthy volunteers; thus, extrapolation across the population is not an issue.

The situation may be more complex for HIV drugs. There are cases for which pharmacokinetic parameters are similar for HIV-infected patients and healthy volunteers; however, differences have been documented for some drugs, including saquinavir *(9)* and atazanavir *(10)*. The differences may be caused by decreased absorption in HIV patients, differences in metabolism, or the presence of concomitant medications. There is some evidence that CYP3A activity is more variable in patients infected with HIV *(11)*, which is important because of the contribution of CYP3A to protease inhibitor and nonnucleoside reverse transcriptase inhibitor metabolism. In the face of differences between healthy volunteers and the relevant patient population, one should consider the objective of the study when selecting the study population (Table 2).

When drug interaction studies are conducted in healthy volunteers and there is a question regarding the applicability to the relevant population, sparse sampling in clinical efficacy trials that include patients taking the two drugs can be useful *(4,12)*.

## Choice of Interacting Drugs

As discussed in the section "When In Vivo Drug Interaction Studies Are Necessary," it is appropriate to conduct interaction studies with probe inhibitors and substrates to demonstrate the in vivo magnitude of interactions with a specific enzyme. If a study with a probe inhibitor or substrate indicates the drug may significantly affect other drugs (inhibition or induction) or may be affected by other drugs, the next step is to consider several factors:

- Important drugs in the target population that may interact
- Narrow therapeutic index drugs that may be affected
- Relevant potent enzyme inhibitors or inducers that may affect the NME
- Commonly used drugs that may interact

**Table 2**
**Selection of Study Population**

| Study Objective | Population |
| --- | --- |
| • Answer scientific question: "Does NME inhibit CYP3A in vivo?" | Healthy volunteers provide the least complicated evaluation. |
| • Determine whether a dose adjustment is needed when the NME is administered with another drug, but a dose adjustment will not be incorporated into the study. | Either population is acceptable, but healthy volunteers may be easier to study. |
| • Determine the appropriate dose adjustment for the NME or other drug when the two are coadministered. | It is most appropriate to conduct the study in patients. If prior knowledge indicates that the pharmacokinetics of both drugs are similar in healthy volunteers and patients, then either population may be used. Also, if the study may result in subtherapeutic concentrations of the HIV drug for a prolonged period of time, it is best to conduct the study in healthy volunteers. |

These criteria can help guide the conduct of further interaction studies. In each case, it is important to consider the worst-case scenario (maximum magnitude of interaction) and use knowledge of exposure–response relationships (safety and efficacy) to determine the need for specific interactions. In some cases, it may be appropriate not to study a combination but recommend the drugs not be coadministered if the combination is likely to result in excessive or subtherapeutic concentrators and a dose adjustment is not possible.

### Analytes Measured in Drug Interaction Studies

The objective of a drug interaction study and the characteristics of the metabolites dictate whether it is necessary to measure parent drug, metabolite(s), or both. When the substrate drug has an active or toxic metabolite, the metabolite usually should be measured. When the metabolites are not active, measuring some metabolites may help explain the mechanism of an interaction.

The HIV nucleoside reverse transcriptase inhibitors (NRTIs) present a unique drug interaction issue. A majority of the NRTIs do not undergo extensive metabolism in the plasma. However, all of the NRTIs undergo anabolic phosphorylation by intracellular kinases to form the active triphosphates that competitively inhibit viral reverse transcriptase *(13)*. Most HIV treatment regimens include two NRTIs in addition to a non-nucleoside reverse transcriptase inhibitor or protease inhibitor. In some cases, the combination of two NRTIs may interfere with the intracellular phosphorylation of at least one of the compounds, even though no interaction is observed in the plasma.

Knowledge of the enzymes that catalyze phosphorylation for two NRTIs helps determine whether an interaction is likely. For example, the same enzyme catalyzes phosphorylation of zidovudine and stavudine, and coadministration of the two NRTIs leads to reduced formation of stavudine triphosphate *(13)*. Knowledge of phosphorylation pathways, in addition to in vitro combination studies, helps determine whether two

NRTIs may interact with one another. If an interaction is possible, a drug interaction study that evaluates intracellular triphosphate concentrations should be conducted prior to administering the two drugs together in clinical trials. These interaction studies are more difficult than interaction studies that evaluate the parent drug in plasma. The studies that evaluate intracellular triphosphate concentrations are affected by cellular kinase activity, exposure to the enzyme, and difficult analytic techniques.

## IN VIVO DRUG INTERACTION COCKTAIL STUDIES

Cocktail studies involve the administration of two or more probe substrates for different enzymes (cocktail) to characterize changes in pharmacokinetics when the study drug is administered *(14–17)*. There is debate regarding the utility of this approach to the evaluation of drug interactions during drug development. Some believe that the information from cocktail studies provides in vivo confirmation of in vitro study results before definitive in vivo drug interaction studies are conducted. Others believe that the cocktail studies are not necessary if adequate in vitro drug metabolism studies are conducted. Some investigators do not support the use of cocktail studies as stand-alone evidence that an interaction will not occur. This lack of support is largely because of the potential for the probe substrates to interact with each other *(6)*.

Some of the newer cocktail mixtures were developed in response to the concerns regarding the substrates used in the earlier cocktails. If there are adequate data that the probe substrates are sensitive and do not interact with one another across a wide range of concentrations, the study design is acceptable, and the sample size provides adequate power, the results of a cocktail study can serve as stand-alone evidence that an interaction will not occur. Thus, the cocktail studies are useful if in vitro studies are not conducted or if in vitro results are not definitive. If a cocktail study indicates that an interaction is likely, it is typically necessary to conduct additional in vivo studies with substrates of the affected enzyme.

## INTERPRETATION OF IN VIVO STUDY RESULTS

The 1999 in vivo drug interaction guidance included an extensive discussion of the interpretation of in vivo drug interaction study results *(4)*. Most studies evaluate pharmacokinetic end points, such as the exposure measures AUC and $C_{max}$. For many anti-infective and antiviral drugs, trough concentration ($C_{min}$) is an important exposure measure.

The results of drug interaction studies should be reported as 90% confidence intervals about the geometric mean ratio of the pharmacokinetic measure of the substrate with and without the interacting drug *(18)*. Confidence intervals are informative because they provide an estimate of the distribution of the change in exposure to the substrate drug. Tests of significance, such as *t*-tests and the resulting *p* values, are not appropriate because consistent exposure changes can be statistically significant but not clinically relevant *(4)*.

Once the 90% confidence interval of the effect is determined, the clinical significance must be determined. To aid interpretation of interaction studies, investigators should determine no-effect boundaries for the substrate drug. No-effect boundaries define the interval within which a change in systemic exposure measure is considered not clinically meaningful *(4)*. No-effect boundaries can be based on dose or concentration–response relationships for the substrate drug. For example, consider an NME that was evaluated at doses ranging from 50 to 400 mg once daily; all doses were safe and well tolerated, but 200 mg once daily was selected because it was on the plateau of the dose–response curve. In this case, an interacting drug that doubles the systemic exposure to the NME is not a concern because concentrations associated with double the dose (assuming dose proportional pharmacokinetics) were safe. If no-effect boundaries are not defined for a substrate drug, the default no-effect range is 80 to 125%.

## CURRENT THOUGHTS ON DRUG INTERACTIONS RELATED TO DRUG TRANSPORTERS

Our knowledge of the relevance of drug transporters to pharmacokinetics, drug disposition, and drug interactions is emerging. However, it is clear that ruling out the potential for CYP-mediated drug interactions does not rule out the potential for clinically significant interactions via other mechanisms. In addition, the significant overlap between CYP3A and P-glycoprotein (P-gp) for substrates, inhibitors, and inducers makes interpretation of in vivo interaction studies challenging *(19)*. It is also clear that transporters other than P-gp, including organic anion transporting polypeptide, contribute to drug interactions.

In some cases, there may be an interaction when no interaction is expected. Based on drug metabolism information, CYP3A inhibitors should not increase fexofenadine or digoxin concentrations. However, ketoconazole increased fexofenadine concentrations, and itraconazole increased digoxin concentrations. It is presumed that these observed in vivo interactions are because of inhibition of intestinal P-gp, organic anion transporting polypeptide, or other transporters.

Numerous transporters play a role in permeability across the gastrointestinal tract, penetration of the blood–brain barrier, and transport into the liver and kidney cells. Interactions can occur at any of the sites *(20)*. Thus, information about interactions with drug transporters can aid in the prediction and identification of drug interactions. However, it is difficult to recommend methods to investigate the potential for interactions with drug transporters. In vitro methods for evaluation of a drug as a P-gp substrate and inhibitor are available, but the methods are not standardized. In vivo probes are evolving. However, it is currently assumed that if a drug does not alter digoxin concentrations, it does not alter P-gp activity. There is no consensus on the evaluation of interaction with drug transporters other than P-gp.

### CASE STUDY: INDINAVIR AND RIFABUTIN

The example of indinavir (CYP3A substrate and inhibitor) and rifabutin (CYP3A substrate and inducer) indicates that several in vivo studies may be needed to determine appropriate dose adjustment instructions.

When indinavir was approved, results for one drug interaction study with rifabutin were available. The study evaluated the approved dose of indinavir (800 mg every 8 hours) with the approved dose of rifabutin (300 mg every day). Results indicated indinavir concentrations were reduced by approx 32%, and rifabutin concentrations were increased by approx 200% when the drugs were coadministered. Based on the results, a dose reduction of rifabutin to 150 mg daily was recommended. The dose adjustment was expected to result in lower rifabutin plasma concentrations and possibly less induction of CYP3A, resulting in less reduction of indinavir concentrations *(21)*.

A subsequent interaction study evaluated the recommended regimen. The lower dose of rifabutin in combination with indinavir did result in lower rifabutin concentrations than the previous combination (~60% higher than 300 mg rifabutin alone). However, the indinavir concentrations were practically identical to those for 800 mg indinavir every 8 hours plus 300 mg rifabutin daily. The dose adjustment recommendations were revised to recommend an increase in the indinavir dose to 1000 mg every 8 hours when administered with 150 mg rifabutin daily *(21)*.

One more interaction study was conducted to evaluate the 1000 mg indinavir every 8 hours regimen in combination with 150 mg rifabutin daily. The results indicated that the increased indinavir dose compensated for the effect of rifabutin. The authors concluded that the studied doses were acceptable for clinical use. The authors also indicated that it is important to conduct a confirmatory pharmacokinetic evaluation when dosing recommendations for a combination are based on previous studies that used different doses of the drugs *(22)*. Although confirmatory studies may be ideal, they are not always practical. If the mechanism of the interaction is well understood and there is some margin for error in the resulting concentrations (some increase or decrease in concentrations would be acceptable), a confirmatory study may not be needed.

## LABELING ISSUES

The 1999 FDA guidance on in vivo evaluations of drug interactions indicated that all relevant information on the metabolic pathways and pharmacokinetic interactions should be included in the Clinical Pharmacology section of the label *(4)*. Such information allows the reader to determine the potential for drug interactions beyond those studied and listed in the label. For example, the Viracept label indicates that nelfinavir is a CYP3A inhibitor that increases simvastatin plasma concentrations by approx 500% *(23)*. Because the mechanism of the interaction is stated, the reader can assume that coadministration of nelfinavir with lovastatin would result in an interaction of a similar magnitude because lovastatin is a CYP3A substrate with similar bioavailability as simvastatin *(24)*.

To simplify the interpretation of drug interaction information, labels for antiretroviral drugs summarize drug interaction data in a table. The tables indicate the doses of all drugs used, the size of the study, and the effect on AUC, $C_{max}$, and $C_{min}$. In many cases, the tables indicate whether the study was conducted in healthy volunteers or HIV-infected patients and whether the study design was crossover or parallel.

The 1999 guidance also stated the Precautions, Warnings, and Contraindications section of the label should describe drug interactions of clinical significance and describe any dose adjustments or special monitoring that are needed. Dose adjustments may also be described in the Dosage and Administration section *(4)*.

It is acceptable to include statements in the Precautions, Warnings, and Contraindications section of the label for interactions that are expected because of known mechanisms of interactions, even if the specific drug interaction information is not available. Some examples are shown in Table 3.

**Table 3**
**Drug Interaction Information in Labels, Not Based on a Drug Interaction Study**

| Drug label | Label section and example of information | Basis for inclusion of information in label |
|---|---|---|
| All protease inhibitors (9,10,23,25–29) | Contraindications: Pimozide | The protease inhibitors inhibit CYP3A; pimozide metabolism is highly dependent on CYP3A, and elevated pimozide concentrations could lead to serious and life-threatening events |
| All protease inhibitors (9,10,23,25–29) | Warnings and Precautions: Recommend against coadministration with St. John's wort because protease inhibitor concentrations may decrease and lead to loss of virological response | St. John's wort induces CYP3A; induction of CYP3A affects all protease inhibitors; data are available for indinavir and St. John's wort |
| Kaletra® (lopinavir/ritonavir) (28) | Precautions: Coadministration of Kaletra and itraconazole may lead to increased itraconazole concentrations; High doses of itraconazole are not recommended in combination with Kaletra | Coadministration of Kaletra and ketoconazole leads to increased ketoconazole concentrations; CYP3A-mediated interactions are often similar for ketoconazole and itraconazole |
| Reyataz® (atazanavir) (10) | Precautions: Coadministration of Reyataz and H$_2$-receptor antagonists is expected to reduce atazanavir plasma concentrations; H$_2$-receptor antagonists and atazanavir should be administered as far apart as possible, preferably 12 h apart | H$_2$-receptor antagonists increase gastric pH; atazanavir solubility decreases as pH increases |

## CONSIDERATIONS FOR INTERACTIONS WITH PHARMACOKINETICALLY ENHANCED PROTEASE INHIBITORS

The addition of a low dose of ritonavir to a protease inhibitor regimen can increase concentrations and decrease elimination rate of the protease inhibitor. This practice is known as *pharmacokinetic enhancement* or *ritonavir boosting*.

### Labeling Considerations

The drug labels for a number of protease inhibitors, including atazanavir *(10)*, fosamprenavir *(29)*, and saquinavir *(9)*, specify dosing instructions with and without low-dose ritonavir. The drug label needs to describe the change in drug interaction potential that is caused by the addition of ritonavir to the dosing regimen. The Clinical Pharmacology section of the label should summarize drug interaction results for the protease inhibitor with and without ritonavir, when available. Such information allows the reader to appreciate the differences observed because of the addition of ritonavir. In some cases, the addition of ritonavir to a regimen can counteract the effect of an enzyme inducer. For example, when 600 mg efavirenz once daily is administered with 400 mg atazanavir once daily, atazanavir concentrations are reduced to less than half those typically observed with atazanavir administered alone. However, when 600 mg efavirenz once daily is administered with 300 mg atazanavir once daily plus 100 mg ritonavir once daily, atazanavir concentrations are not decreased *(10)*. The addition of ritonavir to a protease inhibitor regimen may also increase the CYP3A inhibition observed because of the administration of the protease inhibitor with a CYP3A substrate. All sections of the drug label that include drug interaction information (Clinical Pharmacology, Contraindications, Warnings, Precautions) need to indicate in a clear manner which drug interaction information applies to dosing regimens without ritonavir and which information applies to dosing regimens with ritonavir.

### Extrapolation Across Pharmacokinetically Enhanced Regimens

It is well accepted that much of the effect of ritonavir on other protease inhibitors is caused by ritonavir's potent inhibition of CYP3A *(30)*. Some investigators assume that ritonavir will predominate the drug interaction potential of ritonavir-boosted regimens, and the effect will be similar across all regimens that include ritonavir 100 mg twice daily (or across all regimens that include ritonavir 100 mg once daily or 200 mg ritonavir once daily). However, this assumption has not been validated by data.

In addition, the available scientific literature indicates that interactions may not be similar across all regimens that include the same ritonavir dosing regimen. Interactions with ritonavir are complicated because ritonavir inhibits enzymes other than CYP3A, and it induces several enzymes, including CYP3A. Ritonavir induces CYP3A because of its activation of the pregnane X receptor *(31)*. In addition to CYP3A, the pregnane X receptor regulates expression of CYP2B, CYP2C, and numerous transporters *(32,33)*. The effect of ritonavir on other drugs is a complex interplay of inhibition plus induction of numerous enzymes and transporters. It is difficult to predict the net effect of ritonavir-boosted regimens without an in vivo study because the effect on enzymes and transporter is not consistent across the other protease inhibitors. Thus, it is not possible to conclude that drug interactions will be consistent across ritonavir-boosted regimens that include the same ritonavir dose.

## OTHER CONSIDERATIONS

### Current Thoughts on Drug Interactions With Less-Common CYP Enzymes

Investigators often determine whether a drug is metabolized by or affects CYP3A4/5, CYP2D6, CYP2C9, CYP2C19, and CYP1A2. However, an appreciation of the roles of CYP2B6 and CYP2C8 in drug metabolism and the significance of the contribution of CYP3A5 to combined CYP3A4/5 activity is evolving *(34–36)*. Lack of information about CYP2B6, CYP2C8, or CYP3A5 can lead to an incomplete picture of the potential for drug interactions that investigators and regulators must be aware of when evaluating drug interaction information.

### Interactions Via Mechanisms Other Than Drug Metabolism

Although most discussions of drug interactions focus on drug metabolism, with the recent addition of drug transporters, it is important to remember that there are other mechanisms of drug interactions. Ruling out the potential for drug metabolism- or drug transporter-related interactions does not mean there will not be significant interactions with the drug. Pharmacokinetic drug interactions may involve alterations in absorption, transport, distribution, metabolism, or excretion of a drug or a combination of these factors. When developing an NME, it is important to consider all mechanisms of drug interactions.

### Interactions With Dietary Supplements and Dietary Components

Drugs can interact with dietary supplements (St. John's wort, garlic, echinacea), citrus fruit juices (grapefruit juice, Seville orange juice), alcohol, and other food components (cruciferous vegetables, charbroiled meat) in the same way they interact with other drugs *(37,38)*. These interactions can lead to therapeutic failure or adverse events. It is important to recognize the potential for such interactions, understand the science behind the interactions, and make appropriate recommendations in product labels.

### Role of Genetic Polymorphisms

There is genetic variability in the activity of a number of drug-metabolizing enzymes, including CYP2D6, CYP2C9, and CYP2C19 *(39)*. Because of the variability, patients may be categorized as poor metabolizers, extensive metabolizers, or ultrarapid extensive metabolizers for the various enzymes. The magnitude of a metabolism-based drug interaction varies, depending on the individual's baseline enzyme activity. For example, inhibition of CYP2D6 will not have much effect on a CYP2D6 poor metabolizer. Thus, it is important to know the metabolic phenotype of individuals included in a drug interaction study.

## SUMMARY

Scientists in regulatory agencies, the drug industry, and academia are interested in the impact of drug interactions on the safety and efficacy of drugs. Thus, there are guidance documents and position papers that address the topic of drug interactions. There are numerous similarities across these documents because most parties agree on the objectives of a drug interaction program. The specific objectives of a drug interaction program are to determine whether there are any interactions with an NME that necessitate a dose adjustment of the NME or other drugs that with which it might be used or whether an interaction requires a contraindication or special precautions.

The effect of an NME on the pharmacokinetics of other drugs and the effects of other drugs on the pharmacokinetics of an NME should be determined early in drug development so the clinical implications can be assessed adequately in clinical studies. The drug interaction program can include in vitro and in vivo evaluations. Throughout the evaluation of drug interactions, it is important that all studies are conducted using scientifically accepted procedures. The clinical significance of any observed interactions should be assessed based on exposure–response knowledge of the affected drug. Finally, the drug labels need to include complete information about the potential for drug interactions, including instructions for dose adjustments and special monitoring or precautions.

## REFERENCES

1. Senior K. FDA panel rejects common cold treatment. Lancet Infect Dis 2002;2:264.
2. Hayden FG, Herrington DT, Coats TL, et al. Efficacy and safety of oral pleconaril for treatment of colds due to picornaviruses in adults: results of double-blind, randomized, placebo-controlled trials. Clin Infect Dis 2003;33:1523–1532.
3. Center for Drug Evaluation and Research, Center for Biologics Evaluation and Research. Guidance for Industry drug metabolism/drug interaction studies in the drug development process: studies in vitro (April 1997). US Department of Health and Human Services, Food and Drug Administration.
4. Center for Drug Evaluation and Research, Center for Biologics Evaluation and Research. Guidance for Industry in vivo drug metabolism/drug interaction studies—study design, data analysis, and recommendations for dosing and labeling (November 1999). US Department of Health and Human Services, Food and Drug Administration.
5. Tucker GT, Houston B, Huang SM. Optimizing drug development: strategies to assess drug metabolism/transporter interaction potential—toward a consensus. Clin Pharmacol Ther 2001;70:103–114.
6. Bjornsson TD, Callaghan JT, Einolf HJ, et al. The conduct of in vitro and in vivo drug–drug interaction studies: a Pharmaceutical Research and Manufacturers of America (PhRMA) perspective. Drug Metab Dispos 2003;31:815–832.
7. Kivisto KT, Lamberg TS, Kantola T, Neuvonen PJ. Plasma buspirone concentrations are greatly increased by erythromycin and itraconazole. Clin Pharmacol Ther 1997;62: 348–354.
8. LeCluyse EL. Human hepatocyte culture systems for the in vitro evaluation of cytochrome P450 expression and regulation. Eur J Pharmaceut Sci 2001;13:343–368.
9. Saquinavir (Fortovase and Invirase) [package inserts]. Nutley, NJ: Roche Laboratories, 2003.
10. Atazanavir (Reyataz) product information. Princeton, NJ: Bristol Myers Squibb, 2003.
11. Slain D, Pakyz A, Israel DS, Monroe S, Polk R. Variability in activity of hepatic CYP3A4 in patients infected with HIV. Pharmacotherapy 2000;20:898–907.
12. Center for Drug Evaluation and Research, Center for Biologics Evaluation and Research. Guidance for Industry population pharmacokinetics (February 1999). US Department of Health and Human Services, Food and Drug Administration.
13. Stein DS, Moore KHP. Phosphorylation of nucleoside analog antiretrovirals: a review for clinicians. Pharmacotherapy 2001;21:11–34.
14. Frye RF, Matzke GR, Adedoyin A, Porter JA, Branch RA. Validation of the five-drug "Pittsburgh cocktail" approach for assessment of selective regulation of drug-metabolizing enzymes. Clin Pharmacol Ther 1997;62:365–376.

15. Christensen M, Andersson K, Dalen P, et al. The Karolinska cocktail for phenotyping of five human cytochrome P450 enzymes. Clin Pharmacol Ther 2003;73:517–528.

16. Chainuvati S, Nafziger AN, Leeder JS, et al. Combined phenotypic assessment of cytochrome P450 1A2, 2C9, 2C19, 2D6, and 3A, N-acetyltransferase-2, and xanthine oxidase activities with the "Cooperstown 5 + 1 cocktail." Clin Pharmacol Ther 2003;74: 437–447.

17. Blakey GE, Lockton JA, Perrett J, et al. Pharmacokinetic and pharmacodynamic assessment of a five-probe metabolic cocktail for CYPs 1A2, 3A4, 2C9, 2D6, and 2E1. Br J Clin Pharmacol 2004;57:162–169.

18. Schuirman DJ. A comparison of the two one-sided tests procedure and the power approach for assessing the bioequivalence of average bioavailability. J Pharmacokinet Biopharm 1987;15:657–680.

19. Yasuda K, Lan L, Sanglard D, Furuya K, Schuetz JD, Schuetz EG. Interaction of cytochrome P450 3A inhibitors with p-glycoprotein. J Pharmacol Exp Ther 2002;303:323–332.

20. Ayrton A, Morgan P. Role of transport proteins in drug absorption, distribution and excretion. Xenobiotica 2001;31:469–497.

21. Kraft WK, McCrea JB, Winchell GA, et al. Indinavir and rifabutin interactions in healthy volunteers. J Clin Pharmacol 2004;44:305–313.

22. Hamzeh FM, Benson C, Gerber J, et al. Steady-state pharmacokinetic interaction of modified-dose indinavir and rifabutin. Clin Pharmacol Ther 2003;73:159–169.

23. Nelfinavir (Viracept) [package insert]. Thousand Oaks, CA: Agouron Pharmaceuticals, 2003.

24. Williams D, Feely J. Pharmacokinetic-pharmacodynamic drug interactions with HMG-CoA reductase inhibitors. Clin Pharmacokinet 2002;41:343–370.

25. Ritonavir (Norvir) [package insert]. North Chicago, IL: Abbott Laboratories, 2003.

26. Indinavir (Crixivan) [package insert]. West Point, PA: Merck and Co., 2003.

27. Amprenavir (Agenerase) [package insert]. Research Triangle Park, NC: GlaxoSmithKline, 2002.

28. Lopinavir/ritonavir (Kaletra) product information. Abbott Park, IL: Abbott Laboratories, 2003.

29. Fosamprenavir (Lexiva) product information. Research Triangle Park, NC: GlaxoSmith Kline, 2003.

30. Zeldin RK, Petruschke RA. Pharmacological and therapeutic properties of ritonavir-boosted protease inhibitor therapy in HIV-infected patients. J Antimicrob Chemother 2004;53:4–9.

31. Luo G, Cunningham M, Kim S, et al. CYP3A4 induction by drugs: correlation between pregnane X receptor reporter gene assay and CYP3A4 expression in human hepatocytes. Drug Metab Dispos 2002;30:795–804.

32. Wang H, LeCluyse EL. Role of orphan nuclear receptors in the regulation of drug-metabolising enzymes. Clin Pharmacokinet 2003;42:1331–1357.

33. Handschin C, Meyer UA. Induction of drug metabolism: the role of nuclear receptors. Pharmacol Rev 2003;55:649–673.

34. Ward BA, Gorski JC, Jones DR, Hall SD, Flockhart DA, Desta Z. The cytochrome P450 2B6 (CYP2B6) is the main catalyst of efavirenz primary and secondary metabolism: implications for HIV/AIDS therapy and utility of efavirenz as a substrate marker of CYP2B6 catalytic activity. J Pharmacol Exp Ther 2003;306:287–300.

35. Niemi M, Backman JT, Neuvonen PJ. Effects of trimethoprim and rifampin on the pharmacokinetics of the cytochrome P450 2C8 substrate rosiglitazone. Clin Pharmacol Ther 2004;76:239–249.

36. Williams JA, Cook J, Hurst SI. A significant drug-metabolizing role for CYP3A5? Drug Metab Dispos 2003;31:1526–1530.

37. Huang SM, Hall SD, Watkins P, et al. Drug interactions with herbal products and grape-fruit juice: a conference report. Clin Pharmacol Ther 2004;75:1–12.

38. Harris RZ, Jang GR, Tsunoda S. Dietary effects on drug metabolism and transport. Clin Pharmacokinet 2003;42:1071–1088.

39. Rogers JF, Nafziger AN, Bertino JS. Pharmacogenetics affects dosing, efficacy, and toxicity of cytochrome P450-metabolized drugs. Am J Med 2002;113:746–750.

# 5

# Drug Interactions
# With Antiretrovirals for HIV Infection

## Kimberly A. Struble and Stephen C. Piscitelli

## INTRODUCTION

More than 20 years of research in human immunodeficiency virus (HIV) infection has led to remarkable scientific breakthroughs in drug development. Although the use of highly active antiretroviral therapy (HAART) has dramatically altered survival rates, these complex regimens remain challenging to use, even to the experienced practitioner. In no other disease state does the management and exploitation of drug interactions play such a critical role as it does in HIV disease. Because there are so many potential drug interactions in HIV-infected patients, this book includes two chapters pertaining to HIV/AIDS (acquired immunodeficiency syndrome). This chapter describes the clinically important interactions associated with the four classes of antiretrovirals and discusses management strategies to improve patient outcome. Chapter 6 discusses interactions with antiretroviral agents and agents for opportunistic infections.

Currently, four classes of antiretrovirals are approved for the treatment of HIV infection. HAART consists of at least three antiretrovirals. In addition, many patients also take drugs for opportunistic infections, concurrent diseases, symptomatic relief, and supportive care. Although great strides have been made to reduce pill burden and improve dosing convenience and formulations, the problems and issues of drug interactions have grown as several new compounds have been approved.

The potential for drug interactions in this disease is unprecedented. All of the protease inhibitors (PIs) and nonnucleoside reverse transcriptase inhibitors (NNRTIs) are metabolized by the cytochrome P450 (CYP) system, primarily the CYP3A4 isoform, and have either inducing or inhibitory effects. This leads to numerous combinations, each with its own dose modification strategy. Nucleoside reverse transcriptase inhibitors (NRTIs) may have intracellular interactions in terms of their activation pathways; these reactions may be either beneficial or detrimental to the patient. And, some NRTIs, such as tenofovir (TDF), cause pharmacokinetic interactions that are not generally well understood. Food effects, interactions with alternative medicines, and combinations that lead to excessive toxicity or poor antiviral effect also exist with antiretrovirals. Management of these regimens can be overwhelming for the clinician and patient.

From: *Infectious Disease: Drug Interactions in Infectious Diseases, Second Edition*
Edited by: S. C. Piscitelli and K. A. Rodvold © Humana Press Inc., Totowa, NJ

## NUCLEOSIDE REVERSE TRANSCRIPTASE INHIBITORS

NRTIs are the most commonly used agents in HIV treatment and are often part of the regimen "backbone." A listing of NRTI-related drug interactions is given in Table 1. NRTIs are not metabolized via the CYP450 pathway and may be used concomitantly at standard doses with PIs and NNRTIs. These agents are primarily eliminated by the kidneys unchanged, although zidovudine undergoes extensive glucoronidation. Agents that alter this pathway may markedly increase zidovudine concentrations. Valproic acid and probenecid have both been shown to increase the area under the curve (AUC) of zidovudine by 80% *(1,2)*. Fluconazole increased the AUC of zidovudine by 60% in healthy volunteers *(3)*. Such increases may be associated with an increase in zidovudine toxicities. Other moderate changes in NRTI blood concentrations have been reported. Methadone was observed to decrease didanosine (ddI) AUC by 40% and stavudine AUC by 27% in HIV-infected patients *(4)*.

However, the clinical consequences of these changes are likely to be minimal because these agents are prodrugs that must be phosphorylated intracellularly to their active forms. In general, modest changes in plasma concentrations of NRTIs are of limited clinical importance. However, larger increases in NRTI concentrations can lead to toxicity. For example, ddI concentrations are increased over 100% by ganciclovir and allopurinol and require close monitoring or dose reduction *(5,6)*.

TDF, an NRTI, undergoes two phosphorylation steps intracellularly, compared to three steps for other NRTIs. Although this compound is eliminated renally, a number of interesting drug interactions are observed, even with drugs that are hepatically metabolized.

TDF increases ddI plasma AUC by 40 to 60% *(7)*. This interaction is not thought to involve renal elimination of ddI but possibly TDF's effects on ddI cleavage. Patients are recommended to reduce the dose of enteric-coated (EC) ddI (Videx EC) from 400 mg daily to 250 mg daily when used concomitantly. This interaction was observed when these drugs were given simultaneously or when dosing was staggered by 2 hours, suggesting that the interaction is not caused by a change in absorption *(8)*. TDF also decreases the AUC of the PI atazanavir (ATV) by approx 25% whether ATV is given alone or in combination with ritonavir (RTV) (*see* Protease Inhibitors) *(9)*. The mechanism of this interaction is currently unknown.

Clinically significant drug interactions may occur between agents that compete for these intracellular activation pathways. Zidovudine has been postulated to impair the intracellular phosphorylation of stavudine *(10)*. This NRTI combination was associated with a significantly unfavorable outcome compared to other double-nucleoside regimens in a National Institute of Arthritis and Infectious Diseases clinical study *(11)*. Data are also available demonstrating lamivudine inhibits zalcitabine phosphorylation *(12)*. The current US Department of Health and Human Services antiretroviral guidelines recommend the avoidance of zidovudine/stavudine and lamivudine/zalcitabine combinations *(13)*. In vitro data have also suggested that ribavirin interferes with the phosphorylation of zidovudine and stavudine *(14)*.

Data from a clinical trial also showed the combination of abacavir, TDF, and lamivudine and the combination of ddI, TDF, and lamivudine lead to a high rate of early virological nonresponse *(15)*. An intracellular interaction is possible but unlikely because in vitro data have not shown antagonism, and abacavir and TDF do not compete for the same pathway. A pharmacokinetic study examining plasma concentrations

**Table 1**
**Drug–Drug Interactions: Nucleoside Reverse Transcriptase Inhibitors**

| Drug affected | Didanosine (ddI) | Stavudine (d4T) | Tenofovir (TDF) | Zidovudine (ZDV) |
|---|---|---|---|---|
| Atazanavir (ATV) | Buffered ddI + ATV simultaneously: ATV AUC ↓ 87%; take ATV (with food) 2 hours before or 1 hour after buffered ddI | | 400 mg ATV + 300 mg TDF: ATV AUC ↓ 25% and $C_{min}$ ↓ 40%; TDF AUC ↑ 24%; avoid concomitant use | |
| | No interaction expected with ddI EC, because ddI EC is to be given on an empty stomach, and ATV is to be given with food, so they should be administered at different times | | 300/100 mg ATV/RTV qd + 300 mg TDF qd: ATV AUC ↓ 25% and $C_{min}$ ↓ 23%; ATV $C_{min}$ was higher with RTV than ATV without RTV | |
| | | | Give 300/100 mg ATV/RTV qd + 300 mg TDF qd | |
| Didanosine | | Peripheral neuropathy, lactic acidosis and pancreatitis seen with combination; use with caution | ddI AUC ↑ 44%; $C_{max}$ ↑ 28%; TDF ↔ | |
| | | Use with caution during pregnancy and only if potential benefit outweighs potential risks | Monitor for ddI-associated toxicities | |
| | | | For patients > 60 kg, 250 mg/day of ddI-EC is recommended | |
| Hydroxyurea | Increase in ddI-associated side effects; avoid coadministration | | | |

*Continued on next page*

**Table 1 (Continued)**
**Drug–Drug Interactions: Nucleoside Reverse Transcriptase Inhibitors**

| Drug affected | Didanosine (ddI) | Stavudine (d4T) | Tenofovir (TDF) | Zidovudine (ZDV) |
|---|---|---|---|---|
| Lamivudine (3TC) plus abacavir (ABC) or didanosine | | | High rate of early virological nonresponse with 3TC + ABC or ddI + TDF; combination should be avoided | |
| Methadone | ddI ↓41%, methadone unchanged | d4T ↓ 27%; methadone unchanged No dose adjustment | | |
| Nephrotoxic agents: cidofovir, ganciclovir, valganciclovir | ddI + oral ganciclovir: ddI AUC ↑ 111%; ganciclovir AUC ↓21% Appropriate doses for the combination have not been established | | Possibly competes for active tubular secretion with TDF, may increase serum concentrations of these drugs and/or TDF Monitor for dose-related toxicities | Coadministration of ZDV with other bone marrow-suppressive or cytotoxic agents may increase hematological toxicity of ZDV |
| Ribavirin | Coadministration not recommended; ribavirin increases the intracellular levels of active metabolite of ddI and may cause serious toxicities | Ribavirin inhibits phosphorylation of d4T; this combination should be avoided if possible or closely monitor virological response | | Ribavirin inhibits phosphorylation of ZDV; this combination should be avoided if possible or closely monitor virological response |
| Stavudine | | | | Antagonistic in vitro; do not coadminister |
| Zalcitabine | Additive peripheral neuropathy; avoid concomitant use | Additive peripheral neuropathy; avoid concomitant use | | |

*Source:* From refs. *13, 24,* and *80-86.*

has also not shown a significant effect *(16)*. This interaction is probably caused by a low genetic barrier to resistance from this combination, allowing for the emergence of resistance strains in a short period of time.

Other intracellular interactions may potentiate the activity of NRTIs. Clinical trials have examined the enhanced antiviral benefit of certain NRTIs when used with hydroxyurea *(17,18)*. Hydroxyurea is an antimetabolite used for several decades to treat malignancies. Hydroxyurea has been shown to potentiate the antiviral effect of ddI. The likely mechanism is thought to be through decreasing the intracellular pool of deoxyadenosine 5′-triphosphate (dATP), which competes with ddI's affinity for its active metabolite, dideoxyadenosine 5′-triphosphate (ddATP), for incorporation into viral deoxyribonucleic acid (DNA) *(19)*. This favorably alters the intracellular ratio of ddATP/dATP, improving ddI's antiviral potency. In the presence of hydroxyurea, ddI has a competitive advantage of being incorporated into the forming HIV DNA. The use of hydroxyurea has generally fallen out of favor because of toxicities (hepatitis, pancreatitis) and a blunting of the CD4 response *(20,21)*. As a result, coadministration of hydroxyurea should be avoided.

A similar approach has been used with adding mycophenalate acid to abacavir, which may deplete intracellular deoxyguanosine triphosphate. The addition of mycophenalate acid to a failing regimen including abacavir increased carbovir triphosphate, the active moiety of abacavir, and led to a decrease in viral load in some subjects *(22)*. The long-term risk–benefit profile for this approach has not been established.

Other NRTI interactions occur at the site of absorption. The antacid buffer in ddI-buffered formulations may affect the absorption of indinavir and delavirdine, necessitating a separation from ddI by at least 30 minutes *(23)*. The Videx EC may be coadministered with other antiretrovirals. Administration of 200 mg ddI buffered tablets with 400 mg ATV resulted in a decrease in ATV exposure of almost 90% *(24)*. No interaction is expected with ATV and ddI EC, because ddI EC is given on an empty stomach and ATV is given with food; therefore, these agents are administered at different times.

## NONNUCLEOSIDE REVERSE TRANSCRIPTASE INHIBITORS

NNRTIs are an important drug class in the treatment of HIV infection, and agents such as efavirenz are preferred because of optimal and durable efficacy as a first-line regimen. The three available drugs in this class have very different effects on the CYP450 system and thus have differing interaction profiles (Tables 2 and 3). All three are metabolized primarily by the CYP3A4 isozyme, but the direction of drug interaction depends on whether the drug is an inducer, an inhibitor, or a mixed inducer/inhibitor. Delavirdine is a potent inhibitor of CYP3A4 and increases the AUC of saquinavir (SQV) and indinavir fivefold and 40%, respectively *(25,26)*. These studies suggest possible approaches to optimizing PI blood exposure. However, delavirdine is generally not used for this purpose because it involves a full dose for CYP3A4 inhibition, a large pill burden (six per day) and a high incidence of rash.

Delavirdine is associated with complex interactions involving adefovir and SQV *(27)*. Study ACTG (AIDS Clinical Trials Group) 359 was a six-arm study evaluating the pharmacokinetics of SQV/RTV or SQV/nelfinavir with delavirdine, adefovir, or both. Although the mechanism(s) remains unclear, the delavirdine AUC was significantly

# Table 2
## Drug–Drug Interactions: Nonnucleoside Reverse Transcriptase Inhibitors

| Drug name and dosages studied | Effect | | | Clinical comment |
|---|---|---|---|---|
| | $C_{max}$ | AUC | $C_{min}$ | |
| **Delavirdine (DLV) plus** | | | | |
| • Amprenavir (APV) | | | | |
|   • APV 600 mg bid | ↑40% | ↑130% | ↑39% | Coadministration not recommended |
|   • DLV 600 mg bid | ↓47% | ↓61% | ↓88% | |
| • Atazanavir (ATV) | | | | No data |
| • Fosamprenavir (FOS APV) | | | | Coadministration not recommended |
| • Indinavir (IDV) | | | | Reduce IDV to 600 mg tid when coadministered with DLV 400 mg tid |
|   • IDV 600 mg tid | ↔ | ↑53% | ↑298% | |
|   • DLV 400 mg tid) | ↔ | ↔ | ↔ | |
| • Lopinavir/Ritonavir (LPV/RTV) | LPV levels expected to increase | | | Insufficient data for dose recommendations |
| • Nelfinavir (NLV) | | | | Appropriate doses for this combination have not been established |
|   • NLV 750 mg tid | ↑88% | ↑107% | ↑136% | |
|   • DLV 400 mg tid | ↓27% | ↓31% | ↓33% | |
| • Ritonavir (RTV) | | ↑70% | | Limited data for this combination; appropriate doses for this combination have not been established |
| • Saquinavir (SQV) | | | | Appropriate doses of the combination with respect to safety and efficacy have not been established |
|   • SQV 1000 mg tid (given as Fortovase) | ↑98% | ↑121% | ↑199% | SQV effect on DLV is not well established |
|   • SQV 600 mg tid (given as Invirase) | | ↑5-fold | | Invirase/RTV or Fortovase/RTV interaction has not been evaluated |
|   • DLV 400 mg tid | | | | |
| **Efavirenz (EFV) plus** | | | | |
| • Amprevavir (APV) | | | | Administer APV 1200 mg bid + RTV 200 mg bid + EFV 600 mg qd |
|   • APV 1200 mg bid | ↓36% | ↓39% | ↓43% | |
|   • EFV 600 mg qd | ↔ | ↔ | ↔ | |

| Drug | | | | Recommendation |
|---|---|---|---|---|
| **Amprenavir (APV) + nelfinavir (NLV)** | | | | No dose adjustment needed |
| • APV 1200 mg bid | ↓14% | ↑46% | ↓14% | |
| • NLV 750 mg tid | ↕ | ↕ | ↕ | |
| • EFV 600 mg qd | ↕ | ↕ | ↕ | |
| **Amprenavir (APV) + ritonavir (RTV)** | | | | Administer APV 1200 mg bid + RTV 200 mg bid + EFV 600 mg qd |
| • APV 1200 mg bid | | ↑8% | ↑27% | |
| • RTV 200 mg bid | | ↑18% | ↕ | |
| • EFV 600 mg qd | | ↑21% | ↕ | |
| **Atazanavir (ATV)** | | | | ATV without RTV should not be coadministered with EFV |
| • ATV 400 mg qd | ↓59% | ↓74% | ↓93% | |
| • EFV 600 mg qd | | ↕ | ↕ | |
| **Atazanavir (ATV) + Ritonavir (RTV)** | | | | Administer ATV 300 mg qd + RTV 100 mg qd + EFV 600 mg qd with food |
| • ATV 300 mg qd | ↑14% | ↑39% | ↑48% | |
| • RTV 100 mg qd | | ↕ | ↕ | |
| • EFV 600 mg qd | | ↕ | ↕ | |
| **Fosamprenavir (FOS APV) + Ritonavir (RTV)** | | | | See recommendations below |
| • FOS APV 1400 mg qd | | ↓13% | ↓36% | |
| • RTV 200 mg qd | | ↕ | ↕ | |
| • EFV 600 mg qd | | ↕ | ↕ | |
| • FOS APV 1400 mg qd | ↑18% | ↑11% | ↑17% | Administer APV 1400 mg qd + RTV 300 mg qd + EFV 600 mg qd OR FOS APV 700 mg bid + RTV 100 mg bid + EFV 600 mg qd |
| • RTV 300 mg qd | | ↕ | ↕ | |
| • EFV 600 mg qd | | ↕ | ↕ | |
| • FOS APV 700 mg bid | | | ↕ | |
| • RTV 100 mg bid | | | ↕ | |
| • EFV 600 mg qd | | | ↕ | |
| **Lopinavir/ritonavir (LPV/RTV)** | | | | Increase LPV/RTV dose to 533/133 mg bid + EFV 600 mg qd |
| • LPV/RTV 400/100 mg bid | ↓3% | ↓19% | ↓39% | |
| • EFV 600 mg qd | ↓9% | ↓16% | ↓16% | |
| **Indinavir (IDV)** | | | | Increase IDV dose to 1000 mg q8 h + EFV 600 mg qd Or, consider administering SQV/RTV with EFV |
| • IDV 800 mg q8 hours | ↓16% | ↓31% | ↕ | |
| • EFV 200 mg qd | | ↕ | | |

*Continued on next page*

# Table 2 (*Continued*)
## Drug–Drug Interactions: Nonnucleoside Reverse Transcriptase Inhibitors

| Drug name and dosages studied | Effect | | | Clinical comment |
|---|---|---|---|---|
| | $C_{max}$ | AUC | $C_{min}$ | |
| **Efavirenz (EFV) plus (*Continued*)** | | | | |
| • Nelfinavir (NLV) | | | | No dose adjustment |
| ♦ NLV 750 mg q8 hours | ↑21% | ↑20% | | |
| ♦ M8 metabolite | ↓40% | ↓37% | | |
| ♦ EFV 600 mg qd | ↔ | ↔ | | |
| • Ritonavir (RTV) | | | | No dose adjustment |
| ♦ RTV 500 mg q12 hours | ↑14% | ↑21% | | |
| ♦ EFV 600 mg qd | ↑24% | ↑18% | | |
| • Saquinavir (SQV) | | | | SQV should not be used as sole protease inhibitor in combination with EFV. *SQV 1200 mg q8 hours given as Fortovase |
| ♦ SQV 1200 mg q8 hours* | ↓50% | ↓62% | | Consider administering SQV/RTV with EFV; however, appropriate doses of the combination of EFV and Invirase/RTV or Fortovase/RTV have not been established |
| ♦ EFV 600 mg qd | ↓13% | ↓12% | | |
| **Nevirapine (NVP) plus** | | | | |
| • Amprenavir (APV) | APV levels expected to decrease | | | No data |
| • Atazanavir (ATV) | ATV levels expected to decrease | | | No data |
| • Fosamprenavir (FOS APV) | ATV levels expected to decrease | | | No data |
| • Indinavir (IDV) | | | | Consider increasing IDV to 1000 mg q8 hours or administer IDV + RTV + NVP 200 mg bid |
| ♦ IDV 800 mg q8 hours | ↓11% | ↓28% | | |
| ♦ NVP 200 mg bid | ↔ | ↔ | | |
| • Lopinavir/ritonavir (LPV/RTV) | | | | Increase LPV/RTV dose to 533/133 mg bid + NVP 200 mg bid |
| ♦ LPV/RTV 400/100 mg bid | ↓19% | ↓27% | ↓51% | |
| ♦ NVP 200 mg bid | ↔ | ↔ | ↔ | |

*108*

| Drug | Effect | Comment |
|---|---|---|
| • Nelfinavir (NLV)<br>   ♦ NLV 750 mg tid<br>   ♦ NVP 200 mg bid | No significant changes in NLV or NVP concentrations | No dose adjustment needed |
| • Ritonavir (RTV)<br>   ♦ RTV 600 mg bid<br>   ♦ NVP 200 mg bid | No significant changes in RTV or NVP concentrations | No dose adjustment needed |
| • Saquinavir (SQV)<br>   ♦ SQV 600 mg tid*<br>   ♦ NVP 200 mg bid | ↓28%  ↓24% | SQV should not be used as sole protease inhibitor in combination with NVP. *SQV 600 mg tid given as Fortovase Consider administering SQV/RTV with NVP; however, appropriate doses of the combination of NVP and Invirase/RTV or Fortovase/RTV have not been established |

*Source:* From refs. *13,23,24,35,39,49,51,75–79,86.*

**Table 3**
**Drug Interactions Between NNRTIs and Other Drugs**

| | Delavirdine | Efavirenz | Nevirapine |
|---|---|---|---|
| **Antifungals** | | | |
| • Ketoconazole | No data | No data | Do not coadminister<br>Ketoconazole $C_{max}$ ↓ 63% and AUC ↓ 40%<br>NVP ↑ 15–30% possible |
| **Antimycobacterials** | | | |
| • Clarithromycin | Clarithromycin ↑ 100%<br>Dose adjust clarithromycin for patients with renal failure | Clarithromycin ↓ 39%<br>Clinical significance of these changes is unknown<br>No dose adjustment of EFV is recommended | NVP ↑ 26%<br>Clarithromycin ↓ 30%<br>Clinical significance of these changes is unknown |
| • Rifampin | DLV ↓ 97%<br>Do not coadminister | EFV ↓ 25%<br>Consider ↑ EFV dose to 800 mg qd | NVP ↓ 20–58%<br>Use of this combination is not recommended |
| • Rifabutin | DLV ↓ 82%<br>Rifabutin ↑ 100%<br>Do not coadminister | EFV ↔<br>Rifabutin ↓ 35%<br>↑ Rifabutin dose to 450–600 mg qd or 600 mg three times/week | NVP ↓ 16%<br>No dose adjustment required |
| **Anticonvulsants** | | | |
| • Carbamazepine/ phenobarbitol/ phenytoin | No data<br>Use with caution<br>Monitor anticonvulsant levels | No data<br>Use with caution<br>Monitor anticonvulsant levels | No data<br>Use with caution<br>Monitor anticonvulsant levels |
| **Lipid-lowering agents** | | | |
| • Atorvastatin | Use lowest possible starting dose of atorvastatin with careful monitoring | Atorvastatin ↓ 43%<br>EFV ↔<br>May affect the overall antilipid response during therapy, but any dose escalation requires increased monitoring for toxicity and efficacy | No data |

Lipid-lowering agents (Continued)

| | | | |
|---|---|---|---|
| • Lovastatin, simvastatin | Do not coadminister with either lovastatin or simvastatin; risk of rhabdomyolysis, including rhabdomyolysis, may be increased when used in combination | Simvastatin ↓ 43% EFV ↔ May affect the overall antilipid response during therapy, but any dose escalation requires increased monitoring for toxicity and efficacy | No data |
| • Pravastatin | No data | No data | No data |
| Methadone | No data ↑Methadone expected | Methadone ↓ significantly Monitor for withdrawal and consider ↑ methadone dose if needed | NVP ↔ Monitor for withdrawal and consider ↑ methadone dose if needed |
| Oral contraceptives | No data | Ethinyl estradiol ↑ 37% Use alternative or additional methods | Ethinyl estradiol ↓ 20% Use alternative or additional methods |
| Sildenafil | ↑ Sildenafil expected Do not exceed a maximum single dose of 25 mg sildenafil in a 48-hour period | No data | No data |
| Tadalafil | No data but ↑ tadalafil expected Do not exceed a maximum single dose of 10 mg tadalafil once every 72 hours | No data | No data |
| Vardenafil | No data but ↑ vardenafil expected Start with 2.5-mg dose of vardenafil and do not exceed a single 2.5-mg dose in 24 hours | No data | No data |

*Source*: From refs. *13, 39, 75, 76, 85,* and *88.*

111

decreased in the presence of adefovir. These data is difficult to interpret owing to the small sample sizes and the complexity of the multidrug regimens. However, it demonstrated that "real-world" clinical situations may exhibit unpredictable drug interactions. Interestingly, adefovir was not shown to interact with SQV, indinavir, efavirenz, delavirdine, or lamivudine in controlled, single-dose, normal volunteer studies *(28)*.

Nevirapine and efavirenz are inducers of CYP3A4 and can decrease the exposure of certain PIs. Concomitant administration with indinavir, amprenavir, or SQV results in a decrease in the PI AUC of approx 30% *(29–32)*. The most common management strategy is to add low-dose RTV to this regimen, which increases the PI concentration and negates or reduces the induction effect of nevirapine or efavirenz *(33,34)* (*see* Table 2). Kaletra, a combination of the PIs lopinavir (LPV) and RTV, demonstrated a modest decrease in plasma LPV concentration with efavirenz and nevirapine, and dosage increases to 533 mg LPV and 133 mg RTV are recommended for all patients *(35)*.

Nelfinavir and RTV are not significantly affected by nevirapine, suggesting CYP3A4 is not the only available pathway of metabolism for these agents *(36)*. Efavirenz is a mixed inducer/inhibitor and can inhibit CYP3A4, depending on the specific concomitant drug. Efavirenz will modestly (approx 20%) raise the AUC of RTV and nelfinavir, although dosage adjustments are not required *(37,38)*. The mechanism for the increases is unclear but may involve inhibition of CYP2C9 or CYP2C19 pathways *(28,29)*. Efavirenz also increases plasma ethinyl estradiol concentrations, possibly by inhibiting its metabolism and clearance *(39)*.

The enzyme-inducing effects of both nevirapine and efavirenz may be problematic for patients receiving methadone maintenance therapy. A case series showed that methadone concentrations were markedly reduced in the presence of nevirapine, precipitating symptoms of withdrawal *(40)*. Nevirapine and efavirenz should be used with caution in patients on methadone, and dosage increases should be anticipated to control symptoms.

The combination of two NNRTIs is relatively uncommon. However, data are available suggesting that nevirapine concentrations are unaltered in the presence of efavirenz; the efavirenz AUC is reduced by 22% in the presence of nevirapine. The decrease in efavirenz exposure is most likely not clinically significant *(41)*.

## PROTEASE INHIBITORS

The advent of the PIs signaled a new era in HIV therapy, demonstrating never-before-seen decreases in viral load and improved clinical outcomes. Their large potential for drug interactions has been a double-edged sword. They require careful monitoring, education, and continuous review of concomitant medications. However, the use of RTV as pharmacokinetic enhancer to increase plasma concentrations of other antiretrovirals has redefined the usage of PIs. RTV-"boosted" PIs are now considered by many a first-line therapy.

All PIs approved by the US Food and Drug Administration are metabolized primarily by CYP3A4 and have inhibitory effects on this metabolic pathway *(42)*. Clinically significant interactions with PIs are shown in Tables 4 and 5.

Because of their effects on CYP3A4, a number of drugs are contraindicated with PIs because of the potential for serious or life-threatening toxicity (Table 6). The combination with pimozide and cisapride should be avoided because of the potential for cardiac arrhythmia *(43)*. Similarly, some antiarrhythmics and PI combinations should be avoided (*see* Table 6). The use of PIs with ergot derivatives can lead to serious peripheral ischemia because of the potent vasoconstricting effects of this class. A case report described the use of rifampin to treat PI-induced ergotamine toxicity *(44)*. The rifampin was employed to increase the elimination of the PI via enzyme induction and thus decrease the effects of ergotamine. As most PIs cause increases in triglyceride and cholesterol, many HIV-infected individuals require lipid-lowering agents. Simvastatin and lovastatin are contraindicated because of the risk of myopathy, including rhabdomyolysis. Pravastatin can be used because it is not metabolized primarily by CYP3A4. Atorvastatin is also an option if low doses are used and patients are closely monitored. Oversedation is a potential complication when PIs are administered with certain benzodiazepines (midazolam, triazolam). However, many clinicians will give one to two doses of midazolam prior to a surgical procedure as long as the patient is closely monitored.

Other contraindications are caused by the effect of the concomitant drug on plasma PI concentrations. Rifampin and products containing St. John's wort markedly reduce PI exposure and must be avoided *(45,46)*. Although not contraindicated, many antiepilepsy drugs (phenytoin, phenobarbital, carbamazepine) could also reduce PI concentrations and require close monitoring.

The availability of three agents for erectile dysfunction has led to new drug interaction recommendations. Sildenafil, vardenafil, and tadalafil are used in patients to improve or enhance sexual performance. When combined with SQV or indinavir, a three- to fourfold increase in the sildenafil AUC *(47,48)* is seen. Concomitant use with RTV results in an 11-fold increase, with concentrations 24 hours after dosing still markedly elevated *(47)*. Vardenavil AUC is increased 16-fold and 49-fold with indinavir and fosamprenavir, respectively *(23,49)*. Similar increases for tadalafil are expected. Because of the potential for an increase in adverse effects, patients should start with a low dose and not exceed a maximum single dose over a 48- to 72-hour period, depending on the specific agent (*see* Table 5).

The same precautions and contraindications also apply to delavirdine, as delavirdine is also a potent CYP3A4 inhibitor.

The AUC of the oral contraceptives ethinyl estradiol and progesterones are decreased approx 40% by nelfinavir, RTV and LPV/RTV *(50,51)*. Conversely, ATV, fosamprenavir, and indinavir increase the concentrations of these hormones. In general, clinicians should counsel patients that alternative or additional forms of birth control are recommended when PIs are used. Amprenavir concentrations are markedly decreased in the presence of ethinyl estradiol/norethindrone. Therefore, this may lead to a loss of virological response and possible resistance to amprenavir. Alternative methods of nonhormonal contraception are recommended when amprenavir is used.

RTV is primarily used as a CYP3A4 inhibitor to increase concentrations of other PIs. All PIs, with the exception of nelfinavir and ATV, are concomitantly used with RTV to reduce the pill burden, extend frequency of dosing, and simplify the regimen. Nelfinavir concentrations are increased with RTV coadministration, but this combination is not well tolerated *(52)*. For ATV, the dosing frequency (daily) and pill burden (two capsules) remain the same with or without RTV.

**Table 4**
**Drug–Drug Interactions: Alteration in Dose or Regimen Recommended for Protease Inhibitors**

| Drug name and dosages studied | Effect | | | Clinical comment |
|---|---|---|---|---|
| | $C_{max}$ | AUC | $C_{min}$ | |
| **Amprevanir (APV) plus** | | | | |
| • Atazanavir (ATV) | | | | No data |
| • Indinavir (IDV) | | | | IDV levels based on historical data |
| ♦ IDV 800 mg tid (fasted) | ↓ 22% | ↓ 38% | ↓ 27% | |
| ♦ APV 750 or 800 mg tid (fasted) | ↑ 18% | ↑ 33% | ↑ 25% | Appropriate doses for this combination have not been established |
| • Lopinavir/ritonavir (LPV/RTV) | | | | APV concentrations in combination with LPV/RTV are compared to APV 1200 mg bid alone |
| ♦ APV 750 mg bid | ↓ 12% | ↑ 1.7-fold | ↑ 4.5-fold | |
| ♦ LPV/RTV 400/100 mg bid | ↓ 28% | ↓ 38% | ↓ 57% | Increase Kaletra dose to 533/133 mg and decrease amprenavir dose to 750 mg bid when coadministered |
| • Nelfinavir (NLV) | | | | NLV levels based on historical data |
| ♦ NLV 750 mg tid (fed) | ↑ 12% | ↑ 15% | ↑ 14% | |
| ♦ APV 750 or 800 mg tid (fed) | ↓ 14% | ↔ | ↑ 189 | Appropriate doses for this combination have not been established |
| • Ritonavir (RTV) | | | | Dose: APV 600 + RTV 100 mg bid or APV 1200 mg qd + RTV 200 mg qd |
| ♦ RTV 100 mg bid | ↔ | ↔ | ↔ | |
| ♦ APV 600 mg bid | ↓ 30% | ↑ 64% | ↑ 508% | |
| ♦ RTV 200 mg bid | ↔ | ↔ | ↔ | |
| ♦ APV 1200 mg qd | ↔ | ↑ 62% | ↑ 319% | |
| • Saquinavir (SQV) | | | | SQV levels based on historical data |
| ♦ SQV 800 mg tid (fed) | ↓ 21% | ↓ 19% | ↓ 48% | |
| ♦ APV 750 or 800 mg tid (fed) | ↓ 37% | ↓ 32% | ↓ 14% | Appropriate doses for this combination have not been established |
| **Atazanavir (ATV) plus** | | | | |
| • Fosamprenavir (FOS APV) | | | | No data |
| • Indinavir (IDV) | | | | Coadministration is not recommended because of potential for additive hyperbilirubinemia |
| • Lopinavir/ritonavir (LPV/RTV) | | | | No data |
| • Nelfinavir (NLV) | | | | No data |

| | | | | |
|---|---|---|---|---|
| • Ritonavir (RTV) | | | | |
| ◆ RTV 100 mg qd | | | | |
| ◆ ATV 300 mg qd | ↑18% | ↑103% | ↑671% | ATV concentrations in combination with RTV are compared to ATV 400 qd alone (historical data) |
| • Saquinavir (SQV) | | | | |
| ◆ SQV 1200 mg qd | ↑79% | ↔ | | SQV concentrations in combination with ATV are compared to SQV 1200 mg tid alone |
| ◆ ATV 400 mg qd | ↑4.4-fold | ↑5.5-fold | ↑6.7-fold | No formal recommendation; ATV/SQV resulted in inadequate efficacy compared to ATV/RTV and LPV/RTV in experienced subjects |
| **Fosamprenavir (FOS APV) plus** | | | | |
| • Indinavir (IDV) | | | | IDV was studied with APV; however, appropriate doses for APV or FOS APV + IDV have not been established |
| • Lopinavir/ritonavir (LPV/RTV) | | | | In a three-arm, randomized, crossover study involving healthy volunteers, APV pharmacokinetics were compared after administration of FOS APV 1400 mg bid + LPV/RTV 533 mg/133 mg bid for 2 weeks vs FOS APV 700 mg bid + RTV 100 mg bid for 2 weeks; ↓APV with the regimen containing LPV/RTV: $C_{max}$ ↓ 13%, AUC ↓ 26%, $C_{min}$ ↓ 42%; In the same study, LPV PK were compared after administration of FOS APV 1400 mg bid + LPV/RTV 533 mg/133 mg bid for 2 weeks vs LPV/RTV 400 mg/100 mg bid for 2 weeks, and LPV concentrations were similar (less than 10% change in $C_{max}$, AUC, and $C_{min}$ values) with these 2 regimens |
| ◆ LPV/RTV 400/100 mg bid | ↑30% | ↑37% | ↑52% | |
| ◆ FOS APV 700 mg bid + RTV 100 mg bid | ↓58% | ↓63% | ↓65% | Appropriate doses for have not been established |
| | | | | An increased rate of adverse events has been observed with coadministration of these medications |
| • Nelfinavir (NLV) | | | | NLV was studied with APV; however, appropriate doses for APV or FOS APV + NLV have not been established |
| • Ritonavir (RTV) | | | | FOS APV concentrations in combination with RTV are compared to FOS APV 1400 mg bid alone |
| ◆ FOS APV 1400 mg + RTV 200 mg qd | ↑66% | ↑48% | ↑24% | Treatment-naïve patients: FOS APV 1400 mg qd + RTV 200 mg qd or FOS APV 700 mg bid + RTV 100 mg bid |
| ◆ FOS APV 700 mg + RTV 100 mg bid | ↑79% | ↑42% | ↑16% | PI-experienced patients: 700 mg bid + RTV 100 mg bid |
| | | | | FOS APV + RTV qd is not recommended in PI-experienced patients |

Continued on next page

**Table 4 (*Continued*)**
**Drug–Drug Interactions: Alteration in Dose or Regimen Recommended for Protease Inhibitors**

| Drug name and dosages studied | Effect | | | Clinical comment |
|---|---|---|---|---|
| | $C_{max}$ | AUC | $C_{min}$ | |
| Fosamprenavir (FOS APV) plus (*Continued*) | | | | |
| • Saquinavir (SQV) | | | | SQV was studied with APV; however, appropriate doses for APV or FOS APV + SQV have not been established |
| Indinavir (IDV) plus | | | | |
| • Lopinavir/ritonavir (LPV/RTV) | | | | IDV concentrations in combination with LPV/RTV are compared to IDV 800 mg tid |
| ◆ LPV/RTV 400/100 mg bid | ↕ | ↕ | | |
| ◆ IDV 600 mg bid | ↓ 29% | ↕ | ↑ 3.5-fold | Decrease IDV dose to 600 mg BID + LPV/RTV 400/100 mg bid |
| • Nelfinavir (NLV) | | | | Appropriate doses for combination are not established |
| ◆ NLV 750 mg tid | ↑ 83% | ↑ 31% | NA | Limited data for IDV 1200 mg bid + NLV 1250 mg bid with low-fat snack and on empty stomach |
| ◆ IDV 800 mg single dose | ↑ 51% | ↓ 10% | NA | |
| • Ritonavir (RTV) | | | | Appropriate doses for combination not established Limited data on the following regimens: <br>• IDV 400 mg bid + RTV 400 mg bid; similar IDV concentrations compared to IDV 800 mg q8 hour but higher $C_{min}$ <br>• IDV/RTV 600/100 mg bid or 800/100 mg bid or 800/200 mg bid Caution: renal events may be increased with higher IDV concentrations |
| • Saquinavir (SQV) | | | | |
| ◆ SQV 800 mg single dose (Fortovase) | ↑ 551% | ↑ 620% | NA | Appropriate doses of the combination have not been established Invirase/RTV, Fortovase/RTV interaction has not been evaluated |
| ◆ SQV 1200 mg single dose (Fortovase) | ↑ 299% | ↑ 364% | NA | SQV effect on IDV is not well established |
| ◆ SQV 600 or 1200 mg single dose (Invirase) | NA | ↑ 5-fold | NA | |
| ◆ IDV 800 mg q8 hour | ↕ | ↕ | ↕ | |

| Drug | | | | Comments |
|---|---|---|---|---|
| **Lopinavir/ritonavir (LPV/RTV) plus** | | | | |
| • Nelfinavir (NLV) | | | | Increase LPV/RTV dose to 533/133 mg and decrease NLV dose to 1000 mg BID when coadministered |
| ◦ NLV 1000 mg bid | ↔ | ↔ | ↑ 86% | |
| ◦ LPV/RTV 400/100 mg bid | ↓ 21% | ↓ 27% | ↓ 38% | |
| • Ritonavir (RTV) | | | | Appropriate doses of additional RTV have not been established |
| • Saquinavir (SQV) | | | | SQV concentrations in combination with LPV/RTV are compared to SQV 1200 mg tid alone |
| ◦ SQV 800 mg bid | ↑ 6.3-fold | ↑ 9.6-fold | ↑ 16.7-fold | Decrease SQV dose to 800 mg bid when coadministered with LPV/RTV 400/100 mg bid |
| ◦ LPV/RTV 400/100 mg bid | ↔ | ↔ | ↔ | |
| **Nelfinavir (NLV) plus** | | | | |
| • Ritonavir (RTV) | | | | Appropriate doses for combination are not established |
| ◦ RTV 500 mg single dose | ↔ | ↔ | NA | Consider RTV 400 mg bid + NLV 500–750 mg bid |
| ◦ NLV 750 mg tid | ↑ 152% | ↑ 44% | NA | |
| • Saquinavir (SQV) | | | | SQV 1200 mg bid + NLV 1250 mg bid results in adequate plasma drug concentrations for both protease inhibitors |
| ◦ SQV 1200 mg tid (Fortovase) | ↑ 179% | ↑ 392% | NA | Invirase/RTV and Fortovase/RTV interaction has not been evaluated |
| ◦ NLV 750 mg single dose | ↔ | ↑ 18% | NA | |
| **Ritonavir (RTV) plus** | | | | |
| • Saquinavir (SQV) | | | | SQV concentrations in combination with RTV 100 mg bid are compared to SQV 1200 mg tid alone |
| ◦ Saquinavir 1000 mg bid (Fortovase) + RTV 100 mg bid | ↑ 153% | ↑ 176% | | SQV 1000 mg bid + RTV 100 mg bid or SQV 400 mg bid + RTV 400 mg bid |
| ◦ SQV 400 mg bid (Fortovase) | ↑ 64% | ↑ 121% | | |
| ◦ RTV 400 mg bid | ↔ | | | |

*Source: From refs. 13, 23, 24, 35, 49, 51, 77–79, 85.*
NA, not available.

## Table 5
### Drug Interactions Between Protease Inhibitors and Other Drugs[a]

| Drug affected | Amprenavir (APV) | Atazanavir (ATV) | Fosamprenavir (FOS APV) | Indinavir (IDV) |
|---|---|---|---|---|
| **Antifungals** | | | | |
| • Ketoconazole (keto) | APV ↓ 31% Keto ↑ 44% No dose adjustment | ATV and keto ↔ No dose adjustment | ↑ Keto and FOS APV expected Decrease keto (and itraconazole) for patients receiving more than 400 mg keto (or itraconazole) per day FOS APV/RTV - keto or itraconazole doses >200 mg/day are not recommended | IDV ↓ 66% Decrease IDV dose to 600 mg tid |
| **Antimycobacterials** | | | | |
| • Rifampin | Do not coadminister APV ↓ 82% | Do not coadminister ↓ ATV expected | Do not coadminister APV ↓ 82% | Do not coadminister IDV ↓ 89% |
| • Rifabutin | APV ↓ 15% Rifabutin ↑ 193% Decrease rifabutin dose to 150 mg qod or 3 times per week | Rifabutin ↑ 2.1-fold Decrease rifabutin dose to 150 mg qod or 3 times per week | APV ↓ 15% Rifabutin ↑ 193% Decrease rifabutin dose to 150 mg qod or 3 times per week | IDV ↓ 32% Rifabutin ↑ 2× Decrease rifabutin dose to 150 mg qod or 3 times per week Increase IDV dose to 1000 mg tid |
| • Clarithromycin (clari) | APV ↑ 18% No dose adjustment | ATV ↑ 28% ↓ Clari active metabolite Clari ↑ 94% Increase in clari levels may cause QTc prolongation Decrease clari dose by 50% or consider alternative treatment | APV ↑ 18% No dose adjustment | Clari ↑ 53% No dose adjustment |

| | | | | |
|---|---|---|---|---|
| **Anticonvulsants** | | | | |
| • Carbamazepine | Monitor anticonvulsant levels ↓ APV possible | Monitor anticonvulsant levels ↓ ATV possible | Monitor anticonvulsant levels ↓ APV possible | Monitor anticonvulsant levels ↓ APV possible | Carbamazepine markedly decreases IDV levels; consider alternative treatment |
| • Phenobarbitol | | | | |
| • Phenytoin | | | | |
| **Erectile dysfunction agents** | | | | |
| • Sildenafil | Sildenafil ↑ 2- to 11-fold Do not exceed 25 mg in a 4-hour period; monitor for sildenafil adverse effects | ↑ Sildenafil expected Do not exceed 25 mg in a 48-hour period; monitor for sildenafil adverse effects | ↑ Sildenafil expected Do not exceed 25 mg in a 48-hour period; monitor for sildenafil adverse effects | ↑ Sildenafil Do not exceed 25 mg in a 48-hour period; monitor for sildenafil adverse effects | Sildenafil ↑ threefold Do not exceed 25 mg in a 48-hour period; monitor for sildenafil adverse effects |
| • Tadalafil | No data, but ↑ tadalafil expected; do not exceed a maximum single dose of 10 mg tadalafil once every 72 hours | No data, but ↑ tadalafil expected; do not exceed a maximum single dose of 10 mg tadalafil once every 72 hours | No data, but ↑ tadalafil expected; do not exceed a maximum single dose of 10 mg tadalafil once every 72 hours | No data, but ↑ tadalafil expected; do not exceed a maximum single dose of 10 mg tadalafil once every 72 hours | No data, but ↑ tadalafil expected; do not exceed a maximum single dose of 10 mg tadalafil once every 72 hours |
| • Vardenafil | ↑ Vardenafil expected Do not exceed 2.5 mg in a 24-hour period; do not exceed 2.5 mg in a 72-hour period if administered with RTV | ↑ Vardenafil expected Do not exceed 2.5 mg in a 24-hour period; do not exceed 2.5 mg in a 72-hour period if administered with RTV | ↑ Vardenafil expected Do not exceed 2.5 mg in a 24-hour period; do not exceed 2.5 mg in a 72-hour period if administered with RTV | ↑ Vardenafil expected Do not exceed 2.5 mg in a 24-hour period; do not exceed 2.5 mg in a 72-hour period if administered with RTV | Vardenafil ↑ 16-fold Do not exceed 2.5 mg in a 24-hour period; do not exceed 2.5 mg in a 72-hour period if administered with RTV |
| **Lipid-lowering agents** | | | | |
| • Atorvastatin | ↑ Atorvastatin expected Use lowest possible starting dose of atorvastatin with careful monitoring | ↑ Atorvastatin expected Use lowest possible starting dose of atorvastatin with careful monitoring | ↑ Atorvastatin expected Use lowest possible starting dose of atorvastatin with careful monitoring | ↑ Atorvastatin 130–153% Use ≤ 20 mg/day with careful monitoring or consider alternative treatment | ↑ Atorvastatin expected Use lowest possible starting dose of atorvastatin with careful monitoring |
| • Pravastatin | No data Significant interaction not expected | No data Significant interaction not expected | No data Significant interaction not expected | No data Significant interaction not expected | No data Significant interaction not expected |
| • Simvastatin, lovastatin | Do not coadminister Large ↑ statin levels expected Potential for serious reactions, such as myopathy, including rhabdomyolysis | Do not coadminister Large ↑ statin levels expected Potential for serious reactions, such as myopathy, including rhabdomyolysis | Do not coadminister Large ↑ statin levels expected Potential for serious reactions, such as myopathy, including rhabdomyolysis | Do not coadminister Large ↑ statin levels expected Potential for serious reactions, such as myopathy, including rhabdomyolysis | Do not coadminister Large ↑ statin levels expected Potential for serious reactions, such as myopathy, including rhabdomyolysis |

*Continued on next page*

**Table 5 (*Continued*)**
**Drug Interactions Between Protease Inhibitors and Other Drugs[a]**

| Drug affected | Amprenavir (APV) | Atazanavir (ATV) | Fosamprenavir (FOS APV) | Indinavir (IDV) |
|---|---|---|---|---|
| Methadone | ↓ Methadone 13–40% ↓ APV APV may be less effective because of ↓ APV levels when given with methadone; alternative antiretroviral therapy should be considered | No data | ↓ Methadone expected Dosage of methadone may need to be increased | No change in methadone levels |
| Oral contraceptives (OC) | ↓ APV May lead to loss of virological response and possible resistance to APV; alternative methods of nonhormonal contraception are recommended | Ethinyl estradiol ↑ 48%, norethindrone ↑ 110% Use lowest effect dose of OC or alternative methods | ↑ Ethinyl estradiol Alternative methods of non-hormonal contraception are recommended FOS APV/RTV + OC not studied | No dose adjustment Norethindrone ↑ 26% Ethinylestradiol ↑ 24% |
| Other | | Antacids and buffered agents: • May ↓ ATV levels • Give ATV 2 hour before or 1 hour after these medications Calcium channel blockers • Use with caution • Dose titration of calcium channel blockers and electrocardiogram monitoring are recommended Diltiazem • ↑125% • Reduce Diltiazem by 50% with electrocardiogram monitoring H₂ receptor antagonists • May ↓ ATV levels • Separate dosing by 12 hours | H$_2$ receptor antagonists and proton pump inhibitors • Use with caution • May ↓ FOS APV levels | |

| Drug affected | Lopinavir/ritonavir (LPV/RTV) | Nelfinavir (NLV) | Ritonavir (RTV) | Saquinavir (SQV) |
|---|---|---|---|---|
| **Antifungals** | | | | |
| • Ketoconazole | LPV ↓ 13%<br>Keto ↑ 3×<br>Use with caution; do not exceed 200 mg keto daily | No dose adjustment | Keto ↑ 3×<br>Use with caution; do not exceed 200 mg keto daily | SQV ↑ 3×<br>If keto > 200 mg/day, monitor for excessive diarrhea, nausea, abdominal discomfort; SQV doses may need to be adjusted |
| **Antimycobacterials** | | | | |
| • Rifampin | Do not coadminister<br>LPV ↓ | Do not coadminister<br>NLV ↓ 82% | RTV ↓ 35%<br>No dose adjustment if given with RTV 600 mg bid; increased liver toxicity possible | Do not coadminister<br>SQV ↓ 84% |
| • Rifabutin | Rifabutin ↑ 3×<br>Decrease rifabuin dose to 150 mg qod or 3 times per week | Rifabutin ↑ 2×<br>NLV ↓ 32%<br>Decrease rifabuin dose to 150 mg qod or 3 times per week<br>Increase NLV to 1000 mg tid | Rifabutin ↑ 4×<br>Decrease rifabutin dose to 150 mg qod or 3 times per week | SQV ↓ 40%<br>No rifabutin dose adjustment unless using SQV/RTV, then decrease rifabutin dose to 150 mg qod or 3 times per week |
| • Clarithromycin | Clari ↑ 77%<br>Adjust clari dose for moderate and severe renal impairment | No data | Clari ↑ 77%<br>Adjust clari dose for moderate and severe renal impairment | Clari and SQV ↑<br>No dose adjustment for clari 500 mg bid + Fortovase 1200 mg tid for 7 days<br>Adjust clari for renal impairment |

*Continued on next page*

**Table 5 (Continued)**
**Drug Interactions Between Protease Inhibitors and Other Drugs[a]**

| Drug affected | Lopinavir/ritonavir (LPV/RTV) | Nelfinavir (NLV) | Ritonavir (RTV) | Saquinavir (SQV) |
|---|---|---|---|---|
| **Anticonvulsants** | | | | |
| • Carbamazepine<br>• Phenobarbitol<br>• Phenytoin | ↑Carbamazepine when given with RTV; use with caution and monitor anticonvulsant levels<br><br>Phenytoin ↓ LPV/RTV levels and ↓ phenytoin levels when given together<br>Avoid concomitant use | Monitor anticonvulsant levels<br>↓ NLV expected | Monitor anticonvulsant levels<br>↓ RTV possible<br>↑ Carbamazepine | Monitor anticonvulsant levels<br>↓ SQV expected |
| **Erectile dysfunction agents** | | | | |
| • Sildenafil | Sildenafil ↑ 11-fold<br>Do not exceed 25 mg in a 48-hour period; monitor for sildenafil adverse effects | Sildenafil ↑ 2- to 11-fold<br>Use 25 mg starting dose of sildenafil<br>Monitor for sildenafil adverse effects | Sildenafil ↑ 11-fold<br>Do not exceed 25 mg in a 48-hour period<br>Monitor for sildenafil adverse effects | Sildenafil ↑ twofold<br>Use 25 mg starting dose of sildenafil<br>Monitor for sildenafil adverse effects |
| • Tadalafil | No data but ↑ tadalafil expected; do not exceed a maximum single dose of tadalafil 10 mg once every 72 hours | No data but ↑ tadalafil expected; do not exceed a maximum single dose of tadalafil 10 mg once every 72 hours | No data but ↑ tadalafil expected; do not exceed a maximum single dose of tadalafil 10 mg once every 72 hours | No data but ↑ tadalafil expected; do not exceed a maximum single dose of tadalafil 10 mg once every 72 hours |
| • Vardenafil | ↑ Vardenafil expected<br>Do not exceed 2.5 mg in a 72-hour period if administered with RTV | ↑ Vardenafil expected<br>Do not exceed 2.5 mg in a 24-hour period; do not exceed 2.5 mg in a 72-hour period if administered with RTV | Vardenafil ↑ 49-fold<br>Do not exceed 2.5 mg in a 24-hour period; do not exceed 2.5 mg in a 72-hour period if administered with RTV | ↑ Vardenafil expected<br>Do not exceed 2.5 mg in a 24-hour period; do not exceed 2.5 mg in a 72-hour period if administered with RTV |

Lipid-lowering agents

| | | | | |
|---|---|---|---|---|
| • Atorvastatin | Atorvastatin ↑ 5.88-fold Use lowest possible starting dose of atorvastatin with careful monitoring | Atorvastatin ↑ 74% Use lowest possible starting dose of atorvastatin with careful monitoring | Atorvastatin ↑ 450% when given with RTV/SQV Use lowest possible starting dose of atorvastatin with careful monitoring | Atorvastatin ↑ 450% when given with RTV/SQV Use lowest possible starting dose of atorvastatin with careful monitoring |
| • Pravastatin | No data Significant interaction not expected | No data Significant interaction not expected | Pravastatin ↓ 50% when given with RTV/SQV No dose adjustment | Pravastatin ↓ 50% when given with RTV/SQV No dose adjustment |
| • Simvastatin, lovastatin | Do not coadminister Large ↑ statin levels expected Potential for serious reactions, such as myopathy, including rhabdomyolysis | Do not coadminister Large ↑ statin levels expected Potential for serious reactions, such as myopathy, including rhabdomyolysis | Do not coadminister Large ↑ statin levels expected Potential for serious reactions, such as myopathy, including rhabdomyolysis | Do not coadminister Large ↑ statin levels expected Potential for serious reactions, such as myopathy, including rhabdomyolysis |
| Methadone | Methadone ↓ 53% Monitor for withdrawal and consider ↑ methadone dose if needed | NLV may ↓ methadone levels Monitor for withdrawal and consider ↑ methadone dose if needed | Methadone ↓ 37% Monitor for withdrawal and consider ↑ methadone dose if needed | No data |
| Oral contraceptives | Ethinyl estradiol ↓ 42% Use alternative or additional methods | Norethindrone ↓ 18% Ethinyl estradiol ↓ 47% Use alternative or additional methods | Ethinyl estradiol ↓ 40% Use alternative or additional methods | No data |
| Other | | | Many possible interactions Desipramine ↑ 145%; reduce dose of desipramine Theophylline ↓ 47%; monitor theophylline levels | |

*Source:* From refs. *13, 23, 24, 35, 49, 51, 77–79, 85.*
[a]Increases or decreases in concentrations refer to AUC unless otherwise stated.

**Table 6**
**Drugs Contraindicated or Not Recommended for Use With Protease Inhibitors and NNRTIs**

| Drug class/drug name | Drugs that should not be coadministered | Clinical comment |
|---|---|---|
| Antiarrhythmics: amiodarone, quinidine | Ritonavir | *Contraindicated* because of potential for serious and/or life-threatening reactions such as cardiac arrhythmias secondary to increases in plasma concentrations of antiarrhythmics |
| Antiarrhythmics: flecainide, propafenone | Fosamprenavir + ritonavir; ritonavir | *Contraindicated* because of potential for serious and/or life-threatening reactions such as cardiac arrhythmias secondary to increases in plasma concentrations of antiarrhythmics |
| Antimycobacterials: rifampin | Amprenavir, atazanavir, fosamprenavir, indinavir, lopinavir/ritonavir, nelfinavir, saquinavir Delavirdine, efavirenz, nevirapine | May lead to loss of virological response and possible resistance to each agent or to the class |
| Anticancer: irinotecan | Atazanavir | ATV inhibits UGT and may interfere with the metabolism of irinotecan, resulting in increased irinotecan toxicities |
| Ergot derivatives: dihydroergotamine, ergonovine, ergotamine, methylergonovine | Amprenavir, atazanavir, fosamprenavir, indinavir, lopinavir/ritonavir, nelfinavir, saquinavir Delavirdine, efavirenz | *Contraindicated* because of potential for serious and/or life-threatening events such as acute ergot toxicity characterized by peripheral vasospasm and ischemia of the extremities and other tissues |
| Garlic capsules | Saquinavir | Garlic capsules should not be used while taking saquinavir (Fortovase) as the sole protease inhibitor because of the risk of decreased saquinavir plasma concentrations<br>No data are available for the coadministration of Invirase/ritonavir or Fortovase/ritonavir and garlic capsules |
| Gastrointestinal: cisapride | Amprenavir, atazanavir, fosamprenavir, indinavir, lopinavir/ritonavir, nelfinavir, saquinavir Delavirdine | *Contraindicated* because of potential for serious and/or life-threatening reactions such as cardiac arrhythmias |

| | | |
|---|---|---|
| Herbal products: St. John's wort (*Hypericum perforatum*) | Amprenavir, atazanavir, fosamprenavir, indinavir, lopinavir/ritonavir, nelfinavir, saquinavir Delavirdine, efavirenz, nevirapine | May lead to loss of virological response and possible resistance to each agent or to the class |
| HMG Co-reductase inhibitors: lovastatin, simvastatin | Amprenavir, atazanavir, fosamprenavir, indinavir, lopinavir/ritonavir, nelfinavir, saquinavir Delavirdine | Potential for serious reactions, such as risk of myopathy, including rhabdomyolysis |
| Neuroleptic: pimozide | Amprenavir, atazanavir, fosamprenavir, indinavir, lopinavir/ritonavir, nelfinavir, saquinavir | *Contraindicated* because of potential for serious and/or life-threatening reactions, such as cardiac arrhythmias |
| NNRTIs: delavirdine | Amprenavir Fosamprenavir | May lead to loss of virological response and possible resistance to delavirdine |
| Oral contraceptives: ethinyl estradiol/norethindrone | Amprenavir | May lead to loss of virological response and possible resistance to amprenavir; alternative methods of nonhormonal contraception are recommended |
| Protease inhibitors: indinavir | Atazanavir | Both atazanavir and indinavir are associated with indirect hyperbilirubinemia Coadministration is not recommended because of potential for additive hyperbilirubinemia |
| Proton pump inhibitors | Atazanavir | Coadministration of atazanavir with proton pump inhibitors is expected to substantially decrease atazanavir plasma concentrations and reduce its therapeutic effect |
| Sedative/hypnotics: alprazolam | Delavirdine | *Contraindicated* because of potential for serious and/or life-threatening events, such as prolonged or increased sedation or respiratory depression |
| Sedative/hypnotics: midazolam, triazolam | Amprenavir, atazanavir, fosamprenavir, indinavir, lopinavir/ritonavir, nelfinavir, saquinavir Delavirdine | *Contraindicated* because of potential for serious and/or life-threatening events, such as prolonged or increased sedation or respiratory depression |

*Source:* From refs. *13, 23, 24, 35, 39, 49, 51, 75–79, 85.*

A variety of dosing regimens involving "boosted" PIs have been evaluated (*see* Table 4). LPV even requires coformulation with RTV because LPV alone has a short half-life and poor bioavailability. Given in combination with low-dose RTV (100 mg twice daily), the LPV AUC increases more than 20-fold *(53)*. Fosamprenavir, the prodrug of amprenavir, can be administered either once or twice daily with RTV, but daily dosing should not be used for treatment-experienced patients *(49)*. Once-daily SQV and RTV has also been explored *(54)*. A twice-daily SQV/RTV regimen was approved by the Food and Drug Administration. The new dosing regimen is 1000 mg SQV twice daily coadministered with 100 mg RTV twice daily. For Invirase, the RTV-boosted regimen replaces a previously approved regimen (600 mg three times a day). Invirase should never be used without RTV. For Fortovase, the RTV-boosted regimen allows a reduced pill burden and ease of administration compared to the previously approved regimen (1200 mg three times daily). Unboosted Fortovase remains a dosage option for patients who are unable to tolerate RTV. Low-dose RTV with other PIs is used as a first-line treatment by many clinicians.

Many advantages exist for the use of RTV boosted regimens, specifically dosing convenience, elimination of food effect, and improved pharmacokinetics. However, RTV-related adverse events are a concern with these regimens. Effects on lipids or gastrointestinal intolerance may be more apparent when RTV is added. Also, clinicians need to be aware of additional drug interactions when RTV is added to the regimen.

Although most PI combinations are predictable, some regimens result in interactions that are unexpected. The coadministration of LPV/RTV with amprenavir leads to a decrease in plasma concentrations of both drugs *(55–58)*. More recently, 700 mg fosamprenavir twice daily and 400/100 mg LPV/RTV twice daily also demonstrated a significant reduction (48–69%) in both amprenavir and LPV exposure *(59)*. Studies to better define this interaction have examined increased doses of both fosamprenavir and lopinavri/RTV, which still resulted in decreased amprenavir concentrations *(60)*. Separation of the two by 4 or 12 hours did not negate the interaction *(61)*. In addition, this combination was associated with increased incidence of gastrointestinal symptoms, rash, and headache *(60)*. The mechanism remains unknown but is likely to involve a complex interaction between metabolic induction and inhibition and possibly the involvement of transport processes. Dosing recommendations for this combination have not been established.

Another unexpected interaction occurred with the investigational PI tipranavir. Similar to LPV, tipranavir requires concurrent dosing with RTV to provide adequate plasma concentrations for antiviral activity. The concomitant RTV was also thought to attenuate the CYP3A4-inducing effects of tipranavir. In clinical trials, tipranavir/RTV (500/200 mg) twice daily was added to three different boosted protease regimens in patients with multiple PI mutations *(62)*. Coadministration of tipranvir resulted in decreases in the $C_{min}$ of SQV (81%), amprenavir (56%), and LPV (55%). Despite the concomitant use of RTV, tipranavir led to significant decreases in exposure of the other PI, demonstrating further that not all drug interactions can be predicted based on historical or in vitro data.

## ENTRY INHIBITORS

Enfuvirtide (ENF) is the first of a new class of drugs that inhibits the process of HIV fusion and entry. ENF is a peptide and must be administered twice daily by subcutaneous injection. Because ENF undergoes catabolism and not metabolism by CYP450, ENF does not demonstrate drug interactions with other antiretrovirals. A trial showed no clinically relevant interactions with SQV and RTV, RTV alone (200 mg twice daily), or rifampin, one of the most potent inducers of the CYP3A4 *(63)*.

## DRUG–FOOD INTERACTIONS

A more complete review of drug–food interactions is provided in Chapter 12. A number of formulation changes over the past few years have occurred, but drug-food interactions remain a problem for some antiretrovirals. Specific drug–food interactions for antiretrovirals are shown in Table 7. Didanosine (buffered formulation and ED) and indinavir are recommended to be given on an empty stomach, although indinavir can be given with a low-fat (<2 g) meal *(23)*. The addition of RTV to indinavir removes this food restriction and decreases administration of indinavir to twice daily *(64)*. The once-daily dosing indication for ddI makes administration on an empty stomach easier to manage. However, ddI administration is complicated for some patients, especially when ddI is used as part of a once-daily regimen with other once daily-agents that must be administered with food. Efavirenz is also taken on an empty stomach because food increases exposure, which may result in a higher frequency of adverse events.

ATV, nelfinavir, LPV/RTV, and SQV all require administration with food, which increases their exposure compared to the fasting state. All these drugs are given once or twice daily, so administration can coincide with meals, which also may improve adherence.

Concomitant grapefruit juice increases the AUC of SQV by 50–200%, presumably because of its large degree of metabolism by gastrointestinal CYP3A4 *(65)*. However, because the amounts of flavonoids and other substances vary widely in a natural product such as grapefruit juice, the interaction shows large variability. Therefore, the use of grapefruit juice should not be relied on as a substitute for RTV to increase SQV concentrations. Grapefruit juice also possesses inhibitory effects on P-glycoprotein-mediated gut transport *(66)*. Whether or not these P-glycoprotein effects compensate or dominate, CYP3A4 inhibition is dependent on the specific PI. Indinavir AUC was moderately reduced by grapefruit juice in a single dose in healthy volunteers *(23)* and was unchanged in a multiple-dose study in patients *(67)*.

## ALTERNATIVE MEDICINES

Complementary and alternative medicines are widely used by the HIV-infected population despite limited knowledge of their pharmacology and potential for drug interactions. Of note, St. John's wort, a popular herbal dietary supplement, was shown to markedly decrease the AUC of indinavir by 57% and the $C_{min}$ by 81% *(46)*. These decreases are large enough to be clinically significant, and this product should be avoided in patients receiving PIs. Many HIV-infected patients take garlic for its theoretical effects on lipids. Garlic tablets have been shown to decrease the AUC of SQV by 51% *(68)*. The mechanism of this interaction is unknown. As SQV is usually given along with RTV, the results of this study cannot be extrapolated to standard usage. Milk thistle (silymarin) is an alternative medication that is used for both therapy and prevention of hepatic disease. Two clinical studies in healthy volunteers with silymarin and indinavir failed to demonstrate a difference in indinavir exposure *(69,70)*.

**Table 7**
**Drug–Food Interactions**

| Drug | Food effect | Recommendation |
|---|---|---|
| Nucleoside reverse transcriptase inhibitors | | |
| • Abacavir | No significant difference in systemic exposure in fed and fasted states | Can be taken without regard to meals |
| • Didanosine | EC formulation: In the presence of food, the $C_{max}$ and AUC were reduced by approx 46% and 19%, respectively, compared to the fasted state | Take on empty stomach 1 hour before or 2 hours after a meal |
| • Emtricitabine | AUC was unaffected, but $C_{max}$ decreased by 29% when given with food | Can be taken without regard to meals |
| • Lamivudine | Food has no effect on the extent of absorption | Can be taken without regard to meals |
| • Stavudine | Food has no effect on the extent of absorption | Can be taken without regard to meals |
| • Tenofovir DF | A high-fat meal (40–50% fat) increases the oral bioavailability, with an increase in AUC of approx 40% and an increase in $C_{max}$ of approx 14% <br> A light meal did not have a significant effect when compared to the fasted state | Can be taken without regard to meals |
| • Zalcitabine | Administration with food decreases AUC by 14% | Can be taken without regard to meals |
| • Zidovudine | The extend of zidovudine absorption (AUC) was similar when a single dose of zidovudine was administered with food | Can be taken without regard to meals |
| Nonnucleoside reverse transcriptase inhibitors | | |
| • Delavirdine | Concentrations similar in fed and fasted states | Can be taken without regard to meals; patients with achlorhydria should take delavirdine with an acidic beverage (e.g., orange or cranberry juice) |
| • Efavirenz | Capsules: A high-fat/high-calorie meal or a reduced-fat/normal caloric meal was associated with a mean increase of 22 and 17% in AUC and a mean increase of 39 and 51% in $C_{max}$, respectively, relative to fasted state | Take on empty stomach, preferably at bedtime; increased efavirenz concentrations following a meal may lead to an increase in frequency of adverse events |

| Drug | Effect of food | Recommendation |
|---|---|---|
| • Efavirenz (Continued) | Tablets: A high-fat/high-calorie meal was associated with a 28% increase in AUC and a 79% increase in $C_{max}$ relative to fasted state | |
| • Nevirapine | Absorption not affected by food | Can be taken without regard to meals |
| **Protease inhibitors** | | |
| • Amprenavir | Administration with high-fat meal increases AUC and $C_{max}$ | Can be taken without regard to meals; however, avoid high-fat meals |
| • Atazanavir | Administration with food enhances bioavailability and reduces pharmacokinetic variability<br>A light meal resulted in a 70% increase in AUC and 57% increase in $C_{max}$ relative to fasted state<br>A high-fat meal resulted in 35% increase in AUC and no change in $C_{max}$ relative to fasted state | Take with food |
| • Fosamprenavir | Concentrations similar in fed and fasted states | Can be taken without regard to meals |
| • Indinavir | Administration with high-fat meal decreased $C_{max}$ by 84% and decreased AUC by 77%<br>A light meal resulted in little or no change in AUC or $C_{max}$ or $C_{min}$ | Should be administered without food but with water 1 hour before or 2 hours after a meal<br>May be given with other liquids, such as skim milk, juice, coffee, or tea, or with a light meal (e.g., dry toast with jelly, juice, and coffee with skim milk and sugar or corn flakes with skim milk and sugar)<br>If given with ritonavir, can be taken without regard to meals |
| • Lopinavir/ritonavir | A high-fat meal increased AUC and $C_{max}$ by 97 and 43, respectively, for capsules and 130 and 56%, respectively, for oral solution relative to fasted state | Take with food |
| • Nelfinavir | $C_{max}$ and AUC increased three- to fivefold under fed vs fasted conditions | Take with a meal |
| • Ritonavir | The extent of absorption was 13% higher for the capsules when administered with a meal | Take with meals if possible |
| • Saquinavir | Administration of food increases AUC | Take with a meal or up to 2 hours after a meal |

*Source:* From refs. *13, 23, 24, 35, 39, 49, 51, 75–83, 86,* and *87.*

The pharmacological properties of many complementary and alternative medicines are unknown. Thus, HIV-infected individuals should use these products with caution. HIV clinicians should include alternative therapies in their drug history along with prescription and over-the-counter medications.

---

### CASE STUDY 1

P.J. is a 39-year-old white male recently diagnosed with HIV infection. He contracted his disease several years ago from intravenous drug abuse and currently is in a methadone treatment program. On presentation, his CD4 count was 151 cells/m$^3$, and his viral load was 250,000 copies/mL. He was prescribed 600 mg efavirenz at bedtime and Combivir (zidovudine/lamivudine) twice daily, along with trimethoprim/sulfamethoxazole (TMP/SMX) DS tablet daily. After 3 days, the patient began to have symptoms of opiate withdrawal and returned to his methadone clinic. The enzyme-inducing properties of efavirenz significantly decreased his methadone concentrations, leading to a withdrawal reaction. He required an increase in his methadone dose by 30% to attenuate these symptoms.

The patient developed a rash on day 11 of therapy, necessitating discontinuation of efavirenz. He was prescribed 1400 mg Fosamprenavir twice daily and continued the Combivir. After 2 weeks of therapy, the viral load had significantly declined, but the subject requested to take his PI only once daily. The prescriber added RTV and changed the fosamprenavir to 1400 mg once daily with 200 mg RTV once daily. The addition of RTV inhibits metabolism of fosamprenavir, increasing its concentrations and allowing for once daily dosing.

---

### CASE STUDY 2

R.I. is a 25-year-old black male diagnosed with HIV infection 4 years ago and has never initiated treatment. At his last clinic visit, his CD4 count had dropped to 170 cells/m$^3$, and his viral load was 110,000 copies/mL. He and his physician decided that treatment was now warranted. He was prescribed 600 mg efavirenz at bedtime, 300 mg TDF daily, and 300 mg lamivudine daily. After 1 month on this regimen, a viral load test demonstrated a decrease in HIV to 450 copies/mL. However, the patient complained of dizziness, confusion, and vivid dreams, and efavirenz was discontinued. The patient wanted to keep a once-daily regimen, and 400 mg ATV daily replaced the efavirenz. The patient tolerated this regimen well, but a viral load examination performed 1 month later showed a level of 15,000 copies/mL. TDF has been shown to decrease ATV AUC and $C_{min}$ by 25% and 40%, respectively. As a result, the decreased concentrations led to therapeutic failure and viral breakthrough.

These cases demonstrate that interactions between antiretrovirals and drugs can be both beneficial and harmful.

---

## PERSPECTIVE

The evaluation of potential drug interactions is a critical component of the care of the HIV-infected patient. Management of interactions can prevent toxicity, delay the development of resistance, and provide convenient dosing. Although the amount of literature is staggering, a number of Web sites, charts, and reviews are available to clinicians to manage drug interactions in HIV-infected patients (71–74).

A number of interesting twists have occurred over the more than 15 years of HIV therapy. RTV was originally released as a treatment but now serves primarily as an inhibitor of metabolism to improve exposure to other drugs. Intracellular interactions have been identified demonstrating that not all combinations are possible and reminding us that concentrations in plasma are not always informative. Although drug interactions are still a concern, they are now generally manageable and often beneficial.

Most interactions can be easily explained based on the mechanism, but others are unpredictable. Drug development of new antiretrovirals employs an extensive drug interaction program that attempts to address possible interactions and provide dosing recommendations. But despite our extensive knowledge, some interactions are only discovered after administration to HIV-infected subjects. Clearly, more data on interactions with antiretrovirals and commonly used agents for other concomitant diseases such as seizure and mental health disorders are needed. Unfortunately, not all possible interactions are evaluated before a new drug is approved; however, clinicians and researchers can help identify clinically important interactions for further research and evaluation. Remarkable efforts have been made thus far in our understanding of complex drug–drug interactions for the treatment of HIV infection, and there is still much more to learn.

## NOTE

No official support or endorsement of this article by the Food and Drug Administration is intended or should be inferred.

## REFERENCES

1. Lertora JJ, Rege AB, Greenspan DL, et al. Pharmacokinetic interaction between zidovudine and valproic acid in patients infected with human immunodeficiency virus. Clin Pharmacol Ther 1994;56:272–278.
2. De Miranda P, Good SS, Yarchoan R, et al. Alteration of zidovudine pharmacokinetics by probenecid in patients with AIDS or AIDS-related complex. Clin Pharmacol Ther 1989;46:494–500.
3. Sahai J, Gallicano K, Pakuts A, et al. Effect of fluconazole on zidovudine pharmacokinetics acid in patients infected with human immunodeficiency virus. J Infect Dis 1994; 169:1103–1107.
4. Rainey PM, McCance EF, Mitchell SM, Jatlow P, Andrews L, Friedland G. Interaction of methadone with didanosine and stavudine. Sixth Conference on Retroviruses and Opportunistic Infections, Chicago, IL, January 31–February 4, 1999. Abstract 371.
5. Jung D, Griffy K, Dorr A, et al. Effect of high-dose oral ganciclovir on didanosine disposition in human immunodeficiency virus (HIV)-positive patients. J Clin Pharmacol 1998;38:1057–1062.
6. Boelaert JR, Dom GM, Huitema AD, et al. The boosting of didanosine by allopurinol permits a halving of the didanosine dosage. AIDS 2002;16:2221–2223.
7. Flaherty J, Kearney B, Wolf J, et al. Coadministration of tenofovir DF and didanosine: a pharmacokinetic and safety evaluation. Forty-first Interscience Conference on Antimicrobial Agents and Chemotherapy, Chicago, IL, December 16–19, 2001. Abstract.
8. Kearney BP, Isaacson E, Sayre J, et al. Didanosine and tenofovir DF drug-drug interaction: assessment of didanosine dose reduction. Tenth Conference on Retroviruses and Opportunistic Infections, Boston, MA, February 10–14, 2003. Abstract 533.

9. Kaul S, Bassi K, Damle B, et al. Pharmacokinetic evaluation of the combination of atazanavir, enteric coated didanosine, and tenofovir disoproxil fumarate for a once-daily antiretroviral regimen. Forty-third Interscience Conference on Antimicrobial Agents and Chemotherapy, Chicago, IL, September 14–17, 2003. Abstract A-1616.

10. Hoggard PG, Kewn S, Barry MG, Khoo SH, Back DJ. Effects of drugs on 2′,3′-dideoxy-2′,3′-didehydrothymidine phosphorylation in vitro. Antimicrob Agents Chemother 1997;41:1231–1236.

11. NIAID Division of AIDS Press Release. Important therapeutic information on the combination of zidovudine and stavudine in patients who have previously taken zidovudine. National Institutes of Health, Bethesda, MD, November 22, 1996.

12. Veal GJ, Hoggard PG, Barry MG, Khoo S, Back DJ. Interaction between lamivudine and other nucleoside analogues for intracellular phosphorylation. AIDS 1996;10:546–548.

13. Panel on Clinical Practices for Treatment of HIV Infection. Guidelines for the use of antiretroviral agents in HIV-infected adults and adolescents. Department of Health and Human Services and Henry J. Kaiser Family Foundation, November 10, 2003. Available at: www.aidsinfo.nih.gov. Date accessed: March 11, 2005.

14. Sim SM, Hoggard PG, Sales SD, et al. Effect of ribavirin on zidovudine efficacy and toxicity in vitro: concentration-dependent interaction. AIDS Res Hum Retroviruses 1998;14:1661–1667.

15. Gallant JE, Rodriguez AE, Weinberg W, et al. Early Non-response to tenofovir DF (TDF) + abacavir (ABC) and lamivudine (3TC) in a Randomized trial compared to efavirenz (EFV) + ABC and 3TC: ESS30009 unplanned interim analysis. Oral late-breaker presented at the 43rd Annual Interscience Conference on Antimicrobial Agents and Chemotherapy, Chicago, IL, September 14–17, 2003. Abstract H-1722a.

16. Kearney BP, Isaacson E, Sayre J, et al. The pharmacokinetics of abacavir, a purine nucleoside analogue, are not affected by tenofovir DF. Forty-third Interscience Conference on Antimicrobial Agents and Chemotherapy, Chicago, IL, September 14–17, 2003. Abstract A-1615.

17. Rutschmann OT, Opravil M, Iten A, et al. A placebo-controlled trial of didanosine plus stavudine, with and without hydroxyurea, for HIV infection. The Swiss HIV Cohort Study. AIDS 1998;12:F71–F77.

18. Frank I, Boucher H, Fiscus S, et al. Phase I/II dosing study of once-daily hydroxyurea alone vs didanosine alone vs didanosine + hydroxyurea. Sixth Conference on Retroviruses and Opportunistic Infections, Chicago, IL, January 31–February 4, 1999. Abstract 402.

19. Palmer S, Shafer RW, Merigan TC. Hydroxyurea enhances the activities of didanosine, 9-[2-(phosphonylmethoxy)ethyl]adenine, and 9-[2-(phosphonylmethoxy)propyl]adenine against drug-susceptible and drug-resistant human immunodeficiency virus isolates. Antimicrob Agents Chemother 1999;43:2046–2050.

20. Weissman SB, Sinclair GI, Green CL, Fissell WH. Hydroxyurea–induced hepatitis in human immunodeficiency virus-positive patients. Clin Infect Dis 1999;29:223,224.

21. Rutschmann OT, Opravil M, Iten A, et al. A placebo-controlled trial of didanosine plus stavudine, with and without hydroxyurea, for HIV infection. The Swiss HIV Cohort Study. AIDS 1998;12:F71–F77.

22. Margolis DM, Kewn S, Coull JJ, et al. The addition of mycophenalate mofetil to antiretroviral therapy including abacavir is associated with depletion of intracellular deoxyguanosine triphosphate and a decrease in plasma HIV-1 RNA. J Acquir Immune Defic Syndr 2002;31:45–49.

23. Indinavir (Crixivan) [package insert]. West Point, PA: Merck and Co., 2003.

24. Reyataz (Atazanavir) product information. Princeton, NJ: Bristol Myers Squibb, 2003.

25. Ferry JJ, Herman BD, Cox SR, et al. Delavirdine and indinavir: a pharmacokinetic drug-drug interaction study in healthy adult volunteers. Fourth Conference on Retroviruses and Opportunistic Infections, Washington, DC, January 22–26, 1997. Abstract 121.

26. Cox SR, Batts DH, Stewart F, et al. Evaluation of the pharmacokinetic interaction between saquinavir and delavirdine in healthy volunteers. Presented at the Fourth Conference on Retroviruses and Opportunistic Infections, Washington, DC, January 22–26, 1997. Abstract 381.

27. Acosta EP, Gulick R, Katzenstein D, et al. Pharmacokinetic evaluation of saquinavir soft gel capsule/ritonavir or SQV/nelfinavir in combination with delavirdine and/or adefovie dipoxil-ACTG 359. Sixth Conference on Retroviruses and Opportunistic Infections, Chicago, IL, January 31–February 4, 1999. Abstract 365.

28. Kearney BP, Reul T, Coleman R, et al. Pharmacokinetics of adefovir in combination with saquinavir, indinavir, efavirenz, delavirdine, didanosine, or lamivudine in normal volunteers. Seventh Conference on Retroviruses and Opportunistic Infections, San Francisco, CA, January 30–February 2, 2000. Abstract 86.

29. Murphy RL, Sommadossi JP, Lamson M, Hall DB, Myers M, Dusek A. Antiviral effect and pharmacokinetic interaction between nevirapine and indinavir in persons infected with human immunodeficiency virus type 1. J Infect Dis 1999;179:1116–1123.

30. Sahai J, Cameron W, Salgo M, et al. Drug interaction study between saquinavir and nevirapine. Fourth Conference on Retroviruses and Opportunistic Infections, Washington, DC, January 22–26, 1997. Abstract 496.

31. Fiske WD, Mayers D, Wagner K, et al. Pharmacokinetics of DMP 266 and indinavir multiple oral doses in HIV-1 infected individuals. Fourth Conference on Retroviruses and Opportunistic Infections, Washington, DC, January 22–26, 1997. Abstract 535.

32. Piscitelli S, Vogel S, Sadler S, et al. Effect of efavirenz on the pharmacokinetics of 141W94 in HIV-infected patients. Fifth Conference on Retroviruses and Opportunistic Infections, Chicago, IL, February 1–5, 1998. Abstract 346.

33. Piscitelli SC, Bechtel C, Sadler B, Falloon J. The addition of a second protease inhibitor (PI) eliminates amprenavir-efavirenz drug interactions and increases plasma amprenavir concentrations. Seventh Conference Retroviruses and Opportunistic Infections, San Francisco, CA, January 30–February 2, 2000.

34. Hendrix CW, Fiske WD, Fuchs EJ, et al. Pharmacokinetics of the triple combination of saquinavir. Ritonavir, and efavirenz in HIV-positive patients. Seventh Conference on Retroviruses and Opportunistic Infections, San Francisco, CA, January 30–February 2, 2000. Abstract 79.

35. Kaletra (lopinavir/ritonavir) product information. Abbott Park, IL: Abbott Laboratories, 2003.

36. Skowron G, Leoung G, Dusek A, et al. Stavudine, nelfinavir, and nevirapine preliminary safety, activity, and pharmacokinetic interactions. Fifth Conference on Retroviruses and Opportunistic Infections, Chicago, IL, February 1–5, 1998. Abstract 350.

37. Fiske WD, Benedek IH, White SJ, et al. Pharmacokinetic interaction between efavirenz and nelfinavir mesylate in healthy volunteers. Fifth Conference on Retroviruses and Opportunistic Infections, Chicago, IL, February 1–5, 1998. Abstract 349.

38. Fiske WD, Benedek IH, Joseph JL, et al. Pharmacokinetics of efavirenz and ritonavir after multiple oral doses in healthy volunteers. Twelfth World AIDS Conference, Geneva, Switzerland, June 28–July 3, 1998. Abstract 42269.

39. Sustiva (efavirenz) product information. Princeton, NJ: Bristol Myers Squibb, 2003.

40. Altice FL, Cooney E, Friedland GH. Nevirapine induced methadone withdrawal: implications for antiretroviral treatment of opiate dependent HIV infected patients. Sixth Conference on Retroviruses and Opportunistic Infections, Chicago, IL, January 31–February 4, 1999. Abstract 37.

41. Veldkamp AI, Harris M, Montaner JS, et al. The steady-state pharmacokinetics of efavirenz and nevirapine when used in combination in human immunodeficiency virus type 1-infected persons. J Infect Dis 2001;184:37–42.

42. Piscitelli SC, Gallicano KD. Interactions among drugs for HIV and opportunistic infections. N Engl J Med 2001;344:984–996.

43. Monahan BP, Ferguson CL, Killeavy ES, et al. Torsades de pointes occurring in association with terfenadine use. JAMA 1990;264:2788–2790.

44. Richardson JD, Sorenson S. Rifampin to treat ritonavir-ergotamine drug interaction [abstract]. Clin Infect Dis 1999;29:1002.

45. Centers for Disease Control and Prevention. Updated guidelines for the use of rifabutin or rifampin for the treatment and prevention of tuberculosis among HIV-infected patients taking protease inhibitors or nonnucleoside reverse transcriptase inhibitors. MMWR Morb Mortal Wkly Rep 2000;49:185–189.

46. Piscitelli SC, Burstein AH, Chaitt D, et al. Indinavir concentrations and St. John's wort. Lancet 2000;355:547,548.

47. Muirhead GJ, Wulff MB, Fielding A, Kleinermans D., Faulkner S, Buss N. Pharmacokinetic interactions between protease inhibitors ritonavir and saquinavir and Viagra (sildenafil citrate). Thirty-ninth Interscience Conference on Antimicrobial Agents and Chemotherapy, San Francisco, CA, September 26–29, 1999. Abstract 659.

48. Merry C, Barry MG, Ryan M, et al. Interaction of sildenafil and indinavir when co-administered to HIV-positive patients. AIDS 1999;13:F101–F107.

49. Lexiva (Fosamprenavir) product information. Research Triangle Park, NC: GlaxoSmithKline, 2003.

50. Ouellet D, Hsu A, Qian J, et al. Effect of ritonavir on the pharmacokinetics of ethinyl oestradiol in healthy female volunteers. Br J Clin Pharmacol 1998;46:111–116.

51. Nelfinavir (Viracept) package insert. Thousand Oaks, CA: Agouron Pharmaceuticals, 2003.

52. Raines CP, Flexner C, Sun E. Safety, tolerability, and antiretroviral effects of ritonavir-nelfinavir combination therapy administered for 48 weeks. J Acquir Immune Defic Syndr 2000;25:322–328.

53. Sham HL, Kempf DJ, Molla A, et al. ABT-378, a highly potent inhibitor of the human immunodeficiency virus protease. Antimicrob Agents Chemother 1998;42:3218–3224.

54. Kilby JM, Sfakianos G, Gizzi N, et al. Safety and pharmacokinetics of once-daily regimens of soft-gel capsule saquinavir plus minidose ritonavir in human immunodeficiency virus-negative adults. Antimicrob Agents Chemother 2000;44:2672–2678.

55. Bertz R, Foit C, Ashbrenner E, et al. Effect of amprenavir on the steady-state pharmacokinetics of lopinavir/ritonavir in HIV+ and healthy subjects. In: Abstracts of the 42nd Interscience Conference on Antimicrobial Agents and Chemotherapy, San Diego, CA, September 27–30, 2002. Abstract A-1823.

56. Hsu A, Bertz R, Ashbrenner E, et al. Interaction of ABT-378/ritonavir with protease inhibitors in healthy volunteers. In: Abstracts of the First International Workshop on Clinical Pharmacology of HIV Therapy, Noordwijk, The Netherlands, March 30–April 1, 2000. Abstract 2.4.

57. Meynard JL, Poirier JM, Guiard-Schmid JB, et al. Impact of ABT 378/r on the amprenavir plasma concentrations in HIV-experienced patients treated by the association of APV-ABT 378/r. In: Abstracts of the 41st Interscience Conference on Antimicrobial Agents and Chemotherapy, December 16–19, 2001, Chicago, IL. Abstract 1736.

58. Solas C, Quinson AM, Couprie C, et al. Pharmacokinetic interaction between lopinavir/r and amprenavir in salvage therapy. Ninth Conference on Retroviruses and Opportunistic Infections, Seattle, WA, February 24–28, 2002. Abstract 440-W.

59. Kashuba ADM, Tierney C, Downey GF, et al. Combining GW433908 (fosamprenavir) with lopinavir/ritonavir in HIV-1 infected adults' results in substantial reductions in amprenavir and lopinavir concentrations: pharmacokinetic results from Adult ACTG protocol A5143. Forty-third Interscience Conference on Antimicrobial Agents and Chemotherapy, Chicago, IL, September 14–17, 2003. Abstract H-855A.

60. Wire MB, Naderer O, Masterman AL, Lou Y, Stein DS. The pharmacokinetic interaction between GW433908 and lopinavir/ritonavir (APV10011 and APV 10012). Eleventh Con-

ference on Retroviruses and Opportunistic Infections, San Francisco, CA, February 8–13, 2004. Abstract 612.

61. Corbett AH, Davidson L, Park JJ, et al. Dose separation strategies to overcome the pharmacokinetic interaction of a triple protease inhibitor regimen containing fosamprenavir, lopinavir, and ritonavir. Eleventh Conference on Retroviruses and Opportunistic Infections, San Francisco, CA, February 8–13, 2004. Abstract 611.

62. Leith J, Walmsley S, Katlama C, et al. Pharmacokinetics and safety of tipranavir/ritonavir alone or in combination with saquinavir, amprenavir, or lopinavir: interim analysis of BI1182.51. Fifth International Workshop on Clinical Pharmacology of HIV Therapy, Rome, Italy, April 1–3, 2004. Abstract 5.1.

63. Boyd M, Ruxrungtham K, Zhang X, et al. Evfuvirtide-investigations on the drug interaction potential in HIV-infected patients. Tenth Conference on Retroviruses and Opportunistic Infections, Boston, MA, February 10–14, 2003. Abstract 541.

64. Saah AJ, Winchell G, Seniuk M, Deutsch P. Multiple-dose pharmacokinetics and tolerability of indinavir ritonavir combinations in healthy volunteers. Sixth Conference on Retroviruses and Opportunistic Infections, Chicago, IL, January 31–February 4, 1999. Abstract 362.

65. Kupferschmidt HH, Fattinger KE, Ha HR, Follath F, Krahenbuhl S. Grapefruit juice enhances the bioavailability of the HIV protease inhibitor saquinavir in man. Br J Clin Pharmacol 1998;45:355–359.

66. Wacher VJ, Silverman JA, Zhang Y, Benet LZ. Role of P-glycoprotein and cytochrome P450 3A in limiting oral absorption of peptides and peptidomimetics. J Pharm Sci 1998; 87;1322–1330.

67. Wynn H, Shelton MJ, Bartos L, Difrancesco R, Hewitt R. Grapefruit juice increases gastric pH but does not affect indinavir exposure in HIV patients [abstract]. In: Program and Abstracts of the 39th Interscience Conference on Antimicrobial Agents and Chemotherapy, San Francisco, CA, September 26–29, 1999. p. 25.

68. Piscitelli SC, Burstein AH, Welden N, Gallicano KD, Falloon J. The effect of garlic supplements on the pharmacokinetics of saquinavir. Clin Infect Dis 2002;34:234–238.

69. Piscitelli SC, Formentini E, Burstein AH, et al. Effect of milk thistle on the pharmacokinetics of indinavir in healthy volunteers. Pharmacotherapy. 2002;22:551–556.

70. DiCenzo R, Shelton M, Jordan K , et al. Coadministration of milk thistle and indinavir in healthy subjects. Pharmacotherapy 2003;23:866–870.

71. HIV Insite Website. Available at: hivinsite.ucsf.edu. Date accessed: March 11, 2005.

72. Johns Hopkins AIDS Service Website. Available at: www.hopkins-aids.edu. Date accessed: March 11, 2005.

73. Medscape Website. Available at: www.medscape.com. Date accessed: March 11, 2005.

74. HIV/AIDS Treatment Information Service Website. Available at: www.hivatis.org. Date accessed: March 11, 2005.

75. Nevirapine (Viramune) [package insert]. Columbus, OH: Roxane Laboratories, 2003.

76. Delavirdine (Rescriptor) [package insert]. La Jolla, CA: Agouron Pharmaceuticals, 2001.

77. Amprenavir (Agenerase) [package insert]. Research Triangle Park, NC: GlaxoSmithKline, 2002.

78. Saquinavir (Fortovase and Invirase) [package inserts]. Nutley, NJ: Roche Laboratories, 2003.

79. Ritonavir (Norvir) [package insert]. North Chicago, IL: Abbott Laboratories, 2003.

80. Zidovudine/lamivudine (COMBIVIR) [package insert]. Research Triangle Park, NC: GlaxoSmithKline, 2003.

81. Didanosine (Videx EC) [package insert]: Princeton, NJ: Bristol-Myers Squibb, 2003.

82. Stavudine (Zerit) [package insert]. Princeton, NJ: Bristol-Myers Squibb, 2002.

83. Tenofovir disporoxil fumerate (Viread) [package insert]. Foster City, CA: Gilead Sciences, 2003.

84. Reyataz Dear Health Care Professional Letter, Princeton, NJ: Bristol-Myers Squibb, August 8, 2003.

85. Tseng A. AIDS/HIV: drugs for opportunistic infections. In: Piscitelli S, Rodvold K, eds. Drug Interactions in Infectious Diseases. Totowa, NJ: Humana Press, 2001, pp. 61–107.

86. Zalcitabine (HIVID) [package insert]. Nutley, NJ: Roche Laboratories, 2002.

87. Emtricitabine (Emtrivia) [package insert]. Foster City, CA: Gilead Sciences, 2003.

88. Gerber JC, Fichtenbaum CJ, Rosenkranz S, et al. Efavirenz (EFV) is a significant inducer of simvastatin (SIM) and atorvastatin (ATV) metabolism: results of ACTG A5108 Study. Eleventh Conference on Retroviruses and Opportunistic Infections, San Francisco, CA, February 8–11, 2004. Abstract 603.

# 6

# Drugs for HIV-Related Opportunistic Infections

## Alice Tseng

## INTRODUCTION

As outlined in Chapter 5, drug interactions in human immunodeficiency virus (HIV) are encountered frequently, particularly with protease inhibitors and nonnucleoside reverse transcriptase inhibitors (NNRTIs). In a retrospective chart review of 165 HIV patients newly prescribed a protease inhibitor, at least one potential drug interaction was identified in 82 (49.7%) of the patients (1). In total, 111 interactions were identified, but only 22 (19.8%) were recognized at the time of protease inhibitor therapy initiation. An additional 12 drug interactions were later identified at follow-up, but 77 (69.3%) were never recognized. At the time this study was conducted, only three protease inhibitors (saquinavir, ritonavir, and indinavir) were available. More recently, in a chart review of 189 ambulatory HIV patients, 466 interactions were identified in 153 subjects for an average of 2.46 interactions per patient (2).

With the continual emergence of new agents and drug classes, the potential for significant interactions will continue to be of concern. Although the overall incidence of opportunistic infections has declined (3–5), concurrent therapy for prophylaxis, treatment, or suppression of opportunistic infections is often still required (6–8). Thus, polypharmacy remains an important risk factor for multiple and complex drug interactions. This chapter focuses primarily on drug interactions between antiretroviral medications and agents commonly used for the prevention and management of opportunistic infections.

### General Approach/Considerations

In general, drug interactions may be considered as either pharmacokinetic or pharmacodynamic. Drug absorption, distribution, metabolism, or elimination may be affected by pharmacokinetic interactions, resulting in an alteration of the amount or concentration of one or both agents in the body. Such changes are especially undesirable when the disposition of an agent with a narrow therapeutic index is affected. Pharmacokinetic drug–drug interactions are encountered frequently, particularly with protease inhibitors and NNRTIs. For instance, ritonavir is an extremely potent inhibitor of many cytochrome P450 (CYP) isoenzymes, including CYP3A, CYP2D6, CYP2C9, CYP2C19, and others, and thus has the potential to interact with a multitude of agents metabolized via similar

From: *Infectious Disease: Drug Interactions in Infectious Diseases, Second Edition*
Edited by: S. C. Piscitelli and K. A. Rodvold © Humana Press Inc., Totowa, NJ

routes *(9)*. Agents such as indinavir, nelfinavir, atazanavir, and delavirdine have moderate inhibitory effects on CYP3A, and saquinavir is a weak inhibiting agent. Nevirapine and tipranavir, in contrast, are moderate inducers of CYP3A, and efavirenz and amprenavir are associated with both enzyme-inducing and -inhibiting properties.

With pharmacodynamic interactions, additive, synergistic, or antagonistic drug combinations may affect pharmacological parameters, such as efficacy and toxicity. Pharmacodynamic drug–drug interactions are often desirable to enhance clinical efficacy when agents with complementary mechanisms of action are administered. For example, the combination of zidovudine plus lamivudine has greater effects on improving immunological and viral markers of HIV disease compared to either agent alone *(10)*. Some drug combinations may be used to reduce patient toxicity. To minimize the risk of isoniazid-induced peripheral neuropathy, pyridoxine can be coadministered. In contrast, certain combinations may be undesirable if antagonism or additive toxicity occurs. For example, lamivudine and zalcitabine share structural similarities, and both are initially phosphorylated by the same enzyme, deoxycitidine kinase. Lamivudine and zalcitabine have been shown to interact negatively in vitro, likely via competition for intracellular phosphorylation *(11)*, and thus should not be coadministered. Similar concern exists regarding the combination of zidovudine and stavudine (12).

The clinical significance of an interaction depends on several factors, including the magnitude of change in pharmacokinetic parameters and the efficacy and toxicity of the affected agent(s). Achieving adequate drug concentrations is a very significant factor in determining the success or failure of current as well as future highly active combination antiretroviral therapies. Many antiretroviral agents, particularly protease inhibitors and NNRTIs, have narrow therapeutic indices, and maintenance of minimum drug concentrations may be necessary to achieve optimal therapeutic benefit *(13–15)*. This is of particular concern because within-class cross-resistance is not uncommon *(16)*. Patients who fail therapy with one protease inhibitor often do not experience sustained benefit by switching to another protease inhibitor, even one with different in vitro resistance mutations *(17–20)*.

Furthermore, interactions may result in excessively elevated drug concentrations, which in turn may be associated with increased toxicity. For example, in a study by Preston et al. *(1)*, 82 of 165 patients (49.7%) had at least one potential drug interaction at the time of protease inhibitor therapy initiation. Of those, 29 (35.4%) had at least one potentially serious/life-threatening interaction, 22 (26.8%) had at least one potentially serious interaction with therapeutic drug monitoring available, and 49 (59.8%) had at least one non-life-threatening interaction. Overall, 42.4% of serious or life-threatening interactions were recognized at the time of protease inhibitor therapy initiation. The researchers concluded that patients who were starting protease inhibitors had a high likelihood of concurrently receiving an agent with a potentially serious drug interaction, and that increased awareness and recognition of potential interactions was needed.

### Predicting Pharmacokinetic Interactions With Antiretroviral Agents

Because new therapeutic agents are continually being developed, keeping abreast of potential interactions is extremely challenging. Often, there are little or no pharmacokinetic interaction data available for certain combinations of drugs. In such situations, familiarity with the basic pharmacokinetic and pharmacodynamic characteristics of the agents involved may help practitioners predict the likelihood of interactions. All protease inhibitors and NNRTIs are substrates of the CYP system and possess enzyme-inhibiting or -inducing properties. In addition, many of the drugs used for the management of opportunistic infections may possess either overlapping side-effect profiles or effects on the CYP system (Table 1) *(21–27)*. Careful consideration of all available pharmacological and pharmacokinetic information is necessary to anticipate possible interactions and to optimize therapeutic efficacy and minimize drug toxicity *(28–30)*. These principles and strategies are reviewed extensively in Chapters 2, 3, and 14 of this volume.

This chapter discusses clinically important interactions of drugs commonly used for the prevention and management of opportunistic infections in HIV disease. The focus is on interactions between these classes of drugs and antiretroviral medications. For more detailed and comprehensive information regarding general drug interactions with each of the different antibacterial classes, refer to the specific chapters in this volume.

## ANTIPARASITICS

Antiparasitic drugs such as trimethoprim-sulfamethoxazole (TMP-SMX), dapsone, atovaquone, clindamycin, primaquine, pentamidine, sulfadiazine, and pyrimethamine are used for the management of various opportunistic and bacterial infections. Patients with advanced HIV disease may be at risk of developing *Pneumocystis carinii* pneumonia (PCP) or toxoplasmosis encephalitis, which are associated with significant morbidity and mortality. In severely immunocompromised individuals, antiparasitic drugs may be administered at high doses, often intravenously, for acute treatment of these serious infections; in addition, prolonged oral therapy for prevention or secondary suppression of illness is routinely indicated in susceptible patients *(6)*.

Interactions involving this class of drugs may occur secondary to pharmacokinetic and/or pharmacodynamic mechanisms (Table 2).

### Absorption Interactions

For many years, clinicians were reluctant to coadminister dapsone and didanosine because of concerns that dapsone absorption would be adversely affected. This widespread assumption originated from unexpected findings in a retrospective case series report. Metroka et al. *(31)* noted that in 57 patients enrolled in investigational new drug and open-label studies of didanosine, PCP developed in 11 of 28 patients receiving dapsone prophylaxis vs 1 of 12 patients receiving aerosolized pentamidine and none of 17 patients receiving cotrimoxazole. The mean time to PCP development after initiation of didanosine therapy was 66 days. The authors suggested that because previous studies in humans had shown that dapsone was insoluble at neutral pH, the most likely mechanism for dapsone failure was malabsorption caused by the citrate-phosphate buffer in the didanosine formulation. However, factors such as patient adherence, doses of dapsone, timing of drug administration (i.e., when dapsone doses were taken in relation to daily didanosine), and plasma dapsone concentrations were not assessed. Information on concomitant medications and diseases was also lacking. Subsequently, in a controlled pharmacokinetic study involving both healthy volunteers and HIV-infected individuals, Sahai et al. did not observe a significant drug interaction between didanosine and dapsone *(32)*. Therefore, dapsone and didanosine may be administered concomitantly *(33)*.

**Table 1**
**Summary of Primary Interaction Mechanisms**
**With Antiretrovirals and Antibacterials Commonly**
**Used for the Management of Opportunistic Infections in HIV**

| Drug | Absorption interactions | | Metabolic interactions | | Main side effects |
|---|---|---|---|---|---|
| | Food effect | Gastric pH | Inhibition | Induction | |
| **Antiretrovirals** | | | | | |
| • Nucleoside and nucleotide reverse transcriptase inhibitors | Take on empty stomach (didanosine); take with food (tenofovir) | Needs alkaline pH (didanosine); avoid antacids (zalcitabine) | | | Peripheral neuropathy, pancreatitis (didanosine, stavudine, zalcitabine); hematotoxicity (zidovudine); lactic acidosis (rare for all) |
| • Nonnucleoside reverse transcriptase inhibitors (NNRTIs) | | Needs acidic pH (delavirdine) | CYP3A4—moderate (delavirdine); CYP2C9/19, 3A4—efavirenz (although induction effect usually predominates) | CYP3A4—moderate (efavirenz, nevirapine) CYP2B6 (nevirapine) | Rash (all); CNS toxicity (efavirenz); hepatotoxicity |
| • Protease inhibitors | Empty stomach (indinavir); meal (atazanavir, lopinavir/ritonavir, nelfinavir, saquinavir) | Needs acidic pH (indinavir); decreased solubility (and absorption) in alkaline pH environment (atazanavir) | Potent inhibition of CYP3A4 > 2D6 > 2C9 > 2C19 >> 2A6 > 2E1 (ritonavir); CYP3A4 (moderate for amprenavir, atazanavir, indinavir, nelfinavir; weak for saquinavir); CYP1A2, 2C9 (atazanavir) | Glucuronyl transferase (nelfinavir, ritonavir); CYP1A2, CYP2C9 (ritonavir); CYP3A4 (amprenavir, ritonavir) | Gastrointestinal, increased lipids, hepatotoxicity, changes in body composition (all); nephrolithiasis (indinavir); hyperbilirubinemia (atazanavir, indinavir) |

Antibacterials

| | | | | |
|---|---|---|---|---|
| • Antifungals | Take with food (itraconazole, ketoconazole); take on empty stomach (voriconazole) | Require acidic pH (itraconazole capsules, ketoconazole) | CYP3A4 (ketoconazole > itraconazole > fluconazole > voriconazole); CYP2C9 (fluconazole, voriconazole); CYP2C19 (voriconazole); P-glycoprotein (itraconazole, ketoconazole) | Hepatotoxicity (azoles); nephrotoxicity (amphotericin); hematotoxicity (flucytosine, amphotericin) |
| • Antimycobacterials | Empty stomach (azithromycin capsules, isoniazid, rifampin); take rifapentine with food | Avoid antacids (ethambutol, isoniazid, quinolones) | Moderate CYP3A4 (clarithromycin); CYP1A2 (quinolones); CYP3A4 (rifampin > rifapentine > rifabutin); CYP1A2, CYP2C, glucuronyl transferase (rifampin) | Hepatotoxicity (all); peripheral neuropathy (isoniazid); uveitis (rifabutin) |
| • Antiparasitics | Take with food (atovaquone) | | | Pancreatitis, nephrotoxicity (pentamidine); rash (trimethoprim-sulfamethoxazole, dapsone, sulfadiazine, clindamycin); blood dyscrasias (pyrimethamine, dapsone, TMP-SMX, primaquine) |
| • Antivirals | Take with food (oral ganciclovir, valganciclovir) | Antivirals renally eliminated | | Hematotoxicity (ganciclovir); nephrotoxicity (cidofovir, foscarnet); uveitis (cidofovir, fomivirsen) |

**Table 2**
**Antiparasitic Interactions**

| Primary drug | Interacting drug | Mechanism | Effects | Comments/management |
|---|---|---|---|---|
| Atovaquone | Didanosine | Interference with didanosine absorption | 24% decrease in didanosine AUC; pharmacokinetics of atovaquone not affected (151) | Concomitant therapy not expected to produce clinically significant results; however, didanosine should be given on an empty stomach; atovaquone is administered with food; routine dosage adjustments not recommended |
| | Rifampin | Rifampin induces atovaquone clearance | >50% decrease atovaquone AUC; >0% increase in rifampin AUC (35) | Avoid combination because of potential therapeutic failure of atovaquone |
| | Zidovudine | Atovaquone may be a substrate or competitive inhibitor of zidovudine glucuronidation | 35% increase in zidovudine AUC; likely not clinically significant (34,152) | No dosage adjustment recommended; monitor for zidovudine toxicity |
| | Ritonavir, lopinavir/ ritonavir | Possible induction of glucuronidation | Potential for decreased atovaquone levels (9,153) | Clinical significance unknown; monitor for efficacy; atovaquone dosage adjustment may be necessary |
| Dapsone | Didanosine | Overlapping side-effect profile | No kinetic interaction; additive neuropathy | Monitor for signs and symptoms of peripheral neuropathy |
| | Pyrimethamine | Pyrimethamine may inhibit dapsone clearance | Increased dapsone concentrations (154) | Potential for increased bone marrow toxicity; monitor complete blood count (CBC) |
| | Primaquine | Overlapping side-effect profile | Increased risk of hemolytic anemia, methemoglobinemia (155) | Potential for increased bone marrow toxicity; monitor CBC |
| | Rifampin | Rifampin induces dapsone metabolism | Increased dapsone clearance (156) | Higher dapsone doses may be necessary; monitor for dapsone efficacy |
| | Stavudine | Overlapping side-effect profile | Additive neuropathy | Monitor for signs and symptoms of peripheral neuropathy |
| | Trimethoprim (TMP) | Trimethoprim inhibits clearance of dapsone and vice versa | Dapsone and TMP levels both increased by 40% (157) | Consider reducing the dose of TMP in patients with baseline anemia or if anemia develops; monitor CBC |

| Drug | Interacting drug | Mechanism | Effect | Management |
|---|---|---|---|---|
| | Zalcitabine | Zalcitabine decreases oral clearance of dapsone | 20% decrease in dapsone clearance, but no change in AUC (126) | Potential for additive neuropathy |
| | Zidovudine | Additive toxicity | Potential for increased hemato-toxicity with combination | Monitor for toxicity when using combination |
| Pentamidine | Amphotericin B | Additive toxicity | Increased risk of hypomagnesemia, increased risk of nephrotoxicity (158) | Caution warranted with combination; monitor as above but more frequently for interacting parameters (i.e., three times weekly) |
| | Foscarnet | Additive toxicity | Increased risk of hypocalcemia and hypomagnesemia, nephrotoxicity (159) | Strongly consider alternatives before combining these drugs; aggressive pretherapy hydration may reduce nephrotoxicity; monitor as above but more frequently for interacting parameters (i.e., three times weekly) |
| | Other nephrotoxins (e.g., cidofovir, aminoglycosides) | Additive toxicity | Potential for increased nephro-toxicity with combination | Avoid combination if possible; monitor renal function regularly |
| | Pancreatoxins (e.g., didanosine, stavudine, zalcitabine, alcohol, corticosteroids) | Additive toxicity | Increased risk of pancreatitis (39) | Avoid combination if possible; because of prolonged half-life of pentamidine, do not restart nucleosides until 1 week after pentamidine therapy is concluded (44); monitor amylase, lipase monthly |
| Sulfadiazine/ pyrimethamine | Zidovudine | Antagonistic antibacterial effect | In vitro and in vivo observations that zidovudine antagonizes the toxoplasmacidal effect of pyrimethamine plus sulfadoxine (37); zidovudine clearance also decreased, which may increase risk of bone marrow toxicity (37,160) | The clinical significance of this is unclear; may wish to consider replacing zidovudine with an alternative antiretroviral during therapy for toxoplasmosis; 10–50 mg folinic acid daily is recommended to reduce the risk of pyrimethamine toxicity |

*Continued on next page*

143

**Table 2 (*Continued*)**
**Antiparasitic Interactions**

| Primary drug | Interacting drug | Mechanism | Effects | Comments/management |
|---|---|---|---|---|
| Trimethoprim-sulfamethoxazole (TMP-SMX) | Lamivudine | Trimethoprin inhibits renal tubular secretion of lamivudine | 43% reduction in lamivudine AUC (*36*) | No dosage adjustment required unless patient is renally impaired; monitor for lamivudine side-effects (i.e., gastrointestinal, headache, fatigue, myalgias, neutropenia) |
| | Pyrimethamine | Additive inhibition of dihydrofolate reductase | Megaloblastic anemia, leucopenia (*161*) | Use together in low dosages; folinic acid should be given with pyrimethamine, but is not effective in reducing TMP-SMX hematotoxicity; monitor CBC with differential weekly |
| | Zalcitabine | Trimethoprin inhibits renal tubular secretion of zalcitabine | 37% increase in zalcitabine AUC (*162*) | Clinical significance unclear. Monitor for zalcitabine toxicity, such as peripheral neuropathy, headache, oral ulcers, pancreatitis. |
| | Zidovudine | Trimethoprin inhibits renal tubular secretion of zidovudine | 23% increase in zidovudine AUC because of TMP component; may be more pronounced in hepatic failure; monitor for zidovudine toxicity; risk of increased anemia, neutropenia (*40*) | Consider holding zidovudine during acute therapy for PCP with high-dose TMP-SMX; monitor CBC with differential weekly |
| Trimethoprim-sulfamethoxazole, dapsone, sulfadiazine, clindamycin | Abacavir, NNRTIs (delavirdine, nevirapine, efavirenz), amprenavir, probenecid | Overlapping side effects | Rash may occur with all listed agents | When possible, do not initiate antiparasitic therapy and antiretrovirals at same time; if rash occurs, attempt to determine most likely causative agent so that other drugs are not discontinued unnecessarily |

## Metabolism

Atovaquone may be administered for either prevention or treatment of mild-to-moderate acute PCP episodes. It is administered orally, usually at a dose of 750 mg twice daily (for treatment) or 1500 mg once daily (for prophylaxis) with meals. Atovaquone is a napthoquinone that first undergoes reduction by DT-diaphorase to hydroquinone conjugates; these conjugates may then undergo further glucuronide or sulfate conjugate reactions. Interactions may occur when atovaquone is used in combination with other agents that can affect these metabolic pathways. In an open, randomized, crossover study, 14 HIV-infected subjects received 600 mg zidovudine daily and 1500 mg atovaquone daily, each alone or in combination *(34)*. When these drugs were administered together, a significant increase in zidovudine area under the curve (AUC) of 33% was observed, along with a corresponding decrease in zidovudine clearance and zidovudine glucuronide (GZDV) formation. However, these changes are not expected to be clinically significant.

In contrast, a significant interaction has been observed when atovaquone is given in the presence of rifampin *(35)*. Atovaquone concentrations were reduced by more than 50%, which could potentially lead to therapeutic failure. Therefore, this combination should be avoided if possible. If rifampin is used as part of *Mycobacterium tuberculosis* therapy, clinicians may wish to consider switching to rifabutin (refer to discussion of rifamycins). Alternatively, atovaquone may be replaced by another antiparasitic, depending on patient tolerance and cost considerations.

## Renal Elimination

Renal elimination of lamivudine is impaired in the presence of TMP via competition for renal excretion in the organic cationic transport system of the kidneys. Lamivudine concentrations may increase significantly; however, dosage adjustment is not routinely indicated unless the patient also has renal dysfunction *(36)*. Because of the pharmacological similarities between lamivudine and emtricitabine, it is possible that TMP may exert a similar effect on emtricitabine excretion. Although this combination has not been studied, the clinical significance of such an effect would also likely be negligible.

## Antagonism

In vitro and in vivo observations suggest that zidovudine antagonizes the toxoplasmacidal effect of pyrimethamine-sulfadoxine *(37)*. Sulfadoxine may also inhibit the glucuronidation of zidovudine *(38)*, but this has not been tested in vitro with human liver microsomes, and the clinical significance of these data is unclear. Antiretroviral therapy is usually desirable along with antitoxoplasmosis treatment because it may help to improve immunologic function and subsequently contribute to recovery and improved clinical outcome. If clinicians are concerned about this interaction, zidovudine may be replaced with an alternative agent during treatment for toxoplasmosis encephalitis.

## Overlapping Toxicity

Many agents, such as TMP-SMX, dapsone, pyrimethamine, and primaquine, may cause adverse hematologic effects, including neutropenia, anemia, thrombocytopenia, and, rarely, hemolysis or methemoglobinemia *(39)*. Because these drugs often are administered for a prolonged duration for prophylaxis or suppression of infection, caution is warranted if concomitant administration of zidovudine or ganciclovir is desired *(40)*. Close monitoring is suggested if these drugs are to be coadministered; alternatively, different antiviral agents may be considered.

Pentamidine may be administered by inhalation or given parenterally to treat or prevent episodes of PCP. It is often reserved for severe or refractory cases because of the high frequency of associated toxicities. Systemic pentamidine exposure may cause serious adverse effects, including nephrotoxicity, pancreatitis, and changes in blood glucose. Many of these same side effects may occur with antivirals and antiretrovirals. Didanosine, stavudine, and zalcitabine have been associated with pancreatitis *(41)*, foscarnet and cidofovir can frequently cause nephrotoxicity, and hyperglycemic changes have been observed with protease inhibitor therapy *(42)*. Again, caution is warranted if any of these drugs are to be used in combination.

Finally, rash is a frequent side effect of TMP-SMX, sulfadiazine, dapsone, and clindamycin. The incidence of sulfonamide rash and hypersensitivity is significantly higher in the HIV population compared to healthy individuals and even to other immunosuppressed patient groups *(43)*. Unfortunately, rash is also commonly associated with other medications, including NNRTIs, amprenavir, abacavir, and probenecid. With the majority of these medications, the onset of rash falls within a similar time frame, usually within the first few weeks of therapy. Therefore, when clinically feasible, it may be helpful to initiate treatment with one class of drugs (e.g., antiparasitics) first and then add other regimens, such as combination antiretrovirals, at a subsequent date. In this manner, if a rash occurs, it may be easier to determine the causative agent and thus avoid unnecessary discontinuation of other needed medications.

## CASE STUDY 1

Jared is a 41-year-old flight attendant who works for a major international airline. He was diagnosed with HIV infection 6 years ago but was not interested in taking antiretrovirals because of concerns about side effects and confidentiality at work. When his CD4 count dropped below 200 cells a year and a half ago, he began prophylaxis for PCP, but he experienced severe allergic reactions to both TMP-SMX and dapsone. He also experienced a rash and nausea with atovaquone and was finally placed on monthly aerosolized pentamidine.

Four weeks ago, he returned from an extended work tour of Europe and Asia and developed symptoms of fever, malaise, and dry cough. He initially thought he had the flu, but his symptoms persisted, and he began experiencing chills, sweats, and exertional dyspnea. His symptoms progressed to the point at which he was unable to speak without stopping to rest, and his roommate rushed him to the emergency room on the weekend. On examination, Jared admitted that he had missed the last two or three doses of his monthly pentamidine appointments because of work, and he was shortly diagnosed with moderate-severe PCP. Jared was started on intravenous pentamidine and corticosteroids 3 days ago and has slowly started to improve. His physician would also like to initiate antiretroviral therapy. Given Jared's hectic work schedule and the potential for nonadherence, the physician would like to prescribe a once-daily regimen of 400 mg didanosine, 300 mg tenofovir, and 300 mg atazanavir/100 mg ritonavir.

Labs (normal range)

CD4: 22 cells/µL

AST: 36 (<34 U/L)

ALT: 45 (<39 U/L)

ALP: 130 (<109 U/L)

Amylase: 71 (<115 U/L)

LDH 352 (105–333 IU/L)

Albumin: 34 (38–50 g/L)

$PaO_2$: 67 mmHg (room air)

Viral ribonucleic acid (RNA): 310,000 copies/mL

Hemoglobin: 81 (140–180 g/L)

WBC: 2.3 $(4.0–11.0 \times 10^9/L)$

MCV: 81.7 (80–95 fL)

Platelets: 116 $(150–400 \times 10^9/L)$

ANC: 1.2 $(2.5–7.5 \times 10^9/L)$

Lymph: 0.7 $(1.5–3.5 \times 10^9/L)$

Creatinine: 102 (60–100 µmol/L)

### ASSESSMENT

Ideally, Jared should receive 21 days of pentamidine and prednisone to complete PCP treatment. Following this, he should receive secondary prophylaxis to prevent a recurrence of PCP. Initiation of highly active antiretroviral therapy (HAART) would improve Jared's immune function and may eventually allow discontinuation of secondary PCP prophylaxis if he experiences a significant and sustained immunological and virological response. The regimen the physician is interested in prescribing is an effective and convenient combination because it may be administered once daily and has a relatively low pill burden. However, there is an additive risk of pancreatitis between pentamidine and didanosine. This risk may be further increased as didanosine concentrations are elevated with concomitant tenofovir administration. To minimize the risk of pancreatic toxicity, the following approaches may be considered:

1. *Delay HAART.* To avoid overlapping toxicity, one strategy is to complete PCP therapy with pentamidine before initiating HAART. By minimizing the number of new medications started within the same time frame, clinicians will be better able identify the cause of any potential side effects that may occur. Also, if Jared delays HAART until his acute illness has improved, he may be in better condition to tolerate his antiretrovirals. Because of the extremely long half-life of pentamidine, it is recommended that therapy with a regimen including didanosine be delayed until 1 week after the completion of PCP treatment *(44)*.

2. *Change PCP treatment.* Another alternative for treating PCP is the combination of intravenous trimetrexate and oral leucovorin. In contrast to pentamidine, this regimen is not associated with pancreatoxic effects. However, treatment with trimetrexate may lead to other significant side effects, including neutropenia, thrombocytopenia, anemia, and transaminase and alkaline phosphatase elevations. Administration of trimetrexate requires concomitant use of an expensive rescue agent, leucovorin, and patients need to be closely monitored for toxicity.

3. *Change HAART regimen.* If HAART if considered urgently needed, an antiretroviral combination that minimizes overlapping toxicity may be selected. Because Jared is antiretroviral naïve, many options are available. Although dosage adjustment guidelines are available to manage the didanosine–tenofovir interaction (i.e., reducing didanosine to 250 mg daily), one may still wish to avoid use of a nucleoside component that has been associated with pancreatitis. Therefore, stavudine should also be avoided. Other nucleoside choices include zidovudine, lamivudine, abacavir, and emtricitabine.

### MANAGEMENT SUGGESTION

Based on the above considerations, one management strategy is to complete Jared's course of pentamidine and prednisone before initiating HAART. He has already started to respond to PCP treatment, so potent antiretroviral therapy may be started a few weeks later. This will reduce the number of concurrent drugs, minimize the risk of overlapping toxicities, and simplify medication adherence. Jared should be closely monitored for adverse effects of pentamidine, and his viral load and CD4 should be assessed within 4–6 weeks of starting his antiretrovirals to ensure that his regimen is working effectively.

## ANTIFUNGALS

Azole antifungals (ketoconazole, fluconazole, itraconazole) are commonly used for the management of oral-esophageal *Candida* infections in immunosuppressed HIV-positive patients *(6,45,46)*. These agents are highly efficacious and are usually well tolerated and convenient to take. Voriconazole is a newer triazole antifungal available in both injection and oral formulations for the treatment of invasive aspergillosis. It is also indicated for the treatment of refractory infections caused by *Scedosporium apiospermum* and *Fusarium* spp. and has demonstrated efficacy in the management of oropharyngeal candidiasis. Azoles may be administered for short courses of treatment or long term for chronic suppression of fungal infections in severely immunocompromised patients. In addition to oral antifungal therapy, individuals with advanced HIV disease may be receiving numerous antiretrovirals, as well as treatment or prophylaxis for other concurrent opportunistic infections *(47)*. Consequently, the potential exists for significant interactions between azoles and antiretrovirals, as well as other anti-infectives, particularly those used in the management of pulmonary tuberculosis (TB) or disseminated *Mycobacterium avium* complex (MAC) disease *(48)*. These interactions primarily involve alterations in drug absorption or metabolism via the CYP system (Table 3).

### Absorption Interactions

Optimal dissolution and absorption of ketoconazole and itraconazole capsules occur in an acidic gastric environment in which pH is less than 3.0 *(49)*. Therefore, these agents should not be administered simultaneously with regular didanosine tablets (Videx) because its alkaline buffer may significantly decrease azole absorption *(50–52)*. In a randomized, crossover, volunteer study, coadministration of 200 mg itraconazole and 300 mg didanosine resulted in undetectable itraconazole concentrations in all subjects. Itraconazole absorption was not impaired when administered alone *(53)*. Such interactions may be quite clinically significant; relapse of cryptococcal meningitis was reported in a 35-year-old HIV patient receiving 200 mg itraconazole twice daily and concurrent didanosine *(52)*.

These absorption interactions are now easily avoided with the advent of delayed-release didanosine capsules (Videx EC). These capsules contain enteric-coated (EC) beadlets of didanosine, which protect the active drug from degradation by stomach acid. Because this formulation does not contain an antacid buffer, gastric acidity is not affected, and hence Videx EC may be safely coadministered with itraconazole *(54)* and ketoconazole *(55)*.

In the rare circumstances when only the buffered didanosine tablet formulation is available (i.e., because of formulary, health maintenance organization, or third-party drug insurance restrictions), options to manage azole absorption interactions include the following:

- *Spacing.* Ketoconazole and itraconazole capsules should be administered 2 hours apart from buffered didanosine to avoid this interaction *(56).* However, it is important to remember that additional dosing times may be associated with greater patient inconvenience and possibly reduced adherence.

- *Changing antifungal agent.* In contrast to the other azoles, fluconazole does not require an acidic medium for optimal absorption *(49).* Itraconazole oral suspension also does not require acidic gastric pH for absorption. Therefore, another option is either to switch to the itraconazole suspension formulation or to change to fluconazole, both of which may be coadministered with buffered didanosine *(48).*

- *Changing antiretroviral.* Alternatively, one may also consider substituting didanosine with another antiretroviral agent. Again, issues such as prior antiretroviral experience, risk of cross-resistance, cost, adherence, and side effects need to be considered when attempting to substitute one drug in a current antiretroviral regimen.

### Metabolic Interactions

#### CYP System

As mentionedpreviously, all protease inhibitors and NNRTIs are CYP3A4 substrates and have enzyme-inducing or -inhibiting effects. Similarly, ketoconazole, itraconazole, and fluconazole are also substrates and inhibitors of CYP3A4, with fluconazole generally a less-potent inhibitor compared to ketoconazole and itraconazole *(57).* Fluconazole also may inhibit CYP2C9. Voriconazole is primarily metabolized by CYP2C19, as well as CYP2C9 and CYP3A4; it also inhibits these isoenzymes. The metabolism of voriconazole is saturable; hence, the drug exhibits nonlinear kinetics.

In addition, agents such as rifamycins and macrolides, which are frequently used for the management of other opportunistic infections, are also influenced by the CYP system. Therefore, the potential for significant interactions exists when any of these classes of drugs are coadministered. Metabolic interactions may often be managed by adjusting the dose or dosing interval of one or both agents. Management options may depend on factors such as the clinical consequences of the interaction, availability of therapeutic alternatives, patient convenience, and cost. Some examples include the following:

- *Dose adjustment.* The presence of ketoconazole increases indinavir AUC by 68%; to avoid indinavir-related toxicity such as nephrolithiasis, the product monograph recommends that indinavir dosage should be reduced to 600 mg every 8 hours with concomitant ketoconazole therapy *(58).* However, given the wide intersubject variability in indinavir trough levels and the importance of maintaining adequate indinavir concentrations *(14,59),* many clinicians may choose not to reduce the indinavir dose with ketoconazole unless nephrolithiasis occurs. Rifampin is a potent enzyme inducer and will significantly reduce plasma concentrations of many drugs that are metabolized. If rifampin is to be given to a patient who is also taking fluconazole or itraconazole for maintenance therapy of cryptococcal meningitis, empirically increasing the azole dose to compensate for an interaction may be desirable to minimize the serious consequences of a possible disease relapse.

- *Substitution of an alternative agent.* In some cases, metabolic interactions cannot be adequately managed by dose adjustments. For instance, nevirapine reduces ketoconazole concentrations by 63% *(60).* Patients who are stabilized on nevirapine should be prescribed an alternative antifungal if such therapy is required.

**Table 3**
**Antifungal Interactions**

| Primary drug | Interacting drug | Mechanism | Effects | Comments/management |
|---|---|---|---|---|
| Amphotericin | • Flucytosine | Amphotericin may decrease the renal elimination of flucytosine | Synergistic antifungal activity, but potential for increased flucytosine toxicity (163) | Monitor serum creatinine, urea, flucytosine levels |
| | • Nephrotoxins: aminoglycosides, cidofovir, foscarnet, intravenous pentamidine, high-dose acyclovir | Overlapping side-effect profiles | Additive nephrotoxicity if combined (74) | Cautious use of combinations is warranted; adjust dose and/or dosing interval of amphotericin as well as nephrotoxin(s) in renal failure; monitor serum creatinine, urea three times weekly |
| | • Zidovudine | Overlapping side-effect profiles | Potential for increased bone marrow toxicity with combination (40,127) | Monitor CBC weekly |
| Caspofungin | • Anticonvulsants (carbamazepine, phenytoin) | Increased caspofungin clearance, possibly via enzyme induction | Potential for significant reductions in caspofungin concentrations (81) | Consider increased maintenance dosage of 70 mg iv caspofungin daily |
| | • NNRTIs (efavirenz, nevirapine) | Increased caspofungin clearance, possibly via enzyme induction | Potential for significant reductions in caspofungin concentrations (81) | Consider increased maintenance dosage of 70 mg iv caspofungin daily |
| | • Protease inhibitor: nelfinavir | Increased caspofungin clearance, possibly via enzyme induction | Potential for significant reductions in caspofungin concentrations (81) | Consider increased maintenance dosage of 70 mg iv caspofungin daily |
| | • Rifampin | Increased caspofungin clearance, possibly via enzyme induction | 30% ↓ caspofungin trough levels (81) | Consider increased maintenance dosage of 70 mg iv caspofungin daily |
| Fluconazole | • NNRTIs: delavirdine, efavirenz | Drugs do not affect metabolism of each other | No significant effect on kinetics of NNRTIs (25–27) | May be coadministered without dosage adjustment |

| Drug | Mechanism | Effect | Recommendation |
|---|---|---|---|
| • NNRTI: nevirapine | Fluconazole may inhibit metabolism of nevirapine; nevirapine may increase clearance of fluconazole | Potential for increased nevirapine concentrations and/or decreased fluconazole concentrations | Monitor for nevirapine toxicity and antifungal efficacy |
| • Protease inhibitors: atazanavir, indinavir, lopinavir/ritonavir, nelfinavir, ritonavir, saquinavir | Fluconazole does not affect metabolism of listed protease inhibitors | No significant effect on kinetics of protease inhibitors (9,58,153,164,165) | May be coadministered without dosage adjustment |
| • Rifabutin | Fluconazole inhibits metabolism of rifabutin | 80% increase in rifabutin concentrations; cases of uveitis reported; no significant effect on fluconazole concentrations (166,167) | Do not exceed 300 mg rifabutin daily while on combination; monitor for signs and symptoms of uveitis |
| • Rifampin | Rifampin induces metabolism of fluconazole | 25% decrease in fluconazole AUC (168–170); relapse of cryptococcal meningitis reported in patients receiving combination (169) | Increase fluconazole dosage if necessary and monitor for fluconazole efficacy (e.g., adequate antifungal prophylaxis or suppression) |
| • Zidovudine | Fluconazole inhibits the metabolism of zidovudine to its glucuronide metabolite | 74% increase in zidovudine AUC when given with 400 mg fluconazole (63) | Clinical significance unclear; interaction may be less significant with lower doses of fluconazole; monitor for zidovudine-related toxicity such as neutropenia and anemia; ketoconazole or itraconazole does not affect zidovudine kinetics |
| Itraconazole • Didanosine | Decreased itraconazole capsule absorption because of increase in gastric pH | Undetectable itraconazole concentrations (52,117) | Give itraconazole capsules 2 hours before or after didanosine; alternatively, use itraconazole oral suspension |
| • NNRTIs: delavirdine, nevirapine, efavirenz | Itraconazole may inhibit metabolism of listed NNRTIs; potential for nevirapine and efavirenz to increase itraconazole metabolism | Potential for increased NNRTI concentrations and/or decreased itraconazole concentrations | Clinical significance unknown; monitor for antiretroviral toxicity and antifungal efficacy |

*Continued on next page*

**Table 3 (*Continued*)**
**Antifungal Interactions**

| Primary drug | Interacting drug | Mechanism | Effects | Comments/management |
|---|---|---|---|---|
| | • Indinavir | Itraconazole inhibits indinavir metabolism | Increased indinavir concentrations | Use 600 mg indinavir every 8 hours with 200 mg itraconazole twice daily (58) |
| | • Protease inhibitors: amprenavir, saquinavir | Itraconazole may inhibit metabolism of listed protease inhibitors | Potential for increased protease inhibitor concentrations | Clinical significance unknown; monitor for antiretroviral efficacy and toxicity |
| | • Lopinavir/ritonavir | Lopinavir/ritonavir inhibits itraconazole metabolism | Potential for increased itraconazole concentrations (153) | Avoid itraconazole doses >200 mg per day |
| | • Protease inhibitor: ritonavir | Ritonavir inhibits metabolism of itraconazole | Potential for large (threefold) increase in itraconazole AUC (9) | Caution with combination of ritonavir and itraconazole; may require dosage reduction of itraconazole |
| | • Rifabutin | Rifabutin induces metabolism of itraconazole, and itraconazole may inhibit metabolism of rifabutin | 74% decreased AUC, 71% decreased $C_{max}$ of itraconazole (171); uveitis also reported with combination (172) | Avoid combination; use an alternate antifungal if necessary |
| | • Rifampin | Rifampin induces metabolism of itraconazole | Undetectable concentrations of itraconazole; may remain undetectable until 3–5 days after rifampin discontinuation (173) | Avoid combination |
| Ketoconazole | • Amprenavir | Amprenavir inhibits metabolism of ketoconazole, and vice versa | 32% increased amprenavir AUC, 44% increase in ketoconazole AUC (174) | Clinical significance unclear; monitor for amprenavir and ketoconazole toxicity; dose reduction of ketoconazole (to <400 mg/day) may be required if symptomatic (175) |

| Drug | Mechanism | Effect | Recommendation |
|---|---|---|---|
| • Didanosine | Decreased ketoconazole absorption because of increased gastric pH | May decrease ketoconazole concentrations (176) | Give ketoconazole 2 hours before or after didanosine |
| • Isoniazid | Isoniazid induces ketoconazole metabolism | Decreased ketoconazole concentrations (177); higher doses of ketoconazole may be needed | Monitor for efficacy of ketoconazole (e.g., adequate antifungal prophylaxis or suppression) |
| • Indinavir | Ketoconazole inhibits indinavir metabolism | 68% increase in indinavir AUC (58) | Reduce indinavir dose to 600 mg every 8 hours |
| • Lopinavir/ ritonavir | Lopinavir/ritonavir inhibits ketoconazole metabolism. | 3-fold increase in ketoconazole AUC (153) | Avoid ketoconazole doses >200 mg per day |
| • Nelfinavir | Ketoconazole inhibits nelfinavir metabolism | 35% increase in nelfinavir AUC (178) | No dosage adjustment required |
| • Nevirapine | Nevirapine induces ketoconazole metabolism; ketoconazole inhibits nevirapine metabolism (to a lesser extent) | Ketoconazole levels significantly reduced (63% reduction AUC, 40% reduction $C_{max}$); 15–20% increase in nevirapine concentrations (60) | Consider alternative antifungal if patient is stabilized on nevirapine |
| • Rifampin | Rifampin increases ketoconazole metabolism; ketoconazole may possibly decrease rifampin absorption | >80% reduction in ketoconazole concentrations (179); reduced concentration of rifampin noted in one study (may explain apparent ketoconazole and rifampin failure) (180) | Avoid combination if possible; consider using alternative rifamycin (e.g., rifabutin) and/or alternate antifungal such as fluconazole |
| • Saquinavir | Ketoconazole inhibits saquinavir metabolism | 1.5-fold increase in saquinavir AUC (181) | Dosage adjustment not necessary |
| • Saquinavir + ritonavir | Ketoconazole may inhibit p-glycoprotein-mediated transport of saquinavir and ritonavir | Increased plasma and CSF concentrations of both saquinavir and ritonavir (73) | Clinical significance of combination unknown |

*Uridine Diphosphate-Glucuronosyl Transferase*

In humans, zidovudine is transformed by uridine diphosphate-glucuronosyl transferase (UDPGT) to its major metabolite, GZDV. In vitro, the azoles have demonstrated inhibitory effects on zidovudine metabolism, possibly by lowering UDPGT activity and acting as competitive substrates for UDPGT-binding sites *(61,62)*. In a randomized, two-period, two-treatment, crossover study, 12 HIV-infected men received either zidovudine (200 mg every 8 hours) alone or in combination with 400 mg fluconazole daily for 7 days *(63)*. When the two agents were coadministered, significant decreases in the total oral clearance of zidovudine and the metabolism to GZDV were observed, and the molar ratio of GZDV to zidovudine recovered in the urine was reduced by 34%. In addition, the AUC of zidovudine was increased by 74%, and its half-life increased by 128% in the presence of fluconazole. The clinical significance of this interaction is unclear; the authors suggested that a lesser impact on zidovudine metabolism may be observed with lower, more commonly used doses of fluconazole (e.g., 100–200 mg daily for prophylaxis of fungal infections) because such inhibitory effects are usually dose dependent. Because the clinical impact of this interaction has not been fully defined, hematologic parameters should be closely monitored when these drugs are coadministered. If a patient begins to exhibit signs and symptoms of zidovudine toxicity, such as extreme fatigue, malaise, anemia, or neutropenia, one may consider replacing zidovudine with another antiretroviral agent.

*P-Glycoprotein*

P-Glycoprotein is an adenosine triphosphate (ATP)-dependent efflux membrane transporter present in tissues, including the epithelial cells of the gastrointestinal tract, liver, and kidney; the blood–brain barrier; and in subsets of $CD4^+$ T lymphocytes. P-Glycoprotein can actively transport drug from cells, resulting in decreased drug absorption, enhanced elimination into bile and urine, and prevention of drug entry into the central nervous system. P-Glycoprotein has broad substrate specificity and appears to play a role in the transport of many natural substances and xenobiotics. It is now increasingly recognized as having a role in pharmacokinetics of many medications, including protease inhibitors *(59,64–66)*. For example, the oral bioavailability of saquinavir is significantly limited by many factors, such as the presence of CYP3A4 in the gastrointestinal tract and liver, as well as P-glycoprotein, which may transport the absorbed drug back into the intestinal lumen *(67)*. MDR1 (multidrug resistance 1; the substrate that encodes P-glycoprotein) genotype has been associated with differences in pharmacokinetic disposition and antiviral dynamic response to various protease inhibitors *(68–70)*.

Furthermore, P-glycoprotein may play a significant role in limiting the penetration of many protease inhibitors into the brain and other tissue compartments *(70,71)*. Consequently, an area of current intense interest centers on the potential use of P-glycoprotein inhibitors to augment protease inhibitor concentrations in various compartments. Preliminary data suggest that this may indeed be possible. It was observed that addition of ketoconazole, a potent P-glycoprotein inhibitor *(72)*, to patients stabilized on a combination of ritonavir and saquinavir resulted in increased cerebrospinal fluid (CSF) and plasma concentrations of both protease inhibitors *(73)*. The clinical significance of this is still unclear, and the usual considerations regarding the addition of a new agent to an already complex regimen must be taken into account. A complete review of transport proteins in provided in Chapter 3.

### Amphotericin B and Flucytosine

Amphotericin B and flucytosine are antifungal agents that are usually reserved for life-threatening, systemic fungal infections such as cryptococcal meningitis, aspergillosis, and histoplasmosis. These agents are eliminated renally and are associated with potentially significant side effects. In addition, amphotericin B must be administered parenterally. Interactions with these two agents are primarily pharmacodynamic *(74)* (Table 3).

#### Overlapping Toxicity

Amphotericin B is associated with nephrotoxicity, hypokalemia, and blood dyscrasias. Concomitant administration with other potentially nephrotoxic agents, such as aminoglycosides, intravenous pentamidine, foscarnet, cidofovir, or high-dose acyclovir should be avoided whenever possible *(6,29,74)*. Flucytosine may cause hematologic toxicity, and caution is recommended when patients are receiving treatment with other hematotoxic drugs, such as zidovudine or ganciclovir *(74)*.

#### Decreased Renal Function Requiring Dosage Adjustment

Amphotericin B can often cause nephrotoxicity, especially with high doses and long-term administration. Patients receiving this drug should have their renal function routinely monitored. Significant declines in renal function may necessitate the dosage adjustment of other renally eliminated medications, such as flucytosine, antiviral agents, and nucleoside reverse transcriptase inhibitors (NRTIs).

#### Synergistic/Antagonistic Antifungal Activity

There is some evidence of a synergistic antifungal effect between amphotericin and flucytosine. In a randomized, controlled trial for the initial treatment of acquired immunodeficiency syndrome (AIDS)-associated cryptococcal meningitis, the addition of flucytosine to amphotericin B was associated with an increased rate of CSF sterilization and decreased mortality at 2 weeks, as compared with regimens used in previous studies *(75)*. However, as mentioned in Overlapping Toxicity, amphotericin B may reduce the renal clearance of flucytosine; therefore, patients receiving this combination should be closely monitored for renal dysfunction and blood dyscrasias. Periodic measurement of flucytosine plasma concentrations may also be helpful.

Theoretically, amphotericin B and azoles are antagonistic, but this has not been demonstrated conclusively *(76–79)*. In one case, a non-HIV-infected woman with cryptococcal meningitis was successfully treated with a combination of fluconazole and amphotericin B. She had not responded to amphotericin B alone and could not tolerate amphotericin B plus flucytosine *(80)*. If amphotericin B is coadministered with an azole, careful monitoring of safety and efficacy parameters is recommended.

### Caspofungin

Caspofungin is an echinocandin antifungal administered systemically for the treatment of *Candida* esophagitis and refractory invasive aspergillosis. Caspofungin undergoes *N*-acetylation and hydrolysis, as well as spontaneous chemical degradation to an open-ring chemical compound. Caspofungin does not exhibit enzyme-inhibiting or

-inducing properties. It is considered a poor substrate for CYP enzymes and is not a P-glycoprotein substrate *(81)*. Nevertheless, caspofungin may be susceptible to interactions with certain enzyme-inducing drugs.

In healthy volunteers, coadministration of caspofungin and rifampin led to a 30% reduction in caspofungin trough levels. Furthermore, regression analyses of pharmacokinetic data involving small numbers of patients suggested that caspofungin levels may be reduced in the presence of efavirenz, nevirapine, nelfinavir, phenytoin, dexamethasone, and carbamazepine *(81)*. Although these data require substantiation through further controlled interaction studies, the manufacturer recommends that an increased caspofungin dose be considered when coadministration with any of the aforementioned inducers is necessary.

## ANTIMYCOBACTERIALS

Although infection with MAC has declined in the HIV-infected population *(3,5)*, the frequency of *M. tuberculosis* infections, including multidrug-resistant tuberculosis, has been increasing *(82–85)*. Factors contributing to this increase include nonadherence to treatment or prevention programs and an accelerating or amplifying effect of HIV infection. Disease caused by *M. tuberculosis* or MAC usually requires lengthy treatment with multiple agents *(6,86)*. Drugs often used in combination to treat mycobacterial infections include macrolides, rifamycins, quinolones, isoniazid, ethambutol, and pyrazinamide. These agents are associated with pharmacokinetic interactions of absorption and metabolism, as well as pharmacodynamic interactions of overlapping toxicities.

The potential for interactions increases significantly if patients are also receiving combination therapy for HIV infection. Certain antimycobacterials can significantly decrease protease inhibitor and NNRTI drug concentrations, which may lead to suboptimal viral suppression and possible viral resistance. Conversely, antimycobacterial therapy may be compromised by concomitant antiretrovirals. Patients with HIV may already be at risk of antimycobacterial malabsorption *(87–89)*, and this has occasionally been associated with clinical failure and development of drug resistance *(90)*. Further lowering of drug levels secondary to induction by nevirapine or efavirenz may increase the potential for breakthrough of pulmonary TB, which has serious infectious implications. On the other hand, elevated antimycobacterial concentrations may increase the risk of dose-related toxicities if appropriate dosage adjustments are not made.

Therefore, in addition to factors such as individual CD4 count, viral load, stage of HIV disease, previous antiretroviral history, pathogen sensitivity profile, and antimycobacterial absorption, clinicians must consider the potential for interactions between the different classes of drugs when treating patients with concurrent HIV and mycobacterial infection *(91)*.

### Rifamycins

Rifamycins are often key components of antimycobacterial regimens. Interactions with rifamycins are primarily pharmacokinetic or pharmacodynamic.

#### Metabolic Interactions

Rifamycins are potent inducers of the CYP enzyme system and may dramatically decrease protease inhibitor and NNRTI concentrations. Rifampin is the most potent inducer of CYP3A4, followed by rifapentine; rifabutin is the least-potent inducer *(91)*. Rifampin also induces glucuronyl transferase activity *(92)*. In addition, antiretroviral agents may also increase rifamycin concentrations and thus increase the risk of toxicity. These principles have been reviewed extensively in the literature *(29,91,93,94)*. Recommendations on treatment of concomitant HIV and tuberculosis infection have been published *(86,94–96)*. Options to manage potential rifamycin pharmacokinetic interactions include the following:

- *Select a rifamycin with less potent effects on the CYP system.* Rifampin induces enzyme activity to such an extent that the doses of many susceptible antiretrovirals usually cannot be increased sufficiently to compensate for the interaction. This effect of rifampin likely exists with both daily and intermittent dosing *(91)*. In clinical trials, 6-month rifabutin-containing regimens were found to be as safe and effective as similar regimens including rifampin *(86)*. In addition, rifabutin may offer other advantages compared to rifampin when used in the HIV-infected population. These potential advantages include more reliable absorption in patients with advanced HIV disease, better tolerance in those with rifampin-induced hepatotoxicity, and potential for less-significant drug interactions because rifabutin is a less-potent enzyme inducer *(86)*. Therefore, rifabutin may be substituted for rifampin. The usual dosage of rifabutin is 300 mg daily but may be reduced to 150 mg daily depending on the concurrent antiretroviral agent used (Table 4).
- *Adjust dosage of rifamycin or antiretroviral.* The NRTIs tenofovir and enfuvirtide are not substrates of CYP3A4 and thus may be given at their usual dosages with rifamycins *(96)*. With protease inhibitors and NNRTIs, interactions with rifamycins may often be managed by appropriate dosage adjustment. Protease and NNRTI agents that may be coadministered with full or adjusted-dose rifabutin include amprenavir, fosamprenavir, atazanavir, indinavir, nelfinavir, ritonavir, efavirenz, and nevirapine. Rifabutin may be coadministered with ritonavir-boosted protease inhibitor combinations, including lopinavir/ritonavir. Preliminary data suggest that rifabutin may be safely administered at a dose of 150 mg every 3 days to patients stabilized on a combination of 400 mg saquinavir plus 400 mg ritonavir twice daily *(97)*. In addition, the potential impact of dosage manipulation on patient adherence should be carefully considered. This in turn may depend on the drug formulations available, existing pill burden and dosing schedule, and cost. For instance, to adjust adequately for the interaction between indinavir and rifabutin, indinavir should be increased to 1 g every 8 hours, and rifabutin should be decreased to 150 mg daily or 300 mg three times per week *(58,96)*. This can be done with no additional dosing times and minimal increase in pill burden (i.e., three additional 200-mg indinavir capsules and one less 150-mg rifabutin capsule per day). Some antiretroviral combinations that may possibly be administered with rifampin include efavirenz, nevirapine, ritonavir, or dual protease inhibitor combinations of ritonavir/saquinavir or lopinavir/ritonavir (at therapeutic doses of 400 mg of each protease inhibitor rather than boosted doses) plus two NRTIs or triple NRTI regimens *(95,96)*.
- *Change antiretroviral agent.* In other situations, metabolic interactions cannot be adequately compensated by dosage adjustment. For example, delavirdine concentrations are virtually undetectable in the presence of rifampin *(98)*. With rifabutin, delavirdine concentrations are decreased by 50 to 60% *(99)*. Cox et al. *(100)* attempted to determine whether higher doses of delavirdine were able to compensate for the inductive effects of rifabutin. Even with a median delavirdine dose of 600 mg three times daily (range 400 mg to 1 g three times daily), trough concentrations were often still not adequate, and rifabutin concentrations were significantly elevated *(100)*. Thus, the investigators concluded that this combination should be avoided because of lower-than-normal delavirdine concentrations and the possibility of toxicity related to increased rifabutin exposure. Resistance may develop extremely rapidly with NNRTIs *(101,102)*; therefore, it is imperative to avoid concomitant therapy with agents such as rifamycins that may reduce NNRTI concentrations to subtherapeutic concentrations.

**Table 4**
**Mycobacterial Interactions**

| Primary drug | Interacting drug | Mechanism | Effects | Comments/management |
|---|---|---|---|---|
| Azithromycin | Nelfinavir | Nelfinavir inhibits azithromycin metabolism | Azithromycin AUC and $C_{max}$ increased | Monitor for dose-related azithromycin toxicity, such as hearing loss or elevated liver function tests (182) |
| | Rifabutin | Azithromycin does not inhibit rifabutin metabolism | No pharmacokinetic interaction noted with combination; However, increased incidence of neutropenia observed compared to rifabutin alone (113) | Monitor for development of neutropenia, especially within first 2 weeks of combination therapy |
| | Zidovudine | Lack of azithromycin effect on metabolism of zidovudine | No significant effect on zidovudine pharmacokinetics (183) | No dosage adjustment recommended |
| Clarithromycin | Amprenavir | Amprenavir decreases formation of clarithromycin active metabolite, presumably via inhibition of CYP3A4; clarithromycin may inhibit clearance of amprenavir via inhibition of CYP3A4 | Multidose trial in healthy volunteers using 1200 mg amprenavir bid + 500 mg clarithromycin bid: 18% increase amprenavir AUC, 10% decrease clarithromycin $C_{max}$, $C_{max}$, 35% decrease AUC of clarithromycin-OH metabolite (184) | No dosage adjustment necessary for either drug |
| | Atazanavir | Atazanavir inhibits formation of active clarithromycin metabolite | Clarithromycin AUC increased 94%, clarithromycin-OH AUC decreased by 70% (165) | Recommend 50% dosage reduction of clarithromycin because QTC prolongations have been reported with elevated clarithromycin levels; consider alternate agent for infections other than MAC because clarithromycin metabolite levels reduced (165) |
| | Delavirdine | Delavirdine decreases formation of clarithromycin active metabolite, presumably via inhibition of CYP3A4 | Clarithromycin concentrations doubled (25); inhibition of clarithromycin-OH metabolite observed (data on file, Pharmacia & Upjohn); no effect on delavirdine levels | Inhibition of clarithromycin-OH metabolite may result in reduced Gram-negative (including Haemophilus influenzae) activity (data on file, Pharmacia & Upjohn); adjust dosage of clarithromycin in renal impairment |

| Drug | Mechanism | Effect | Recommendation |
|---|---|---|---|
| Didanosine | Clarithromycin does not affect didanosine absorption or metabolism | No effect of clarithromycin on didanosine pharmacokinetics (*111*); didanosine buffer should not affect clarithromycin absorption | Drugs may be administered together |
| Efavirenz | Efavirenz increases clearance of clarithromycin parent drug via CYP3A4 induction and increases formation of clarithromycin active metabolite; clarithromycin may inhibit clearance of efavirenz via inhibition of CYP3A4 | 39% decrease in clarithromycin AUC, 34% increase in clarithromycin-OH AUC; 11% increase in efavirenz AUC observed; however, increased incidence of rash observed; no significant interaction with azithromycin (*185*) | Clinical significance unknown; however, because of increased incidence of rash observed, may wish to consider alternatives to clarithromycin, such as azithromycin |
| Indinavir | Metabolism of both drugs is inhibited because of effects on CYP3A4 | 29% increase indinavir AUC, 53% increase clarithromycin AUC (*58*) | No dose modification necessary |
| Lopinavir/ritonavir | Decreased clarithromycin metabolism via inhibition of CYP3A4 and reduced formation of clarithromycin active metabolite | Potential for increased clarithromycin and decreased clarithromycin metabolite levels (*153*) | Reduce clarithromycin dose only if renal failure; inhibition of clarithromycin-OH metabolite may result in reduced Gram-negative (including *H. influenzae*) activity |
| Nevirapine | Nevirapine increases clearance of clarithromycin parent drug via CYP3A4 induction and increases formation of clarithromycin active metabolite | Interaction study of nevirapine 200 mg bid + clarithromycin 500 mg bid: significant reduction in clarithromycin concentrations with 29.5% decrease in AUC, 20.8% decrease in $C_{max}$, 46% decrease in $C_{min}$; also 27% increase in AUC of clarithromycin-OH metabolite (*186*) | Because increase in metabolite is of approximately the same magnitude as decrease in parent drug, dosage adjustment of clarithromycin likely not necessary with nevirapine |
| Rifabutin | Rifabutin increases clearance of clarithromycin via CYP3A4 induction; clarithromycin decreases rifabutin metabolism via inhibition of CYP3A4 | Significant bidirectional interaction observed: 44% decrease in clarithromycin AUC, 57% increase clarithromycin-OH metabolite AUC, along with 99% increase in rifabutin AUC and 375% increase in AUC of rifabutin metabolite (*112*) | Increased frequency of adverse events (including gastrointestinal and neutropenia) noted with combination; monitor for clinical efficacy of clarithromycin and dose-related rifabutin toxicities (e.g., myalgia, uveitis, neutropenia); may also consider switching to azithromycin, which has no enzyme-inhibiting effects |

*Continued on next page*

**Table 4 (Continued)**
**Mycobacterial Interactions**

| Primary drug | Interacting drug | Mechanism | Effects | Comments/management |
|---|---|---|---|---|
| | Rifampin | Rifampin increases clarithromycin clearance via CYP3A4 induction | 87% decrease in clarithromycin AUC with concomitant rifampin (187) | Clinical significance unclear; may consider changing to azithromycin |
| | Ritonavir | Ritonavir decreases clarithromycin metabolism via inhibition of CYP3A4 and reduces formation of clarithromycin active metabolite | 77% increase in AUC of clarithromycin; reduce dose only if renal failure; inhibition of clarithromycin-OH metabolite (188) | Reduce clarithromycin dose only if renal failure; inhibition of clarithromycin-OH metabolite may result in reduced Gram-negative (including *H. influenzae*) activity |
| | Saquinavir | Metabolism of both drugs is inhibited because of effects on CYP3A4 | 177% increase in saquinavir-sgc AUC; 45% increase in clarithromycin AUC (189) | Dose adjustment likely not needed given the wide therapeutic index of saquinavir |
| | Zalcitabine | Clarithromycin does not affect zalcitabine metabolism | No clinically significant interaction (190) | Drugs may be coadministered |
| | Zidovudine | Clarithromycin reduces zidovudine absorption (presumed) | 41% decrease in $C_{max}$, 25% decrease in AUC of zidovudine when coadministered with clarithromycin (191); however, in vitro phosphorylation of zidovudine not affected by clarithromycin (192) | May wish to separate doses of zidovudine and clarithromycin by 4 h, but because clinical significance of this interaction is unclear, such spacing may not be necessary |
| Ethambutol | Aluminum salts | Decreased ethambutol absorption | 10% decrease in AUC, 28% decrease in $C_{max}$ of ethambutol (118,119) | Separate aluminum salts from ethambutol by at least 2 hours |
| | Didanosine | Didanosine buffer may interfere with ethambutol absorption | Potential for decreased ethambutol concentrations | Clinical significance unclear; avoid concomitant administration if possible |
| Ethionamide | Protease inhibitors, delavirdine, azoles, clarithromycin | Listed drugs may inhibit metabolism of ethionamide | Potential for increased ethionamide concentrations (91) | Clinical significance unclear; monitor for development of ethionamide toxicity |
| Isoniazid | Aluminum salts | Decreased isoniazid absorption | Up to 19% decrease in isoniazid AUC. (39,193) | Separate aluminum salts from isoniazid by at least 2 hours |

160

| Drug | Interacting drug | Mechanism | Effect | Recommendation |
|---|---|---|---|---|
| | Didanosine | No effect of didanosine buffer on isoniazid absorption | The antacids in two didanosine placebo tablets had no significant effect on the plasma pharmacokinetics of a single oral dose of 300 mg isoniazid administered to 12 healthy volunteers (194) | These results suggest that isoniazid bioavailability will be unaffected by the antacids in didanosine tablets when the two medications are administered simultaneously to HIV-seropositive patients; monitor for peripheral neuropathy |
| | Indinavir | Indinavir does not inhibit indinavir metabolism | No evidence of pharmacokinetic interaction (120) | Combination may be coadministered |
| | Neurotoxins (e.g., didanosine, stavudine, zalcitabine, vincristine, dapsone, ethambutol) | Overlapping toxicity profile | Increased risk of peripheral neuropathy | Consider administration of 25–50 mg pyridoxine daily with isoniazid; monitor for signs and symptoms of peripheral neuropathy |
| | Rifampin | Overlapping toxicity profile | Increased risk hepatoxocitiy (195) | Monitor for signs and symptoms of hepatotoxicity |
| | Zalcitabine | Lactose in zalcitabine formulation may form hydrazone derivatives with isoniazid | Potential for decreased isoniazid absorption (196) | Separate doses by at least 1 hour |
| Quinolones | Antacids, didanosine, iron, aluminum, calcium zinc, magnesium sucralfate, enteral feeds, vitamins with minerals | Decreased quinolone absorption because of formation of chelation complexes with di-trivalent cations | 98% decrease in ciprofloxacin AUC | Best to avoid combination; if necessary, administer listed products 6 hours before or 2 hours after quinolones (56); monitor for quinolone efficacy (e.g., clinical status) |
| Rifabutin | Amprenavir/ fosamprenavir | Rifabutin increases clearance of amprenavir via CYP3A4 induction; amprenavir decreases rifabutin metabolism via inhibition of CYP3A4 | 14% decrease in amprenavir concentrations, three- to sixfold increase in rifabutin $C_{min}$ | Decrease dose of rifabutin to 150 mg daily or 300 mg three times per week to avoid toxicity (97,179,197) |
| | Amprenavir/ fosamprenavir plus ritonavir | Potential for increased rifabutin concentrations secondary to ritonavir inhibition | | Reduce rifabutin dose to 150 mg every 2 days or three times per week (96) |

*Continued on next page*

161

**Table 4 (Continued)**
**Mycobacterial Interactions**

| Primary drug | Interacting drug | Mechanism | Effects | Comments/management |
|---|---|---|---|---|
| | Atazanavir | Rifabutin increases clearance of atazanavir via CYP3A4 induction; atazanavir decreases rifabutin metabolism via inhibition of CYP3A4 | No change in atazanavir levels with rifabutin 150 mg daily, 2.5-fold increase in rifabutin and metabolite exposure (vs standard 300-mg dose) (198) | Reduce rifabutin dosage by at least 75% (i.e., maximum 150 mg every 2 days or 3 times/ week); monitor for adverse events and further decrease rifabutin dose if necessary (165) |
| | Atazanavir plus ritonavir | Potential for increased rifabutin concentrations secondary to ritonavir inhibition | | Reduce rifabutin dose to 150 mg every 2 days or three times per week (96) |
| | Clarithromycin | Rifabutin increases clearance of clarithromycin via CYP3A4 induction; clarithromycin decreases rifabutin metabolism via inhibition of CYP3A4 | Significant bidirectional interaction observed: 44% decrease in clarithromycin AUC, 57% increase of clarithromycin-OH metabolite AUC, along with 99% increase rifabutin AUC and 375% increase AUC of rifabutin metabolite (112) | Increased frequency of adverse events (including gastrointestinal and neutropenia) noted with combination; monitor for clinical efficacy of clarithromycin and dose-related rifabutin toxicities (e.g., myalgia, uveitis, neutropenia); may also consider switching to azithromycin, which has no enzyme inhibiting effects |
| | Delavirdine | Rifabutin increases clearance of delavirdine via CYP3A4 induction; delavirdine decreases rifabutin metabolism via inhibition of CYP3A4 | 50–60% decrease in delavirdine concentrations (99) (not adequately compensated with 600 mg tid dose); also >200% increase in rifabutin AUC (100) | Avoid concomitant use |
| | Didanosine | It has been suggested that didanosine may undergo hepatic metabolism; rifabutin is an inducer of drug metabolism | Phase I, open-label, pharmacokinetic, and safety drug interaction study between 300–600 mg rifabutin and didanosine ($N = 12$); no statistically significant differences in $C_{max}$, AUC, half-life of either drug when coadministered; also, no significant changes in laboratory values or electrocardiograms (199) | Based on the safety and pharmacokinetic assessments, rifabutin did not appear to interact with didanosine; drugs may be coadministered |

162

| | | | |
|---|---|---|---|
| Efavirenz | Rifabutin may increase clearance of efavirenz via CYP3A4 induction; efavirenz may increase or decrease metabolism of rifabutin | 38% decrease in rifabutin AUC (200) | Increase rifabutin to 450 mg/day or 600 mg three times per week with concomitant efavirenz (86,91,96) |
| Fluconazole | Fluconazole inhibits metabolism of rifabutin | 80% increase in rifabutin concentrations; cases of uveitis reported; no significant effect on fluconazole concentrations (166,167) | Do not exceed 300 mg/day rifabutin while on combination; monitor for signs and symptoms of uveitis |
| Indinavir | Rifabutin increases clearance of indinavir via CYP3A4 induction; indinavir decreases rifabutin metabolism via inhibition of CYP3A4 | Interaction study of half-dose rifabutin + indinavir: 155% increase in rifabutin AUC, 33% decrease in indinavir AUC (58) | Thus, increase indinavir to 1000 mg every 8 hours and reduce rifabutin to 150 mg daily or 300 mg three times per week (96) |
| Indinavir plus ritonavir | Potential for increased rifabutin concentrations secondary to ritonavir inhibition | | Reduce rifabutin dose to 150 mg every 2 days or three times per week (96) |
| Itraconazole | Rifabutin induces metabolism of itraconazole, and itraconazole may inhibit metabolism of rifabutin | 74% decrease in AUC, 71% decrease in $C_{max}$ of itraconazole (171); uveitis also reported with combination (172) | Avoid combination; use an alternate antifungal if necessary |
| Lopinavir/ritonavir | Lopinavir/ritonavir inhibits metabolism of rifabutin | Rifabutin $C_{max}$, AUC, and $C_{min}$ increased significantly (153) | Reduce rifabutin dosage by at least 75% (i.e., maximum 150 mg every 2 days or three times/week); monitor for adverse events and further decrease rifabutin dose if necessary |
| Nelfinavir | Rifabutin increases clearance of nelfinavir via CYP3A4 induction; nelfinavir decreases rifabutin metabolism via inhibition of CYP3A4 | 32% decrease in nelfinavir AUC, threefold increase in rifabutin AUC (178) | Reduce rifabutin dose to 150 mg daily or 300 mg three times per week; increase nelfinavir to 1000 mg every 8 hours (96) or possibly 1250 mg bid (201) |
| Nevirapine | Rifabutin increases clearance of nevirapine via CYP3A4 induction | 16% decrease in nevirapine AUC (26) | Administer rifabutin at 300 mg daily or three times per week (96) |
| Saquinavir | Rifabutin increases clearance of saquinavir via CYP3A4 induction | 40% decrease in saquinavir AUC (202) | Avoid combination if using saquinavir as sole protease inhibitor |

*Continued on next page*

**Table 4 (Continued)**
**Mycobacterial Interactions**

| Primary drug | Interacting drug | Mechanism | Effects | Comments/management |
|---|---|---|---|---|
| | Saquinavir/ritonavir | Potential for inhibition of rifabutin metabolism via CYP3A4 | Adequate rifabutin concentrations achieved when administered 300 mg weekly or 150 mg every 3 days to patients stabilized on 400 mg ritonavir /400 mg saquinavir bid (97) | Administer 150 mg rifabutin every 2 days or three times per week (96) |
| | Ritonavir | Ritonavir decreases rifabutin metabolism via inhibition of CYP3A4 | 400% increase in rifabutin AUC, risk of toxicity (9) | *Avoid combination* if possible; otherwise, reduce rifabutin dose to 150 mg every 2 days or three times per week (96) |
| | Zidovudine | Lack of significant effect on zidovudine pharmacokinetics | Except for a statistically significant decrease (28%) in the terminal half-life of zidovudine, concurrent administration of rifabutin had no statistically significant effects on zidovudine plasma and urine pharmacokinetic parameters (152) | Treatment with rifabutin is unlikely to influence the effectiveness of treating HIV-infected patients with zidovudine because of any pharmacokinetic interaction between these drugs |
| Rifampin | Amprenavir | Rifampin increases clearance of amprenavir via CYP3A4 induction | 81% decrease in AUC and 91% decrease in $C_{min}$ of amprenavir (197) | *Avoid combination* |
| | Atovaquone | Rifampin induces atovaquone clearance | >50% reduction of atovaquone AUC, >30% increase in rifampin AUC (35) | *Avoid combination* because of potential therapeutic failure of atovaquone |
| | Clarithromycin | Rifampin increases clarithromycin clearance via CYP3A4 induction | 87% decrease in clarithromycin AUC with concomitant rifampin (187) | Clinical significance unclear; may consider changing to azithromycin |
| | Delavirdine | Rifampin increases clearance of delavirdine via CYP3A4 induction | Virtually undetectable delavirdine concentrations (98) | *Combination contraindicated* |
| | Efavirenz | Rifampin increases clearance of efavirenz via CYP3A4 induction | 26% decrease in AUC, 20% decrease in $C_{max}$ of efavirenz; clinical significance unknown (203) | Rifampin dosage adjustment not necessary; increase dose of efavirenz to 800 mg daily (96,103) |

| Drug | Mechanism | Effect | Recommendation |
|---|---|---|---|
| Fluconazole | Rifampin increases clearance of fluconazole via CYP3A4 induction | 25% decrease in fluconazole AUC (168–170); relapse of cryptococcal meningitis reported in patients receiving combination (169) | Increase fluconazole dosage if necessary and monitor for fluconazole efficacy (e.g., adequate antifungal prophylaxis or suppression) |
| Indinavir | Rifampin increases clearance of indinavir via CYP3A4 induction | Indinavir concentrations reduced 89% (58) | *Avoid combination* |
| Ketoconazole | Rifampin increases clearance of ketoconazole via CYP3A4 induction | >80% reduction in ketoconazole concentrations (179); reduced concentration of rifampin noted in one study (may explain apparent ketoconazole and rifampin failure (180) | Avoid combination if possible; consider using alternative rifamycin (e.g., rifabutin) or alternate antifungal such as fluconazole |
| Lopinavir/ritonavir | Rifampin increases clearance of lopinavir/ritonavir | Lopinavir AUC decreased by 75% (153) | May consider 400 mg lopinavir/400 mg ritonavir twice daily; however, limited clinical experience with this combination and potential for increased hepatotoxicity (96) |
| Nelfinavir | Rifampin increases clearance of nelfinavir via CYP3A4 induction | 82% decrease in nelfinavir AUC (178) | *Avoid combination* |
| Nevirapine | Rifampin increases clearance of nevirapine via CYP3A4 induction | No change in rifampin AUC or $C_{max}$; 58% reduction of nevirapine average concentrations, 68% reduction in $C_{min}$ (125) | Limited data for efficacy of 200 mg nevirapine bid dose; could also consider 300 mg bid if close monitoring available (96); however, potential for additive hematotoxicity; *avoid combination if possible (103)* |
| Ritonavir | Rifampin increases clearance of ritonavir via CYP3A4 induction | 35% reduction of ritonavir AUC (9) | May need to increase ritonavir dose |
| Saquinavir | Rifampin increases clearance of saquinavir via CYP3A4 induction | 80% reduction in saquinavir AUC (181) | *Avoid combination* |
| Saquinavir/ritonavir | Ritonavir may offset induction effect of rifampin | | Limited clinical experience with 400 mg/400 mg bid dose (96) |
| Zidovudine | Rifampin increases clearance of zidovudine via induction of glucuronyl transferases | 42–47% reduction zidovudine $C_{max}$ and AUC (204) | Dose adjustment of zidovudine may be necessary during rifampin therapy; effects may last until approx 2 weeks after discontinuation of rifampin; monitor clinical efficacy of zidovudine (e.g., symptomatic improvement, CD4, viral load) |

Rifabutin should also not be coadministered with saquinavir when it is used as a single protease inhibitor in a regimen because of significant reductions in saquinavir plasma concentrations *(96)*. In such situations, alternative antiretroviral or antimycobacterial agents need to be considered.

Selection of a specific management strategy will depend partly on the patient's response to current antiretroviral treatment. For patients who are satisfactorily treated with a regimen that includes a protease inhibitor or NNRTI, appropriate dosage adjustment of the affected antiretroviral or rifabutin should be made (Table 4). If the potential rifamycin–antiretroviral interaction cannot be adequately compensated for by dose adjustment, then an alternate antiretroviral agent should be substituted. For example, if a patient is currently virologically suppressed on a regimen that includes delavirdine, it may be replaced by another NNRTI such as nevirapine or efavirenz if concomitant rifabutin is necessary.

On the other hand, in a setting of incomplete viral suppression, changing at least two or all components of an antiretroviral regimen is recommended *(103)*. When possible, one should attempt to include agents in the new regimen that may be safely combined with rifabutin. Appropriate dosage adjustments should be made to compensate for concomitant antimycobacterial therapy.

### Overlapping Toxicity

Rifamycins may also be associated with pharmacodynamic interactions, primarily those involving additive side effects. For instance, hepatotoxicity has been reported with antiretroviral use, including protease inhibitors and NNRTIs. It is also a serious side effect of rifampin and isoniazid. Furthermore, coinfection with hepatitis B or C may also compromise hepatic activity. If these classes of agents are used in combination, patients should be closely monitored for changes in liver function. Most antiretrovirals are metabolized by the liver; hence, dosage reductions may be indicated in moderate-to-severe hepatic impairment to avoid excessive toxicity *(104,105)*. Alternatively, substitution of one or more agents by drugs with less-hepatotoxic potential may be necessary.

Another example involves the combination of rifabutin and cidofovir; both agents have been associated with uveitis *(106–109)*. Therefore, patients who receive treatment with both drugs should be closely monitored for development of this adverse event. If uveitis occurs, one or both drugs should be discontinued and replaced with other medications. Topical symptomatic therapy may also be required until resolution of symptoms.

### Macrolides

The advent of newer macrolide agents, specifically azithromycin and clarithromycin, has had a significant impact on the ability to successfully treat and prevent disseminated MAC infection in HIV-infected patients. Treatment for this debilitating opportunistic infection involves long-term multidrug therapy, of which the macrolides are a cornerstone *(6)*. They are also effective when administered as primary prophylaxis for MAC disease. In general, interactions of greatest clinical significance usually occur between macrolides and other agents used for managing opportunistic infections in HIV.

*Absorption*

When azithromycin was administered with a dose of aluminum/magnesium antacid, the peak concentration, but not the AUC, of azithromycin was reduced *(110)*. This interaction is likely of little significance, and azithromycin may be coadministered with antacids or didanosine. Similarly, no interaction has been observed between clarithromycin and didanosine *(111)*.

*Metabolism*

Clarithromycin is often combined with rifabutin for MAC treatment or prophylaxis. Each agent is a substrate of CYP3A4, and they have opposite effects on the CYP system: clarithromycin inhibits CYP3A4, and rifabutin is a moderate inducer. When these agents are coadministered, a significant bidirectional interaction is observed. Concentrations of clarithromycin are considerably reduced (with a corresponding increase in metabolite levels); concentrations of rifabutin and its desacetyl metabolite are substantially elevated *(112)*. An increased frequency of adverse events, primarily gastrointestinal toxicity and neutropenia, was also observed with this combination *(113)*. Patients receiving these drugs in combination should be monitored for clinical efficacy and dose-related rifabutin toxicities, such as myalgia, uveitis, and neutropenia. It is not advisable to use increased doses of clarithromycin because this may have an even more pronounced inhibitory effect on rifabutin metabolism. If a patient is not tolerating this combination, one may consider substituting clarithromycin with azithromycin, which has no effects on the CYP system and does not interact with rifabutin. However, patients should still be closely monitored for development of neutropenia with this regimen *(113)*.

*Overlapping Toxicity*

Hepatotoxicity has been reported with macrolide use. Therefore, careful monitoring of liver function is recommended when these drugs are administered with other potentially hepatotoxic agents, such as protease inhibitors, NNRTIs, azoles, rifamycins, isoniazid, pyrazinamide, and TMP-SMX *(6)*.

## Quinolones, Ethambutol

Quinolone interactions usually involve either an inhibition of quinolone absorption or quinolone-induced inhibition of drug metabolism via cytochrome P4501A2 enzymes. With respect to concomitant antiretroviral therapy, clinically significant interactions primarily involve absorption. The oral bioavailability of fluoroquinolones has been shown to be significantly compromised by coadministration with dairy products *(114)*, elemental minerals *(115)*, or nutritional supplements *(116)* because of formation of nonabsorbable cation complexes. Similar effects have been demonstrated with didanosine buffered tablets (Videx). In a cohort of 12 healthy volunteers, the simultaneous administration of ciprofloxacin with didanosine placebo resulted in a 98% reduction in ciprofloxacin AUC and a 93% reduction in peak concentrations *(117)*. These alterations would likely lead to therapeutic failure; therefore, quinolones should be administered either 2 hours before or at least 6 hours after such compounds *(56)*. This interaction does not apply to the delayed-release enteric formulation of didanosine (Videx EC), and this drug may be safely coadministered with ciprofloxacin *(55)*. A similar interaction exists between antacids and ethambutol, and these drugs should also be spaced accordingly *(118)*.

## Isoniazid

Isoniazid is usually a cornerstone of TB treatment-and-prevention regimens *(95)*. Drug interactions of clinical significance primarily involve absorption, metabolism, or overlapping toxicity.

### Absorption

In general, isoniazid should be taken on an empty stomach because food may significantly decrease absorption. Thus, it may need to be administered apart from certain protease inhibitors, such as atazanavir, lopinavir/ritonavir, nelfinavir, and saquinavir, which require food for adequate absorption. Aluminum hydroxide also decreases the bioavailability of isoniazid, and these products should be separated by at least 2 hours *(118,119)*. In addition, isoniazid is not stable in the presence of certain sugars, including glucose and lactose. It should not be given with beverages, foods, or drugs that contain high amounts of these sugars. For example, zalcitabine tablets contain high amounts of lactose and should not be coadministered with isoniazid *(91)*.

### Metabolism

Isoniazid inhibits hepatic isoenzyme activity, including CYP2E1, CYP1A2, CYP2C9, and CYP3A; it may also act as an enzyme inducer *(92)*. Isoniazid is generally considered to be a mild inhibitor of CYP3A, and hence the potential for significant metabolic interactions with antiretrovirals is likely to be low *(91)*. The combination of indinavir and isoniazid revealed no evidence of an interaction *(120)*.

### Overlapping Toxicity

Peripheral neuropathy can develop with prolonged isoniazid therapy, particularly in patients who are slow acetylators, malnourished, or at increased risk of neuropathy secondary to other conditions such as diabetes mellitus or HIV *(39)*. The risk of peripheral neuropathy can be minimized by the daily administration of pyridoxine *(121)*. Certain NRTIs (e.g., didanosine, stavudine, zalcitabine) can also cause peripheral neuropathy. The mechanism of NRTI-associated neuropathy is different from isoniazid-induced neuropathy and is thought to involve direct mitochondrial toxicity *(41,122)*. Therefore, additional administration of pyridoxine will not be helpful for this antiretroviral complication. In fact, high-dose pyridoxine can itself cause neuropathy *(123, 124)*. Patients taking these medications in combination should be carefully monitored for signs and symptoms of neurological complications. If such toxicities occur, the offending agents may need to be discontinued.

As mentionedpreviously, isoniazid may be associated with hepatotoxicity *(39)*. Therefore, similar pharmacodynamic interactions may occur when isoniazid is administered with other medications that are also known to have adverse hepatic effects.

## Miscellaneous Antimycobacterials

Many other drugs in this class are also hepatically metabolized, which raises the possibility of pharmacokinetic interactions with antiretrovirals. However, most of these agents were approved for use decades ago, and specific information regarding metabolic properties and pharmacokinetics is often lacking. In such situations, clinicians need to rely on in vitro and in vivo information to predict or anticipate possible interactions *(92)*. Ethionamide is primarily metabolized by CYP3A and hence is the only agent that may have potential for interaction with protease inhibitors or NNRTIs *(91)*.

Patients receiving protease inhibitor or NNRTI therapy plus ethionamide should be closely monitored for antimycobacterial efficacy or development of dose-related ethion-amide toxicity.

## CASE STUDY 2

Jim is a 36-year-old Caucasian male (5 feet 10 inches, 68 kg) who has been HIV positive for 3 years. At the time of diagnosis, he was asymptomatic with a CD4 count of 330 cells/μL and a viral load of 80,000 copies/mL. He has been incarcerated for the last 2 years and began antiretroviral therapy last year with 400 mg didanosine, 300 mg lamivudine, and 400 mg nevirapine, all once daily. He has responded well to his regimen and has achieved a viral load less than 50 copies/mL and CD4 count of 720 cells/μL.

Recently, an outbreak of TB occurred in the prison, and Jim had a positive tuber-culin skin test (10 mm increase in the diameter of the induration). The prison physi-cian would like to initiate treatment for latent TB infection. Treatment options include (1) a 9-month course of daily or twice-weekly isoniazid; (2) a 4-month course of daily rifampin or rifabutin; or (3) a 2-month course of pyrazinamide and rifampin or rifabutin. Jim is scheduled to be released in 6 months.

### ASSESSMENT

Jim requires appropriate treatment for his latent TB infection to prevent the occurrence of active disease. His antiretroviral therapy should also be continued to maintain his excellent virological suppression and immunological response.

The three treatment options for latent TB considered by the physician are all efficacious *(95)*. However, each regimen is associated with various advantages and disadvantages (Table 5). Selecting an appropriate treatment for latent TB requires consideration of many factors, including potential side effects, drug interactions, adherence, drug cost, and quality of life.

Daily or twice weekly isoniazid with pyridoxine is the first choice for treating latent TB infection *(6)*. This option should not be associated with any significant pharmacokinetic interactions with Jim's antiretroviral regimen and has the advan-tage of low pill burden and low cost. However, there is additive risk of peripheral neuropathy with didanosine. In addition, the duration of isoniazid therapy is quite long and exceeds Jim's remaining time in prison, where he is able to receive all of his medications under direct observation. If the full course of isoniazid treatment is not completed, there is a risk of developing active TB disease.

The shortest course of therapy for latent TB is with the combination of pyrazi-namide plus a rifamycin. However, there have been reports of severe and fatal hepatotoxicity with this combination in HIV-negative individuals *(6)*; the risk of hepatotoxicity may be further exacerbated by the nevirapine component of Jim's antiretroviral regimen. Therefore, it may be best to avoid using this regimen if possible.

Rifamycin or rifabutin are potent enzyme inducers and may interact with many antiretrovirals. With respect to Jim's regimen, rifamycin significantly reduces nevirapine concentrations; this interaction could theoretically be compensated for by increasing the nevirapine dose by 50% (i.e., 300 mg twice daily) *(125)*. This

**Table 5**
**Treatment Options for Latent Tuberculosis**

|  | Isoniazid | Rifampin or rifabutin | Rifampin/rifabutin plus pyrazinamide |
|---|---|---|---|
| Pharmacokinetic interactions | Isoniazid is a weak enzyme inhibitor; significant interaction not expected with nevirapine | Rifamycins and nevirapine are potent enzyme inducers; risk of negative bidirectional interactions | Rifamycins and nevirapine are potent enzyme inducers; risk of negative bidirectional interactions |
| Side effects | Overlapping risk of peripheral neuropathy with didanosine | Potential hepatotoxicity | Risk of hepatotoxicity with this combination; risk may be further exacerbated with concomitant nevirapine |
| Other | Low cost Adherence concerns: Will patient still need to complete 3 months of treatment after release from prison? | Rifabutin is more expensive than rifampin, particularly if increased dose adjustments are necessary | Shortest course of therapy |

approach is not practical and may also increase the risk of hepatotoxicity. Therefore, rifamycin should not be used with nevirapine. Rifabutin may be prescribed without dosage adjustment.

Alternatively, if rifabutin is not available and rifampin is the only rifamycin agent available, another option would be to modify Jim's antiretroviral regimen. Because he is virologically suppressed on his current regimen, it is possible to replace one component of the regimen with another agent. In this case, nevirapine could be replaced by efavirenz, which may be coadministered with rifampin (efavirenz should be offered at a higher dose of 800 mg once daily to achieve therapeutic concentrations in the presence of rifampin).

*MANAGEMENT SUGGESTION*

Based on the above considerations, the most appropriate treatment option would be to use 300 mg rifabutin once daily for 4 months. This approach does not require any modifications to Jim's current antiretroviral regimen, which is conveniently associated with once-daily dosing and low pill burden. The duration of rifabutin therapy also allows Jim to receive all treatment doses under direct observation, thus ensuring optimal adherence.

## ANTIVIRALS

Antiviral agents are often used to treat infections of the herpes virus family, including herpes simplex virus (HSV) type 1 and HSV-2, varicella zoster virus, and cytomegalovirus (CMV) infections. Oral acyclovir, famciclovir, and valacyclovir are used primarily for the treatment or suppression of HSV infections; these agents are relatively well tolerated and usually have little effect on the disposition or tolerance of concomitant antiretroviral therapy *(126)*.

Fomivirsen is an antisense oligonucleotide indicated for the treatment and maintenance of CMV retinitis in AIDS patients. Fomivirsen is administered via intravitreal injection, and systemic absorption is minimal; hence, the risk of pharmacokinetic drug interactions is negligible. Of more concern are the systemic medications indicated for treatment or suppression of CMV disease, such as ganciclovir, valganciclovir, foscarnet, and cidofovir. These antiviral drugs are usually administered for prolonged periods of time and are associated with various significant toxicities. Hence, the potential for clinically significant interaction with antiretroviral drugs is higher. The most pertinent types of antiviral–antiretroviral interactions involve either overlapping or synergistic efficacy or toxicity or interference with renal elimination (Table 6).

## Overlapping Toxicity

Both zidovudine and ganciclovir are associated with hematologic side effects, including neutropenia and anemia. Not surprisingly, a high rate of intolerance is observed when zidovudine is administered concurrently with ganciclovir *(40,127)*. Concomitant administration of 600–1200 mg of zidovudine daily and 5 mg/kg of ganciclovir once or twice daily resulted in hematologic toxicity in 82% of AIDS patients, with neutropenia occurring in 55% (128). In a controlled pharmacokinetic study, administration of 100 mg zidovudine orally every 4 hours, five times daily, with 1 g of oral ganciclovir every 8 hours resulted in a 14.5% increase in zidovudine AUC ($p = 0.032$) *(129)*. Changes in hematologic parameters were not assessed in this study. In an open-label clinical trial, 113 patients (80 with AIDS, 33 with AIDS-related complex) were treated with 200 mg zidovudine orally every 4 hours for a median duration of 152 days (range 5–386 days) *(127)*. Multiple regression analysis indicated that concurrent ganciclovir was associated with an increased risk of anemia and thrombocytopenia.

Because of the potential for additive hematotoxicity, concomitant therapy with these two agents is usually discouraged *(130)*. However, if systemic ganciclovir therapy is necessary in a patient with acute CMV retinitis who is already stabilized on a regimen including zidovudine, options to manage this pharmacodynamic interaction include the following:

- *Discontinue one drug.* In certain situations, one approach is to discontinue one medication, either temporarily or permanently. Options that were often suggested in the past included either temporarily reducing the zidovudine dosage *(126)* or holding zidovudine therapy *(131)* during the period of acute ganciclovir induction therapy *(128,132)*. However, one must consider the therapeutic consequences of temporarily or permanently discontinuing one component of an antiretroviral regimen. These practices were most commonly followed prior to the evolution of knowledge regarding the principles of HIV viral dynamics and development of drug resistance. Current standards of practice do not support the use of suboptimal antiretroviral dosing or the removal of a component of a multidrug antiretroviral regimen *(103)*. Therefore, this approach would no longer be considered appropriate.
- *Change one agent.* A more favorable option is to switch one of the interacting agents to another medication with a different side-effect profile. For example, zidovudine could be replaced by another antiretroviral agent, such as abacavir, stavudine, or tenofovir (NB: didanosine would not be a first choice replacement because of a separate interaction with ganciclovir). Factors such as the comparative efficacy, side effects, cost, availability, and other drug interactions associated with the new agent need to be considered. In addition, issues such as prior antiretroviral experience, risk of cross-resistance, cost,

adherence, and side effects need to be considered when attempting to substitute one drug in a current antiretroviral regimen. Alternatively, one could consider replacing ganciclovir with another antiviral agent, such as foscarnet or cidofovir. However, given the relative toxicity profiles of these drugs, it may be more desirable to consider antiretroviral replacements for zidovudine first.

- *Add another agent to counteract the effect of interaction.* If treatment with both ganciclovir and zidovudine are absolutely necessary, a colony-stimulating factor such as filgrastim may be added to combat neutropenia *(133)*. The consequences of adding yet another drug to a patient's regimen (as described previously) must be considered.

### Synergistic or Antagonistic Antiviral Activity

In vitro experiments have demonstrated that ganciclovir can antagonize the antiretroviral effects of zidovudine and didanosine; the combination of foscarnet and zidovudine results in synergistic antiviral activity *(40)*. However, the clinical significance of these observations is unclear. In a trial of 234 patients with AIDS and CMV retinitis, those randomized to receive foscarnet treatment had a median survival advantage of 3 months compared with those treated with ganciclovir, although foscarnet was not tolerated as well *(134,135)*. Although the patients assigned to ganciclovir received less antiretroviral therapy on average than those assigned to foscarnet (presumably because of additive toxicity between ganciclovir and zidovudine), the excess mortality could not be explained entirely by differences in exposure to antiretroviral drugs. Thus, synergistic or antagonistic anti-HIV effects may also have contributed to the difference in outcomes between the foscarnet- and ganciclovir-treated groups. In the era of HAART, these pharmacodynamic anti-HIV effects may be of less clinical importance given the wide selection of available antiretroviral agents as well as the significant reduction in CMV disease *(3,5)*.

Infection with hepatitis C is an increasing concern in the HIV population, particularly among injection drug users, in whom coinfection rates may approach 90% *(136)*. The progression of hepatitis C is accelerated by the presence of HIV, particularly in the context of increasing immunodeficiency *(137)*, and can lead to high rates of morbidity and mortality *(138,139)*. Ribavirin and pegylated interferon are the standards of treatment in the non-HIV-infected population, and preliminary experience in the HIV/HCV coinfected subjects is also promising *(136)*.

Concerns exist regarding the use of ribavirin with nucleoside analogs. Ribavirin is a guanosine analog and inhibits the intracellular phosphorylation of zidovudine, stavudine, and zalcitabine in vitro. This may in turn cause antagonism of anti-HIV effect of the nucleosides, although this has not been observed clinically. Of more immediate concern is the risk of increased toxicity because ribavirin and zidovudine are both associated with dose-dependent anemia.

Ribavirin is also a potent inhibitor of inosine monophosphate dehydrogenase and leads to elevated levels of dideoxyadenosine triphosphate; this didanosine metabolite is considered to be a key culprit involved in mitochondrial toxicity, and there have been numerous reports of pancreatitis and lactic acidosis with this combination *(140–142)*. Currently available treatment guidelines recommend that concomitant use of zidovudine or didanosine with ribavirin be avoided whenever possible. If coadministration is absolutely necessary, close monitoring for nucleoside toxicity (including lactic acidosis and pancreatitis) is recommended *(143)*.

**Table 6**
**Antiviral Interactions**

| Primary drug | Interacting drug | Mechanism | Effects | Comments/management |
|---|---|---|---|---|
| Acyclovir | Zidovudine | Synergistic antiretroviral activity? | Combination suggested to have some favorable effects on survival, but this has not consistently demonstrated (205–209) | Clinical significance unclear in era of potent combination antiretroviral therapy; combination is usually well tolerated; no pharmacokinetic interaction observed (210) |
| | Zidovudine | Unknown | Increased lethargy reported with combination ($N = 1$) (211) | Combination is usually well tolerated; no pharmacokinetic interaction demonstrated (210) |
| | Probenecid | Probenecid inhibits renal tubular secretion of acyclovir | 40% increase in acyclovir AUC (212) | Unlikely to be clinically significant unless using high doses of acyclovir |
| | Nephrotoxins: aminoglycosides, amphotericin B, cidofovir, foscarnet, intravenous pentamidine | Overlapping side-effect profiles | Additive nephrotoxicity if combined with high-dose intravenous acyclovir (213) | Cautious use of combinations is warranted; adjust dose or dosing interval of acyclovir as well as nephrotoxin(s) in renal failure; Monitor serum creatinine, urea three times weekly |
| Cidofovir | Nephrotoxins: aminoglycosides, amphotericin B, foscarnet, intravenous pentamidine | | Risk of additive nephrotoxicity (214) | Avoid concomitant administration if possible; monitor serum creatinine, urea, urine protein prior to each cidofovir dose |
| | Probenecid | Probenecid blocks active renal tubular secretion of cidofovir. NB: Probenecid may interact with metabolism or renal tubular excretion of many drugs (see the following page for additional interactions with probenecid) | Decreased risk of cidofovir-induced nephrotoxicity | Administer 2 g probenecid orally 3 hours prior to cidofovir dose and 1 g orally at 2 and 8 hours after completion of cidofovir infusion (total 4 g probenecid) (214); serum creatinine, urea, urine protein prior to each cidofovir dose; monitor for adverse reactions to probenecid such as rash (usually appear after second or third dose); attempt to treat with antihistamine |

*Continued on next page*

173

**Table 6 (*Continued*)**
**Antiviral Interactions**

| Primary drug | Interacting drug | Mechanism | Effects | Comments/management |
|---|---|---|---|---|
| | Rifabutin | Similar side effects | Both agents may be associated with uveitis (*106–109*) | Administer cidofovir with probenecid to minimize risk of toxicity; reduce dose of rifabutin or change to another agent if this is the causative drug |
| Probenecid (with cidofovir) | Zalcitabine | Probenecid inhibits renal tubular secretion of zalcitabine | 50% increase in zalcitabine AUC (*215*) | Monitor for zalcitabine toxicity; may require zalcitabine dose reduction |
| | Zidovudine | Probenecid may inhibit zidovudine glucuronidation or renal tubular secretion | 75–115% increase in zidovudine AUC (*144,145*) | Monitor for zidovudine toxicity, rash, and flulike symptoms |
| Ganciclovir, valganciclovir | Didanosine | Increased didanosine concentration and decreased ganciclovir concentration (mechanism unknown) | With po ganciclovir: increase in didanosine concentration >100%; decreased ganciclovir concentration 20% (with sequential administration) With intravenous ganciclovir: didanosine concentration increased >70% Potential for increased didanosine toxicity and decreased ganciclovir efficacy (*28,148*) | Administer oral ganciclovir before/with didanosine to minimize effect on ganciclovir absorption; monitor for didanosine toxicity (e.g., diarrhea, pancreatitis, peripheral neuropathy) and progression of CMV disease |
| | Zidovudine | Additive bone marrow toxicity | Increased risk of neutropenia, anemia (*128,132*) | Hold zidovudine during induction therapy with ganciclovir; reinstitute with caution during maintenance or switch to alternative antiretroviral with different side-effect profile; monitor CBC with differential three times weekly initially, then once weekly |
| | Antineoplastics, amphotericin B, dapsone, flucytosine, intravenous pentamidine, primaquine, pyrimethamine, TMP-SMX, trimetrexate | Increased risk of bone marrow toxicity | Cautious use of combinations is warranted (*130,216*) | Monitor closely for blood dyscrasias |

174

| | Drug | Mechanism | Effect | Comment |
|---|---|---|---|---|
| | Imipenem | | Increased risk of seizures (217) | Do not exceed 2 g/day imipenem; dose adjust *both* agents in renal failure; serum creatinine, urea |
| | Probenecid | Probenecid inhibits ganciclovir clearance | Increase in ganciclovir AUC of 50% | Avoid concomitant use because of potential for increased risk of dose-related ganciclovir toxicities, risk of probenecid side effects (e.g., headache, gastrointestinal upset, rash, etc.), and interference with renal elimination of other drugs a patient may be taking concomitantly |
| Foscarnet | Nephrotoxins | Overlapping side-effect profiles | Additive nephrotoxicity (213) | Cautious use of combinations is warranted; adjust dosages of both drugs in renal failure; serum creatinine, urea three times weekly |
| | Didanosine | Potential for drugs to compete for renal tubular secretion | No pharmacokinetic interaction observed (126) | Drugs may be coadministered without dosage adjustment |
| | Zalcitabine | Potential for drugs to compete for renal tubular secretion | No apparent pharmacokinetic interaction observed (218) | Drugs may be coadministered without dosage adjustment |
| | Zidovudine | Synergistic anti-HIV effect | Additive/synergistic antiretroviral activity observed in vitro (219,220) | Clinical significance unclear in era of potent combination antiretroviral therapy; no pharmacokinetic interaction observed (221); may be increased risk of anemia |
| Ribavarin | Didanosine | Enhanced phosphorylation of didanosine | Potential for increased didanosine toxicity | Cases of pancreatitis, fatal and nonfatal lactic acidosis reported with combination (222); avoid concomitant use whenever possible; if coadministration is necessary, routine (monthly) monitoring of serum lactate and amylase levels is recommended (136,143) |
| | Zidovudine | Inhibition of zidovudine phosphorylation (223); overlapping risk of anemia | May antagonize anti-HIV effect of zidovudine and lead to zidovudine toxicity | Potential for reduced activity and increased toxicity of zidovudine *Avoid combination* whenever possible; if coadministration is necessary, regular monitoring of hemoglobin is recommended (143) |

## Competition for Renal Elimination

Probenecid is routinely administered with cidofovir to minimize renal toxicity; however, probenecid may in turn affect the clearance of reverse transcriptase inhibitors and other renally excreted agents. For instance, probenecid inhibits the liver metabolism and renal tubular secretion of zidovudine, resulting in 80–100% increases in zidovudine AUC *(144,145)*. However, the clinical significance of increased plasma zidovudine concentrations is unclear because efficacy and dosing frequency are based on intracellular zidovudine levels. Although it may be theoretically appealing to use probenecid to allow administration of lower zidovudine dosages at increased intervals with subsequent increased convenience and lowered costs, it is generally not recommended to combine these drugs for this purpose because the concomitant effect on intracellular zidovudine concentrations has not been determined. In addition, probenecid may interact unfavorably with other medications, and use of this combination may also be associated with a higher incidence of probenecid-related hypersensitivity reactions in patients with AIDS *(146)*.

## Decreased Renal Function Requiring Dosage Adjustment

Foscarnet and cidofovir can often cause nephrotoxicity, especially with high doses and long-term administration *(131,147)*. Patients receiving either of these agents should have their renal function monitored routinely. Significant declines in renal function may necessitate the dosage adjustment of concomitant therapy. In addition, coadministration of other nephrotoxic agents, such as intravenous pentamidine or aminoglycosides, is not advised *(39)*.

## Unknown Mechanism

Occasionally, unpredictable interactions may be observed, as with the case of didanosine and ganciclovir. In a multiple-dose crossover pharmacokinetic interaction study, 13 HIV-positive patients received 1 g ganciclovir every 8 hours orally and 200 mg didanosine every 12 hours orally *(129)*. Ganciclovir and didanosine were administered both sequentially (i.e., didanosine 2 hours before oral ganciclovir) and simultaneously to evaluate the effect of the didanosine buffer on the absorption of ganciclovir. In the presence of ganciclovir, significant increases in didanosine AUC were noted with both sequential and simultaneous administration (114.6 and 107.7%, respectively, $p < 0.001$). In addition, the AUC of ganciclovir was decreased by 21.4% ($p = 0.002$) when administered 2 hours after didanosine; no significant changes in renal clearance of either drug were observed *(129)*.

Similar results were observed when didanosine was coadministered with intravenous ganciclovir *(148)*. In the presence of ganciclovir, both the mean AUC and peak serum concentration of didanosine increased significantly (70.4%, $p < 0.001$, and 49.3%, $p = 0.024$, respectively). No significant changes in time to maximum serum concentrations $T_{max}$, half-life, or renal clearance of didanosine were observed. In the presence of didanosine, a modest increase in ganciclovir AUC (6.2%, $p = 0.018$) was noted *(148)*. The mechanism for this interaction is unknown. Patients receiving both didanosine and ganciclovir should be closely monitored for ganciclovir efficacy as well as the development of didanosine-related toxicities *(129,148)*.

It should be noted that, although the buffered tablet formulation of didanosine (Videx) was used in these studies, a comparable effect with the EC capsule formulation of didanosine (Videx EC) cannot be ruled out *(149)*. Similarly, because valganciclovir is rapidly converted to ganciclovir, interactions associated with ganciclovir are expected to occur with valganciclovir *(150)*. The optimal doses for coadministering ganciclovir and didanosine regarding safety and efficacy have not been determined. Therefore, clinicians are advised to use this combination with caution regardless of the formulations of either drug prescribed.

## SUMMARY

Given the increasing complexity of HIV therapy, the potential for drug interactions is extremely high. Clinicians need to be aware of the potential for interactions between antiretrovirals and other medications used for the management or prevention of opportunistic infections. Some drug combinations may result in clinically beneficial interactions, such as increasing drug concentrations for agents with demonstrated dose-related efficacy, decreasing toxicity, or reducing pill burden or dosing frequency. The increasing popularity of boosted protease inhibitor therapy reflects the potential benefits of desirable drug interactions. However, many interactions are associated with potentially detrimental or even life-threatening effects. For instance, treatment of concurrent HIV and pulmonary TB infection can be quite complex. Certain antimycobacterials can significantly decrease protease inhibitor and NNRTI drug concentrations, which may lead to suboptimal viral suppression and possible viral resistance. Conversely, antimycobacterial therapy may be compromised by concomitant antiretrovirals; reduced drug levels may result in TB breakthrough, and increased antimycobacterial concentrations may increase the risk of dose-related toxicities if appropriate dosage adjustments are not made.

To avoid compromising therapeutic efficacy or increasing drug toxicity, practitioners need to be aware of potential interactions within complex individual drug regimens. Absorption interactions can usually be avoided by separating drug administration times; metabolic interactions may often be managed by adjusting drug dosages or dosing intervals. Interactions involving overlapping or synergistic toxicities may require the substitution of one drug by another with a different side-effect profile.

In the absence of specific data, being familiar with the pharmacokinetic and pharmacodynamic characteristics of the particular agents may assist clinicians in predicting the likelihood of possible interactions. Management options will depend on factors such as the mechanism and the clinical significance of the interaction, the availability of therapeutic alternatives, patient convenience, and cost.

## REFERENCES

1. Preston SL, Postelnick M, Purdy BD, Petrolati J, Aasi H, Stein DS. Drug interactions in HIV-positive patients initiated on protease inhibitor therapy [letter]. AIDS 1998;12: 228–230.
2. Mur Lalaguna MA, Cobo Campos R, Hurtado Gomez MF, Martinez Tutor MJ. [Study of interactions between anti-retroviral agents and concomitant drugs]. Farmacia Hospitalaria 2003;27:84–92.

3. Palella FJJ, Delaney KM, Moorman AC, et al. Declining morbidity and mortality among patients with advanced human immunodeficiency virus infection. HIV Outpatient Study Investigators. N Engl J Med 1998;338:853–860.

4. Moore RD, Keruly JC, Chaisson RE. Decline in CMV and other opportunistic disease with combination antiretroviral therapy. Fifth Conference on Retroviruses and Opportunistic Infections, Chicago, IL, February 1–5, 1998, p. 113. Abstract 184.

5. Holtzer CD, Jacobson MA, Hadley WK, et al. Decline in the rate of specific opportunistic infections at San Francisco General Hospital, 1994–1997 [letter]. AIDS 1998;12:1931–1933.

6. United States Public Health Services/Infectious Diseases Society of America (USPHS/IDSA) Prevention of Opportunistic Infections Working Group. 2001 USPHS/IDSA guidelines for the prevention of opportunistic infections in persons infected with human immunodeficiency virus. November 28, 2001. USPHS/IDSA, Washington, DC

7. Michelet C, Arvieux C, Francois C, et al. Opportunistic infections occurring during highly active antiretroviral treatment. AIDS 1998;12:1815–1822.

8. Horowitz HW, Telzak EE, Sepkowitz KA, Wormser GP. Human immunodeficiency virus infection, Part II. Disease-A-Month 1998;44:677–716.

9. Abbott Laboratories Limited Canada. Norvir (ritonavir) prescribing information. Saint-Laurent, QC: 2001.

10. Eron JJ, Benoit SL, Jemsek J, et al. Treatment with lamivudine, zidovudine, or both in HIV-positive patients with 200 to 500 CD4$^+$ cells per cubic millimeter. N Engl J Med 1995;333:1662–1669.

11. Veal GJ, Hoggard PG, Barry MG, Khoo S, Back DJ. Interaction between lamivudine (3TC) and other nucleoside analogues for intracellular phosphorylation [letter]. AIDS 1996;10:546–548.

12. Back D, Haworth S, Hoggard P, Khoo S, Barry M. Drug interactions with d4T phosphorylation in vitro [abstract]. Eleventh International Conference on AIDS, Vancouver, Canada, July 1996.

13. Fletcher CV, Anderson PL, Kakuda TN, et al. Concentration-controlled compared with conventional antiretroviral therapy for HIV infection. AIDS 2002;16:551–560.

14. Acosta EP, Henry K, Baken L, Page LM, Fletcher CV. Indinavir concentrations and antiviral effect. Pharmacotherapy 1999;19:708–712.

15. Harris M, Durakovic C, Rae S, et al. Virologic response to indinavir/nevirapine/3TC correlates with indinavir trough concentrations. Thirty-seventh Interscience Conference on Antimicrobial Agents and Chemotherapy, Toronto, September 28–October 1, 1997. Abstract I-173.

16. Hertogs K, Mellors JW, Schel P, et al. Patterns of cross-resistance among protease inhibitors in 483 clinical HIV-1 isolates. Fifth Conference on Retroviruses and Opportunistic Infections, Chicago, IL, February 1–5, 1998. Abstract 395.

17. Patick AK, Mo H, Markowitz M, et al. Antiviral and resistance studies of AG1343, an orally bioavailable inhibitor of human immunodeficiency virus protease. Antimicrob Agents Chemother 1996;40:292–297.

18. Sampson MS, Barr MR, Torres RA, Hall G. Viral load changes in nelfinavir treated patients switched to a second protease inhibitor after loss of viral suppression. Thirty-seventh Interscience Conference on Antimicrobial Agents and Chemotherapy, Toronto, September 28–October 1, 1997. Abstract LB-5.

19. Deeks S, Grant R, Horton C, Simmonds N, Follansbee S, Eastman S. Virologic effect of ritonavir plus saquinavir in subjects who have failed indinavir. Thirty-seventh Interscience Conference on Antimicrobial Agents and Chemotherapy, Toronto, September 28–October 1, 1997. Abstract I-205.

20. Sampson M, Torres RA, Stein AJ, et al. Ritonavir-saquinavir combination treatment in protease inhibitor experienced patients with advanced HIV disease. Thirty-seventh

Interscience Conference on Antimicrobial Agents and Chemotherapy, Toronto, September 28–October 1, 1997. Abstract I-104.

21. Woolley J, Studenberg S, Boehlert C, Bowers G, Sinhababu A, Adams P. Cytochrome P-450 isozyme induction, inhibition, and metabolism studies with the HIV protease inhibitor, 141W94. Thirty-seventh Interscience Conference on Antimicrobial Agents and Chemotherapy, Toronto, September 28–October 1, 1997. Abstract A-60.

22. Yeh KC, Deutsch PJ, Haddix H, et al. Single-dose pharmacokinetics of indinavir and the effect of food. Antimicrob Agents Chemother 1998;42:332–338.

23. Eagling VA, Back DJ, Barry MG. Differential inhibition of cytochrome P450 isoforms by the protease inhibitors, ritonavir, saquinavir and indinavir. Br J Clin Pharmacol 1997; 44:190–194.

24. Lee CA, Liang BH, Wu EY, et al. Prediction of nelfinavir mesylate (VIRACEPT) clinical drug interactions based on in vitro human P450 metabolism studies. Fourth National Conference on Retroviruses and Opportunistic Infections, Washington, DC, January 22–26, 1997.

25. Agouron Pharmaceuticals Canada. Rescriptor (delavirdine) prescribing information. Mississauga, Ontario, Canada, 2001

26. Boehringer Ingelheim Pharmaceuticals. Viramune (nevirapine) product monograph. Ridgefield, CT, September 4, 2003.

27. Bristol-Myers Squibb Company. Sustiva (efavirenz) prescribing information. Princeton, NJ, 2003.

28. Tseng AL, Foisy MM. Significant interactions with new antiretrovirals and psychotropic drugs. Ann Pharmacother 1999;33:461–473.

29. Tseng AL, Foisy MM. Management of drug interactions in patients with HIV. Ann Pharmacother 1997;31:1040–1058.

30. Piscitelli SC, Flexner C, Minor JR, Polis MA, Masur H. Drug interactions in patients infected with HIV. Clin Infect Dis 1996;23:685–693.

31. Metroka CE, McMechan MR, Andrada R, Laubenstein LJ, Jacobus DP. Failure of prophylaxis with dapsone in patients taking dideoxyinosine [letter]. N Engl J Med 1991; 325:737.

32. Sahai J, Garber G, Gallicano K, Oliveras L, Cameron DW. Effects of the antacids in didanosine tablets on dapsone pharmacokinetics. Ann Intern Med 1995;123:584–587.

33. Bristol-Myers Squibb Company. Videx (didanosine) prescribing information. Princeton, NJ, February 2003.

34. Lee BL, Tauber MG, Sadler B, Goldstein D, Chambers HR. Atovaquone inhibits the glucuronidation and increases the plasma concentrations of zidovudine. Clin Pharmacol Ther 1996;59:14–21.

35. Sadler BM, Caldwell P, Scott JD, Rogers M, Blum MR. Drug interaction between rifampin and atovaquone in HIV+ asymptomatic volunteers [abstract]. Thirty-fifth Interscience Conference on Antimicrobial Agents and Chemotherapy, San Francisco, September 17–20, 1995.

36. Moore KHP, Yuen GJ, Raasch RH, et al. Pharmacokinetics of lamivudine administered alone and with trimethoprim-sulfamethoxazole. Clin Pharmacol Ther 1996;59:550–558.

37. Israelski DM, Tom C, Remington JS. Zidovudine antagonizes the action of pyrimethamine in experimental infection with *Toxoplasma gondii*. Antimicrob Agents Chemother 1989;33:30–34.

38. Harvey WD, Holzman RS, Avramis V, Bawdon R, Fall H, Feinberg J. Clinical and pharmacokinetic interactions of combined zidovudine therapy and sulfadoxine-pyrimethamine (Fansidar) prophylaxis in post-PCP AIDS patients (ACTG 021). Fifth International Conference on AIDS, Montreal, June 1989. Abstract TBP46.

39. Lee BL, Safrin S. Interactions and toxicities of drugs used in patients with AIDS. Clin Infect Dis 1992;14:773–779.

40. Burger DM, Meenhorst PL, Koks CHW, Beijnen JH. Drug interactions with zidovudine. AIDS 1993;7:445–460.

41. Brinkman K, ter Hofstede HJ, Burger DM, Smeitink JA, Koopmans PP. Adverse effects of reverse transcriptase inhibitors: mitochondrial toxicity as common pathway [editorial]. AIDS 1998;12:1735–1744.

42. Kaufman MB, Simionatto C. A review of protease inhibitor-induced hyperglycemia. Pharmacotherapy 1999;19:114–117.

43. Gordin FM, Simon GL, Wofsy CB, Mills J. Adverse reactions to trimethoprim-sulfamethoxazole in patients with the acquired immunodeficiency syndrome. Ann Intern Med 1984;100:495–499.

44. Foisy MM, Slayter KL, Hewitt RG, Morse GD. Pancreatitis during intravenous pentamidine therapy in an AIDS patient with prior exposure to didanosine. Ann Pharmacother 1994;28:1025–1028.

45. Darouiche RO. Oropharyngeal and esophageal candidiasis in immunocompromised patients: treatment issues. Clin Infect Dis 1998;26:259–274.

46. Vasquez JA. Options for the management of mucosal candidiasis in patients with AIDS and HIV infection. Pharmacotherapy 1999;19:76–87.

47. Greenblatt RM, Hollander H, McMaster JR, et al. Polypharmacy among patients attending an AIDS clinic: utilization of prescribed, unorthodox, and investigational treatments. J Acquir Immune Defic Syndr 1991;4:136–143.

48. Lomaestro BM, Piatek MA. Update on drug interactions with azole antifungal agents. Ann Pharmacother 1998;32:915–928.

49. Blum RA, D'Andrea DT, Florentino BM, et al. Increased gastric pH and the bioavailability of fluconazole and ketoconazole. Ann Intern Med 1991;114:755–757.

50. Hardin TC, Sharkey-Mathis PK, Rinaldi MG, Graybill JR. Evaluation of the pharmacokinetic interaction between itraconazole and didanosine in HIV-infected subjects [abstract]. Thirty-fifth Interscience Conference on Antimicrobial Agents and Chemotherapy, San Francisco, CA, September 17–20, 1995.

51. Knupp CA, Brater C, Relue J, Barbhaiya RH. Pharmacokinetics of didanosine and ketoconazole after coadministration to patients seropositive for the human immunodeficiency virus. J Clin Pharmacol 1993;33:912–917.

52. Moreno F, Hardin TC, Rinaldi MG, Graybill JR. Itraconazole-didanosine excipient interaction [letter]. JAMA 1993;269:1508.

53. May DB, Drew RH, Yedinak KC, Bartlett JA. Effect of simultaneous didanosine administration on itraconazole absorption in healthy volunteers. Pharmacotherapy 1994;14:509–513.

54. Damle B, Hess H, Kaul S, Knupp C. Absence of clinically relevant drug interactions following simultaneous administration of didanosine-encapsulated, enteric-coated bead formulation with either itraconazole or fluconazole. Biopharm Drug Dispos 2002;23:59–66.

55. Damle BD, Mummaneni V, Kaul S, Knupp CA. Lack of effect of simultaneously administered didanosine encapsulated enteric bead formulation (Videx EC) on oral absorption of indinavir, ketoconazole, or ciprofloxacin. Antimicrob Agents Chemother 2002;46:385–391.

56. Sahai J. Avoiding the ciprofloxacin-didanosine interaction [letter]. Ann Intern Med 1995;123:394–395.

57. Ervine CM, Matthew DE, Brennan B, Houston JB. Comparison of ketoconazole and fluconazole as cytochrome P450 inhibitors. Use of steady-state infusion approach to achieve plasma concentration-response relationships. Drug Metab Dispos 1996;24:211–215.

58. Merck and Co. Crixivan (indinavir) prescribing information. Whitehouse Station, NJ, January 2003.

59. Back DJ, Gatti G, Fletcher C, et al. Therapeutic drug monitoring in HIV infection: current status and future directions. AIDS 2002;16:S5–S37.

60. Lamson M, Robinson P, Gigliotti M, Myers M. The pharmacokinetic interactions of nevirapine and ketoconazole. Twelfth World AIDS Conference, Geneva, Switzerland, June 28–July 3, 1998. Abstract 12218.

61. Asgari M, Back DJ. Effect of azoles on the glucuronidation of zidovudine by human liver UDP-glucuronosyltransferase [letter; comment]. J Infect Dis 1995;172:1634–1636.

62. Sampol E, Lacarelle B, Rajaonarison JF, Catalin J, Durand A. Comparative effects of antifungal agents on zidovudine glucuronidation by human liver microsomes. Br J Clin Pharmacol 1995;40:83–86.

63. Sahai J, Gallicano K, Pakuts A, Cameron DW. Effect of fluconazole on zidovudine pharmacokinetics in patients infected with human immunodeficiency virus [see comments]. J Infect Dis 1994;169:1103–1107.

64. Washington CB, Duran GE, Man MC, Sikic BI, Blaschke TF. Interaction of anti-HIV protease inhibitors with the multidrug transporter P-glycoprotein (P-gp) in human cultured cells. J Acquir Immune Defic Syndr Hum Retrovirol 1998;19:203–209.

65. Alsenz J, Steffen H, Alex R. Active apical secretory efflux of the HIV protease inhibitors saquinavir and ritonavir in Caco-2 cell monolayers [published erratum appears in Pharm Res 1998;15:958]. Pharm Res 1998;15:423–428.

66. Lee CG, Gottesman MM, Cardarelli CO, et al. HIV-1 protease inhibitors are substrates for the MDR1 multidrug transporter. Biochemistry 1998;37:3594–3601.

67. Kim AE, Dintaman JM, Waddell DS, Silverman JA. Saquinavir, an HIV protease inhibitor, is transported by P-glycoprotein. J Pharmacol Exp Ther 1998;286:1439–1445.

68. Anderson PL, Lamba J, Schuetz E, Fletcher CV. MDR1 genotypes associated with antiviral dynamics and indinavir (IDV) disposition in HIV-infected patients. Fourth International Workshop on Clinical Pharmacology of HIV Therapy, Cannes, France, March 27–29, 2003. Abstract 2.1.

69. Fellay J, Marzolini C, Meaden ER, et al. Response to antiretroviral treatment in HIV-1-infected individuals with allelic variants of the multidrug resistance transporter 1: a pharmacogenetics study.[comment]. Lancet 2002;359:30–36.

70. Kim RB. Drug transporters in HIV therapy. Topics HIV Med 2003;11:136–139.

71. Kim RB, Fromm MF, Wandel C, et al. The drug transporter P-glycoprotein limits oral absorption and brain entry of HIV-1 protease inhibitors. J Clin Invest 1998;101:289–294.

72. Takano M, Hasegawa R, Fukuda T, Yumoto R, Nagai J, Murakami T. Interaction with P-glycoprotein and transport of erythromycin, midazolam and ketoconazole in Caco-2 cells. Eur J Pharmacol 1998;358:289–294.

73. Khaliq Y, Gallicano K, Venance S, et al. Effect of the p-glycoprotein and cytochrome P450 3A4 inhibitor ketoconazole, on ritonavir and saquinavir plasma and cerebrospinal fluid concentrations. Eighth Annual Canadian Conference on HIV/AIDS Research, Victoria, British Columbia, Canada, May 1–4, 1999. Abstract B205.

74. Albengres E, Le Louet H, Tillement JP. Systemic antifungal agents. Drug interactions of clinical significance. Drug Safety 1998;18:83–97.

75. van der Horst CM, Saag MS, Cloud GA, et al. Treatment of cryptococcal meningitis associated with the acquired immunodeficiency syndrome. National Institute of Allergy and Infectious Diseases Mycoses Study Group and AIDS Clinical Trials Group. N Engl J Med 1997;337:15–21.

76. Lewis RE, Lund BC, Klepser ME, Ernst EJ, Pfaller MA. Assessment of antifungal activities of fluconazole and amphotericin B administered alone and in combination against *Candida albicans* by using a dynamic in vitro mycotic infection model. Antimicrob Agents Chemother 1998;42:1382–1386.

77. Ghannoum MA, Fu Y, Ibrahim AS, et al. In vitro determination of optimal antifungal combinations against *Cryptococcus neoformans* and *Candida albicans*. Antimicrob Agents Chemother 1995;39:2459–2465.

78. Scheven M, Schwegler F. Antagonistic interactions between azoles and amphotericin B with yeasts depend on azole lipophilia for special test conditions in vitro. Antimicrob Agents Chemother 1995;39:1779–1783.

79. Scheven J, Scheven ML. Interaction between azoles and amphotericin B in the treatment of candidiasis [letter]. Clin Infect Dis 1995;20:1079.

80. Clark AB, Lobo BL, Gelfand MS. Fluconazole and amphotericin B for cryptococcal meningitis. Ann Pharmacother 1996;30:1408–1410.

81. Merck and Co. Cancidas (caspofungin) prescribing information. Whitehouse Station, NJ, September 2002.

82. Chin DP, DeRiemer K, Small PM, et al. Differences in contributing factors to tuberculosis incidence in U.S. -born and foreign-born persons. Am J Resp Crit Care Med 1998;158: 1797–1803.

83. Murray JF. Tuberculosis and HIV infection: a global perspective. Respiration 1998;65: 335–342.

84. Pilheu JA. Tuberculosis 2000: problems and solutions. Int J Tuberculosis Lung Dis 1998; 2:696–703.

85. Snyder DC, Mohle-Boetani JC, Chandler A, Oliver G, Livermore T, Royce S. A population-based study determining the incidence of tuberculosis attributable to HIV infection. J Acquir Immune Defic Syndr Hum Retrovirol 1997;16:190–194.

86. Prevention and treatment of tuberculosis among patients infected with human immunodeficiency virus: principles of therapy and revised recommendations. Centers for Disease Control and Prevention. MMWR Recomm Rep 1998;47:1–58.

87. March F, Garriga X, Rodriguez P, et al. Acquired drug resistance in *Mycobacterium tuberculosis* isolates recovered from compliant patients with human immunodeficiency virus-associated tuberculosis. Clin Infect Dis 1997;25:1044–1047.

88. Sahai J, Gallicano K, Swick L, et al. Reduced plasma concentrations of antituberculosis drugs in patients with HIV infection. Ann Intern Med 1997;127:289–293.

89. Peloquin CA, Nitta AT, Burman WJ, et al. Low antituberculosis drug concentrations in patients with AIDS. Ann Pharmacother 1996;30:919–925.

90. Patel KB, Belmonte R, Crowe HM. Drug malabsorption and resistant tuberculosis in HIV-infected patients [letter]. N Engl J Med 1995;332:336–337.

91. Burman WJ, Gallicano K, Peloquin C. Therapeutic implications of drug interactions in the treatment of human immunodeficiency virus-related tuberculosis. Clin Infect Dis 1999;28:419–430.

92. Bertz RJ, Granneman GR. Use of in vitro and in vivo data to estimate the likelihood of metabolic pharmacokinetic interactions. Clin Pharmacokinet 1997;32:210–258.

93. de Maat MM, Ekhart GC, Huitema AD, Koks CH, Mulder JW, Beijnen JH. Drug interactions between antiretroviral drugs and comedicated agents. Clin Pharmacokinet 2003;42: 223–282.

94. Burman WJ, Jones BE. Treatment of HIV-related tuberculosis in the era of effective antiretroviral therapy. Am J Resp Crit Care Med 2001;164:7–12.

95. Centers for Disease Control and Prevention. Treatment of tuberculosis. American Thoracic Society, CDC, and Infectious Diseases Society of America. MMWR Morbid Mortal Wkly Rep 2003;52:1–88.

96. Centers for Disease Control and Prevention. Updated guidelines for the use of rifamycins for the treatment of tuberculosis among HIV-infected patients taking protease inhibitors or nonnucleoside reverse transcriptase inhibitors [version 1.20.04]. MMWR Morbid Mortal Wkly Rep 2004;53:37.

97. Gallicano K, Khaliq Y, Carignan G, Tseng A, Walmsley S, Cameron DW. A pharmacokinetic study of intermittent rifabutin dosing with a combination of ritonavir and saquinavir in patients infected with human immunodeficiency virus. Clin Pharmacol Ther 2001;70:149–158.

98. Borin MT, Chambers JH, Carel BJ, Gagnon S, Freimuth WW. Pharmacokinetic study of the interaction between rifampin and delavirdine mesylate. Clin Pharmacol Ther 1997;61.

99. Borin MT, Chambers JH, Carel BJ, Freimuth WW, Aksentijevich S, Piergies AA. Pharmacokinetic study of the interaction between rifabutin and delavirdine mesylate in HIV-1 infected patients. Antiviral Res 1997;35:53–63.

100. Cox SR, Herman BD, Batts DH, Carel BJ, Carberry PA. Delavirdine and rifabutin: pharmacokinetic evaluation in HIV-1 patients with concentration-targeting of delavirdine. Fifth Conference on Retroviruses and Opportunistic Infections, Chicago, IL, February 1–5, 1998. Abstract 344.

101. de Jong MD, Vella S, Carr A, et al. High-dose nevirapine in previously untreated human immunodeficiency virus type 1-infected persons does not result in sustained suppression of viral replication. J Infect Dis 1997;175:966–970.

102. Cheeseman SH, Havlir D, McLaughlin MM, et al. Phase I/II evaluation of nevirapine alone and in combination with zidovudine for infection with human immunodeficiency virus. J Acquir Immune Defic Syndr 1995;8:141–151.

103. Panel on Clinical Practices for Treatment of HIV Infection convened by the Department of Health and Human Services (DHHS). Guidelines for the use of antiretroviral agents in HIV-infected adults and adolescents. Federal Register, November 10, 2003.

104. Hilts AE, Fish DN. Dosage adjustment of antiretroviral agents in patients with organ dysfunction. Am J Health Syst Pharm 1998;55:2528–2533.

105. Maserati R, Villani P, Seminari E, Pan A, Lo Caputo S, Regazzi MB. High plasma levels of nelfinavir and efavirenz in two HIV-positive patients with hepatic disease. AIDS 1999; 13:870–877.

106. Tseng AL, Walmsley SL. Rifabutin-associated uveitis. Ann Pharmacother 1995;29: 1149–1155.

107. Davis JL, Taskintuna I, Freeman WR, Weinberg DV, Feuer WJ, Leonard RE. Iritis and hypotony after treatment with intravenous cidofovir for cytomegalovirus retinitis. Arch Ophthalmol 1997;115:733–737.

108. Palau LA, Tufty GT, Pankey GA. Recurrent iritis after intravenous administration of cidofovir. Clin Infect Dis 1997;25:337–338.

109. Tseng AL, Mortimer CB, Salit IE. Iritis associated with intravenous cidofovir. Ann Pharmacother 1999;33:167–171.

110. Foulds G, Hilligoss DM, Henry EB, Gerber N. The effects of an antacid or cimetidine on the serum concentrations of azithromycin. J Clin Pharmacol 1991;31:164–167.

111. Gillum JG, Bruzzese VL, Israel DS, Kaplowitz LG, Polk RE. Effect of clarithromycin on the pharmacokinetics of 2′,3′-dideoxyinosine in patients who are seropositive for human immunodeficiency virus. Clin Infect Dis 1996;22:716–718.

112. Hafner R, Bethel J, Power M, et al. Tolerance and pharmacokinetic interactions of rifabutin and clarithromycin in human immunodeficiency virus-infected volunteers. Antimicrob Agents Chemother 1998;42:631–639.

113. Apseloff G, Foulds G, LaBoy-Goral L, Willavize S, Vincent J. Comparison of azithromycin and clarithromycin in their interactions with rifabutin in healthy volunteers. J Clin Pharmacol 1998;38:830–835.

114. Neuvonen PJ, Kivisto KT, Lehto P. Interference of dairy products with the absorption of ciprofloxacin. Clin Pharmacol Ther 1991;50:498–502.

115. Polk RE, Healy DP, Sahai J, Drewal L, Racht E. Effect of ferrous sulfate and multivitamins with zinc on absorption of ciprofloxacin in normal volunteers. Antimicrob Agents Chemother 1989;33:1841–1844.

116. Mueller BA, Abel SR, Brierton DG. Fluoroquinolone bioavailability in patients receiving nutritional supplements. Am J Health Syst Pharm 1995;52:892–893.

117. Sahai J, Gallicano K, Oliveras L, Khaliq S, Hawley-Foss N, Garber G. Cations in the didanosine tablet reduce ciprofloxacin bioavailability. Clin Pharmacol Ther 1993;53: 292–297.

118. Peloquin CA, Bulpitt AE, Jaresko GS, Jelliffe RW, Nix DE. Effect of food and antacids on the pharmacokinetics of ethambutol and pyrazinamide. Thirty-seventh Interscience Conference on Antimicrobial Agents and Chemotherapy, Toronto, September 28–October 1, 1997. Abstract A-3.

119. Mattila MJ, Linnoila M ST, Koskinen R. Effect of aluminium hydroxide and glycopyrrhonium on the absorption of ethambutol and alcohol in man. Br J Clin Pharmacol 1978;5:161–166.

120. The Indinavir (MK 639) Pharmacokinetic Study Group. Indinavir (MK 639) drug interaction studies. Eleventh International Conference on AIDS, Vancouver, July 7–12, 1996, p. 18. Abstract Mo.B.174.

121. Snider DE Jr. Pyridoxine supplementation during isoniazid therapy. Tubercle 1980;61: 191–196.

122. Simpson DM, Tagliati M. Nucleoside analogue-associated peripheral neuropathy in human immunodeficiency virus infection. J Acquir Immune Defic Syndr Hum Retrovirol 1995;9:153–161.

123. Dalton K, Dalton MJ. Characteristics of pyridoxine overdose neuropathy syndrome. Acta Neurol Scand 1987;76:8–11.

124. Snodgrass SR. Vitamin neurotoxicity. Mol Neurobiol 1992;6:41–73.

125. Robinson P, Lamson M, Gigliotti M, Myers M. Pharmacokinetic interaction between nevirapine and rifampin. Twelfth World AIDS Conference, Geneva, Switzerland, June 28–July 3, 1998. Abstract 60623.

126. Taburet A, Singlas E. Drug interactions with antiviral drugs. Clin Pharmacokinet 1996;30: 385–401.

127. Pinching AJ, Helbert M, Peddle B, Robinson D, Janes K, Gor D. Clinical experience with zidovudine for patients with acquired immune deficiency syndrome and acquired immune deficiency syndrome-related complex. J Infect 1989;18(suppl 1):33–40.

128. Hochster H, Dieterich D, Bozzette S, et al. Toxicity of combined ganciclovir and zidovudine for cytomegalovirus disease associated with AIDS. Ann Intern Med 1990;113: 111–117.

129. Gaines K, Wong R, Jung D. Pharmacokinetic interactions with oral ganciclovir: zidovudine, didanosine, probenecid [abstract]. Tenth International Conference on AIDS, Yokohama, Japan, August 1994.

130. Hoffmann-LaRoche Limited. Cytovene (ganciclovir) prescribing information. Nutley, NJ, September 2000.

131. Morris DJ. Adverse effects and drug interactions of clinical importance with antiretrovirals. Drug Safety 1994;10:281–291.

132. Millar AB, Miller RF, Patou G, Mindel A, Marsh R, Semple SJG. Treatment of cytomegalovirus retinitis with zidovudine and ganciclovir in patients with AIDS: outcome and toxicity. Genitourin Med 1990;66:156–158.

133. Hermans P, Rozenbaum W, Jou A, et al. Filgrastim to treat neutropenia and support myelosuppressive medication dosing in HIV infection. G-CSF 92105 Study Group. AIDS 1996;10:1627–1633.

134. Studies of Ocular Complications of AIDS Research Group in collaboration with the AIDS Clinical Trials Group. Mortality in patients with the acquired immunodeficiency syndrome treated with either foscarnet or ganciclovir for cytomegalovirus retinitis. N Engl J Med 1992;326:213–220.

135. Studies of Ocular Complications of AIDS Research Group in collaboration with the AIDS Clinical Trials Group. Morbidity and toxic effects associated with ganciclovir or foscarnet therapy in a randomized cytomegalovirus retinitis trial. Arch Intern Med 1995;155:65–74.

136. Rockstroh JK. Management of hepatitis B and C in HIV co-infected patients. J Acquir Immune Defic Syndr 2003;34:S59–S65.

137. Soto B, Sanchez-Quijano A, Rodrigo L, et al. Human immunodeficiency virus infection modifies the natural history of chronic parenterally-acquired hepatitis C with an unusually rapid progression to cirrhosis. J Hepatol 1997;26:1–5.

138. Garcia-Samaniego J, Rodriguez M, Berenguer J, et al. Hepatocellular carcinoma in HIV-infected patients with chronic hepatitis C. Am J Gastroenterol 2001;96:179–183.

139. Darby SC, Ewart DW, Giangrande PL, et al. Mortality from liver cancer and liver disease in haemophilic men and boys in UK given blood products contaminated with hepatitis C. UK Haemophilia Centre Directors' Organisation. Lancet 1997;350:1425–1431.

140. Lafeuillade A, Hittinger G, Chadapaud S. Increased mitochondrial toxicity with ribavirin in HIV/HCV coinfection. Lancet 2001;357:280–281.

141. Salmon-Ceron D, Chauvelot-Moachon L, Abad S, Silbermann B, Sogni P. Mitochondrial toxic effects and ribavirin [comment]. Lancet 2001;357:1803–1804.

142. Kakuda TN, Brinkman K. Mitochondrial toxic effects and ribavirin [comment]. Lancet 2001;357:1802–1803.

143. Soriano V, Sulkowski M, Bergin C, et al. Care of patients with chronic hepatitis C and HIV co-infection: recommendations from the HIV-HCV International Panel. AIDS 2002; 16:813–828.

144. de Miranda P, Good SS, Yarchoan R, et al. Alteration of zidovudine pharmacokinetics by probenecid in patients with AIDS or AIDS-related complex. Clin Pharmacol Ther 1989; 46:494–500.

145. Kornhauser DM, Petty BG, Hendrix CW, et al. Probenecid and zidovudine metabolism. Lancet 1989;2:473–475.

146. Petty BG, Kornhauser DM, Lietman PS. Zidovudine with probenecid: a warning [letter]. Lancet 1990;335:1044–1045.

147. Lalezari JP, Kuppermann BD. Clinical experience with cidofovir in the treatment of cytomegalovirus retinitis. J Acquir Immune Defic Syndr Hum Retrovirol 1997;14:S27–S31.

148. Frascino RJ, Gaines Griffy K, Jung D, Yu S. Multiple dose crossover study of IV ganciclovir induction dose (5 mg/kg iv q 12 h) and didanosine (200 mg po q 12 h) in HIV-infected persons. Thirty-fifth Interscience Conference on Antimicrobial Agents and Chemotherapy, San Francisco, September 17–20, 1995. Abstract A-27.

149. Bristol-Myers Squibb Co. Videx EC (didanosine enteric coated) prescribing information. Princeton, NJ, February 2003.

150. Hoffmann-LaRoche Laboratories. Valcyte (valganciclovir) prescribing information. Nutley, NJ, September 2003.

151. Glaxo Wellcome. Data on file, RM1996/00090/00. Personal communication, 1996.

152. Gallicano K, Sahai J, Swick L, Seguin I, Pakuts A, Cameron DW. Effect of rifabutin on the pharmacokinetics of zidovudine in patients infected with human immunodeficiency virus. Clin Infect Dis 1995;21:1008–1011.

153. Abbott Laboratories. Kaletra (lopinavir/ritonavir) prescribing information. North Chicago, IL: January 2003.

154. Falloon J, Lavelle J, Ogata-Arakaki D, et al. Pharmacokinetics and safety of weekly dapsone and dapsone plus pyrimethamine for prevention of pneumocystis pneumonia. Antimicrob Agents Chemother 1994;38:1580–1587.

155. McEvoy GK, ed. American Hospital Formulary Service Drug Information. Bethesda, MD: American Society of Health-System Pharmacists, 1995.

156. Zuidema J, Hilbers-Modderman ESM, Merkus FWHM. Clinical pharmacokinetics of dapsone. Clin Pharmacokinet 1986;11:299–315.

157. Lee BL, Medina I, Benowitz NL, Jacob P, Wofsy CB, Mills J. Dapsone, trimethoprim and sulfamethoxazole plasma levels during treatment of *Pneumocystis* pneumonia in patients with acquired immunodeficiency syndrome: evidence of drug interactions. Ann Intern Med 1989;110:606–611.

158. Aventis Pharma Inc.. Pentacarinat product monograph. Laval, Canada: 2002.

159. Youle MS, Clarbour J, Gazzard B, Chanas A. Severe hypocalcemia in AIDS patients treated with foscarnet and pentamidine [letter]. Lancet 1988;1:1455–1456.
160. Collaborative AZT Study Group. Tolerance of AZT in association with trimethoprim-sulfamethoxazole, pyrimethamine, or rifampin [abstract]. Fourth International Conference on AIDS, Stockholm, June 12–16, 1988.
161. GlaxoSmithKline. Daraprim (pyrimethamine) prescribing information. Research Triangle Park, NC, March 2003.
162. Lee BL, Tuber MG, Chambers HR, Gambertoglio J, Delahunty T. The effect of trimethoprim on the pharmacokinetics of zalcitabine in HIV-infected patients [abstract]. Thirty-fifth Interscience Conference on Antimicrobial Agents and Chemotherapy, San Francisco, CA, September 17–20, 1995.
163. Squibb. Fungizone intravenous product monograph. Montreal, Canada, 1996.
164. Kerr B, Yuen G, Daniels R, Quart B, Anderson R. Strategic approach to nelfinavir mesylate (NFV) drug interactions involving CYP3A metabolism. Fourth National Conference on Retroviruses and Opportunistic Infections, Washington, DC, January 1997.
165. Bristol-Myers Squibb Co. Reyataz (atazanavir) prescribing information. Princeton, NJ, June 2003.
166. Trapnell CB, Narang PK, Li R, Lavelle JP. Increased plasma rifabutin levels with concomitant fluconazole therapy in HIV-infected patients. Ann Intern Med 1996;124:573–576.
167. Trapnell CB, Lavelle JP, O'Leary CR, et al. Rifabutin does not alter fluconazole pharmacokinetics [abstract PII-106]. Clin Pharmacol Ther 1993;52:196.
168. Lazar JD, Wilner KD. Drug interactions with fluconazole. Rev Infect Dis 1990;12(suppl 3):S327S333.
169. Coker RJ, Tomlinson DR, Parkin J, Harris JRW, Pinching AJ. Interaction between fluconazole and rifampicin [letter]. BMJ 1990;301:818.
170. Apseloff G, Hilligoss DM, Gardner MJ, et al. Induction of fluconazole metabolism by rifampin: in vivo study in humans. J Clin Pharmacol 1991;31:358–361.
171. Smith JA, Hardin TC, Patterson TF, Rinaldi MG, Graybill JR. Rifabutin decreases itraconazole plasma levels in patients with HIV infection. Second National Conference on Human Retroviruses and Related Infections, Washington, DC, January 29–February 2, 1995. Abstract 126.
172. Lefort A, Launay O, Carbon C. Uveitis associated with rifabutin prophylaxis and itraconazole therapy [letter]. Ann Intern Med 1996;125:939–940.
173. Drayton J, Dickinson G, Rinaldi MG. Coadministration of rifampin and itraconazole leads to undetectable levels of serum itraconazole [letter]. Clin Infect Dis 1994;18:266.
174. Polk RE, Crouch M, Israel DS, et al. Pharmacokinetic interaction between ketoconazole and amprenavir after single doses in healthy men. Pharmacotherapy 1999;19:1378–1384.
175. GlaxoSmithKline. Agenerase (amprenavir) prescribing information. Research Triangle Park, NC, October 2002.
176. Lelawongs P, Barone JA, Colaizzi JL, et al. Effect of food and gastric acidity on absorption of orally administered ketoconazole. Clin Pharm 1988;7:228–235.
177. Pilheu JA, Galati MR, Yunis AS, et al. Interaccion farmacocinetica entre ketconazol, isoniacida y rifampicina [Pharmacokinetic interaction of ketoconazole, isoniazid, and rifampicin]. Medicina 1989;49:43–47.
178. Kerr B, Lee C, Yuen G, et al. Overview of in-vitro and in-vivo drug interaction studies of nelfinavir mesylate, a new HIV-1 protease inhibitor. Fourth Conference on Retroviruses and Opportunistic Infections, Washington, DC, January 22–26, 1997. Abstract 373.
179. Tucker RM, Denning DW, Hanson LH, et al. Interaction of azoles with rifampin, phenytoin, and carbamazepine: in vitro and clinical observations. Clin Infect Dis 1992;14:165–174.
180. Engelhard D, Stutman HR, Marks MI. Interaction of ketoconazole with rifampin and isoniazid. N Engl J Med 1984;311:1681–1683.

181. Hoffmann-La Roche. Invirase (saquinavir) prescribing information. Nutley, NJ, July 2002.
182. Agouron Pharmaceuticals. Viracept (nelfinavir) prescribing information. La Jolla, CA, August 2003.
183. Chave JP, Munafo A, Chatton JY, Dayer P, Glauser MP, Biollaz J. Once-a-week azithromycin in AIDS patients: tolerability, kinetics, and effects on zidovudine disposition. Antimicrob Agents Chemother 1992;36:1013–1018.
184. Sadler BM, Gillotin C, Chittick GE, Symonds WT. Pharmacokinetic drug interactions with amprenavir. Twelfth World AIDS Conference, Geneva, Switzerland, June 28–July 3, 1998. Abstract 12389.
185. Benedek IH, Joshi A, Fiske WD, et al. Pharmacokinetic interaction studies in healthy volunteers with efavirenz and the macrolide antibiotics, azithromycin and clarithromycin. Fifth Conference on Retroviruses and Opportunistic Infections, Chicago, IL, February 1–5, 1998. Abstract 347.
186. Robinson P, Gigliotti M, Lamson M, Azzam S, MacGregor T. Effect of the reverse transcriptase inhibitor, nevirapine, on the steady-state pharmacokinetics of clarithromycin in HIV-positive patients. Sixth Conference on Retroviruses and Opportunistic Infections, Chicago, IL, January 31–February 4, 1999. Abstract 374.
187. Wallace RJ Jr, Brown BA, Griffith DE, Girard W, Tanaka K. Reduced serum levels of clarithromycin in patients treated with multidrug regimens including rifampin or rifabutin for *Mycobacterium avium–M. intracellulare* infection. J Infect Dis 1995;171:747–750.
188. Ouellet D, Hsu H, Mukherjee D, Locke C, Leonard JM. Assessment of the pharmacokinetic interaction between ritonavir and clarithromycin [Abstract PI-58]. Clin Pharmacol Ther 1996;59:143..
189. Buss N. Saquinavir soft gel capsule (Fortovase): pharmacokinetics and drug interactions. Fifth Conference on Retroviruses and Opportunistic Infections, Chicago, IL, February 1–5, 1998. Abstract 354.
190. Pastore A, Van Cleef G, Risher EJ, Gillum JG, LeBel M, Polk RE. Dideoxycytidine pharmacokinetics and interaction with clarithromycin in patients seropositive for HIV [abstract]. Fourth National Conference on Retroviruses and Opportunistic Infections, Washington, DC, January 1997.
191. Polis MA, Piscitelli SC, Vogel S, et al. Clarithromycin lowers plasma zidovudine levels in persons with human immunodeficiency virus infection. Antimicrob Agents Chemother 1997;41:1709–1714.
192. Rana KZ, Darnowski JW, Strayer AH, Dudley MN. Clarithromycin does not affect phosphorylation of zidovudine in vitro. Antimicrob Agents Chemother 1996;40:1945–1947.
193. Hurwitz A, Scholzman DL. Effects of antacids on gastrointestinal absorption of isoniazid in rat and man. Am Rev Resp Dis 1974;109:41–47.
194. Gallicano K, Sahai J, Zaror-Behrens G, Pakuts A. Effect of antacids in didanosine tablet on bioavailability of isoniazid. Antimicrob Agents Chemother 1994;38:894–897.
195. Sarma GR, Kailasam S, Nair NGK, Narayana ASL, Tripathy SP. Effect of prednisone and rifampin on isoniazid metabolism in slow and rapid inactivators of isoniazid. Antimicrob Agents Chemother 1980;18:661–666.
196. Lee BL, Tauber MG, Chambers HF, Gambertoglio J, Delahunty T. The effect of zalcitabine on the pharmacokinetics of isoniazid in HIV-infected patients. Thirty-fourth Interscience Conference on Antimicrobial Agents and Chemotherapy, New Orleans, LA, October 4–7, 1994, p. 3. Abstract A4.
197. Polk RE, Brophy DF, Israel DS, et al. Pharmacokinetic interaction between amprenavir and rifabutin or rifampin in healthy males. Antimicrob Agents Chemother 2001;45:502–508.
198. Agarwala S, Mummaneni V, Randall D, Geraldes M, Stoltz R, O'Mara E. Pharmacokinetic effect of rifabutin on atazanavir with and without ritonavir in healthy subjects. Ninth Conference on Retroviruses and Opportunistic Infections, Seattle, WA, February 24–28, 2002, p. 221. Abstract 445-W.

199. Sahai J, Narang PK, Hawley-Foss N, Li RC, Kamal M, Cameron DW. A phase I evaluation of concomitant rifabutin and didanosine in symptomatic HIV-infected patients. J Acquir Immune Defic Syndr Hum Retrovirol 1995;9:274–279.

200. Benedek IH, Fiske WD, White SJ, Stevenson D, Joseph JL, Kornhauser DM. Pharmacokinetic interaction between multiple doses of efavirenz and rifabutin in healthy volunteers [abstract]. Clin Infect Dis 1998;27:1008.

201. Kerr BM, Daniels R, Clendeninn N. Pharmacokinetic interaction of nelfinavir with half-dose rifabutin. Eighth Annual Canadian Conference on HIV/AIDS Research, Victoria, British Columbia, Canada, May 1–4, 1999. Abstract B203.

202. Sahai J, Stewart F, Swick L, et al. Rifabutin reduces saquinavir plasma levels in HIV-infected patients. Thirty-sixth Interscience Conference on Antimicrobial Agents and Chemotherapy, New Orleans, LA, September 1996. Abstract A027.

203. Benedek IH, Joshi A, Fiske WD, et al. Pharmacokinetic interaction between efavirenz and rifampin in healthy volunteers. Twelfth World AIDS Conference, Geneva, Switzerland, June 28–July 3, 1998. Abstract 42280.

204. Gallicano KD, Sahai J, Shukla VK, et al. Induction of zidovudine glucuronidation and amination pathways by rifampicin in HIV-infected patients. Br J Clin Pharmacol 1999;48:168–179.

205. Gallant JE, Moore RD, Keruly J, Richman DD, Chaisson RE. Lack of association between acyclovir use and survival in patients with advanced human immunodeficiency virus disease treated with zidovudine. Zidovudine Epidemiology Study Group. J Infect Dis 1995;172:346–352.

206. Stein DS, Graham NM, Park LP, et al. The effect of the interaction of acyclovir with zidovudine on progression to AIDS and survival. Analysis of data in the Multicenter AIDS Cohort Study. Ann Intern Med 1994;121:100–108.

207. Cooper DA, Pehrson PO, Pedersen C, et al. The efficacy and safety of zidovudine alone or as cotherapy with acyclovir for the treatment of patients with AIDS and AIDS-related complex: a double-blind randomized trial. European-Australian Collaborative Group. AIDS 1993;7:197–207.

208. Pedersen C, Cooper DA, Brun-Vezinet F, et al. The effect of treatment with zidovudine with or without acyclovir on HIV p24 antigenaemia in patients with AIDS or AIDS-related complex. AIDS 1992;6:821–825.

209. Cooper DA, Pedersen C, Aiuti F, et al. The efficacy and safety of zidovudine with or without acyclovir in the treatment of patients with AIDS-related complex. The European-Australian Collaborative Group. AIDS 1991;5:933–943.

210. Tartaglione TA, Collier AC, Opheim K, Gianola FG, Benedetti J, Corey L. Pharmacokinetic evaluations of low- and high-dose zidovudine plus high-dose acyclovir in patients with symptomatic human immunodeficiency virus infection. Antimicrob Agents Chemother 1991;35:2225–2231.

211. Bach MC. Possible drug interaction during therapy with azidothymidine and acyclovir for AIDS [letter]. N Engl J Med 1987;317:547.

212. Laskin OL, de Miranda P, King DH, et al. Effects of probenecid on the pharmacokinetics and elimination of acyclovir in humans. Antimicrob Agents Chemother 1982;21:804–807.

213. Reines ED, Gross PA. Antiviral agents. Med Clin North Am 1988;72:691–715.

214. Gilead Sciences. Vistide product monograph. Foster City, CA, 1996.

215. Massarella JW, Nazareno LA, Passe S, Min B. The effect of probenecid on the pharmacyokinetics of zalcitabine in HIV-positive patients. Pharm Res 1996;13:449–452.

216. Freitas VR, Fraser-Smith EB, Matthews TR. Efficacy of ganciclovir in combination with other antimicrobial agents against cytomegalovirus in vitro and in vivo. Antiviral Res 1993;20:1–12.

217. Faulds D, Heel RC. Ganciclovir—a review of its antiviral activity, pharmacokinetic properties and therapeutic efficacy in cytomegalovirus infections. Drugs 1990;39:597–638.

218. Aweeka FT, Brody SR, Jacobson M, Botwin K, Martin-Munley S. Is there a pharmacokinetic interaction between foscarnet and zalcitabine during concomitant administration? Clin Ther 1998;20:232–243.
219. Koshida R, Vrang L, Gilljam G, Harmenberg J, Oberg B, Wahren B. Inhibition of human immunodeficiency virus in vitro by combinations of 3′-azido-3′-deoxythymidine and foscarnet. Antimicrob Agents Chemother 1989;33:778–780.
220. Eriksson BF, Schinazi RF. Combinations of 3′-azido-3′-deoxythymidine (zidovudine) and phosphonoformate (foscarnet) against human immunodeficiency virus type 1 and cytomegalovirus replication in vitro. Antimicrob Agents Chemother 1989;33:663–669.
221. Aweeka FT, Gambertoglio JG, van der Horst C, Raasch R, Jacobson MA. Pharmacokinetics of concomitantly administered foscarnet and zidovudine for treatment of human immunodeficiency virus infection (AIDS Clinical Trials Group protocol 053). Antimicrob Agents Chemother 1992;36:1773–1778.
222. Butt AA. Fatal lactic acidosis and pancreatitis associated with ribavirin and didanosine therapy. AIDS Reader 2003;13:344–348.
223. Vogt MW, Hartshorn KL, Furman PA, et al. Ribavirin antagonizes the effect of azidothymidine on HIV replication. Science 1987;235:1376–1379.

# 7

# Drugs for Tuberculosis

## Rocsanna Namdar, Steven C. Ebert, and Charles A. Peloquin

### INTRODUCTION

Tuberculosis (TB) remains one of the most prevalent infectious killers on the planet. Given the broad range of interactions associated with rifamycins, it is highly likely TB patients will be at risk of drug interactions. Since TB and human immunodeficiency virus (HIV) often co-exist as infections, it is inevitable that drug interactions will occur in this population.

### STANDARD TREATMENTS FOR TUBERCULOSIS

The treatment of TB can be highly successful, even in HIV-positive patients, when published guidelines are carefully followed (1,2). These references are recommended to the interested reader who is likely to face patients with TB on a regular basis because they provide additional detail not found in this chapter. When fully susceptible or only monoresistant TB is likely, an initial regimen of isoniazid (INH), rifampin (RIF), pyrazinamide (PZA), and ethambutol (EMB) is used. Because of the inconvenience of parenteral administration and the rising rates of streptomycin (SM) resistance along the Pacific Rim, SM is now considered a second-line agent. As discussed in this chapter, rifabutin (RBN) may be considered as an alternative to RIF when hepatic enzyme induction will severely disrupt concurrent treatments, such as treatment with the HIV protease inhibitors. The fourth drug (usually EMB) can be discontinued if the isolate is found to be fully drug susceptible. PZA can be discontinued in patients who respond normally after 8 weeks of treatment (1,2). Thereafter, INH and the rifamycin (RIF or RBN) are continued for an additional 4 months or longer if the patient is slow to respond.

Multidrug-resistant tuberculosis (MDR-TB, defined as resistance to at least INH and RIF) is much more difficult to treat (1,2). There is no standard treatment for this condition. Further, the drugs used for MDR-TB generally are weaker and more toxic than INH and RIF, and the duration of treatment for MDR-TB is much longer (24 months or more). Therefore, the period over which interactions can occur is greatly extended, and because these second-line drugs are not as effective as first line, interactions that reduce bioavailability can adversely affect the outcome of treatment.

From: *Infectious Disease: Drug Interactions in Infectious Diseases, Second Edition*
Edited by: S. C. Piscitelli and K. A. Rodvold © Humana Press Inc., Totowa, NJ

## ORAL ABSORPTION ISSUES
## WITH THE TUBERCULOSIS DRUGS

### Interactions With Food

INH and RIF show marked decreases in the maximum serum concentration ($C_{max}$, 51 and 36%, respectively), and lesser decreases in area under the serum concentration–time curve (AUC, 9 and 10%, respectively) when given with high-fat meals (Table 1) *(3,4)*. EMB shows modest decreases in $C_{max}$ (17%) but not AUC; PZA only shows a modest delay in absorption when these drugs are given with high-fat meals *(5,6)*. High-fat meals do not adversely affect the absorption of ethionamide (ETA), but decrease the $C_{max}$ of cycloserine (CS) by 27% (AUC decreases by only 5%) *(7,8)*. Orange juice also decreases the $C_{max}$ of CS by about 13% (AUC decreases by only 3%), and presumably this would occur with other acidic beverages *(8)*. In contrast, high-fat meals increase the $C_{max}$ of clofazimine (CF) and *p*-aminosalicylic acid (PAS) granules *(9,10)*.

### Interactions With Antacids

Of the four most frequently used TB drugs, only EMB appears to be significantly affected by coadministration with antacids (Mylanta®; Table 1) *(3–6)*. Conflicting data exist for INH, with our recent investigation showing no significant effect when Mylanta was given 9 hours before INH, at the time of dosing, and then with lunch and dinner following dosing. Antacids produced little change in the absorption of CS, ETA, PAS, and CF, although food would be preferred with the latter two *(7–10)*.

### Interactions With H₂ Antagonists

RIF is not affected by the coadministration of ranitidine *(4)*. Data are not available for the other TB drugs.

### Malabsorption in Selected Patient Populations

Patients with known or suspected gastroenteropathies may have difficulty absorbing some of the TB drugs normally. RIF and EMB appear to be more prone to malabsorption, with lower $C_{max}$ and AUC *(11–17)*. RBN fares somewhat better in patients with acquired immunodeficiency syndrome (AIDS) than RIF, as does rifapentine (RPNT) *(18–20)*. In one publication, INH had few problems being absorbed by AIDS patients, although diarrhea can decrease the $C_{max}$ by 39% *(11)*. Still, newer studies showed that INH absorption problems may lead to treatment failures and the selection of drug resistance, and that this may occur more commonly among AIDS patients compared to others *(21,22)*. PZA's AUC is somewhat lower among patients with low CD4 counts and diarrhea, but PZA is otherwise well absorbed *(11,12)*.

The precise reasons for drug malabsorption in AIDS patients are not known but may include HIV-related achlorhydria, HIV enteropathy, and opportunistic infections of the gastrointestinal (GI) tract, such as cryptosporidiosis *(23–27)*. There also is some anecdotal experience suggesting that patients with cystic fibrosis and diabetes mellitus may be susceptible to similar absorption problems. When TB patients do not respond as expected to drug treatment, therapeutic drug monitoring (TDM) may be used to identify the problem and to guide the dose adjustments *(17)*.

**Table 1**
**Effects of Food and Antacids on the Absorption of Antituberculous Drugs**

| Drug | Effect of food | Effect of antacids | Clinical implications |
|---|---|---|---|
| Aminosalicylic acid (PAS) granules | Acidic beverage or yogurt prevents release in stomach, thus reducing nausea; food increases absorption | Small decrease in absorption | Give PAS granules with acidic beverage or with food; avoid antacids if possible |
| Ciprofloxacin | Delayed $T_{max}$, but minimal effect on AUC | Large decrease in $C_{max}$ and AUC | Do not coadminister with di- and trivalent cations, including antacids |
| Cycloserine | Food decreases $C_{max}$ 17%; no effect on AUC | Antacids slightly increase $C_{max}$ | Do not coadminister with food if possible |
| Ethambutol | Delayed $T_{max}$, 16% decrease in $C_{max}$, but minimal effect on AUC | 28% decrease in $C_{max}$ and 10% decrease in AUC | May be given with food; do not coadminister with antacids |
| Ethionamide | No significant effect | No significant effect | Can be coadministered with food and antacids |
| Isoniazid | Food, especially carbohydrate-based meals, significantly reduces isoniazid $C_{max}$ and AUC | 0–19% decrease in AUC | Do not coadminister with meals; do not coadminister with antacids whenever possible |
| Levofloxacin | No significant effect | Large decreases in $C_{max}$ and AUC | Do not coadminister with di- and trivalent cations, including antacids |
| Pyrazinamide | Delayed $T_{max}$; no effect on AUC | No significant effect | May be given with food or antacids |
| Rifabutin | No significant effect | Unknown, not affected by didanosine | May be given with food; do not coadminister with antacids until studied |
| Rifampin | Delayed $T_{max}$, 15–36% decrease in $C_{max}$, and 4–23% decrease in AUC | No significant change in serum concentrations, 30% decrease in 24-hour urinary excretion | Do not coadminister with food; may be given with ranitidine; avoid coadministration with antacids whenever possible |

*Source*: References *3–10*. Adapted from ref. 27 with permission.
AUC, area under the serum concentration–time curve; $C_{max}$, peak (maximal) serum concentration; $T_{max}$, time from drug ingestion to peak (maximal) serum concentration.

## DRUG AND DISEASE STATE INTERACTIONS
## IN PATIENTS WITH TUBERCULOSIS

### INH Interactions

INH is cleared by *N*-acetyltransferase 2 (NAT2) to the microbiologically inactive metabolite acetylisoniazid and subsequently to mono- and di-acetyl-hydrazine *(21,28)*. Because of its rapid hepatic clearance, INH is not substantially removed by hemodialysis *(29)*. INH does have a few clearly established drug interactions. The most significant involve phenytoin and carbamazepine. INH has been associated with elevated concentrations of both anticonvulsant agents. Phenytoin is a cytochrome P450 (CYP) 2C9 substrate; carbamazepine appears to be cleared by CYP3A4 and either CYP2C8 or CYP2C9. INH also has been described as inhibiting the clearance of diazepam (CYP3A4 and CYP2C19), primidone (enzyme not reported), chlorzoxazone (CYP2E1), and warfarin (CYP1A2, CYP2C9, CYP2C19, CYP3A4) *(30–34)*.

Desta and colleagues showed that INH inhibits CYP2C19 and CYP3A4 in a concentration-dependent manner *(35)*. In their human liver microsome system, inhibition was not demonstrated for CYP2C9 and CYP1A2 whereas INH was considered a weak noncompetitive inhibitor of CYP2E1 and a competitive inhibitor of CYP2D6 *(35)*. Given INH's inhibitory effects on several P450 enzymes, it is somewhat surprising that a longer list of interacting agents has not been identified for INH.

INH causes an initial inhibition, followed by induction of CYP2E1 *(33)*. Therefore, INH can alter the clearance of ethanol. INH may inhibit or promote the conversion of acetaminophen to its putative toxic intermediate metabolite, *N*-acetyl-*p*-benzoquinone imine, depending on the timing of the doses *(33)*. Therefore, high-dose acetaminophen should be avoided with INH *(33,36,37)*.

A few studies have examined oral bioavailability interactions between INH and other drugs. The oral bioavailability of RIF was reduced by an average of 32% in volunteers who were administered an INH-RIF fixed-dose combination (FDC) product compared with RIF alone *(38)*. The decrease in bioavailability appears to be a function of the FDC formulation and not directly caused by an interaction between INH and RIF. This is compensated by giving a slightly higher dose of RIF (in milligrams) as the FDC product. Coadministration of ciprofloxacin and INH results in a delay (but not a reduction in the extent) of INH absorption *(39)*.

### Rifamycin Interactions

The available rifamycins include RIF, RBN, and RPNT. Rifalazil (KRM-1648) is an investigational agent. All of these drugs share a similar mechanism of action and in general show cross-resistance. They are primarily cleared by esterases to the 25-desacetyl derivatives, which retain most of the parent drugs' activities against mycobacteria. Most of the parent compounds and metabolites are cleared through the biliary tract, with small amounts showing up in the urine *(4,28,37)*. In the case of 25-desacetyl RBN, subsequent metabolism appears to take place via CYP3A4. Because of its rapid hepatic clearance and large molecular size, RIF is not substantially removed by hemodialysis *(29)*. With the exception of rifalazil, rifamycins are among the most potent known inducers of the hepatic CYP enzyme system, with most marked effect on isoforms CYP3A4 and CYP2C8/9 *(27,40)*.

RIF intracellular concentrations and the extent by which RIF is able to induce CYP3A has been strongly correlated with P-glycoprotein levels *(41)*. The gene that encodes this protein is the multidrug resistance 1 (MDR1) gene. Patients with specific polymorphisms of MDR1 have been shown to demonstrate significantly different levels of P-glycoprotein activity *(42)*. This may partially explain the wide interpatient variability in CYP3A induction by RIF. The relative inductive potency toward CYP3A is RIF > RPNT >> RBN *(43)*. For certain drug substrates and metabolic pathways, the extent of induction by rifamycins might be increased by increasing the dose and decreased by extending the administration interval between constant doses of the rifamycin. As a practical matter, drugs cleared by CYP3A4 can be assumed to be maximally induced by standard 600-mg doses of RIF. Induction of CYP3A is greater when RPNT is given daily than when it is given every 3 days *(44)*. Enzyme induction with rifamycins reaches a maximum after approx 7 days of administration. Effects persist for 7–14 days after dosing is stopped, and the pharmacodynamic effects of the affected drug generally return to baseline levels within 2 weeks after discontinuing rifamycin therapy *(44,45)*.

The potent enzyme induction of CYP3A4 and CYP2C8/9 can affect the metabolism of many other drugs when administered concomitantly, especially if they are substrates for CYP3A4 and to a lesser degree CYP2C8/9, CYP2C19, and CYP2D6. Most hepatically metabolized drugs will have shorter half-lives and are likely to display lower plasma concentrations in the presence of RIF, RBN, or RPNT. The list of drug interactions will continue to grow as new drugs are introduced and as the pathways for drug clearance are better defined.

RBN induces and is partly metabolized by CYP3A. As a result, complex bidirectional interactions with RBN can occur *(27,40)*. The CYP3A-inducing effect of RBN results in decreased concentrations of drugs. Coadministration of CYP3A inhibitors increase the concentrations of RBN, especially 25-*O*-desacetyl RBN, sometimes leading to RBN toxicity *(27,40)*. Unlike RBN, RPNT does not offer any advantage in sparing the drug interactions and is similar to RIF regarding drug interactions. However, because both RPNT and RIF are not substrates for CYP enzymes, they are not the objects of drug interactions, as is the case with RBN.

Significant variability exists among patients in the expression of the various drug-metabolizing enzymes *(17,27,40,46)*. Therefore, even without drug interactions, significant interpatient variability in pharmacokinetics can be seen. Most available drug interaction data come from small studies of healthy volunteers and focus on bidirectional interactions involving only two drugs. More complex interactions commonly are seen in the clinical setting, sometimes involving four, five, or even six drugs simultaneously, making it difficult, if not impossible, to anticipate the final outcomes. Patients who receive three or more interacting drugs likely would benefit from individualized dosing of these various drugs. Further, some of these patients have conditions, such as HIV, that have been associated with more erratic drug absorption *(17,46)*. TDM is available for the various TB drugs, including the rifamycins, and for the HIV protease inhibitors and nonnucleoside reverse transcriptase inhibitors (NNRTIs), as well as the azole antifungals and macrolide antibiotics. It is not uncommon for HIV-positive patients to receive all of these classes of drugs simultaneously. TDM should be considered whenever the failure to achieve an immediate therapeutic response would put the patients in danger of adverse clinical outcomes or when the expected clinical responses have not been seen after several weeks of therapy *(17,46)*.

A review of rifamycin drug interactions with antimicrobials is described next. A summary is provided in Table 2 *(11,47–49)*.

### Azoles

RIF has significant pharmacokinetic interactions with itraconazole. Concomitant administration in both healthy volunteers and in AIDS patients has shown a reduction (64–88%) in AUC and has also resulted in undetectable itraconazole concentrations *(50,51)*. Antifungal therapy with itraconazole during RIF administration has been ineffective *(51)*. RIF has also been shown to significantly reduce (82%) the AUC of ketoconazole in healthy volunteers *(52)*. Based on these data, the concurrent use of RIF and itraconazole or ketoconazole should be avoided because of the risk of therapeutic failure. Alternative antifungal therapies should be considered in patients taking RIF.

The magnitude of the effect of RIF on fluconazole has not been well established. Data suggest that the coadministration results in increased rates of clearance and reduction in the AUC (23–52%) of fluconazole *(53,54)*. Antifungal treatment failures have also been reported with the concurrent administration of fluconazole and RIF *(55)*. Based on current data, fluconazole can be used with rifamycins, but the dose of fluconazole may have to be increased *(1,56,57)*. There is no significant effect of fluconazole on RIF pharmacokinetics *(58)*.

RBN has demonstrated bidirectional interactions when administered with cytochrome P450 (CYP) 3A inhibitors. The effects of fluconazole on the pharmacokinetics of RBN showed an increase (76%) in AUC of RBN *(59)*. The concentration of RBN's active metabolite, 25-desacetyl RBN, also was markedly increased. The concurrent use of fluconazole with RBN is not recommended because of the increased risk of RBN-associated adverse effects.

### Chloramphenicol

Several case reports have described decreased chloramphenicol serum concentrations when patients were concomitantly treated with RIF. The dose of chloramphenicol could be increased to maintain serum concentrations; however, this would put the patient at greater risk for aplastic anemia. Alternative therapies should be considered in patients taking RIF *(60,61)*.

### Dapsone

RIF and RBN have been associated with a significant increase (50–70%) in the clearance of dapsone *(19,62)*. The clinical significance of this interaction has not been determined. However, higher dapsone AUCs have been associated with a lower risk of *Pneumocystis carinii* pneumonia *(62)*. Dosage adjustments for patients taking dapsone with RBN or RIF may be necessary. Patients should be monitored closely and TDM should be considered.

### Doxycycline

Treatment failures have been reported in patients with brucellosis treated with doxycycline and RIF. Patients receiving RIF and doxycycline had decreased doxycycline AUCs (59%) and higher clearances when compared to the doxycycline-plus-SM combination. Alternatives to doxycycline should be considered in patients taking RIF *(63)*.

**Table 2**
**Rifamycin Drug Interactions With Anti-Infective Agents**

| Drug class | Drugs with concentrations that are substantially decreased by rifamycins | Comments |
|---|---|---|
| Anti-Infectives | HIV-1 protease inhibitors (saquinavir, indinavir, nelfinavir, amprenavir, ritonavir, lopinavir/ritonavir) | Can be used with rifabutin. Ritonavir, 400–600 mg twice daily, probably can be used with rifampin. The combination of saquinavir and ritonavir can also be used with rifampin. |
| | Nonnucleoside reverse transcriptase inhibitors (delavirdine, nevirapine, efavirenz) | Delavirdine should not be used with any rifamycin. Doses of nevirapine and efavirenz need to be increased if given with rifampin; no dose increase needed if given with rifabutin. |
| | Fluoroquinolones | Based on current data, no adjustments necessary. |
| | Metronidazole | Limited data; ↑ clearance. |
| | NRTI (zidovudine, lamivudine) | No significant clinical effect. |
| | SMX–TMP | Reduced concentrations of SMX/TMP; clinical effects unknown. |
| | Macrolide antibiotics (clarithromycin, erythromycin) | Avoid concomitant administration of clarithromycin and rifampin or rifabutin. Azithromycin has no significant interaction with rifamycins. |
| | Doxycycline | May require use of a drug other than doxycycline. |
| | Azole antifungal agents (ketoconazole, itraconazole, voriconazole) | Itraconazole, ketoconazole, and voriconazole concentrations may be subtherapeutic with any of the rifamycins. Fluconazole can be used with rifamycins, but the dose of fluconazole may have to be increased. |
| | Atovaquone, dapsone Chloramphenicol | Consider alternative *Pneumocystis carinii* treatment or prophylaxis. Consider an alternative antibiotic. |

*Source:* Adapted from ref. *49* with permission.

*Fluoroquinolones*

Limited data exist regarding the interaction between fluoroquinolones and rifamycins. Currently, there is no evidence for significant pharmacokinetic or pharmacodynamic interactions in humans. Total plasma clearance may be increased, but peak/minimum inhibition concentration (MIC) ratios and efficacy are not significantly affected *(64,65)*. Based on current data, dosage adjustment of either agent is not necessary.

*Macrolides*

The combination of clarithromycin and RIF resulted in reduced mean peak clarithromycin concentrations (87%) when compared to clarithromycin monotherapy *(59)*. The concentrations of the active metabolite of clarithromycin, 14-OH clarithromycin, were not affected. Based on current data, RIF can decrease the efficacy of clarithromycin by reducing serum concentrations. Concomitant treatment may reduce clarithromycin's efficacy .

Macrolide drug interactions with RBN are complex. The CYP3A-inducing effect of RBN results in decreased concentrations of the macrolides; the macrolides, CYP3A inhibitors, increase the concentration of RBN and its active metabolite, leading to increased risk of RBN toxicity. The reduced affinity of azithromycin for CYP results in fewer clinically significant interactions. However, studies evaluating the combination of azithromycin and RBN resulted in unusually high rates of neutropenia *(66)*.

The pharmacokinetics of clarithromycin plus RBN has been evaluated in healthy volunteers and in HIV-positive patients *(59,66,67)*. The concomitant administration of the two drugs resulted in an increase in the serum concentration (76%) and AUC (99%) of RBN and its active metabolite, 25-*O*-desacetyl RBN, when compared to each agent alone. Effects of RBN on clarithromycin have demonstrated a 44% reduction in AUC and an increase in concentrations of clarithromycin's active metabolite, 14-OH clarithromycin. Reports of significant adverse reactions, including neutropenia, fever, myalgia, and uveitis, have been associated with the combination of clarithromycin plus RBN *(66,67)*. Based on current data, the combination of RBN and clarithromycin should be avoided when feasible and used cautiously when necessary. Azithromycin can be considered if macrolide therapy is necessary. TDM should be used to monitor for efficacy and risk of adverse effects.

*Metronidazole*

Limited data have shown that RIF increases the clearance of metronidazole and decreases the AUC *(68)*.

*Nonnucleoside Reverse Transcriptase Inhibitors*

Table 3 summarizes the effects of RIF and RBN on the AUC of NNRTIs *(27,57,69)*. Because of the bidirectional interaction with RBN and the significant reduction in AUC caused by RIF, delavirdine should not be used with any rifamycin *(1,56,57,70,71)*. Nevirapine and efavirenz can be used with either RBN or RIF; dosage adjustments may be necessary if given with RIF *(72)*. RBN doses may also need to be adjusted to 450 and more likely 600 mg per dose when used together with efavirenz.

*Nucleoside Reverse Transcriptase Inhibitors*

Zidovudine and lamivudine are not metabolized by the CYP enzymes. The efficacy of these drugs is correlated with the intracellular concentrations of the active derivative.

**Table 3**
**Coadministration Rifabutin and Rifampin With Currently Approved Nonnucleoside Reverse Transcriptase Inhibitors: Effect on the Area-Under-the-Curve (AUC) of Each Drug**

| NNRTI | Rifabutin | | Rifampin[a] | |
|---|---|---|---|---|
| | Effect of rifabutin on NNRTI | Effect of NNRTI on rifabutin (predicted)[b] | Effect of rifampin on NNRTI | Effect of NNRTI on rifampin (predicted)[b] |
| Nevirapine | ↓ 16% | NR (↓) | ↓ 37% | NR (unchanged) |
| Delavirdine | ↓ 80% | ↑ 342% | ↓ 96% | Unchanged |
| Efavirenz | ↓ 10% | ↓ 38% | ↓ 13% | Unchanged |

*Source:* Refs. *27,57,69*. Adapted from ref. 27 with permission.
[a] Rifapentine produces approx 85% of the effects seen with rifampin.
[b] Predicted using existing knowledge regarding metabolic pathways for the two drugs.
NR, not reported.

199

The coadministration.of RIF with zidovudine resulted in a decrease (43%) in $C_{max}$ and AUC (47%) of zidovudine. Decreased plasma concentrations have not been shown to reduce the concentration of the intracellular metabolite *(73)*. Therefore, RIF has not been proven to impact the clinical effect and antiviral activity of zidovudine *(45)*.

### Protease Inhibitors

The protease inhibitors are CYP3A substrates and inhibitors and therefore exhibit a bidirectional interaction. Table 4 summarizes the effects of RIF and RBN on the AUC of protease inhibitors *(27,57,70)*. Because of the profound effects of RIF and RPNT on the AUCs of saquinavir, indinavir, nelfinavir, and amprenavir, concomitant administration is discouraged *(74–79)*. RBN should be used if combination therapy is necessary *(80,81)*. However, because of the bidirectional interaction and the potential for intolerance, RBN or protease inhibitor dosage adjustments may be warranted *(77,79,82)*. The effects of RIF on the AUC of ritonavir and the combination of saquinavir and ritonavir are less pronounced. Based on current data, ritonavir or saquinavir and ritonavir can be used in combination with RIF *(1,56,57)*. TDM may help to optimize regimens for the coadministration of these agents.

Drug doses for persons with HIV coinfection who are under treatment with highly active antiretroviral therapy often must be adjusted when rifamycins are used concurrently. Many interaction effects are drug specific, and an effort should be made to obtain expert consultation and the latest available information to guide dosing.

### Trimethoprim and Sulfamethoxazole

The effect of RIF on concentrations of trimethoprim/sulfamethoxazole (TMP/SMX) was evaluated in HIV-positive patients *(83)*. A decrease (23%) in mean AUC of TMP/SMX was observed. The clinical significance of this interaction has not been established, but reduced efficacy of TMP/SMX may be of concern.

Rifamycins interact with several other classes of drugs beyond those listed. Additional information regarding rifamycin interactions can be found in the article by Niemi et al. *(84)* and in several other papers *(85–87)*.

## PZA Interactions

PZA is metabolized to pyrazinoic acid and 5-hydroxypyrazinoic acid, which are subsequently cleared renally *(6,28,37)*. PZA is removed by hemodialysis *(29)*. It is not associated with a large number of drug interactions. Because PZA can compete with uric acid for excretion, patients will accumulate uric acid while on PZA. In most cases, this is not a clinically significant problem, but in the case of patients at risk for gout, this may precipitate a flare-up of the disease. Therefore, PZA must be used cautiously in those patients. Allopurinol inhibits the clearance of PZA's primary metabolite, pyrazinoic acid, thereby exacerbating the metabolite's inhibition of uric acid secretion *(88,89)*. Further, probenecid may be significantly less effective as a uricosuric agent in the presence of PZA *(90)*. Thus, the most effective management of PZA-induced elevations of uric acid and arthralgias may be to hydrate the patient and withhold PZA.

It has been shown that the combination of RIF and PZA in the absence of INH leads to an unexpectedly high incidence of hepatotoxicity *(91–94)*. It is important to stress that this was seen in the context of 2-month regimens of RIF and PZA for latent TB

**Table 4**
**Coadministration of Rifabutin and Rifampin With HIV-1 Protease Inhibitors (PIs): Effect on the Area-Under-the-Curve (AUC) of Each Drug**

| PI | Rifabutin | | Rifampin[a] | |
|---|---|---|---|---|
| | Effect of rifabutin on PI | Effect of PI on rifabutin | Effect of rifampin on PI | Effect of PI on rifampin |
| Saquinavir | ↓ 45% | ↑ 44% | ↓ 80% | NR |
| Ritonavir[b] | NR | ↑ 293% | ↓ 35% | Unchanged |
| Indinavir | ↓ 34% | ↑ 173% | ↓ 92% | NR |
| Nelfinavir | ↓ 32% | ↑ 207% | ↓ 82% | NR |
| Amprenavir | ↓ 14% | ↑ 200% | ↓ 82% | Unchanged |
| Atazanavir | NR | ↑ 250% | NR (↓ predicted) | NR |
| Lopinavir/ritonavir | NR | ↑ 303% | ↓ 75% | NR |

*Source:* Refs. 27,57,69. Adapted from ref. 27 with permission.

*Note:* (1) These are average changes, but the effect of these interactions in an individual patient may be substantially different. (2) Rifampin is a potent inducer of CYP3A, but is not itself a CYP3A substrate. For example, concomitant delavirdine, a moderate CYP3A inhibitor, does not change serum concentrations of rifampin. Therefore, although there are very few data at present, it is likely that protease inhibitors will not substantially increase the serum concentrations of rifampin (the same is true of rifapentine). (3) There are no data regarding the magnitude of these bidirectional interactions when the rifamycin is administered twice or three times weekly.

NR, not reported.

[a] Rifapentine produces approx 85% of the effects seen with rifampin.
[b] Data from only two subjects.

infection and not during the treatment of active TB disease with INH, RIF, PZA, and EMB. Therefore, this 2-month regimen generally should no longer be used *(93)*. Presently, there are insufficient data from patients treated for active TB disease with PZA but not INH to comment on the rate of hepatotoxicity under those conditions. The precise reason for this is unknown, but it is under investigation (C. Peloquin, unpublished data). It is possible that INH or one of its metabolites blocks the formation of a hepatotoxic PZA metabolite or blocks the interaction between PZA or its metabolites and key receptors in the liver.

Another combination of PZA that appears to have a high incidence of patient intolerance is PZA combined with ofloxacin or levofloxacin for latent TB infection because of multidrug-resistant TB *(95–97)*. It is possible that PZA or its metabolites compete with quinolones for renal tubular secretion, although this has not been proven to date. This regimen also cannot be recommended at this time.

## EMB Interactions

EMB is cleared both hepatically and renally *(5,28,37)*. EMB is not significantly removed by hemodialysis *(29)*. The specific pathways involved in its hepatic clearance are not known. Like PZA, EMB has few documented interactions. The affect of concurrent antacids was described in a separate section. Because EMB can cause optic neuritis, patients receiving other potential ocular toxins (RBN, cidofovir) should be monitored carefully. Although RBN and cidofovir are associated with uveitis and not optic neuritis, additive effects may adversely affect vision *(31,98,99)*. Based on current data, unlike the situation involving INH and PZA, the absence of EMB in regimens used to treat TB does not seem to influence significantly the incidence of hepatotoxicity.

## Aminoglycoside and Polypeptide Interactions

The aminoglycosides amikacin, kanamycin, SM, as well as the polypeptides capreomycin and viomycin, are all primarily cleared renally *(28,100,101)*. Aminoglycosides are partially removed by hemodialysis *(28,100)*. However, under clinical conditions, especially in the intensive care setting, hemodialysis removal may be more limited. All aminoglycosides and polypeptides can adversely affect vestibular, auditory, and renal function. Reported differences in the incidence of these toxicities among the agents reflect, in part, differences in the sizes and frequencies of doses studied. Elevated serum creatinine values caused by nonoliguric acute tubular necrosis are usually reversible; renal wasting of cations also may occur *(28,37,100)*. Periodic monitoring (every 2–4 weeks) of the serum urea nitrogen, creatinine, calcium, potassium, and magnesium should be considered, especially if other nephrotoxins (such as amphotericin B) are used *(1)*. Note that more frequent monitoring is necessary when using aminoglycosides in the intensive care unit.

Vestibular changes may be noted on physical exam, and may occur independently of, or in conjunction with, tinnitus and auditory changes. The former can be detected using heel-to-toe walking, Romberg testing, and lateral nystagmus testing *(102)*. Auditory changes are best detected by monthly audiograms for those patients requiring prolonged treatment or those receiving concurrent potential ototoxins (clarithromycin, ethacrynic acid, furosemide) *(1,102)*. Aminoglycosides and polypeptides can potentiate the neuromuscular blocking agents or may precipitate neuromuscular blockade in patients with myasthenia gravis *(37,100)*. Therefore, these drugs should be used cautiously in those settings.

## CS Interactions

There are relatively few articles published regarding CS *(103)*. Therefore, there is little known regarding the potential for drug interactions with CS. This drug is renally cleared, and there are no known metabolites *(28,103)*. CS is cleared by hemodialysis *(104)*. It can cause a variety of central nervous system (CNS) disturbances, among them anxiety, confusion, memory loss, dizziness, lethargy, and depression, including suicidal tendencies *(28)*. Other agents associated with any of these effects (INH, ETA, and quinolones) may have additive CNS toxicities. CS should be used cautiously in patients with a history of depression or psychosis or those receiving treatment for these conditions.

It is not clear if CS can alter the potential for seizures in patients predisposed to these events. Caution is advised, as is TDM, to ensure that concentrations do not exceed the recommended range of 20–35 µg/mL *(17,103)*. Older literature suggested that CS may decrease the clearance of phenytoin, possibly leading to toxicity *(37)*. More recent mouse model work suggested that such a combination may actually improve seizure control *(105)*. CS is undergoing active research efforts to determine if it has synergistic interactions with other drugs used for a variety of CNS conditions, including opioid withdrawal, schizophrenia, and Alzheimer's disease. Results to date are fairly preliminary *(106–109)*.

## ETA Interactions

ETA is extensively metabolized, including to a sulfoxide metabolite that appears to be active against mycobacteria and that may interconvert with the parent compound *(28,110)*. The specific hepatic microsomal enzymes responsible for this metabolism are not known. Little unchanged drug is excreted in the urine or cleared by hemodialysis *(104,110)*. ETA causes significant GI distress, and this may be additive with other such agents. ETA may cause CNS effects, including headache, drowsiness, giddiness, depression, psychosis, and visual changes, although a causative role has not been established *(37,110)*. Therefore, additive effects with INH, CS, or fluoroquinolones are possible.

ETA may cause peripheral neuritis, so caution should be exercised in patients receiving other agents, such as nucleoside reverse transcriptase inhibitors, that share this toxicity. ETA can cause hepatotoxicity and goiter, with or without hypothyroidism; the latter is worsened by the concurrent use of PAS *(110)*. Thyroid-stimulating hormone concentrations should be monitored periodically in patients receiving ETA. In animal models, ETA combined with gatifloxacin and PZA proved to be a potent combination against TB *(111)*. Human trials are needed to follow up on these findings.

## Para-Aminosalicylic Acid Interactions

PAS is metabolized by *N*-acetyltransferase 1 to acetyl-PAS, which is subsequently cleared renally *(9,28,104,112)*. Little PAS is cleared by hemodialysis, but some of the acetyl-PAS is cleared this way *(104)*. Older forms of PAS were particularly prone to GI toxicity; this is substantially lessened by the granule form of the drug *(112)*. Still, PAS can cause diarrhea, and this can affect the pharmacokinetics of other drugs.

Various types of malabsorption with PAS have been described, including steatorrhea and malabsorption of vitamin $B_{12}$, folate, xylose and iron. With the possible exception of digoxin, it is not known if PAS can cause specific drugs to be malabsorbed *(112)*.

Hypersensitivity reactions with fever, including hepatitis, can occur, and desensitization to PAS-induced hypersensitivity is not recommended *(112)*. PAS is known to produce goiter, with or without myxedema, and this is more frequent with concomitant ETA therapy. This can be prevented or treated with thyroxine. Older tablet forms of PAS that contained bentonite reduced serum RIF concentrations; this should not occur with the granule form *(112)*. The concurrent use of ammonium chloride with PAS is not recommended.

## CF Interactions

CF is a weak anti-TB drug and has a very unusual pharmacokinetic profile *(10,28,37, 101)*. It is highly tissue-tropic and as a result displays a very long elimination half-life. It is primarily excreted nonrenally, but the precise mechanisms have not been described. Little CF is removed by hemodialysis *(104)*. As noted in the section on interaction with foods, oral absorption is improved when CF is given with a high-fat meal.

The most serious adverse reactions associated with CF are dose-related GI toxicities, and these can be additive with other drugs' effects *(28,37,101)*. Skin discoloration may also occur, and other drugs, including amiodarone and RBN, may make this worse. CF can produce a statistically significant increase in the $T_{max}$ of RIF, but this interaction is unlikely to be clinically significant. The large accumulation of CF in macrophages may affect the function of these cells, but this has not been well defined. It is at least theoretically possible that such effects contribute to the worse outcome seen in some AIDS patients who received CF as part of their regimen for disseminated *Mycobacterium avium* complex infection. CF is under study as a potential adjuvant to cancer chemotherapy in the hope that it may reduce or reverse acquired multidrug resistance *(113)*.

## MANAGEMENT OF PATIENTS COINFECTED WITH TUBERCULOSIS AND HUMAN IMMUNODEFICIENCY VIRUS

The Centers for Disease Control and Prevention has published guidelines for the management of TB in patients coinfected with HIV *(1,56,57)*. Clinicians should look for a paradoxical worsening of TB symptoms on the introduction of anti-HIV therapy, presumably caused by the reconstitution of the immune system *(1,56,57)*. In general, the guidelines recommend the use of RBN instead of RIF in an attempt to minimize drug interactions. It is very important to bear in mind that most interaction studies involving the anti-HIV protease inhibitors were performed in small numbers (8 to 10) of healthy volunteers. These volunteers received only two drugs under controlled conditions, and most of the studies were either single-dose or short-term dosing studies.

Table 5 summarizes the current data available on drug interactions between protease inhibitors and antituberculosis drugs other than rifamycins *(27,114)*. How these results compare to what is seen in patients receiving multiple drugs under "real-world" conditions is unknown. It is our practice to "trust but verify" by measuring the serum concentrations of the various drugs (antimycobacterial drugs, oral azole antifungals, and anti-HIV protease inhibitors) to verify adequate dosing *(17,27)*. Further research is required to refine this approach.

**Table 5**

**Predicted Potential for Drug–Drug Interaction Between HIV Protease Inhibitors and Antituberculosis Drugs Other Than Rifamycins**

| Drug | Metabolism | Effect on CYP3A | Effect of drug X on PI (predicted)[a] | Effect of PI on drug X (predicted)[a] |
|---|---|---|---|---|
| Isoniazid | Acetylation > CYP[b] | Mild inhibitor | No change in indinavir | None |
| Pyrazinamide | Deamidase > xanthine oxidase | None known | (None) | (None) |
| Ethambutol | Renal > CYP[b] | None known | (None) | (None) |
| Ethionamide | CYP[b] | None known | Unknown | (Increase) |
| PAS | Acetylation | None known | (None) | (None) |
| Quinolones | Renal > CYP | None known | (None) | (None) |
| Aminoglycosides | Renal | None known | (None) | (None) |

*Source*: Adapted from ref. 27 with permission.

[a] Predicted using existing knowledge regarding metabolic pathways for the two drugs.

[a] Precise hepatic metabolic pathway has not been defined.

# NONTUBERCULOUS MYCOBACTERIAL INFECTIONS

The nontuberculous myobacterial (NTM) infections comprise a substantial list of infections caused by various slow- and rapid-growing mycobacteria. The management of such infections has been summarized elsewhere *(115,116)*. Clinicians should be aware that there are differences between HIV-infected and noninfected hosts as far as disease presentation and management. It is important to consider the drug interactions described above for TB because many of these same drugs are used to treat NTM infections. Advanced-generation macrolides (azithromycin, clarithromycin) are frequently used to treat NTM infections, such as *M. avium* complex, and clarithromycin has been associated with many CYP3A4 interactions *(30,37,86,116)*. In particular, bidirectional interactions involving RBN and clarithromycin should be anticipated *(117)*. RIF causes a more pronounced decline in clarithromycin concentrations than RBN *(118,119)*.

## CASE STUDY 1

R.G. is a 46-year-old homosexual male diagnosed with HIV 2 years ago. His current HIV regimen includes 400 mg delavirdine (Rescriptor®) three times a day orally, 300 mg lamivudine (Epivir®) daily, and zidovudine 300 mg (Retrovir®) orally twice daily. R.G.'s viral load has been below 50 ribonucleic acid (RNA) copies/mL, and his CD4 count was 340 cells/mm$^3$. R.G. was recently admitted to the hospital following complaints of cough, fevers, and night sweats. Sputum cultures were positive for acid-fast bacillus. A rifamycin-containing tuberculosis regimen was initiated and included 300 mg RBN daily, 300 mg INH daily, 1500 mg PZA daily, 800 mg EMB daily. RBN was selected because of its lower interaction potential. Three weeks later, his sputum smears were negative for acid-fast bacillus; however, he developed symptoms consistent with uveitis. RBN was held, and serum drug concentrations were obtained. Results revealed very high RBN concentrations and lowered delavirdine concentrations. R.G.'s NNRTI was changed to 200 mg nevirapine (Viramune®) orally twice a day, and therapy with RBN was restarted to complete the TB treatment course. Nevirapine and efavirenz are the suggested NNRTIs to be used in combination with rifamycins. Dosage adjustments may be necessary.

## CASE STUDY 2

K.J. is a 42-year-old female inpatient being treated for prosthetic valve endocarditis. Past medical history is significant for heroin intravenous drug abuse and cocaine. Cultures were 3-of-3 positive for *Staphylococcus epidermidis*. The following treatment regimen was initiated: 1 g vancomycin intravenously every 12 hours and 300 mg RIF orally every 8 hours for 6 weeks and 70 mg gentamicin intravenously every 8 hours for 14 days. On day 21 of therapy, K.J. began having low-grade fevers. Her white blood cells (WBCs) increased from $10 \times 10^3$/mm$^3$ to $17 \times 10^3$/mm$^3$ and continued to rise. Her serum creatinine also increased to 1.9 mg/dL. Microscopic analysis of urine revealed 60–80 WBCs and the presence of more than $10^5$ CFU/mL *Candida albicans*. One blood culture of 2 was also positive for *C. albicans*. She was started on voriconazole loading dose and then 300 mg intravenously twice a day. Her PICC line was changed, and the vancomycin and RIF were continued. Despite treatment, K.J. continued to have fevers and an elevated WBC count. After further negative workup, it was decided to change antifungal treatment to fluconazole. Itraconazole, ketoconazole, and voriconazole concentrations may be subtherapeutic when concomitantly administered with any of the rifamycins. Fluconazole can be used with rifamycins, but dosage adjustments may be necessary. Treatment courses were completed.

## CONCLUSION

The discussion in this chapter highlights the need for the careful introduction of the TB drugs into existing drug regimens. In particular, rifamycins can seriously disrupt ongoing treatment, with potentially serious consequences. Although the role of TDM remains to be better defined for these situations, it does offer the potential to untangle multidirectional drug interactions.

## REFERENCES

1. American Thoracic Society/Centers for Disease Control and Prevention/Infectious Disease Society of America. Treatment of tuberculosis. Am J Respir Crit Care Med 2003;167: 603–662.
2. Peloquin CA. Tuberculosis. In DiPiro JT, Talbert RL, Yee GC, Matzke GR, Wells BG, Posey LM, eds. Pharmacotherapy: A Pathophysiologic Approach. 5th Ed. New York, NY, McGraw Hill, 2002, pp. 1917–1937.
3. Peloquin CA, Namdar R, Singleton MD, Nix DE. Pharmacokinetics of isoniazid under fasting conditions, with food, and with antacids. Int J Tuberc Lung Dis 1999;3:703–710.
4. Peloquin CA, Namdar R, Singleton MD, Nix DE. Pharmacokinetics of rifampin under fasting conditions, with food, and with antacids. Chest 1999;115:12–18.
5. Peloquin CA, Bulpitt AE, Jaresko GS, Jelliffe RW, Childs JM, Nix DE. Pharmacokinetics of ethambutol under fasting conditions, with food, and with antacids. Antimicrob Agents Chemother 1999;43:568–572.
6. Peloquin CA, Bulpitt AE, Jaresko GS, Jelliffe RW, James GT, Nix DE. Pharmacokinetics of pyrazinamide under fasting conditions, with food, and with antacids. Pharmacotherapy 1998;18:1205–1211.
7. Auclair B, Nix DE, Adam RD, James GT, Peloquin CA. Pharmacokinetics of ethionamide under fasting conditions, with orange juice, food, and antacids. Antimicrob Agents Chemother 2001, 45:810–814.
8. Zhu M, Nix DE, Adam RD, Childs JM, Peloquin CA. Pharmacokinetics of cycloserine under fasting conditions, with orange juice, food, and antacids. Pharmacotherapy 2001; 21:891–897.
9. Peloquin CA, Zhu M, Adam RD, Godo, PG, Nix DE. Pharmacokinetics of *p*-aminosalicylate under fasting conditions, with orange juice, food, and antacids. Ann Pharmacother 2001;35:1332–1338.
10. Nix DE, Zhu M, Adam RD, Godo PG, Peloquin CA. Pharmacokinetics of clofazimine under fasting conditions, with orange juice, food, and antacids. Tuberculosis 2004;84: 365–373.
11. Sahai J, Gallicano K, Swick L, et al. Reduced plasma concentrations of antituberculous drugs in patients with HIV infection. Ann Intern Med 1997;127:289–293.
12. Peloquin CA, Nitta AT, Burman WJ, et al. Low antituberculosis drug concentrations in patients with AIDS. Ann Pharmacother 1996;30:919–925.
13. Berning SE, Huitt GA, Iseman MD, Peloquin CA. Malabsorption of antituberculosis medications by a patient with AIDS [letter]. N Engl J Med 1992;327:1817–1818.

14. Patel KB, Belmonte R, Crowe HM. Drug malabsorption and resistant tuberculosis in HIV-infected patients [letter]. N Engl J Med 1995;332:336–337.

15. Peloquin CA, MacPhee AA, Berning SE. Malabsorption of antimycobacterial medications [letter]. N Engl J Med 1993;329:1122–1123.

16. Gordon SM, Horsburgh CR Jr, Peloquin CA, et al. Low serum levels of oral antimycobacterial agents in patients with disseminated *Mycobacterium avium* complex disease. J Infect Dis 1993;168:1559–1562.

17. Peloquin CA. Therapeutic drug monitoring in the treatment of tuberculosis. Drugs 2002;62:2169–2183.

18. Colborn D, Lewis R, Narang P. HIV disease does not influence rifabutin absorption [abstract]. Thirty-fourth Interscience Conference on Antimicrobial Agents and Chemotherapy, Orlando, FL, October, 1994.

19. Gatti G, Di Biagio A, De Pascalis CR, Guerra M, Bassetti M, Bassetti D. Pharmacokinetics of rifabutin in HIV-infected patients with or without wasting syndrome. Br J Clin Pharmacol 1999;48:704–711.

20. Keung AC, Owens RC Jr, Eller MG, Weir SJ, Nicolau DP, Nightingale CH. Pharmacokinetics of rifapentine in subjects seropositive for the human immunodeficiency virus: a phase I study. Antimicrob Agents Chemother 1999;43:1230–1233.

21. Weiner M, Burman W, Vernon A, et al. Low isoniazid concentration associated with outcome of tuberculosis treatment with once-weekly isoniazid and rifapentine. Am J Respir Crit Care Med 2003;167:1341–1347.

22. Weiner M, Burman B, Khan A, et al. The effect of HIV serostatus on isoniazid pharmacokinetics among patients with active tuberculosis [abstract]. The 100th International Conference of the American Thoracic Society, Orlando, FL, May, 2004.

23. Ehrenpreis ED, Ganger DR, Kochvar GT, Patterson BK, Craig RM. D-Xylose malabsorption: characteristic finding in patients with the AIDS wasting syndrome and chronic diarrhea. J Acquir Immune Defic Syndr 1992;5:1047–1050.

24. Kotler DP, Francisco A, Clayton F, Scholes JV, Orenstein JM. Small intestinal injury and parasitic diseases in AIDS. Ann Intern Med 1990;113:444–449.

25. Kotler DP, Giang TT, Thiim M, Nataro JP, Sordillo EM, Orenstein JM. Chronic bacterial enteropathy in patients with AIDS. J Infect Dis 1995;171:552–558.

26. Blum RA, D'Andrea DT, Florentino BM, et al. Increased gastric pH and the bioavailability of fluconazole and ketoconazole. Ann Intern Med 1991;114:755–757.

27. Burman WJ, Gallicano K, Peloquin, C. Therapeutic implications of drug interactions in the treatment of HIV-related tuberculosis. Clin Infect Dis 1999;28:419–430.

28. Peloquin CA. Antituberculosis drugs: pharmacokinetics. In Heifets, L, ed. Drug Susceptibility in the Chemotherapy of Mycobacterial Infections. Boca Raton, FL, CRC Press, 1991, pp. 59–88.

29. Malone RS, Fish DN, Spiegel DM, Childs JM, Peloquin CA. The effect of hemodialysis on isoniazid, rifampin, pyrazinamide, and ethambutol. Am J Respir Crit Care Med 1999;159:1580–1584.

30. Bertz RJ, Granneman GR. Use of in vitro and in vivo data to estimate the likelihood of metabolic pharmacokinetic interactions. Clin Pharmacokinet 1997;32:210–258.

31. Ochs HR, Greenblatt DJ, Roberts GM, Dengler HJ. Diazepam interaction with antituberculosis drugs. Clin Pharmacol Ther 1981;29:671–678.

32. Sutton G, Kupferberg HJ. Isoniazid as an inhibitor of primidone metabolism. Neurology 1975;25:1179–1181.

33. Zand R, Nelson SD, Slattery JT, et al. Inhibition and induction of cytochrome P4502E1-catalyzed oxidation by isoniazid in humans. Clin Pharmacol Ther 1993;54:142–149.

34. Baciewicz AM, Self TH. Isoniazid interactions. South Med J 1985;78:714–718.

35. Desta Z, Soukhova NV, Flockhart DA. Inhibition of cytochrome P450 (CYP450) isoforms by isoniazid: potent inhibition of CYP2C19 and CYP3A4. Antimicrob Agent Chemother 2001;45:382–392.

36. Nolan CM, Sandblom RE, Thummel KE, Slattery JT, Nelson SD. Hepatotoxicity associated with acetaminophen usage in patients receiving multiple drug therapy for tuberculosis. Chest 1994;105:408–411.

37. McEvoy GK, ed. AHFS Drug Information 2004. American Society of Health-Systems Pharmacists, Bethesda, MD, 2004, 554–560.

38. Shishoo CJ, Shah SA, Rathod IS, Savale SS, Vora MJ. Impaired bioavailability of rifampicin in presence of isoniazid from fixed dose combination (FDC) formulation. Int J Pharm 2001;228:53–67.

39. Ofoefule SI, Obodo CE, Orisakwe OE, et al. Some plasma pharmacokinetic parameters of isoniazid in the presence of a fluoroquinolone antibacterial agent. Am J Ther 2001; 8:243–246.

40. Burman WJ, Gallicano K, Peloquin C. Comparative pharmacokinetics and pharmacodynamics of the rifamycin antibacterials. Clin Pharmacokinet 2001;40:327–341.

41. Schuetz EG, Schinkel AH, Relling MV, Schuetz JD. P-Glycoprotein: a major determinant of rifampicin inducible expression of cytochrome P4503A in mice and humans. Proc Natl Acad Sci U S A 1996;93:4001–4005.

42. Hoffmeyer S, Burk O, von Richter O. Functional polymorphisms of the human multidurg resistance gene: multiple sequence variations and correlation of one allele with P-glycoprotein expression and activity in vivo. Proc Natl Acad Sci U S A 2000;97:3473–3478.

43. Li AP, Reith MK, Rasmussen A, et al. Primary human hepatocytes as a tool for the evaluation of structure-activity relationship in a cytochrome P450 induction potential of xenobiotics: evaluation of rifampin, rifapentine, and rifabutin. Chem Biol Interact 1997; 107:17–30.

44. Keung AC, Reith K, Eller MG. Enzyme induction observed in healthy volunteers after repeated administration of rifapentine and its lack of effect on steady-state rifapentine pharmacokinetics. Int J Tuberc Lung Dis 1999;3:426–436.

45. Gallicano KD, Sahai J, Shukla VK, et al. Induction of zidovudine glucuronidation and amination pathways by rifampicin in HIV-infected patients. Br J Clin Pharmacol 1999; 48:168–179.

46. Peloquin C. What is the right dose of rifampin? Int J Tuberc Lung Dis 2003;7:3–5.

47. Indinavir Pharmacokinetics Study Group. Indinavir (MK 639) drug interactions studies. Program and Abstracts of the XI International AIDS Conference. Vancouver, Canada, July, 1996, p. 18. Abstract MoB174.

48. Grub S, Bryson H, Goggin T, Ludin E, Jorga K. The interaction of saquinavir with ketoconazole, erythromycin and rifampin: comparison of the effect in healthy volunteers and in HIV-infected patients. Eur J Clin Pharmacol 2001;57:115–121.

49. Centers for Disease Control and Prevention. Treatment of tuberculosis. MMWR Morb Mortal Wkly Rep 2003;52:1–77.

50. Jaruratanasirikul S, Sriwiriyajan S. Effect of rifampicin on the pharmacokinetics of itraconazole in normal volunteers and AIDS patients. Eur J Clin Pharmacol 1998;54: 155–158.

51. Drayton J, Dickenson G, Rinaldi MG. Coadministration of rifampin and itraconazole leads to undetectable levels of serum itraconazole. Clin Infect Dis 1994;18:266.

52. Doble N, Shaw R, Rowland-Hill C, Lush M, Warnock DW, Keal EE. Pharmacokinetic study of the interaction between rifampicin and ketoconazole. J Antimicrob Chemother 1998;21:633–635.

53. Nicolau DP, Crowe HM, Nightingale CH, Quintiliani R. Rifampin-fluconazole interaction in critically ill patients. Ann Pharmacother 1995;29:994–996.

54. Apseloff G, Hilligoss DM, Gardner MJ, Henry EB, Inskeep PB, Gerver N. Induction of fluconazole metabolism by rifampin: in vivo study in humans. J Clin Pharmacol 1991;31: 358–361.

55. Coker RJ, Tomlinson DR, Prakin J, Harris JRW, Pinching AJ. Interaction between fluconazole and rifampicin. BMJ 1990;301:818.

56. Centers for Disease Control and Prevention. Updated guidelines for the use of rifabutin or rifampin for the treatment and prevention of tuberculosis among HIV-infected patients taking protease inhibitors or nonnucleoside reverse transcriptase inhibitors. MMWR Morb Mortal Wkly Rep 2000;49:185–189.

57. Centers for Disease Control and Prevention. Updated guidelines for the use of rifamycins for the treatment of tuberculosis among HIV-infected patients taking protease inhibitors or non-nucleoside reverse transcriptase inhibitors. MMWR Morb Mortal Wkly Rep 2004; 53;37.

58. Jaruratanasirikul S, Kleepkaew A. Lack of effect of fluconazole on the pharmacokinetics of rifampicin in AIDS patients. J Antimicrob Chemother 1996;38:877–880.

59. Jordan MK, Polis MA, Kelly G, Narang PK, Masur H, Piscitelli SC. Effects of fluconazole and clarithromycin on rifabutin and 25-O-desacetylrifabutin pharmacokinetics. Antimicrob Agents Chemother 2000;44:2170–2172.

60. Kelly HW, Couch RC, Davis RL, Cushing AH, Knott R. Interaction of chloramphenicol and rifampin. J Pediatr 1988;112:817–820.

61. Prober CG. Effect of rifampin on chloramphenicol levels. N Engl J Med 1985;312: 788–789.

62. Mirochnick M, Cooper E, Capparelli E, et al. Population pharmocokinetics of dapsone in children with human immunodeficiency virus infection. Clin Pharmacol Ther 2001;70: 24–32.

63. Colmenero JD, Fernandez-Gallardo LC, Agundez JAG, Sedeno J, Benitez J, Valverde E. Possible implications of doxycycline-rifampin interaction for treatment of brucellosis. Antimicrob Agents Chemother 1994;38:2798–2802.

64. Temple ME, Nahata MC. Interaction between ciprofloxacin and rifampin. Ann Pharmacother 1999;33:868–870.

65. Chandler MH, Toler SM, Rapp RP, Muder RR, Korvick JA. Multiple dose pharmacokinetics of concurrent oral ciprofloxacin and rifampin therapy in elderly patients. Antimicrob Agents Chemother 1990;34:442–447.

66. Apseloff G, Foulds G, LaBoy-Goral L, Willavize S, Vincent J. Comparison of Azithromycin and clarithromycin in their interactions with rifabutin in healthy volunteers. J Clin Pharmacol 1998;38:830–835.

67. Hafner R, Bethel J, Power M, et al. Tolerance and pharmacokinetic interactions of rifabutin and clarithromycin in human immunodeficiency virus-infected volunteers. Antimicrob Agents Chemother 1998;42:631–639.

68. Djojosaputro M, Mustofa S, Donatus IA, Santoso B. The effects of doses and pre-treatment with rifampicin on the elimination kinetics of metronidazole. Eur J Pharmacol 1990; 183:1870.

69. Viramune product information. Ridgeville, CT, Boehringer Ingelheim Pharmaceuticals, 2002.

70. Borin MT, Chambers JH, Carel BJ, Gagnon S, Freimuth WW. Pharmacokinetic study of the interaction between rifampin and delavirdine mesylate. Clin Pharmacol Ther 1997;61: 544–553.

71. Borin MT, Chambers JH, Carel BJ, Freimuth WW, Aksentijevich S, Piergies AA. Pharmacokinetic study of the interaction between rifabutin and delavirdine mesylate in HIV1 infected patients. Antiviral Res 1997;35:53–63.

72. Lopez-Cortes LF, Ruiz-Valderas R, Viciana P, et al. Pharmacokinetic interactions between efavirenz and rifampicin in HIV infected patients with tuberculosis. Clin Pharmacokinet 2002;41:681–690.

73. Barry M, Mulcahy F, Merry C. Pharmacokinetics and potential interactions amongst antiretroviral agents used to treat patients with HIV infection. Clin Pharmacokinet 1999; 36:289–304.

74. Cato A, Cavanaugh J, Shi H, Hsu A, Leonard J, Granneman GR. The effect of multiple doses of ritonavir on the pharmacokinetics of rifabutin. Clin Pharmacol Ther 1998;63: 414–421.
75. Lillibridge JH, Liang BH, Kerr BM, et al. Characterization of the selectivity and mechanism of human cytochrome P450 inhibition by the human immunodeficiency virus-protease inhibitor nelfinavir mesylate. Drug Metab Dispos. 1998;26:609–616.
76. Kerr BM, Daniels R, Cledeninn N. Pharmacokinetic interaction of nelfinavir with half-dose rifabutin. Can J Infect Dis 1999;10:21B.
77. Moyle J, Buss NE, Goggin T, Snell P, Higgs C, Hawkins DA. Interaction between saquinavir soft-gel and rifabutin in patients infected with HIV. Br J Clin Pharmacol 2002; 54:178–182.
78. Moreno S, Podzamczer D, Blazquez R, et al. Treatment of tuberculosis in HIV-infected patients: safety and antiretroviral efficacy of the concomitant use of ritonavir and rifampin. AIDS 2001;15:1185–1187.
79. Polk RE, Brophy DF, Israel DS, et al. Pharmacokinetic interaction between amprenavir and rifabutin or rifampin in healthy males. Antimicrob Agents Chemother 2001;45: 502–508.
80. Narita M, Stambaugh JJ, Hollender ES, Jones D, Pitchenik AE, Ashkin D. Use of rifabutin with protease inhibitors for human immunodeficiency virus-infected patients with tuberculosis. Clin Infect Dis 2000;30:779–783.
81. Peloquin CA. Tuberculosis drug serum levels [letter]. Clin Infect Dis 2001;33:584–585.
82. Hamzeh FM, Benson C, Gerber J, et al. Steady-state pharmacokinetic interaction of modified-dose indinavir and rifabutin. Clin Pharmacol Ther 2003;73:159–169.
83. Ribera E, Pou L, Fernandez-Sola A, et al. Rifampin reduces concentrations of trimethoprim and sulfamethoxazole in serum in human immunodeficiency virus-infected patients. Antimicrob Agents Chemother 2001;45:3238–3241.
84. Niemi M, Backman JT, Fromm MF, Neuvonen PJ, Kivisto KT. Pharmacokinetic interactions with rifampin: clinical relevance. Clin Pharmacokinet 2003;42:815–850.
85. Mae T, Hosoe K, Yamamoto T, et al. Effect of a new rifamycin derivative, rifalazil, on liver microsomal enzyme induction in rat and dog. Xenobiotica 1998;28:759–766.
86. Lin JH, Lu AYH. Inhibition and induction of cytochrome P450 and the clinical implications. Clin Pharmacokinet 1998;35:361–390.
87. Michalets EL. Update: clinically significant cytochrome P-450 drug interactions. Pharmacotherapy 1998;18:84–112.
88. Lacroix C, Guyonnaud C, Chaou M, Duwoos H, Lafont O. Interaction between allopurinol and pyrazinamide. Eur Respir J 1988;1:807–811.
89. Urban T, Maquarre E, Housset C, Chouaid C, Devin E, Lebeua B. Allopurinol hypersensitivity. A possible cause of hepatitis and mucocutaneous eruptions in a patient undergoing antitubercular treatment. Revue des Maladies Respiratoires 1995;12:314–316.
90. Yu TF, Perel J, Berger L, Roboz J. The effect of the interaction of pyrazinamide and probenecid on urinary uric acid excretion in man. Am J Med 1977;63:723–728.
91. Burman WJ, Reves RR. Hepatotoxicity from rifampin plus pyrazinamide: lessons for policymakers and messages for care providers. Am J Respir Crit Care Med 2001;164: 1112–1113.
92. Jasmer RM, Saukkonen JJ, Blumberg HM, et al. Short-course rifampin and pyrazinamide compared with isoniazid for latent tuberculosis infection: a multicenter clinical trial. Ann Intern Med. 2002;137:640–647.
93. Centers for Disease Control and Prevention (CDC); American Thoracic Society. Update: adverse event data and revised American Thoracic Society/CDC recommendations against the use of rifampin and pyrazinamide for treatment of latent tuberculosis infection—United States, 2003. MMWR Morb Mortal Wkly Rep 2003:52;735–739.

94. Kunimoto D, Warman A, Beckon A, et al. Severe hepatotoxicity associated with rifampin-pyrazinamide preventative therapy requiring transplantation in an individual at low risk for hepatotoxicity. Clin Infect Dis 2003;36:158–161.

95. Ridzon R, Meador J, Maxwell R, Higgins K, Weismuller P, Onorato IM. Asymptomatic hepatitis in persons who received alternative preventive therapy with pyrazinamide and ofloxacin. Clin Infect Dis 1997;24:1264–1265.

96. Papastavros T, Dolovich LR, Holbrook A, Whitehead L, Loeb M. Adverse events associated with pyrazinamide and levofloxacin in the treatment of latent multidrug-resistant tuberculosis. CMAJ 2002;167:131–136.

97. Lou HX, Shullo MA, McKaveney TP. Limited tolerability of levofloxacin and pyrazinamide for multidrug-resistant tuberculosis prophylaxis in a solid organ transplant population. Pharmacotherapy 2002;22:701–704.

98. Tseng AL, Walmsley SL. Rifabutin-associated uveitis. Ann Pharmacother 1995;29: 1149–1155.

99. Tseng AL, Mortimer CB, Salit IE. Iritis associated with intravenous cidofovir. Ann Pharmacother 1999;33:167–171.

100. Nicolau DP, Quintiliani R. Aminoglycosides. In: Yu VL, Merigan TC, Barriere S, White NJ, eds. Antimicrobial Chemotherapy. Baltimore, MD, Williams and Wilkins, 1998, pp. 621–637.

101. Kucers A, Bennett N McK, eds. The Use of Antibiotics. 4th Ed. Philadelphia, PA, Lippincott, 1988.

102. Peloquin CA, Berning SE, Nitta AT, et al. Aminoglycoside toxicity: daily vs thrice-weekly dosing for treatment of mycobacterial diseases. Clin Infect Dis 2004;38:1538–1544.

103. Berning SE, Peloquin CA. Antimycobacterial agents: cycloserine. In: Yu VL, Merigan TC, Barriere S, White NJ, eds. Antimicrobial Chemotherapy. Baltimore, MD, Williams and Wilkins, 1998, pp. 638–642.

104. Malone RS, Fish DN, Spiegel DM, Childs JM, Peloquin CA. The effect of hemodialysis on cycloserine, ethionamide, para-aminosalicylate, and clofazimine. Chest 1999;116: 984–990.

105. Wlaz P, Rolinski Z, Czuczwar SJ. Influence of D-cycloserine on the anticonvulsant activity of phenytoin and carbamazepine against electroconvulsions in mice. Epilepsia 1996;37:610–617.

106. Oliveto A, Benios T, Gonsai K, Feingold A, Poling J, Kosten TR. D-Cycloserine-naloxone interactions in opioid-dependent humans under a novel-response naloxone discrimination procedure. Exp Clin Psychopharmacol 2003;11:237–246.

107. Evins AE, Amico E, Posever TA, Toker R, Goff DC. D-Cycloserine added to risperidone in patients with primary negative symptoms of schizophrenia. Schizophr Res 2002;56:19–23.

108. Butterfield DA, Pocernich CB. The glutamatergic system and alzheimer's disease: therapeutic implications. CNS Drugs 2003;17:641–645.

109. Falk WE, Daly EJ, Tsai GE, Gunther J, Brown P. A case series of D-cycloserine added to donepezil in the treatment of alzheimer's disease. J Neuropsychiatry Clin Neurosci 2002; 14:466–467.

110. Berning SE, Peloquin CA. Antimycobacterial agents: ethionamide. In: Yu VL, Merigan TC, Barriere S, White NJ, eds. Antimicrobial Chemotherapy. Baltimore, MD, Williams and Wilkins, 1998, pp. 650–654.

111. Cynamon MH, Sklaney M. Gatifloxacin and ethionamide as the foundation for therapy of tuberculosis. Antimicrob Agents Chemother 2003;47:2442–2444.

112. Berning SE, Peloquin CA. Antimycobacterial agents: para-aminosalicylic acid. In: Yu VL, Merigan TC, Barriere S, White NJ, eds. Antimicrobial Chemotherapy. Baltimore, MD, Williams and Wilkins, 1998, pp. 663–668.

113. Van Rensburg CE, Anderson R, Myer MS, Joone GK, O'Sullivan JF. The riminophena-zine agents clofazimine and B669 reverse acquired multidrug resistance in a human lung cancer cell line. Cancer Lett 1994;85:59–63.

114. Burman WJ, Peloquin CA. Isoniazid. In: Yu VL, Edwards G, McKinnon PS, Peloquin C, Morse GD, eds. Antimicrobial Chemotherapy and Vaccines. 2nd Ed, vol. II: Antimicro-bial Agents. Esun Technologies, 2005, pp. 539–550.

115. Yu VL, Merigan TC, Barriere S, White NJ, eds. Antimicrobial Chemotherapy. Balti-more, MD, Williams and Wilkins, 2003.

116. American Thoracic Society. Diagnosis and treatment of disease caused by nontuberculous mycobacteria. Am J Respir Crit Care Med 1997;156:S1–S25.

117. Amsden GW. Macrolides vs azalides: a drug interaction update. Ann Pharmacother 1995; 29:906–917.

118. Wallace RJ, Brown BA, Griffith DE. Reduced serum levels of clarithromycin in patients treated with multidrug regimens including rifampin or rifabutin for *Mycobacterium avium-intracellulare* infection. J Infect Dis 1995;171:747–750.

119. Peloquin CA, Berning SE. Evaluation of the drug interaction between clarithromycin and rifampin. J Infect Dis Pharmacother 1996;2:19–35.

# 8

# Quinolones

## David R. P. Guay

## INTRODUCTION

Drug–drug interactions can be categorized into those originating from pharmacokinetic mechanisms and those originating from pharmacodynamic mechanisms. Pharmacokinetic interactions are those that result in alterations of drug absorption, distribution, metabolism, and elimination; pharmacodynamic interactions occur when one drug affects the actions of another drug. This chapter deals only with the pharmacokinetic and pharmacodynamic interactions of fluoroquinolone (hereafter referred to as quinolone) with non-antimicrobial agents. Additive, synergistic, or antagonistic antimicrobial activity interactions between quinolones and other antimicrobials are not discussed.

Some drug interactions can be predicted from the chemical structure of the agent, its pharmacological activity, its toxicological profile, and other characteristics determined in its premarketing evaluation. Other interactions cannot be prospectively predicted and can only be detected through intense, large-scale clinical studies or postmarketing surveillance. The quinolones exhibit drug–drug interactions of both types.

There are a number of problems in the prospective clinical evaluation of drug–drug interactions in humans. First, there may be ethical concerns when administering interacting drug combinations to patients or volunteers, depending on the potential consequences of the interaction. Second, because there are an endless number of drug combinations, doses, and timings of administration that could be investigated, it is economically impossible to fund all possibilities. Third, the prospective evaluation of an interaction in a manageable number of patients is unlikely to uncover a rare interaction. Finally, studies that are carried out in normal volunteers and demonstrate a pharmacokinetic interaction, such as decreased absorption of a drug, may be of uncertain clinical relevance.

Despite these obstacles, delineating the frequencies and types of pharmacokinetic interactions of the quinolones with other drugs is important for several reasons. Because quinolones are often administered orally, absorptive interactions may compromise the efficacy of antimicrobial therapy. Because of their breadth of activity, agents of this class find substantial use in the critically ill and elderly, many of whom receive potentially interacting medications *(1–3)*. Because the elderly have an increased sensitivity

From: *Infectious Disease: Drug Interactions in Infectious Diseases, Second Edition*
Edited by: S. C. Piscitelli and K. A. Rodvold © Humana Press Inc., Totowa, NJ

to drug-induced toxicity and experience more adverse drug reactions, they may also exhibit an increased incidence and severity of drug–drug interactions. Finally, the quinolones are such a structurally diverse group that the extrapolation of drug–drug interactions from one to another of these agents may not be appropriate.

## PHARMACOKINETIC INTERACTIONS

### Absorption Interactions

The deleterious effect of multivalent cations on the oral bioavailability of quinolones was first reported in 1985 (4). Since this pivotal report, numerous investigations have duplicated and extended this observation; these are detailed in Table 1 (4–64).

The concomitant oral administration of magnesium- or aluminum-containing antacids has been found to result in 6- to 10-fold decreases in the absorption of oral quinolones. Even when dose administrations of the agents were separated by two or more hours, substantial reductions in quinolone absorption persisted (3,9,13–15,18,23,24,33,34,39, 41,42,45,46,48–50,65,66). Studies of the oral coadministration of calcium-containing antacids with oral quinolones have produced conflicting results, with some reporting no significant effect (6,9,15–17,19,21,24), and others reporting significant reductions in absorption (8,13,14,17,18,20,22,23,45). Studies have also documented significant reductions in quinolone bioavailability during coadministration with calcium-fortified orange juice and calcium polycarbophil, calcium acetate, and sevelamer hydrochloride (25–29).

Studies have documented substantial reductions in quinolone bioavailability when coadministered with sucralfate. Again, this interaction persisted even when dose administrations of the agents were spaced two or more hours apart (38,45,52,53,55,58,61,64). Further studies have documented substantial reductions in quinolone bioavailability when coadministered with iron preparations or multiple vitamins with minerals such as zinc, magnesium, copper, and manganese (33,34), although one study did not find a significant interaction with iron (9).

It is hypothesized that the reduction in quinolone absorption is caused by the formation of insoluble and hence unabsorbable drug–cation complexes or chelates in the gastrointestinal tract (67–71). This has been confirmed in binding experiments utilizing nuclear magnetic resonance spectroscopy (33,43,72). It appears that the complexation or chelation involves the 4-keto and 3-carboxyl groups of the quinolones. In addition, it appears that the presence of these ions results in impaired dissolution of the quinolones, at least in vitro (73). It is thus not recommended to use magnesium-, aluminum-, or calcium-containing antacids, sucralfate, or iron/vitamin-mineral preparations concomitantly with quinolones. Histamine $H_2$-receptor antagonists such as ranitidine and cimetidine, with the exception of enoxacin (reduced bioavailability), have not been shown to alter quinolone absorption (6,40,44,57,58,74–85). Omeprazole has also not been shown to alter the pharmacokinetics of quinolones to a clinically significant degree (50,86,87). Thus, these agents can be recommended as alternative noninteracting antiulcer therapy. In addition, intensive antacid therapy has been demonstrated not to alter the kinetics of intravenous enoxacin to a clinically significant degree (88).

Agents that alter gastric motility may affect quinolone absorption. Pirenzepine, a gastrointestinal tract-specific anticholinergic not available in the United States, delayed gastric emptying and absorption of ciprofloxacin, thus delaying the time to achievement of maximal serum concentration. However, the extent of absorption was not altered (40,74).

**Table 1**
**Effects of Multivalent Cations on Quinolone Absorption**

| Quinolone | Cation/preparation/schedule | Mean % change in | | Reference |
|---|---|---|---|---|
| | | $C_{max}$ | AUC | |
| Flerox | AlOH/0.5, 12, 24, 36 h postquinolone | $-24^a$ | $-17$ | 5 |
| Levoflox | AlOH/simultaneous with quinolone | $-65^a$ | $-44^a$ | 6 |
| Norflox | AlOH/simultaneous with quinolone | — | $-86^{a,b}$ | 7 |
| Norflox | AlOH/simultaneous with quinolone | $-28^c$ | $-29^c$ | 8 |
| Oflox | AlOH/simultaneous with quinolone | $-29^a$ | $-19$ | 9 |
| Oflox | Al phos/simultaneous with quinolone | $-10$ | $-3$ | 10 |
| Oflox | Al phos/simultaneous with quinolone | — | $-7$ | 11 |
| Norflox | Bi subsalicylate/simultaneous with quinolone | — | $-10^b$ | 7 |
| Cipro | Bi subsalicylate/simultaneous with quinolone | $-13$ | $-13$ | 12 |
| Cipro | Ca carb/simultaneous with quinolone | $-38^a$ | $-41^a$ | 13 |
| Cipro | Ca carb antacid/simultaneous with quinolone | $-47^a$ | $-42^a$ | 14 |
| Cipro | Ca carb antacid/with meals (PO$_4$ binder) | $+13$ | — | 15 |
| Cipro | Ca carb/2 h prequinolone | $+22^a$ | $0$ | 16 |
| Cipro | Ca carb/simultaneous with quinolone | — | $-29^{a,b}$ | 17 |
| Cipro | Ca carb/(tid × 11 doses) 2 h after Dose 10 | $-24^a$ | $-14$ | 18 |
| Gati | Ca carb/simultaneous with quinolone | $-7$ | $-8$ | 19 |
| | 2 hours prequinolone | $-13$ | $-8$ | |
| | 2 hours postquinolone | $+2$ | $0$ | |
| Levoflox | Ca carb/simultaneous with quinolone | $-23$ | $-3$ | 6 |
| Lomeflox | Ca carb/simultaneous with quinolone | $-14^a$ | $-2$ | 20 |
| Moxi | Ca carb/simultaneous with quinolone | $-15^a$ | $-2$ | 21 |
| | +12 and 24 hours postquinolone | | | |
| Gemi | Ca carb/simultaneous with quinolone | $-21^a$ | $-17^a$ | 22 |
| | 2 hours prequinolone | $-11$ | $-10$ | |
| | 2 hours postquinolone | $0$ | $-7$ | |
| Norflox | Ca carb/simultaneous with quinolone | $-28^c$ | $-47^{a,c}$ | 8 |
| Norflox | Ca carb antacid/simultaneous with quinolone | $-66^a$ | $-63^a$ | 23 |
| Norflox | Ca carb antacid/simultaneous with quinolone | $-66$ | $-62$ | 22 |
| Oflox | Ca carb/simultaneous with quinolone | — | $0^b$ | 17 |
| Oflox | Ca carb/simultaneous with quinolone | $-18$ | $+10$ | 9 |
| Oflox | Ca carb antacid/2 hours prequinolone | $+3$ | $-4$ | 24 |
| | 24 hours prequinolone | $+9$ | $-4$ | |
| | 2 hours postquinolone | $+3$ | $-3$ | |
| Cipro | Ca acetate/simultaneous with quinolone | $-50^a$ | $-51^a$ | 25 |
| Cipro | Ca polycarbophil 1200 mg (5.0 mmol Ca)/ | $-64^a$ | $-52^a$ | 26 |
| | Simultaneous with quinolone | | | |
| Cipro | Ca-fortified orange juice/simultaneous with quinolone | $-41^a$ | $-38^a$ | 27 |
| Gati | Ca-fortified orange juice/simultaneous with quinolone | $-14$ | $-12^a$ | 28 |
| Levo | Ca-fortified orange juice/ | $-23^a$ | $-14^a$ | 29 |
| | Ca-fortified orange juice + milk/ | $-24^a$ | $-16^a$ | |
| | (Both simultaneous with ready-to-eat cereal and quinolone) | | | |
| Moxi | Ca lact-gluc + carb/ | | | 21 |
| | Immediately before and 12 + 24 hours after quinolone | $-15^a$ | $-2$ | |
| Cipro | Didanosine (+ cations)/3 doses | | | 30 |
| | (Dose 3 simultaneous with quinolone) | $-93^a$ | $-98^a$ | |

*Continued on next page*

**Table 1 (*Continued*)**
**Effects of Multivalent Cations on Quinolone Absorption**

| Quinolone | Cation/preparation/schedule | Mean % change in | | Reference |
|---|---|---|---|---|
| | | $C_{max}$ | AUC | |
| Cipro | Didanosine (+ cations)/6 doses | −16 | −26[a] | 31 |
| | (Quinolone 2 hours predidanosine) | | | |
| Cipro | Didanosine (− cations)/simultaneous with quinolone | −8 | −9 | 32 |
| Cipro | Fe gluc/600 mg simultaneous with quinolone | −57[a] | −64[a] | 33 |
| Cipro | FeSO$_4$/300 mg simultaneous with quinolone | −33[a] | −42[a] | 33 |
| Cipro | FeSO$_4$/325 mg tid × 7 days | −75[a] | −63[a] | 34 |
| Cipro | FeSO$_4$/simultaneous with quinolone | −54[a] | −57[a] | 35 |
| Gati | FeSO$_4$/simultaneous with quinolone | −52 | −28 | 36 |
| Gati | FeSO$_4$/simultaneous with quinolone | −54[a] | −35[a] | 19 |
| | 2 hours prequinolone | −12 | −10 | |
| | 2 hours postquinolone | −3 | −5 | |
| Levoflox | FeSO$_4$/simultaneous with quinolone | −45[a] | −19[a] | 6 |
| Lomeflox | FeSO$_4$/simultaneous with quinolone | −28[a] | −14 | 20 |
| Moxi | FeSO$_4$/simultaneous with quinolone | −59[a] | −39[a] | 37 |
| Norflox | FeSO$_4$/simultaneous with quinolone | −75[a] | −73[a] | 35 |
| Norflox | FeSO$_4$/simultaneous with quinolone | −97[a,c] | −97[a,c] | 8 |
| Norflox | FeSO$_4$/simultaneous with quinolone | — | −55[a,b] | 7 |
| Oflox | FeSO$_4$/simultaneous with quinolone | — | −10[a,b] | 11 |
| Oflox | FeSO$_4$/simultaneous with quinolone | −36[a] | −25[a] | 35 |
| Oflox | FeSO$_4$/simultaneous with quinolone | +9 | +35 | 9 |
| Gemi | FeSO$_4$/3 hours before quinolone | −20[a] | −11 | 38 |
| | 2 hours after quinolone | −4 | −10 | |
| Norflox | Mg OH/simultaneous with quinolone | — | −90[a,b] | 7 |
| Levoflox | Mg O/simultaneous with quinolone | −38[a] | −22[a] | 6 |
| Norflox | Mg trisilicate/simultaneous with quinolone | −72[a,c] | −81[a,c] | 8 |
| Oflox | Mg trisilicate/simultaneous with quinolone | −2 | +19 | 9 |
| Cipro | Mg/Al antacid/simultaneous with quinolone | −81[a] | −84[a] | 14 |
| Cipro | Mg/Al antacid/5–10 minutes prequinolone | −80[a] | −85[a] | 39 |
| | 2 hours prequinolone | −74[a] | −77[a] | |
| | 4 hours prequinolone | −13 | −30[a] | |
| | 6 hours prequinolone | 0 | +9 | |
| | 2 hours postquinolone | +32[a] | +7 | |
| Cipro | Mg/Al antacid/10 doses over 24 hours prequinolone | −93[a] | −91[a] | 40 |
| Cipro | Mg/Al antacid/with meals (PO$_4$ binder) | −65 | — | 15 |
| Cipro | Mg/Al antacid/24 hours prequinolone | −94[a] | — | 4 |
| Enox | Mg/Al antacid/0.5 hours prequinolone | −70[a] | −73[a] | 41 |
| | 2 hours prequinolone | −38 | −48[a] | |
| | 8 hours prequinolone | −9 | −17 | |
| Gati | Mg/Al antacid/2 hours prequinolone | −45[a] | −42[a] | 42 |
| | Simultaneous with quinolone | −68[a] | −64[a] | |
| | 2 hours postquinolone | −3 | −18[a] | |
| | 4 hours postquinolone | +3 | +1 | |
| Lomeflox | Mg/Al antacid/simultaneous with quinolone | −46[a] | −41[a] | 43 |
| Moxi | Mg/Al antacid/simultaneous with quinolone | −61[a] | −59[a] | 44 |
| | 2 hours postquinolone | −7 | −26[a] | |
| | 4 hours prequinolone | −1 | −23[a] | |

*Continued on next page*

**Table 1** *(Continued)*
**Effects of Multivalent Cations on Quinolone Absorption**

| Quinolone | Cation/preparation/schedule | $C_{max}$ | AUC | Reference |
|---|---|---|---|---|
| | | Mean % change in | | |
| Norflox | Mg/Al antacid/simultaneous with quinolone | $-95^a$ | — | 23 |
| | 2 hours postquinolone | $-24^a$ | $-20$ | |
| Norflox | Mg/Al antacid/simultaneous with quinolone | $-95$ | $-98$ | 45 |
| | 2 hours postquinolone | $-24$ | $-22$ | |
| Oflox | Mg/Al antacid/10 doses over 24 hours prequinolone | $-73^a$ | $-69^a$ | 40 |
| Oflox | Mg/Al antacid/2 hours prequinolone | $-30^a$ | $-21^a$ | 24 |
| | 24 hours prequinolone | $-5$ | $-5$ | |
| | 2 hours postquinolone | $+3$ | $+5$ | |
| Oflox | Mg/Al antacid/simultaneous with quinolone | $-24$ | — | 46 |
| Peflox | Mg/Al antacid/13 doses; Quinolone 1 hour after Dose 10 | $-61^a$ | $-54^a$ | 47 |
| Ruflox | Mg/Al antacid/Simultaneous with quinolone | $-43^a$ | $-38^a$ | 48 |
| | 4 hours postquinolone | $+6$ | $-15^a$ | |
| Tema | Mg/Al antacid/8 doses per day prior to study and 5 doses on study day | $-59^a$ | $-61^a$ | 49 |
| Trovaflox | Mg/Al antacid/10 PM the night before and 1 and 3 hours after meals and at bedtime on the study day and 0.5 hours before quinolone | $-60$ | $-66$ | 50 |
| | 10 PM the night before and 1 and 3 hours after meals and at bedtime on the study day and 2 hours after the quinolone | $-11$ | $-28$ | |
| Gemi | Mg/Al antacid/3 hours before quinolone | $-17^a$ | $-15$ | 51 |
| | 10 minutes after quinolone | $-87^a$ | $-85^a$ | |
| | 2 hours after quinolone | $+10$ | $+3$ | |
| Cipro | Multivit with Zn/once daily × 7 days | $-32^a$ | $-22^a$ | 34 |
| Cipro | Multivit with Fe/Zn/once simultaneous with quinolone | $-53^a$ | $-52^a$ | 33 |
| Norflox | Na HCO$_3$/simultaneous with quinolone | $+5^c$ | $+5^c$ | 8 |
| Cipro | Sevelamer hydrochloride/seven 403-mg caps | | | 25 |
| | Simultaneous with quinolone | $-34^a$ | $-48^a$ | |
| Cipro | Sucralfate/1 g 6 and 2 hours prequinolone | $-30^a$ | $-30^a$ | 52 |
| Cipro | Sucralfate/1 g qid × 1 day then simultaneous with quinolone | $-90^a$ | $-88^a$ | 53 |
| Cipro | Sucralfate/2 g bid × 5 doses | | | 54 |
| | Quinolone simultaneous with Dose 5 | $-95^a$ | $-96^a$ | |
| | Quinolone 2 hours before Dose 5 | $+5$ | $-20$ | |
| | Quinolone 6 hours before Dose 5 | $0$ | $-7$ | |
| Enox | Sucralfate/1 g simultaneous with quinolone | $-91^a$ | $-88^a$ | 55 |
| | 1 g 2 hours prequinolone | $-51^a$ | $-54^a$ | |
| | 1 g 2 hours postquinolone | $0$ | $-8$ | |
| Flerox | Sucralfate/1 g qid × 12 doses Quinolone simultaneous with Dose 5 | $-26^a$ | $-24^a$ | 56 |
| Levoflox | Sucralfate/1 g 2 hours postquinolone | $+14$ | $-5$ | 57 |
| Lomeflox | Sucralfate/1 g 2 hours prequinolone | $-30^a$ | $-25^a$ | 58 |
| Lomeflox | Sucralfate/1 g simultaneous with quinolone | $-65^a$ | $-51^a$ | 20 |
| Moxi | Sucralfate/1 g simultaneous with quinolone + 5, 10, 15, 24 hours postquinolone | $-71^a$ | $-60^a$ | 59 |
| Norflox | Sucralfate/ Simultaneous with quinolone | $-90$ | $-98$ | 45 |
| | 2 hours prequinolone | $-28$ | $-42$ | |

*Continued on next page*

**Table 1** *(Continued)*
**Effects of Multivalent Cations on Quinolone Absorption**

| | | Mean % change in | | |
|---|---|---|---|---|
| Quinolone | Cation/preparation/schedule | $C_{max}$ | AUC | Reference |
| Norflox | Sucralfate/ 1 g simultaneous with quinolone | −92 [a] | −91 [a] | 60 |
| | 1 g 2 hours postquinolone | +9 | −5 | |
| Norflox | Sucralfate/ 1 g simultaneous with quinolone | −90 [a] | −98 [a] | 61 |
| | 1 g 2 hours prequinolone | −28 | −43 | |
| Oflox | Sucralfate/ 1 g simultaneous with quinolone | −70 [a] | −61 [a] | 60 |
| | 1 g 2 hours postquinolone | +7 | −5 | |
| Oflox | Sucralfate/ Fasting + 1 g simultaneous with quinolone | −70 [a] | −61 [a] | 62 |
| | Nonfasting + 1 g simultaneous with quinolone | −39 [a] | −31 [a] | |
| Spar | Sucralfate/1 g qid × 8 doses; | −39 [a] | −47 [a] | 63 |
| | Quinolone 0.5 hours post Dose 8 | | | |
| Spar | Sucralfate/1.5 g bid × 5 doses/ | | | 64 |
| | Quinolone simultaneous with Dose 5 | −52 [a] | −50 [a] | |
| | Quinolone 2 hours before Dose 5 | −30 [a] | −36 [a] | |
| | Quinolone 4 hours before Dose 5 | +3 | −8 | |
| Gemi | Sucralfate/ 2 g 3 hours before quinolone | −69 [a] | −53 [a] | 38 |
| | 2 g 2 hours after quinolone | −2 | −8 | |
| Norflox | Tripotassium citrate/simultaneous with quinolone | −48 [a,b] | −40 [a,c] | 8 |
| Norflox | ZnSO$_4$/simultaneous with quinolone | — | −56 [a,b] | 7 |

% change, change from baseline or placebo control; $C_{max}$, peak serum or plasma concentration; AUC, area under the plasma or serum concentration–time curve; enox, enoxacin; oflox, ofloxacin; cipro, ciprofloxacin; norflox, norfloxacin; carb, carbonate; PO$_4$, phosphate; lomeflox, lomefloxacin; levoflox, levofloxacin; tid, 3 times daily; qid, 4 times daily; bid, twice daily; gluc, gluconate; trovaflox, trovafloxacin; spar, sparfloxacin; gati, gatifloxacin; moxi, moxifloxacin; gemi, gemifloxacin; lact, lactate; multivit, multivitamin.

[a] Statistically significant change from baseline or placebo control.
[b] Based on urinary excretion data.
[c] Based on salivary AUC data.

*N*-Butylscopolamine, another anticholinergic, interacted with oral ciprofloxacin in an identical manner *(76)*. In contrast, absorption of ciprofloxacin was accelerated by the gastrointestinal motility stimulant metoclopramide; again, the extent of absorption was unaltered *(76)*. Similarly, cisapride accelerated the absorption of sparfloxacin, resulting in a significant increase in peak plasma concentration but no significant effect on the extent of absorption *(63)*. These quinolone–drug interactions are thought to be of no clinical importance during usual multiple-dose regimens.

The absorption of temafloxacin and ciprofloxacin has been reported not to be significantly altered in the presence of Osmolite® enteral feedings *(89,90)*. However, other studies have found significant interaction potential between the quinolones and enteral feedings. Concurrent administration of Osmolite and Pulmocare® enteral feedings has been found to significantly reduce single-dose ciprofloxacin bioavailability as assessed using $C_{max}$ (mean −26 and −31%, respectively) and area under the serum concentration-vs-time curve (AUC; mean −33 and −42%, respectively) data *(91)*. Concurrent administration of Sustacal® enteral feeding orally has been found to significantly reduce single-dose ciprofloxacin bioavailability as assessed using $C_{max}$ (mean −43%) and AUC (mean −27%) data. In the same study, continuous administration of Jevity® enteral feeding via gastrostomy and jejunostomy tubes was found to significantly reduce single-dose ciprofloxacin bioavailability as assessed using $C_{max}$ (mean −37 and −59%, respectively) and AUC (mean −53 and −67%, respectively) data *(92)*. Concurrent administration of Ensure® enteral feeding has been found to significantly reduce single-dose ciprofloxacin and ofloxacin bioavailability as assessed using $C_{max}$ (mean −47 and −36%, respectively) and AUC (mean −27 and −10%, respectively) data. However, the extent of the interaction was significantly greater for ciprofloxacin than ofloxacin *(93)*.

The interaction potential between quinolones and dairy products appears to be quinolone specific. Studies have demonstrated no significant interaction between lomefloxacin, fleroxacin, enoxacin, gatifloxacin, moxifloxacin, and ofloxacin and milk (240 or 300 mL) or yogurt (250–300 mL) *(20,36,94–98)*. In contrast, ciprofloxacin and norfloxacin bioavailability is substantially reduced (by 28–58%) by concurrent administration with milk or yogurt *(96,99,100)*.

### Distribution Interactions

The quinolones are plasma protein bound to the extent of only 20–30%. Ciprofloxacin does not displace bilirubin from albumin, which suggests that interactions involving displacement of other drugs from their carrier proteins are unlikely to occur during coadministration of quinolones *(101)*. The absence of such an interaction with the quinolones may be of particular importance to elderly debilitated patients with hypoalbuminemia who receive multiple drugs.

### Metabolism Interactions

The effect of quinolones on the metabolism of antipyrine, a probe drug for hepatic drug metabolism, has been evaluated. Ofloxacin given 200 mg twice daily for 7 days was found not to influence antipyrine metabolism significantly *(102)*. Similarly, 125 mg ciprofloxacin twice daily for 7 or 8 days was found not to influence antipyrine metabolism significantly *(103)*. In contrast, a regimen of 500 mg ciprofloxacin twice daily for 8 to 10 days, a clinically relevant dosing regimen, was associated with a significant mean 39% reduction in antipyrine clearance and mean 58% increase in terminal disposition half-life *(104)*.

A number of case reports have documented a clinically significant drug–drug interaction between ciprofloxacin and theophylline, in some cases leading to death *(105–111)*. A number of the quinolones have been found to reduce the hepatic metabolism of coadministered drugs such as the xanthines theophylline *(112–146)* and caffeine *(147–156)* (Table 2). In contrast to the absorption interactions with multivalent cations, which appear to be generalizable to the entire quinolone drug class, differences do exist between individual quinolones in their propensity to inhibit hepatic xanthine metabolism. A meta-analysis of quinolone–theophylline interaction studies revealed that enoxacin (and, based on ref. *142*, grepafloxacin), ciprofloxacin, and norfloxacin (in descending order) are clinically significant inhibitors of theophylline metabolism; ofloxacin, lomefloxacin, and (based on refs. *120, 125, 126, 137–139, 144–146, 157, 158*) levofloxacin, temafloxacin, trovafloxacin, sparfloxacin, gatifloxacin, moxifloxacin, gemifloxacin, and rufloxacin are clinically insignificant inhibitors *(159)*. Using a simple pharmacokinetic model that allowed cross-comparison between quinolone–caffeine interaction studies, Barnett and colleagues developed a relative potency index of quinolone interaction as follows: enoxacin (100), ciprofloxacin (11), norfloxacin (9), and ofloxacin (0) *(160)*.

**Table 2**
**Effect of Quinolones on Methylxanthine Pharmacokinetics**

| Quinolone | | Mean % change in steady-state concentration | CL | $t_{1/2}$ | Reference |
|---|---|---|---|---|---|
| Theophylline | | | | | |
| • Enox | 400 bid | +109 [a] | 55 [a] | — | 112 |
| • Norflox | 400 bid | — | –8 [a] | +9 [a] | 113 |
| • Norflox | 400 bid | — | 10 | +26 | 114 |
| • Cipro | 750 bid | — | –31[a] | — | 115 |
| • Oflox | 400 bid | +9 [a] | –15[a] | — | 116 |
| • Norflox | 400 bid | — | –15[a] | +13 [a] | 117 |
| • Lomeflox | 400 qd | — | –7 | +4 [a] | 118 |
| • Enox | 25 bid | — | –53 [a] | +35 [a] | 119 |
| | 100 bid | — | –66 [a] | +74 [a] | |
| | 400 bid | — | –73 [a] | +83 [a] | |
| • Enox | 400 bid | +91 [a] | –65 [a] | +187 | 120 |
| • Enox | 400–600 bid | +155 [a] | –42 [a] | — | 120 |
| • Tema | 400 bid | –55 | –10 | +9 | 121 |
| • Enox | 200 tid | +118 [a] | –65 [a] | — | 122 |
| • Enox | 400 bid | +163 [a] | –64 [a] | +159 [a] | 123 |
| • Cipro | 500 bid | +66 [a] | –30 [a] | +42 [a] | 123 |
| • Oflox | 400 bid | +2 | –5 | +2 | 123 |
| • Oflox | 200 tid | — | 0 | +6 | 124 |
| • Ruflox | 200 mg qd | — | +2 | –1 | 125 |
| • Spar | 200 qd | — | –9 | — | 126 |
| • Norflox | 200 tid | — | –7 | +15 | 124 |
| • Enox | 200 tid | — | –50 [a] | +53 [a] | 127 |
| • Oflox | 200 tid | — | 0 | +6 | 127 |
| • Norflox | 200 tid | — | –7 | +15 | 127 |
| • Cipro | 500 bid | — | –27 [a] | — | 128 |
| • Lomeflox | 400 bid | — | –2 | — | 128 |
| • Lomeflox | 400 × 1 dose | +1 | –2 | +1 | 129 |
| | 400 bid | +8 | –7 | +7 | |
| • Flerox | 400 bid | — | –6 [a] | +9 | 130 |
| • Flerox | 200 bid | — | 0 | — | 131 |
| • Enox | 400 bid | +243 [a] | –74 [a] | — | 132 |
| • Lomeflox | 400 bid | — | +7 | +3 | 133 |
| • Norflox | 200 tid | — | –4 | — | 134 |
| • Enox | 200 tid | — | –84 [a] | — | 134 |
| • Oflox | 200 tid | — | –11 | — | 134 |
| • Cipro | 200 tid | — | –22 [a] | — | 134 |
| • Enox | 600 bid | +248 [a] | — | — | 135 |
| • Cipro | 750 bid | +87 [a] | — | — | 136 |
| • Levoflox | 500 bid | — | +3 | –1 | 137 |
| • Trovaflox | 300 qd | — | –8 [a] | +13 [a] | 138 |

*Continued on next page*

**Table 2** *(Continued)*
**Effect of Quinolones on Methylxanthine Pharmacokinetics**

| Quinolone | | Mean % change in | | | |
|---|---|---|---|---|---|
| | | steady-state concentration | CL | $t_{1/2}$ | Reference |
| • Trovaflox | 200 qd | — | −7 | — | 139 |
| • Oflox | 200 bid | — | −5 | +5 | 140 |
| • Cipro | 500 bid | — | −20[a] | +25[a] | 141 |
| • Grepa | 600 qd | — | −52[a] | — | 142 |
| • Gati | 400 bid | — | 0 | — | 143 |
| • Moxi | 200 bid | — | −4 | +4 | 144 |
| • Moxi | 200 bid | — | +5 | +3 | 145 |
| • Gemi | 320 qd | — | −1 | — | 146 |
| Caffeine | | | | | |
| • Peflox | 400 bid | — | −47[a] | +96[a] | 147 |
| • Enox | 400 bid | — | −83[a] | +492[a] | 147 |
| • Norflox | 800 bid | — | −35[a] | +23 | 148 |
| • Cipro | 750 bid | — | −45[a] | +58[a] | 149 |
| • Cipro | 750 bid | +877[a] | −145[a] | +116[a] | 150 |
| • Oflox | 200 bid | — | +2 | −3 | 150 |
| • Norflox | 400 bid | — | −16 | +16[a] | 151 |
| • Cipro | 100 bid | — | −17 | +6 | 151 |
| | 250 bid | — | −57[a] | +15[a] | |
| | 500 bid | — | −58[a] | +26 | |
| • Enox | 100 bid | — | −138[a] | +103[a] | 151 |
| | 200 bid | — | −176[a] | +126[a] | |
| | 400 bid | — | −346[a] | +258[a] | |
| • Enox | 400 bid | — | −79[a] | +475[a] | 152 |
| • Oflox | 200 bid | — | +4 | −3 | 153 |
| • Cipro | 250 bid | — | −33[a] | +15[a] | 153 |
| • Enox | 400 bid | — | −78[a] | +258[a] | 153 |
| • Pip | 400 bid | — | −65[a] | −121[a] | 154 |
| • Lomeflox | 400 qd | −6 | −3 | 0 | 155 |
| • Trovaflox | 200 mg qd | — | −17 | — | 156 |

% change, change from baseline or placebo control; CL, total body clearance; $t_{1/2}$, elimination half-life; enox, enoxacin; norflox, norfloxacin; cipro, ciprofloxacin; lomeflox, lomefloxacin; levoflox, levofloxacin; tema, temafloxacin; oflox, ofloxacin; pip, pipemidic acid; trovaflox, trovafloxacin; ruflox, rufloxacin; spar, sparfloxacin; peflox, pefloxacin; grepa, grepafloxacin; gati, gatifloxacin; moxi, moxifloxacin; gemi, gemifloxacin; qd, once daily; bid, twice daily; tid, three times a day.
[a] Statistically significant difference from baseline or placebo control.

Few other substrates have been examined. Enoxacin decreased the metabolism of the less-active enantiomer of warfarin, R-warfarin, without potentiation of anticoagulant effect *(161)*. In addition, levofloxacin, norfloxacin, temafloxacin, trovafloxacin, grepafloxacin, moxifloxacin, gemifloxacin, sparfloxacin, and ciprofloxacin have been shown not to potentiate the anticoagulant effect of warfarin in healthy subjects and patients requiring long-term anticoagulation *(142,162–171)*. However, case reports have documented quinolone-associated increases in prothrombin time (PT) in patients receiving warfarin concurrently with ciprofloxacin, ofloxacin, norfloxacin, gatiflox-acin, levofloxacin, and moxifloxacin *(172–184a,184b)*. Pending additional informa-tion, patients who are receiving long-term warfarin therapy in whom a quinolone is to be used should be monitored for changes in PT/international normalized ratio (PT/INR). Temafloxacin has been shown not to interact with low-dose heparin as measured by changes in activated factor levels, activated partial thromboplastin time (APTT), PT, and thrombin time (TT) tests *(185)*.

Case reports have suggested that the quinolones may reduce the metabolism of cyclosporin A and hence potentiate the nephrotoxicity of this agent *(186–189)*. In addition, results of one study conducted in pediatric renal transplant recipients sug-gested that norfloxacin may interfere with cyclosporine disposition, as evidenced by the difference in mean daily dose of cyclosporine required to maintain trough blood cyclosporine concentrations of 150–400 ng/mL (4.5 mg/kg/day in norfloxacin recipi-ents vs 7.4 mg/kg/day in nonrecipients) *(190)*. However, numerous formal in vitro and pharmacokinetic studies have not found a significant interaction between cyclosporine and ciprofloxacin, pefloxacin, and levofloxacin *(191–199)*. This suggests that these agents may be used together with routine monitoring. In contrast, high-dose levo-floxacin (1 g/day) significantly increases tacrolimus systemic exposure (mean 26%), and combination therapy would appear to warrant enhanced monitoring *(200)*.

Studies have documented nonsignificant interactions of moxifloxacin, sparfloxacin, gemifloxacin, levofloxacin, and gatifloxacin with digoxin *(201–205)*. Coadministration of oral trovafloxacin and intravenous morphine results in 36 and 46% reductions in trovafloxacin bioavailability (based on AUC and $C_{max}$ data, respectively). Morphine pharmacokinetics and pharmacodynamics are not altered by concurrent administration *(206)*. Similar findings of reduced quinolone bioavailability have been noted with coadministration of oral ciprofloxacin and intramuscular papaveretum *(207)*. In con-trast, oral oxycodone had no significant effect on oral levofloxacin pharmacokinetics *(208a)*. Ciprofloxacin significantly reduced the total body clearance, renal clearance, and nonrenal clearance and increased the terminal disposition half-life and urinary excretion of R(–) and S(+) mexiletine in both smokers and nonsmokers. However, these changes were modest in degree (≤20%) and suggested the absence of a clini-cally-relevent drug interaction between the two agents *(208b)*.

Ciprofloxacin may impair the elimination of diazepam *(209)*, although this is contro-versial *(210)*. Gatifloxacin does not significantly alter the pharmacokinetics of intrave-nous midazolam *(211)*. Waite and coworkers demonstrated that elderly subjects are not more sensitive than younger subjects to the inhibitory effect of ciprofloxacin on hepatic metabolism of antipyrine *(212)*. Similarly, Loi and coworkers demonstrated that eld-erly subjects are not more sensitive to the inhibitory effect of ciprofloxacin on hepatic metabolism of theophylline *(213)*. In addition, Chandler and colleagues showed that rifampin does not induce the metabolism of ciprofloxacin, suggesting that the two agents may be used concomitantly in standard clinical dosing regimens *(214)*.

In contrast, Bernard and colleagues demonstrated that rifampin does induce the metabolism of grepafloxacin, resulting in a statistically significant 25% decrease in ter-minal disposition half-life and a 48% increase in apparent oral clearance *(215)*. In addition, rifampin coadministration significantly enhanced fleroxacin apparent oral clear-ance (mean 15%) and reduced the terminal disposition half-life (mean 19%) by significantly enhancing metabolic clearance by *N*-demethylation (no effect on *N*-oxidation) *(216)*. Examining the rifampin component of the combination, single-dose ciprofloxacin significantly increased the terminal disposition half-life and reduced the $C_{max}$ but had no effect on the AUC, volume of distribution, or urinary excretion of single-dose rifampin *(217a,217b)*. Single-dose pefloxacin significantly increased the terminal disposition half-life, peak plasma concentration, area under the plasma concentration–time curve (from 0–24 hours and 0–∞), volume of distribution, absorption half-life, and urinary excretion of single-dose rifampin *(217c,217d)*.

One case report each has suggested inhibition of clozapine, olanzapine, and methadone metabolism by ciprofloxacin *(218–220)*. In a study conducted in seven patients with schizophrenia, 250 mg ciprofloxacin twice daily caused significant elevations in serum clozapine and *N*-desmethylclozapine concentrations (mean 29 and 31%, respectively) after 1 week of concurrent therapy *(221)*.

Two cases of severe methotrexate toxicity caused by concomitant use of ciprofloxacin have been reported. In both cases, elimination of methotrexate after high-dose therapy for cancer was substantially delayed with resultant dermatological, bone marrow, hepatic, and renal toxicity. The mechanism is unclear but may involve alterations of methotrexate plasma protein binding, reduction in renal function (thus enhancing drug retention), inhibition of hepatic aldolase (thus reducing drug metabolism), or inhibition of renal tubular secretion (again, enhancing retention). Another issue with combination quinolone–high-dose methotrexate therapy is the effect of urinary alkalinization (required for safe high-dose methotrexate use) on the crystalluria risk of the quinolones *(222)*.

A case report of lithium toxicity caused by concurrent levofloxacin use has also been reported. It appears that an acute deterioration in renal function occurred, causing retention of lithium. Whether the deterioration in renal function was caused by the quinolone or the combination of the two drugs is not known *(223)*.

Ciprofloxacin and moxifloxacin have not been found to interact pharmacokinetically and pharmacodynamically with low-dose oral contraceptives (containing 30 μg of ethinyl estradiol and 150 μg desogestrel) *(202,224)*. Levofloxacin does not alter the pharmacokinetics of zidovudine, efavirenz, or nelfinavir, and ciprofloxacin does not alter the pharmacokinetics of didanosine *(30,225,226)*. Ciprofloxacin does not interact pharmacokinetically with metronidazole *(80)* or isoniazid *(227,228)*.

The effect of quinolones on the pharmacokinetics and pharmacodynamics of ethanol are uncertain. One study using healthy volunteers found there was no pharmacokinetic or pharmacodynamic interaction with ciprofloxacin *(229)*. However, another study, again using healthy volunteers, found that 750 mg ciprofloxacin twice daily significantly reduced the ethanol elimination rate (by mean 9%, range 5–18%) and increased the AUC (mean 12%) and time to zero blood ethanol concentration (mean 10%). This pharmacokinetic interaction was felt to be caused by the effect of ciprofloxacin on the ethanol-metabolizing intestinal flora and not its hepatic effects (on enzymes and blood flow) *(230)*. Perhaps the discrepancies between results of these two studies are caused by differences in subject numbers (statistical power), drug doses, or study design (randomized, parallel group vs crossover).

The effects of multiple-dose oral ciprofloxacin on the single-dose pharmacokinetics of intravenous ropivacaine have been evaluated in nine healthy volunteers. The clearance of ropivacaine was significantly reduced (mean 31%) during concurrent therapy, with considerable intersubject variability (range –52 to +39%). The cytochrome P450 (CYP) 1A2-mediated formation of 3-OH-ropivacaine was significantly reduced; the AUC and 24-hour urinary excretion of this metabolite fell 38 and 27%, respectively. In contrast, the CYP3A4-mediated formation of (S)-2′,6′-pipecoloxylidide was significantly enhanced, as manifested by mean increases in AUC and 24-hour urinary excretion of 71 and 97%, respectively *(231)*.

A number of case reports have documented substantial reductions in serum phenytoin concentrations when ciprofloxacin therapy was initiated, an unexpected finding for a drug usually associated with enzyme inhibition and reduced drug clearance *(232–237)*. Indeed, results of a small study revealed that ciprofloxacin cotherapy was associated with nonsignificant reductions in mean steady-state phenytoin $C_{max}$ (4%) and AUC (6%) *(238)*. The mechanism underlying this interaction is unknown. In any case, caution is warranted when coadministering phenytoin and quinolones on the basis of this kinetic interaction as well as the epileptogenic potential of the quinolones (quinolones and nonsteroidal anti-inflammatory drugs).

The effect of combinations of enzyme inhibitors such as ciprofloxacin plus clarithromycin and ciprofloxacin plus cimetidine has been evaluated *(213,239–241)*. Interestingly, clarithromycin (1000 mg twice daily) was not found to significantly augment the effect of ciprofloxacin (500 mg twice daily) on steady-state theophylline pharmacokinetics *(240)*. In contrast, coadministration of cimetidine (400 mg twice daily or 600 mg four times daily) plus ciprofloxacin (500 mg twice daily) exerted a greater inhibitory effect on theophylline elimination than each agent alone, although the combined effect was less than the additive sum produced by the individual drugs *(213,239,241)*.

The mechanism of these metabolic interactions is largely unexplored. It has been suggested that inhibition of metabolism may be related to the 4-oxo metabolites of the quinolones, but more recent data suggest that the sequence $N* - C = N - C - N - C$ (where $N*$ = nitrogen on the piperazine ring) is the entity responsible for metabolic inhibition *(151,242)*. It appears that metabolic inhibition is dose related, at least for enoxacin and ciprofloxacin *(119,151)*.

The structure–activity relationships for in vitro inhibition of human CYP1A2 have been investigated by Fuhr and coworkers. The $3^1$-oxo derivatives had similar or reduced activity and M1 metabolites (cleavage of piperazinyl substituent) had greater inhibitory activity compared with the parent molecule. Alkylation of the 7-piperazinyl substituent resulted in reduced inhibitory potency. Naphthyridines with an unsubstituted piperazinyl group position 7 displayed greater inhibitory potency than did corresponding quinolone derivatives. Molecular modeling studies revealed that the keto group, carboxylate group, and core nitrogen at position 1 are likely to be the most important groups for binding to the active site of CYP1A2. These investigators also developed an equation to estimate *a priori* using quantitative structure–activity relationship analysis the potency of a given quinolone to inhibit CYP1A2 *(243)*. These investigators as well as Sarkar and coworkers also developed in vitro human liver microsome models that may be useful in qualitatively predicting relevant drug interactions between quinolones and methylxanthines *(244,245)*.

Clinically, caution is advised when using any quinolone in combination with a xanthine compound such as theophylline. Close monitoring of serum theophylline concentrations is recommended in any patient receiving these drugs. The clinical significance of inhibited metabolism of other drugs remains unclear at present. Until further data become available, clinicians should be aware of the possibility of reduced drug metabolism resulting in adverse effects whenever the quinolones are coadministered with drugs that depend on hepatic metabolism for their elimination.

### Excretion Interactions

The quinolone antimicrobials are generally excreted into the urine at a rate higher than creatinine clearance, implying that tubular secretion is a prominent excretory pathway. Indeed, the administration of probenecid, a blocker of the anionic renal tubular secretory pathway, substantially reduces the renal elimination of norfloxacin, levofloxacin, gatifloxacin, and ciprofloxacin, reflecting competitive blockade of quinolone tubular secretion *(246–250)*. In contrast, probenecid coadministration does not affect the pharmacokinetics of moxifloxacin *(251)*. In addition, furosemide and ranitidine reduce the renal tubular secretion of lomefloxacin, again reflecting competitive blockade *(252,253)*. There is thus a possibility that other drugs may interact with the quinolones at this site to competitively impair their mutual renal elimination, thus elevating blood concentrations and perhaps enhancing therapeutic or toxic effects.

This in fact has been noted in a study of the interaction between ofloxacin and procainamide in healthy volunteers. Ofloxacin coadministration was associated with 22 and 30% falls in procainamide oral total body and renal clearances, respectively. However, neither the pharmacokinetics of *N*-acetylprocainamide nor the pharmacodynamics of the antiarrhythmic, as assessed by standard 12-lead and signal-averaged electrocardiograms, were affected by ofloxacin coadministration *(254a)*. The 14.4% decrease in garenoxacin clearance in recipients of pseudoephedrine, identified in a population pharmacokinetic analysis of phase II respiratory tract infection clinical trial data (*N* = 721 patients, *N* = 1908 plasma concentrations), was felt to be done due to competition for active tubular secretion *(254b)*.

## PHARMACODYNAMIC INTERACTIONS

### Quinolones and Nonsteroidal Anti-Inflammatory Drugs

Central nervous system toxicity, including tremulousness and seizures, is rare with quinolones *(255–262)*. In some cases, concurrent use of nonsteroidal anti-inflammatory drugs (NSAIDs) have been noted *(258,259,262,263)*. It was the report of multiple cases of seizures associated with the concurrent use of enoxacin and fenbufen (an NSAID unavailable in the United States) to Japanese regulatory authorities that led to a plethora of investigations into the possible interaction between quinolones and NSAIDs *(262,263)*.

Some rat studies have suggested that NSAIDs such as fenbufen may enhance central nervous system uptake of quinolones such as ciprofloxacin, norfloxacin, and ofloxacin *(264,265)*. However, other studies conducted in the same species have documented an absence of a pharmacokinetic interaction between fenbufen and sparfloxacin, ciprofloxacin, enoxacin, and ofloxacin *(266–269)*. In addition, human studies have documented absence of a pharmacokinetic interaction between ciprofloxacin and fenbufen and ketoprofen and pefloxacin or ofloxacin *(270–272)*. Any interaction that occurs between quinolones and NSAIDs is thus probably purely pharmacodynamic.

Numerous in vitro models have been utilized to elucidate the mechanisms underlying the epileptogenic effects of quinolones with or without concurrent NSAID administration: voltage-clamped rat hippocampal or dorsal root ganglion or frog dorsal root ganglion neurons in cell culture, ($^3$H)-muscimol or GABA (γ-aminobutyric acid) binding to rat GABA synaptic receptors, and ($^3$H)-muscimol binding to human GABA synaptic receptors (273-278). Quinolones function as weak, dose-dependent GABA$_A$ receptor antagonists (273,274,277,279). Quinolones vary in their potencies as receptor antagonists (273–278,280–284), probably at least partly because of differences in the degree to which their 7-piperazine substituents look like GABA (275). This receptor antagonism is greatly enhanced by concurrent exposure to fenbufen or its active metabolite, biphenyl acetic acid (274,275,277–279,281,283,285–287). Flurbiprofen, indomethacin, ketoprofen, naproxen, and ibuprofen are much weaker potentiators (277,284); diclofenac and piroxicam do not potentiate quinolone GABA$_A$ receptor binding at all (276,284). This receptor antagonism appears to occur principally in the hippocampus and frontal cortex (278,288). In vivo studies in rats evaluating the epileptogenic potential of quinolones and potentiation by biphenyl acetic acid corroborated these in vitro data (289,290). The mechanism underlying this interaction is not established but does not appear to be mediated via benzodiazepine receptor effects (284). Studies suggested that the mechanism may involve enhanced cerebral glutamate (an excitatory amino acid neurotransmitter) or nitric acid concentrations (291–293).

Although of theoretical interest, the pharmacodynamic interaction between quinolones and NSAIDs is probably of little clinical relevance so long as fenbufen is not concurrently used with a quinolone.

## Quinolones and Electrophysiology

Sparfloxacin, grepafloxacin, levofloxacin, gatifloxacin, and moxifloxacin have been associated with prolongation of the QTc interval on the electrocardiogram, which in a few cases has been associated with the development of polymorphous ventricular tachycardia (torsades de pointes), which in turn can degenerate into ventricular fibrillation (294–303b). One case of levofloxacin-associated torsades de pointes in the absence of QTc interval prolongation has also been reported (304). Grepafloxacin was removed from the market by its manufacturer in October 1999 because of its electrophysiological adverse event profile.

Almost no data are available regarding the relative risk of cardiac arrhythmias with various quinolones. In a retrospective analysis utilizing the Food and Drug Administration adverse event reporting database from January 1, 1996, through May 2, 2001, the rates of torsades de pointes with ciprofloxacin, levofloxacin, and gatifloxacin were 0.3, 5.4, and 27 per 10 million prescriptions, respectively ($p < 0.05$ for all pairwise comparisons) (300). However, the numerous potential problems with study design preclude generalizability of these results (300,301).

Numerous in vitro models have been utilized to elucidate the mechanism underlying the arrhythmogenic effects of these agents: HERG (human ether-a-go-go-related gene) potassium channels, mouse atrial tumor cells, guinea pig myocardium, and canine Purkinje fibers (305–309). The potency of quinolones in inhibiting HERG-mediated outward potassium currents was sparfloxacin > grepafloxacin > moxifloxacin = gatifloxacin > levofloxacin = ciprofloxacin > ofloxacin in one study;

for the other, it was sparfloxacin > moxifloxacin = grepafloxacin >>> ciprofloxacin *(305,309)*. Similar findings were noted for mouse atrial tumor cell potassium channels (sparfloxacin > moxifloxacin >> gatifloxacin = grepafloxacin) *(306)*. In guinea pig ventricular myocardium, prolongation of action potential duration was 41, 25, 24, and 13% for sparfloxacin, moxifloxacin, grepafloxacin, and gatifloxacin, respectively, and the prolongation with levofloxacin, sitafloxacin, trovafloxacin, ciprofloxacin, gemifloxacin, and tosufloxacin was essentially zero *(307)*. Similar findings were noted with canine cardiac Purkinje fibers (sparfloxacin > grepafloxacin = moxifloxacin > ciprofloxacin) *(308)*.

In vivo, quinolones again differed in their propensity to alter cardiac electrophysiology and cause ventricular arrhythmias. In rabbits, the potency of quinolones in prolonging the maximum QT interval was sparfloxacin > moxifloxacin = gatifloxacin = grepafloxacin, and ventricular tachycardia and torsades de pointes were only induced in sparfloxacin-treated animals *(306)*. In dogs receiving 3 and 30 mg/kg iv doses of sparfloxacin, cardiac output and ventricular repolarization and refractory periods rose, and heart rate fell. Blood pressure fell only after the high-dose administration. The increase in repolarization exceeded that of refractoriness, enhancing arrhythmia vulnerability, and the prolongation in repolarization was of a reverse use-dependent type (i.e., prolongation was especially enhanced at lower heart rates) *(310)*. In dogs with complete atrioventricular block and dogs under halothane anesthesia, oral and intravenous levofloxacin produced essentially no adverse electrophysiological and hemodynamic effects, and sparfloxacin had dose-dependent arrhythmogenic, electrophysiological, and negative chronotropic effects *(311)*.

In summary, the in vitro and in vivo (animal) studies revealed that quinolones cause a drug-specific, dose-dependent prolongation in QTc interval by inhibiting outward potassium currents in myocytes. In turn, this prolongation in action potential duration leads to a drug-specific risk of ventricular tachycardia and torsades de pointes. However, the lack of full agreement of the results of evaluations of potassium channel inhibition and QT interval prolongation, in terms of relative drug potencies, suggests that more than potassium channel inhibition may be involved *(306)*.

In healthy volunteers, multiple doses of oral sparfloxacin (200, 400, 800 mg daily for 3 days) produced a dose-dependent prolongation in QTc interval (mean respective increases from baseline on day 1 = 9, 16, 28 milliseconds; day 3 = 7, 12, 26 milliseconds) *(312)*. The pharmacodynamic interaction of sparfloxacin and terfenadine administered in usual therapeutic doses to healthy volunteers, in terms of QTc interval prolongation, was additive in nature (no pharmacokinetic interaction was found) *(313)*. In a retrospective review of 23 patients receiving 500 mg levofloxacin once daily in whom pre- and intratherapy electrocardiograms were available, the QTc prolongation exceeded 30 milliseconds in 4 patients (17%) and 60 milliseconds in 2 patients (9%), with an absolute QT prolongation to more than 500 milliseconds in 4 patients *(314)*. Single oral doses of 400 and 800 mg moxifloxacin caused $4.0 \pm 5.1$ (mean $\pm$ SD) and $4.5 \pm 3.8\%$ prolongation of the QTc interval at rest ($p < 0.05$ for both) in healthy volunteers. Significant QTc interval prolongation occurred at all heart rates and across the entire RR interval range (400–1000 milliseconds). The effect was similar in males and females and did not show dose dependence. No significant reverse rate dependence was seen. Statistically significant but weak correlations existed between moxifloxacin

**Table 3**
**Drugs Prolonging the QTc Interval That May Potentially Interact**
**Pharmacodynamically With Selected Quinolone Antimicrobials**

| | |
|---|---|
| • Cisapride | • Macrolides |
| • Trimethoprim/sulfamethoxazole | (erythromycin, clarithromycin, spiramycin) |
| • Pentamidine | • Chloroquine |
| • Halofantrine | • Phenothiazines |
| • Quinidine | • Tricyclic and tetracyclic antidepressants |
| • Procainamide | • Disopyramide |
| • Ibutilide | • Lidocaine, mexiletine (rare) |
| • β-Blockers (rare) | • Amiodarone (rare) |
| • Bepridil | • Lidoflazine |
| • Sotalol | • Dofetilide |
| • Flecainide | • Encainide |

*Source*: From ref. *317*.

plasma concentrations and QT interval ($r = 0.35$) and change in QT interval vs placebo ($r = 0.72$) *(315a)*.

In another healthy volunteer study, periodic and continuous ECGs were recorded before and after administration of single doses of intravenous levofloxacin 500, 1000, and 1500 mg. Using periodic ECG data, the only significant differences noted were the mean QTc intervals at 1.5 hours after administration of 1500 mg (Bazett formula: 415.33 vs 399.48 milliseconds with placebo; Fredericia correction: 409.67 vs 400.46 milliseconds with placebo) and 2.0 hours after administration of 1500 mg (corresponding values of 414.10 vs 398.92 and 409.58 vs 400.10 milliseconds) (all $p < 0.05$). Using continuous ECG data, significant QTc interval prolongation occurred after administration of 1000 mg (Bazett correction: in 3/4 baseline correction methods, mean change ranged from 2.8 to 3.9 milliseconds [$p \leq 0.05$]; Fredericia correction: in 1/4 baseline correction methods, the mean change was 2.8 milliseconds [$p \leq 0.05$]) and 1500 mg (Bazett correction: in 4/4 baseline correction methods, mean change ranged from 6.4 to 7.7 milliseconds [$p \leq 0.001$]; Fredericia correction: in 4/4 baseline correction methods, mean change ranged from 4.9 to 6.9 milliseconds [$p \leq 0.001$]) *(315b)*.

Only one comparative study of the effect of quinolones on QTc interval in humans has been published. Single oral doses of 1000 mg levofloxacin, 1500 mg ciprofloxacin, and 800 mg moxifloxacin were compared in healthy volunteers. Mean QT and QTc interval prolongation was significantly greater for moxifloxacin compared to placebo for all end points, but it was generally not for levofloxacin and ciprofloxacin (the exception was that the mean postdose QTc and QTc at 1.5, 2, and 2.5 hours postdose, using the Bazett method, were significantly increased for levofloxacin vs placebo). The proportion of subjects with prolongation in QTc interval of 30 milliseconds or greater was higher with moxifloxacin (72–81%) compared to levofloxacin (33–38%) and ciprofloxacin (34–40%) *(316)*.

Caution is warranted with the use of these agents in patients receiving other drugs with similar electrophysiological effects (Table 3) *(317–319)*. In addition, caution is warranted in using these agents in patients with an abnormal pretreatment QT interval, pretreatment electrolyte abnormalities (e.g., hypokalemia, hypomagnesemia, rarely hypocalcemia), starvation/liquid protein fast diets, and a prior or current history of coronary heart disease, bradyarrhythmias, or atrial fibrillation *(317–319)*.

## Quinolones and Immunosupressants

Based on the ability of the quinolones to enhance interleukin 2 production significantly, ex vivo studies have been conducted evaluating the effect of quinolones on lymphocyte proliferation and the ability of tacrolimus and sirolimus to inhibit it. Quinolones had no significant effect on either human lymphocyte proliferation or the ability of tacrolimus or sirolimus to inhibit it. Enoxacin, lomefloxacin, norfloxacin, and ciprofloxacin were the quinolones tested. Thus, no significant pharmacodynamic interaction between the quinolones and tacrolimus/sirolimus appears to exist *(320,321)*.

## Quinolones and Glucose Homeostasis

Case reports have documented pharmacodynamic interactions between quinolones and oral hypoglycemics in patients with type 2 diabetes mellitus, leading to symptomatic, prolonged hypoglycemia. Implicated agents included oral ciprofloxacin with 5 and 2.5 mg glyburide daily *(322a,322b)*; oral gatifloxacin with 0.5 mg repaglinide three times daily, 5 mg glyburide daily plus 30 mg pioglitazone daily, with 3 mg glimepiride daily *(323a)*, 5 mg glyburide daily *(323b)* and insulin plus repaglinide 6 mg/day plus vogilbose 0.6 mg/day *(323c)*. In the cases involving gatifloxacin, the profound hypoglycemia occurred after the first dose of gatifloxacin and persisted until the drug was discontinued. After recovery of the blood glucose, oral hypoglycemic therapy was restarted, and blood glucose values returned to pregatifloxacin baseline levels. Case reports have also documented gatifloxacin-associated hyperglycemia, including hyperosmolar nonketotic hyperglycemia, in patients with no history of diabetes *(323c,323d)*.

During the postmarketing period, reports have been made to the US Food and Drug Administration's Medwatch® program regarding serious disturbances in glucose homeostasis in gatifloxacin recipients. Hypoglycemic episodes, some severe, have been reported in patients with diabetes mellitus treated with either sulfonylurea or nonsulfonylurea oral hypoglycemics. These events frequently occurred on day 1 of therapy and usually within 3 days of initiating gatifloxacin therapy. Hyperglycemic episodes, in some cases severe and associated with hyperosmolar nonketotic hyperglycemic coma, have also been reported in patients with diabetes mellitus, mainly between days 4 and 10 of gatifloxacin therapy. Some of these hypo- and hyperglycemic events were life threatening, and many required hospitalization. Episodes of hyperglycemia, including hyperosmolar nonketotic hyperglycemic coma, have also occurred in patients without prior documented diabetes mellitus. Elderly subjects with age-related reductions in renal function and underlying medical problems or concomitant medications associated with hyperglycemia may be at particular risk *(324a)*.

Glucose homeostasis abnormalities (GHAs) reported to the FDA in the Spontaneous Adverse Event (Medwatch) program from November 1997 to September 2003, inclusive, have been reviewed for the agents ciprofloxacin, gatifloxacin, levofloxacin, and moxifloxacin. These events were identified under 14 unique coding items. Rates were calculated using US retail pharmacy prescriptions as the denominator. These four quinolones accounted for 16,868 adverse event reports (10,025 unique US reports). Of these US reports, 568 were GHA reports and 25 fatal GHA reports. Gatifloxacin was associated with 80% of all GHA reports and 68% of fatal GHA reports. Spontaneous reporting rates were higher for gatifloxacin than the three comparators combined for total GHA reports (477/10 million prescriptions vs 8, $p < 0.0001$) and fatal GHA reports (18 vs 0.6, $p < 0.0001$). GHA reports constituted 24% of gatifloxacin and 1.4% of the combined comparator quinolone adverse event reports. For gatifloxacin, subjects involved in GHA reports were older (median 74 vs 61 years old, $p < 0.0001$) and were likely to be taking antibiotic medications (69 vs 14%, $p < 0.0001$) than subjects with other types of adverse events. Whether or not the true population rate of GHA is 56-fold higher for gatifloxacin compared to the other quinolones can be questioned, based on the multiple biases and limitations of the database. These data need to be accessed in the context of other data in order to establish causality *(324b)*.

Studies have been conducted to evaluate the mechanism of this interaction. Altered pharmacokinetics of oral hypoglycemics do not appear to be the explanation as gatifloxacin and moxifloxacin do not significantly alter glyburide pharmacokinetics *(202,325)*.

Most studies have concentrated on a pharmacodynamic etiology for this interaction. In healthy volunteers treated for 14 days with various doses of once-daily intravenous gatifloxacin (200, 400, 600, 800 mg), a transient, dose-dependent reduction in fasting serum glucose concentration at the end of the infusion without corresponding changes in serum insulin/C-peptide concentrations occurred. No drug-associated effect was noted on predose fasting serum glucose concentrations throughout therapy or on the dynamics of the oral glucose tolerance test (OGTT) at the end of therapy *(326)*.

In patients with type 2 diabetes mellitus stabilized on diet and exercise therapy, multiple oral dose gatifloxacin (400 mg once daily for 10 days) produced no significant effects on the dynamics of the OGTT, fasting serum insulin, and glucose profiles over 6 hour after dosing on study days 1 and 10 and predose fasting insulin, glucose, and C-peptide concentrations on study days 2, 4, 6, 8, and 11 compared to placebo. The only significant drug-associated effect was a significant increase in the 0- to 6-hour postdose fasting serum insulin concentrations on study day 1. In the same study, 500 mg ciprofloxacin twice daily produced virtually identical results except that the significant drug-associated increase in the 0- to 6-hour postdose fasting serum insulin concentrations occurred on study day 10 *(327)*.

In patients with type 2 diabetes mellitus stabilized on metformin or metformin-glyburide combination therapy, 400 mg oral gatifloxacin once daily for 14 days produced an initial hypoglycemia (study days 1 and 2) caused by elevations in serum insulin concentrations, followed by hyperglycemia (study day 4 onward). In some cases, the hyperglycemia was symptomatic, requiring single doses of insulin for correction. Serum glucose concentrations did not always return to baseline, even by 1 month after stopping the drug *(324)*. In a similar patient population treated with glyburide, 10 days of 400 mg gatifloxacin once daily caused serum insulin concentrations to fall by 30 to 40% during OGTT. No significant effect on serum glucose concentrations was noted *(325)*. Last, moxifloxacin has been reported not to alter serum insulin dynamics in patients with type 2 diabetes mellitus stabilized on glyburide therapy. The increases reported in serum glucose 0- to 6-hour postdose AUC (mean 7%) and $C_{max}$ (mean 6%), although statistically significant, were felt to be clinically insignificant *(202)*.

**Table 4**
**Intravenous Fluid and Admixed Drug**
**Incompatibilities With Injectable Quinolones**

| Quinolone | Incompatibilities | |
| | LVP intravenous fluid | Admixed drugs |
| --- | --- | --- |
| Ciprofloxacin | Sodium bicarbonate,[a] sodium phosphate | Amoxicillin, amphotericin B, amoxicillin/clavulanate, clindamycin, floxacillin, flucloxacillin, furosemide,[b] cefepime,[b] ceftazidime, cefuroxime, heparin,[c] metronidazole, propofol,[b] hydrocortisone,[b] potassium phosphates,[b] mezlocillin,[c] ampicillin/sulbactam,[c] piperacillin, ticarcillin, aminophylline,[c] teicoplanin, magnesium,[b] dexamethasone,[b] phenytoin,[b] warfarin,[b] methylprednisolone,[b] TPN[b] |
| Gatifloxacin | None reported | Amphotericin B,[b] cefoperazone,[b] cefoxitin,[b] diazepam,[b] furosemide,[b] heparin,[b] phenytoin,[b] piperacillin,[b] piperacillin/tazobactam,[b] potassium phosphates,[b] vancomycin[b] |
| Levofloxacin | Mannitol, sodium bicarbonate | Acyclovir,[b] alprostadil,[b] furosemide,[b] heparin,[b] indomethacin,[b] insulin,[b] nitroglycerin,[b] nitroprusside,[b] propofol[b] |
| Moxifloxacin | None reported | Not assessed |
| Ofloxacin | None reported[d] | Flucloxacillin, cefepime,[b] amphotericin B,[b] doxorubicin,[b] heparin[b] |
| Trovafloxacin (alatrofloxacin) | Lactated Ringer's, normal saline (with/without other diluents) | Aztreonam,[b] ceftazidime,[b] ceftriaxone,[b] dobutamine,[b] famotidine,[b] furosemide,[b] heparin,[b] insulin,[b] magnesium sulfate,[b] midazolam,[b] morphine,[b] piperacillin/ tazobactam,[b] ticarcillin/clavulanate[b] |

*Source*: From ref. *328*.
LVP, large volume parenteral.
[a] Incompatible on simulated Y-site administration as well as when used as an LVP intravenous fluid.
[b] Incompatible (evaluated only on simulated Y-site administration).
[c] Incompatible on simulated Y-site administration as well as when admixed into an LVP intravenous fluid.
[d] Use caution in light of the issues with mannitol and sodium bicarbonate LVP solutions and levofloxacin.

At present, gatifloxacin appears to be the quinolone most associated with perturbations in glucose homeostasis, especially in patients diagnosed with diabetes mellitus and receiving insulin or oral hypoglycemic therapy. It is probably prudent to avoid the use of gatifloxacin in such patients, considering the variety of alternative antimicrobial agents available. If use of gatifloxacin is desired, more intensive fingerstick blood glucose monitoring is warranted, with alteration of hypoglycemic dosing regimen(s) made based on results.

## PHYSICOCHEMICAL INTERACTIONS

Physicochemical interactions involve physical incompatibilities between injectable quinolones and intravenous fluids and admixed medications. Studies of these types of interactions involve combinations of visual inspection (for precipitation), assessment of pH changes, and quantitation of drug and breakdown products. Table 4 illustrates the known incompatibilities of the injectable quinolones *(328a)*. A case report of an interaction between indomethacin and ciprofloxacin, both administered as eyedrops following phototherapeutic keratectomy, has recently been published. The interaction appeared to be physicochemical in nature, as a precipitate containing both drugs was deposited in the cornea *(328b)*.

| CASE STUDY 1 | |
|---|---|
| HPI: | Mrs. Jones is a 57-year-old obese female presenting with a 1 week history of pain and burning on urination, frequency, and urgency. |
| PMH: | Hypertension |
| | Hyperlipidemia |
| | Type II diabetes |
| | Gastroesophageal reflux disease (GERD) |
| | Nephrolithiasis (struvite (infection) stones) |
| Meds: | Enalapril 10 mg qd po |
| | Simvastatin 20 mg qd po |
| | Glyburide 10 mg qd po |
| | Ranitidine 150 mg bid po |
| | Nitrofurantoin 50 mg hs po |
| Allergies: | Sulfonamides (hives), penicillins (anaphylaxis) |
| PE: | In general, an ill-appearing female in no acute distress |
| | BP (supine) 152/90 mmHg, pulse 104/min, temperature 101.4°F, respirations 18/min |
| HEENT: | PERRLA, EOM intact, fundi with KW II changes, TM clear, oropharynx clear, upper dentures |
| Neck: | No JVD; carotids no bruits |
| Lungs: | Clear to A + P |
| CV: | RRR, S1 + S2 with 1/6 SEM at left upper sternal border, no gallops |
| Abdomen: | Soft, normal BS, no bruits, slight abdominal tenderness in suprapubic area, no masses or hepatosplenomegaly |
| GU and rectal: | Deferred |
| Back: | CVA tenderness bilaterally |
| Extremities: | Good pulses bilaterally |
| Neuro: | Gross motor, sensory, reflex function intact, cranial nerves normal |
| Labs: | GlyHgb 6.8% (WNL) |
| | $K^+$ 4.2 mmol/L (WNL) |
| | BUN/Cr 18/1.4 mg/dL (BUN WNL, Cr slightly ↑) |
| | CBC WBC = 16,400 (slightly ↑) with 4% bands (slightly ↑) |
| | UA: packed WBCs, large LE, nitrite positive, pH 8.0 |
| Assessment: | Recurrent UTI in patient with a history of struvite stones; presumed urease-splitting organism based on urine pH |
| Plan: | Begin empiric therapy after obtaining urine for C + S; plan to begin ofloxacin 200 mg bid po pending C + S results |
| Follow-up: | Culture came back positive for >10$^5$ CFU/mL$^3$ *P. rettgeri*, which was resistant to all tested agents except gentamicin, tobramycin, norfloxacin, and ciprofloxacin. Ofloxacin was to be continued for |

a total 14-day course. Patient's condition did not improve after several days despite presumed adequate dosage regimen and sensitivity of pathogen in vitro. On further questioning, it was determined that Mrs. Jones had been ingesting Maalox TC® (magnesium/aluminum hydroxide) several times per day for a GERD flare. After adjusting her GERD regimen and counseling the patient to avoid all antacids for the duration of quinolone use, her symptoms quickly responded, and a follow-up UC was negative.

### Discussion

Absorption drug–drug interactions may contribute to clinical failure of quinolone therapy. This case illustrates the potential for concurrent cation administration to reduce quinolone bioavailability sufficiently to cause clinical failure, even when the microorganism is sensitive to the agent and the agent concentrates in the infection compartment (i.e., the urinary tract). This list of potential interacting agents is long, and even with spacing of administration of the quinolone with the interacting agent, interactions may not be eliminated. It is best to *avoid* potentially interacting agents during the course of quinolone therapy, if at all possible. It is also important to note that absorption drug–drug interactions appear to be a *class effect*, that is, they occur to a reasonably similar extent with all quinolones.

---

### Case Study 2

| | |
|---|---|
| HPI: | Mr. Doe is a 77-year-old male presenting with a 5-day history of nausea, vomiting, and coarse tremors of the upper extremities. Patient has a recent history of an acute exacerbation of chronic bronchitis. |
| PMH: | Chronic obstruction pulmonary disease (COPD) |
| | Hypertension |
| | Benign prostatic hypertrophy |
| | Type II diabetes |
| | Varicose veins |
| | Kyphoscoliosis |
| | Chronic renal insufficiency |
| | Degenerative joint disease |
| Meds: | Ipratropium MDI 2 puffs qid |
| | Albuterol MDI 2 puffs qid |
| | Theophylline SR 300 mg bid po |
| | Prednisone 10 mg q AM po |
| | Terazosin 10 mg qd po |
| | Acetaminophen 1 g qid po |
| | Ciprofloxacin 750 mg bid po |
| Allergies: | Penicillin (rash), sulfonamides (rash) |
| PE: | BP (supine) 160/95 mmHg, pulse 120/min, temperature 98.2°F, respirations 30/min (labored) |
| HEENT: | PERRLA, horizontal nystagmus, EOM intact, fundi clear, TM clear, oropharynx clear, edentulous |

| Neck: | No JVD, right carotid bruit (left clear) |
| Lungs: | Diffuse bilateral rhonchi and decreased breath sounds, egophony |
| CV: | Irregular rate and rhythm, S1 + S2 with 3/6 SEM left lower sternal border, S3 gallop |
| Abdomen: | Normal BS, generalized guarding, no bruists, no masses or hepatosplenomegaly |
| GU and rectal: | Deferred |
| Back: | Kyphoscoliosis, otherwise WNL |
| Extremities: | Decreased dorsalis pedis and posterior tibial pulses, crepitus and pain on knee flexion bilaterally |
| Neuro: | Coarse tremor bilaterally in upper extremities, gross motor and sensory function intact, cranial nerves normal, generalized hyperreflexia |
| Labs: | Gly Hgb 7.2% (WNL)<br>K$^+$ 5.0 mmol/L (WNL)<br>BUN/Cr 28/1.9 mg/dL (both slightly ↑)<br>CBC WNL<br>Theophylline 38 mg/L (therapeutic range 10–20 mg/L) |
| Assessment: | Theophylline intoxication secondary to a drug–drug interaction. |
| Plan: | Hold theophylline. Follow serial theophylline concentrations. Stop ciprofloxacin. Substitute cefuroxime axetil 500 mg bid po. |
| Follow-up: | Over the next 72 hours, Mr. Doe's nausea/vomiting/course tremor resolved, his serum theophylline concentration fell into the therapeutic range, and his AECB symptoms improved substantially. |

### DISCUSSION

Metabolic drug–drug interactions may contribute to patient morbidity because of potentiation of pharmacological effects of the interacting drug through inhibition of hepatic drug metabolism by quinolone antimicrobials. In contrast to absorption drug–drug interactions, quinolones exhibit drug-specific degrees of inhibition of hepatic drug metabolism. For example, enoxacin, grepafloxacin, ciprofloxacin, and norfloxacin (in descending order of potency) are clinically significant inhibitors of xanthine metabolism; ofloxacin, lomefloxacin, levofloxacin, temafloxacin, trovafloxacin, sparfloxacin, gatifloxacin, moxifloxacin, and rufloxacin are clinically insignificant inhibitors. The choice of quinolone may be predicated on other drugs that the patient is taking. All other things being equal, the clinician should choose a clinically insignificant inhibitor of hepatic drug metabolism when the patient is receiving hepatically metabolized drugs, especially those with a narrow therapeutic margin. Although this is no guarantee of an absence of drug–drug interaction potential, this should still substantially reduce such risk.

## SUMMARY

The quinolone antimicrobials have proven to be important additions to our therapeutic armamentarium based on their broad spectra of activity, favorable pharmacological properties, and ease and cost-efficiency of administration. However, with their widespread use comes the realization that drug–drug interactions will occur with these

**Table 5**
**Clinically Significant Pharmacokinetic Quinolone–Drug Interactions**

| Interacting drug | Results | Comments |
|---|---|---|
| Ca-, Mg-, Al-containing antacids; Ca supplements; iron or mineral preparations; sucralfate; didanosine | Reduced quinolone absorption | Avoid quinolone therapy if possible; otherwise space administrations as far apart as possible |
| Theophylline | Reduced theophylline metabolism | Follow levels if on enoxacin, grepafloxacin, ciprofloxacin, or norfloxacin; watch clinical status if on other quinolones |
| Caffeine | Reduced caffeine metabolism | Reduce consumption of caffeinated foods/beverages, follow clinical status |
| Warfarin | (?) Reduced warfarin metabolism | Follow INR intra- and post-quinolone therapy and adjust warfarin dose accordingly |

agents. It is important that the clinician be aware of clinically significant interactions with these agents and pay attention to other potential interactions with drugs exhibiting narrow therapeutic/toxic dose ratios (Table 5).

## ACKNOWLEDGMENT

I gratefully acknowledge the secretarial assistance of Kari Bunjer.

## REFERENCES

1. Yuk JH, Williams TW Jr. Drug interaction with quinolone antibiotics in intensive care unit patients [letter]. Arch Intern Med 1991;151:619.
2. Lomaestro BM, Lesar TS. Concurrent administration of ciprofloxacin and potentially interacting drugs [letter]. Am J Hosp Pharm 1989;46:1770.
3. Bowes J, Graffunder EM, Lomaestro B, Venezia RA. Concomitant administration of drugs known to decrease the systemic availability of gatifloxacin. Pharmacotherapy 2002; 22:800–801.
4. Hoffken G, Borner K, Glatzel PD, et al. Reduced enteral absorption of ciprofloxacin in the presence of antacids [letter]. Eur J Clin Microbiol 1985;4:345.
5. Shiba K, Saito A, Shimada J, et al. Interactions of fleroxacin with dried aluminum hydroxide gel and probenecid. Rev Infect Dis 1989;11 (suppl 5):S1097–S1098.
6. Shiba K, Sakai O, Shimada J, Okazaki O, Aoki H, Hakusui H. Effects of antacids, ferrous sulfate, and ranitidine on absorption of DR-3355 in humans. Antimicrob Agents Chemother 1992;36:2270–2274.
7. Campbell NRC, Kara M, Hasinoff B, Haddara WM, McKay DW. Norfloxacin interaction with antacids and minerals. Br J Clin Pharmacol 1992;33:115–116.
8. Okhamafe AO, Akerele JO, Chukuka CS. Pharmacokinetic interactions of norfloxacin with some metallic medicinal agents. Int J Pharm 1991;68:11–18.
9. Akerele JO, Akhamafe AO. Influence of co-administered metallic drugs on ofloxacin pharmacokinetics. J Antimicrob Chemother 1991;28:87–94.
10. Sanchez Navarro A, Martinez Cabarga M, Dominguez-Gil Hurle A. Oral absorption of ofloxacin administered together with aluminum. Antimicrob Agents Chemother 1994;38: 2510–2512.

11. Martinez Cabarga M, Sanchez Navarro A, Colino Gandarillas CI, Dominguez-Gil A. Effects of two cations on gastrointestinal absorption of ofloxacin. Antimicrob Agents Chemother 1991;35:2102–2105.
12. Rambout L, Sahai J, Gallicano K, Oliveras L, Garber G. Effect of bismuth subsalicylate on ciprofloxacin bioavailability. Antimicrob Agents Chemother 1994;38:2187–2190.
13. Sahai J, Healy D, Stotka J, Polk R. The influence of chronic administration of calcium carbonate on the bioavailability of oral ciprofloxacin. Br J Clin Pharmacol 1993;35:302–304.
14. Frost DW, Lasseter KC, Noe AJ, Shamblen EC, Lettieri J. Effect of aluminum hydroxide and calcium carbonate antacids on the bioavailability of ciprofloxacin. Antimicrob Agents Chemother 1992;36:830–832.
15. Fleming LW, Moreland TA, Stewart WK, Scott AC. Ciprofloxacin and antacids [letter]. Lancet 1986;2:294.
16. Lomaestro BM, Baillie GR. Effect of staggered dose of calcium on the bioavailability of ciprofloxacin. Antimicrob Agents Chemother 1991;35:1004–1007.
17. Sanchez Navarro A, Martinez Cabarga M, Dominguez-Gil Hurle A. Comparative study of the influence of $Ca^{2+}$ on absorption parameters of ciprofloxacin and ofloxacin. J Antimicrob Chemother 1994;34:119–125.
18. Lomaestro BM, Baillie GR. Effect of multiple staggered doses of calcium on the bioavailability of ciprofloxacin. Ann Pharmacother 1993;27:1325–1328.
19. Lacreta FP, Kaul S, Kollia GD, Duncan G, Randall DM, Grasela DM. Pharmacokinetics (PK) and safety of gatifloxacin in combination with ferrous sulfate or calcium carbonate in healthy volunteers. Proceedings of the 39th Interscience Conference on Antimicrobial Agents and Chemotherapy, San Francisco, CA, September, 1999. Abstract 198.
20. Lehto P, Kivisto KT. Different effects of products containing metal ions on the absorption of lomefloxacin. Clin Pharmacol Ther 1994;56:477–482.
21. Stass H, Wandel C, Delesen H, Moller JG. Effect of calcium supplements on the oral bioavailability of moxifloxacin in healthy male volunteers. Clin Pharmacokinet 2001;40(suppl 1):27–32.
22. Pletz MW, Petzold P, Allen A, Burkhardt O, Lode H. Effect of calcium carbonate on bioavailability of orally administered gemifloxacin. Antimicrob Agents Chemother 2003; 47:2158–2160.
23. Nix DE, Wilton JH, Ronald B, et al. Inhibition of norfloxacin absorption by antacids. Antimicrob Agents Chemother 1990;34:432–435.
24. Flor S, Guay DRP, Opsahl JA, et al. Effects of magnesium-aluminum hydroxide and calcium carbonate antacids on bioavailability of ofloxacin. Antimicrob Agents Chemother 1990;34:2436–2438.
25. Kays MB, Overholser BR, Mueller BA, Moe SM, Sowinski KM. Effects of sevelamer hydrochloride and calcium acetate on the oral bioavailability of ciprofloxacin. Am J Kid Dis 2003;42:1253–1259.
26. Kato R, Ueno K, Imano H, et al. Impairment of ciprofloxacin absorption by calcium polycarbophil. J Clin Pharmacol 2002;42:806–811.
27. Neuhofel AL, Wilton JH, Victory JM, Hejmanowsky LG, Amsden GW. Lack of bioequivalence of ciprofloxacin when administered with calcium-fortified orange juice: a new twist on an old interaction. J Clin Pharmacol 2002;42:461–466.
28. Wallace AW, Victory JM, Amsden GW. Lack of bioequivalence of gatifloxacin when coadministered with calcium-fortified orange juice in healthy volunteers. J Clin Pharmacol 2003;43:92–96.
29. Amsden GW, Whitaker A-M, Johnson PW. Lack of bioequivalence of levofloxacin when coadministered with a mineral-fortified breakfast of juice and cereal. J Clin Pharmacol 2003;43:990–995.
30. Sahai J, Gallicano K, Oliveros L, Khaliq S, Hawley-Foss N, Garber G. Cations in the didanosine tablet reduce ciprofloxacin bioavailability. Clin Pharmacol Ther 1993;53: 292–297.

31. Knupp CA, Barbhaiya RH. A multiple-dose pharmacokinetic interaction study between didanosine (Videx®) and ciprofloxacin (Cipro®) in male subjects seropositive for HIV but asymptomatic. Biopharm Drug Dispos 1997;18:65–77.
32. Damle BD, Mummaneni V, Kaul S, Knupp C. Lack of effect of simultaneously administered didanosine encapsulated enteric bead formulation (Videx EC) on oral absorption of indinavir, ketoconazole, or ciprofloxacin. Antimicrob Agents Chemother 2002;46: 385–391.
33. Kara M, Hasinoff BB, McKay D, Campbell NRC. Clinical and chemical interactions between iron preparations and ciprofloxacin. Br J Clin Pharmacol 1991;31:257–261.
34. Polk RE, Healy DP, Sahai J, et al. Effect of ferrous sulfate and multivitamins with zinc on absorption of ciprofloxacin in normal volunteers. Antimicrob Agents Chemother 1989;33:1841–1844.
35. Lehto P, Kivisto KT, Neuvonen PJ. The effect of ferrous sulphate on the absorption of norfloxacin, ciprofloxacin and ofloxacin. Br J Clin Pharmacol 1994;37:82–85.
36. Shiba K, Sakamoto M, Saito A, et al. Effect of ferrous sulfate, tea, and milk on absorption of AM-1155, a 6-fluoro-8-methyoxy quinolone, in humans. Proceedings of the 35th Interscience Conference on Antimicrobial Agents and Chemotherapy, San Francisco, CA, September, 1995. Abstract A43.
37. Stass H, Kubitza D. Effect of iron supplements on the oral bioavailability of moxifloxacin, a novel 8-methoxyfluoroquinolone, in humans. Clin Pharmacokinet 2001;40(suppl 1):57–62.
38. Allen A, Bygate E, Faessel H, Isaac L, Lewis A. The effect of ferrous sulphate and sucralfate on the bioavailability of oral gemifloxacin in healthy volunteers. Int J Antimicrob Agents 2000;15:283–289.
39. Nix DE, Watson WA, Lener ME, et al. Effects of aluminum and magnesium antacids and ranitidine on the absorption of ciprofloxacin. Clin Pharmacol Ther 1989;46:700–705.
40. Hoffken G, Lode H, Wiley R, et al. Pharmacokinetics and bioavailability of ciprofloxacin and ofloxacin: effect of food and antacid intake. Rev Infect Dis 1988;10(suppl 1):S138–S139.
41. Grasela TH Jr, Schentag JJ, Sedman AT, et al. Inhibition of enoxacin absorption by antacids or ranitidine. Antimicrob Agents Chemother 1989;33:615–617.
42. Lober S, Ziege S, Rau M, et al. Pharmacokinetics of gatifloxacin and interaction with an antacid containing aluminum and magnesium. Antimicrob Agents Chemother 1999;43: 1067–1071.
43. Shimada J, Shiba K, Oguma T, et al. Effect of antacid on absorption of the quinolone lomefloxacin. Antimicrob Agents Chemother 1992;36:1219–1224.
44. Stass H, Bottcher MF, Ochmann K. Evaluation of the influence of antacids and $H_2$ antagonists on the absorption of moxifloxacin after oral administration of a 400 mg dose to healthy volunteers. Clin Pharmacokinet 2001;40(suppl 1):39–48.
45. Nix DE, Wilton JH, Ronald B, et al. Inhibition of norfloxacin absorption by antacids and sucralfate. Rev Infect Dis 1989;11(supp 5):S1096.
46. Maesen FPV, Davies BI, Geraedts WH, Sumajow CA. Ofloxacin and antacids [letter]. J Antimicrob Chemother 1987;19:848–849.
47. Jaehde U, Sorgel F, Stephan U, Schunack W. Effect of an antacid containing magnesium and aluminum on absorption, metabolism, and mechanism of renal elimination of pefloxacin in humans. Antimicrob Agents Chemother 1994;38:1129–1133.
48. Lazzaroni M, Imbimbo BP, Bargiggia S, et al. Effects of magnesium-aluminum hydroxide antacid on absorption of rufloxacin. Antimicrob Agents Chemother 1993;37:2212–2216.
49. Granneman GR, Stephan U, Birner B, et al. Effect of antacid medication on the pharmacokinetics of temafloxacin. Clin Pharmacokinet 1992;22(suppl 1):83–89.
50. Teng R, Dogolo LC, Willavize SA, Friedman HL, Vincent J. Effect of Maalox and omeprazole on the bioavailability of trovafloxacin. J Antimicrob Chemother 1997; 39(suppl B):93–97.

51. Allen A, Vousden M, Porter A, Lewis A. Effect of Maalox® on the bioavailability of oral gemifloxacin in healthy volunteers. Chemotherapy 1999;45:504–511.
52. Nix DE, Watson WA, Handy L, et al. The effect of sucralfate pretreatment on the pharmacokinetics of ciprofloxacin. Pharmacotherapy 1989;9:377–380.
53. Garrelts JC, Godley PJ, Peterie JD, et al. Sucralfate significantly reduces ciprofloxacin concentrations in serum. Antimicrob Agents Chemother 1990;34:931–933.
54. Van Slooten AD, Nix DE, Wilton JH, Love JH, Spivey JM, Goldstein HR. Combined use of ciprofloxacin and sucralfate. DICP Ann Pharmacother 1991;25:578–582.
55. Ryerson B, Toothaker R, Schleyer I, Sedman A, Colburn W. Effect of sucralfate on enoxacin pharmacokinetics. Proceedings of the 29th Interscience Conference on Antimicrobial Agents and Chemotherapy, Houston, TX, September, 1989. Abstract 214.
56. Lubowski TJ, Nightingale CH, Sweeney K, Quintiliani R. Effect of sucralfate on pharmacokinetics of fleroxacin in healthy volunteers. Antimicrob Agents Chemother 1992;36:2758–2760.
57. Lee L-J, Hafkin B, Lee I-D, Hoh J, Dix R. Effects of food and sucralfate on a single oral dose of 500 mg of levofloxacin in healthy subjects. Antimicrob Agents Chemother 1997;41:2196–2200.
58. Nix D, Schentag J. Lomefloxacin (L) absorption kinetics when administered with ranitidine (R) and sucralfate (S). Proceedings of the 29th Interscience Conference on Antimicrobial Agents and Chemotherapy, Houston, TX, September, 1989. Abstract 1276.
59. Stass H, Schuhly U, Moller JG, Delesen H. Effects of sucralfate on the oral bioavailability of moxifloxacin, a novel 8-methoxyfluoroquinolone. Clin Pharmacokinet 2001;40(suppl 1):49–55.
60. Lehto P, Kivisto KT. Effect of sucralfate on absorption of norfloxacin and ofloxacin. Antimicrob Agents Chemother 1994;38:248–251.
61. Parpia SH, Nix DE, Hejmanowski LG, et al. Sucralfate reduces the gastrointestinal absorption of norfloxacin. Antimicrob Agents Chemother 1989;33:99–102.
62. Kawakami J, Matsuse T, Kotaki H, et al. The effect of food on the interaction of ofloxacin with sucralfate in healthy volunteers. Eur J Clin Pharmacol 1994;47:67–69.
63. Zix JA, Geerdes-Fenge HF, Rau M, et al. Pharmacokinetics of sparfloxacin and interaction with cisapride and sucralfate. Antimicrob Agents Chemother 1997;41:1668–1672.
64. Kamberi M, Nakashima H, Ogawa K, Oda N, Nakano S. The effect of staggered dosing of sucralfate on oral bioavailability of sparfloxacin. Br J Clin Pharmacol 2000;49:98–103.
65. Golper T, Hartstein AI, Morthland VH, Christensen JM. Effects of antacids and dialysate dwell times on multiple dose pharmacokinetics of oral ciprofloxacin in patients on continuous ambulatory peritoneal dialysis. Antimicrob Agents Chemother 1987;31:1787–1790.
66. Preheim LC, Cuevas TA, Roccaforte JS, Mellencamp MA, Bittner MJ. Ciprofloxacin and antacids [letter]. Lancet 1986;2:48.
67. Tuncel T, Bergisadi N. In vitro adsorption of ciprofloxacin hydrochloride on various antacids. Pharmazie 1992;47:304–305.
68. Wallis SC, Charles BG, Gahan LR, Filippich LJ, Bredhauer MG, Duckworth PA. Interaction of norfloxacin with divalent and trivalent pharmaceutical cations. In vitro complexation and in vivo pharmacokinetic studies in the dog. J Pharm Sci 1996;85:803–809.
69. Ross DL, Elkington SK, Knaub SR, Riley CM. Physicochemical properties of the fluoroquinolone antimicrobials VI. Effect of metal-ion complexation on octan-1-ol-water partitioning. Int J Pharmaceutics 1993;93:131–138.
70. Ross DL, Riley CM. Physicochemical properties of the fluoroquinolone antimicrobials V. Effect of fluoroquinolone structure and pH on the complexation of various fluoroquinolones with magnesium and calcium. Int J Pharmaceutics 1993;93:121–129.

71. Ross DL, Riley CM. Physicochemical properties of the fluoroquinolone antimicrobials III. complexation of lomefloxacin with various metal ions and the effect of metal ion complexation on aqueous solubility. Int J Pharmaceutics 1992;87:203–213.

72. Helena M, Teixeira SF, Vilas-Boas LS, Gil VMS, Teixeira F. Complexes of ciprofloxacin with metal ions contained in antacid drugs. J Chemother 1995;7:126–132.

73. Sonia Rodriguez Cruz M, Gonzalez Alonso I, Sanchez-Navarro A, Luisa Sayalero Marinero M. In vitro study of the interaction between quinolones and polyvalent cations. Pharm Acta Helv 1999;73:237–245.

74. Hoffken G, Lode H, Wiley P D, et al. Pharmacokinetics and interaction in the bioavailability of new quinolones. Proceedings of the International Symposium of the New Quinolones, Geneva, Switzerland, July, 1986. Abstract 141.

75. Sorgel F, Seelmann R, Granneman G R, Locke C. Effect of cimetidine on the pharmacokinetics of temafloxacin. Clin Pharmacokinet 1992;22(suppl 1):75–82.

76. Wingender W, Foerster D, Beermann D, et al. Effect of gastric emptying time on rate and extent of the systemic availability of ciprofloxacin. Proceedings of the 14th International Congress of Chemotherapy, Kyoto, Japan, June, 1985. Abstract P-37-91.

77. Sorgel F, Mahr G, Uwe Koch H, Stephan U, Wiesemann HG, Malter U. Effects of cimetidine on the pharmacokinetics of pefloxacin in healthy volunteers. Rev Infect Dis 1988;10 (suppl 1):S137.

78. Misiak PM, Eldon MA, Toothaker RD, Sedman AJ. Effects of oral cimetidine or ranitidine on the pharmacokinetics of intravenous enoxacin. J Clin Pharmacol 1993; 33:53–56.

79. Levofloxacin. Data on file (protocol HR 355/1/GB/101). Raritan, NJ: RW Johnson Pharmaceutical Research Institute.

80. Ludwig E, Graber H, Szekely E, Csiba A. Metabolic interactions of ciprofloxacin. Diagn Microbiol Infect Dis 1990;13:135–141.

81. Lebsack ME, Nix D, Ryerson B, et al. Effect of gastric acidity on enoxacin absorption. Clin Pharmacol Ther 1992;52:252–256.

82. Efthymiopoulos C, Bramer SL, Maroli A. Effect of food and gastric pH on the bioavailability of grepafloxacin. Clin Pharmcokinet 1997;33(suppl 1):18–24.

83. Gries JM, Honorato J, Taburet AM, et al. Cimetidine does not alter sparfloxacin pharmacokinetics. Int J Clin Pharmacol Ther Toxicol 1995;33:585–587.

84. Perry CM, Barman Balfour JA, Lamb HM. Gatifloxacin. Drugs 1999;58:683–696.

85. Stass HH, Ochmann K. Study to evaluate the interaction between BAY 12-8039 and ranitidine. Proceedings of the 20th International Congress of Chemotherapy, Sydney, Australia, June–July, 1997. Abstract 3357.

86. Stuht H, Lode H, Koeppe P, Rost KL, Schaberg T. Interaction study of lomefloxacin and ciprofloxacin with omeprazole and comparative pharmacokinetics. Antimicrob Agents Chemother 1995;39:1045–1049.

87. Allen A, Vousden M, Lewis A. Effect of omeprazole on the pharmacokinetics of oral gemifloxacin in healthy volunteers. Chemotherapy 1999;45:496–503.

88. Nix DE, Lebsack ME, Chapelsky M, Sedman AJ, Busch J, Norman A. Effect of oral antacids on disposition of intravenous enoxacin. Antimicrob Agents Chemother 1993;37:775–777.

89. Yuk JH, Nightingale CH, Sweeney KR, et al. Relative bioavailability in healthy volunteers of ciprofloxacin administered through a nasogastric tube with and without enteral feeding. Antimicrob Agents Chemother 1989;33:1118–1120.

90. Lubowski TJ, Nightingale CH, Sweeney K, Quintiliani R. The relative bioavailability of temafloxacin administered through a nasogastric tube with and without enteral feeding. Clin Pharmacokinet 1992;22(suppl 1):43–47.

91. Noer BL, Angaran DM. The effect of enteral feedings on ciprofloxacin pharmacokinetics. Pharmacotherapy 1990;10:254. Abstract 154.

92. Healy DP, Brodbeck MC, Clendenning CE. Ciprofloxacin absorption is impaired in patients given enteral feedings orally and via gastrostomy and jejunostomy tubes. Antimicrob Agents Chemother 1996;40:6–10.

93. Mueller BA, Brierton DG, Abel SR, Bowman L. Effect of enteral feeding with Ensure on oral bioavailabilities of ofloxacin and ciprofloxacin. Antimicrob Agents Chemother 1994;38:2101–2105.

94. Dudley MN, Marchbanks CR, Flor SC, Beals S. The effect of food or milk on the absorption kinetics of ofloxacin. Eur J Clin Pharmacol 1991;41:569–571.

95. Neuvonen PJ, Kivisto KT. Milk and yoghurt do not impair the absorption of ofloxacin. Br J Clin Pharmacol 1992;33:346–348.

96. Hoogkamer JFW, Kleinbloesem CH. The effect of milk consumption on the pharmacokinetics of fleroxacin and ciprofloxacin in healthy volunteers. Drugs 1995;49(suppl 2): 346–348.

97. Lehto P, Kivisto KT. Effects of milk and food on the absorption of enoxacin. Br J Clin Pharmacol 1995;39:194–196.

98. Stass H, Kubitza D. Effects of dairy products on the oral bioavailability of moxifloxacin, a novel 8-methoxyfluoroquinolone, in healthy volunteers. Clin Pharmacokinet 2001;40(suppl 1):33–38.

99. Neuvonen PJ, Kivisto KT, Lehto P. Interference of dairy products with the absorption of ciprofloxacin. Clin Pharmacol Ther 1991;50:498–502.

100. Kivisto KT, Ojala-Karlsson P, Neuvonen PJ. Inhibition of norfloxacin absorption by dairy products. Antimicrob Agents Chemother 1992;36:489–491.

101. Stutman HR, Parker KM, Marks MI. Potential of moxalactam and other new antimicrobial agents of bilirubin-albumin displacement in neonates. Pediatrics 1985;75:294–298.

102. Graber H, Ludwig E, Magyar T, Csiba A, Szekely E. Ofloxacin does not influence antipyrine metabolism. Rev Infect Dis 1989;11(suppl 5):S1093–S1094.

103. Ludwig E, Graber H, Szekely E, Csiba A. Effect of ciprofloxacin on antipyrine metabolism. Rev Infect Dis 1989;11(suppl 5):S1100–S1101.

104. Ludwig E, Szekely E, Csiba A, Graber H. The effect of ciprofloxacin on antipyrine metabolism. J Antimicrob Chemother 1988;22:61–67.

105. Rybak MJ, Bowles SK, Chandrasekar PH, Edwards DJ. Increased theophylline concentrations secondary to ciprofloxacin. Drug Intell Clin Pharm 1987;21:879–881.

106. Duraski RM. Ciprofloxacin-induced theophylline toxicity [letter]. South Med J 1988;81: 1206.

107. Paidipaty B, Erickson S. Ciprofloxacin-theophylline drug interaction [letter]. Crit Care Med 1990;18:685–686.

108. Holden R. Probable fatal interaction between ciprofloxacin and theophylline [letter]. Br Med J 1988;297:1339.

109. Bem JL, Mann RD. Danger of interaction between ciprofloxacin and theophylline [letter]. Br Med J 1988;296:1131.

110. Spivey JM, Laughlin PH, Goss TF, Nix DE. Theophylline toxicity secondary to ciprofloxacin administration. Ann Emerg Med 1991;20:1131–1134.

111. Thomson AH, Thomson GD, Hepburn M, Whiting B. A clinically significant interaction between ciprofloxacin and theophylline. Eur J Clin Pharmacol 1987;33:435–436.

112. Rogge MC, Solomon WR, Sedman AJ, et al. The theophylline-enoxacin interaction: II. changes in disposition of theophylline and its metabolites during intermittent administration of enoxacin. Clin Pharmacol Ther 1989;46:420–428.

113. Davis RL, Kelly HW, Quenzer RW, et al. Effect of norfloxacin on theophylline metabolism. Antimicrob Agents Chemother 1989;33:212–214.

114. Bowles SK, Popovski Z, Rybak MJ, et al. Effect of norfloxacin on theophylline pharmacokinetics at steady state. Antimicrob Agents Chemother 1988;32:510–512.

115. Schwartz J, Jauregui L, Lettieri J, Bachmann K. Impact of ciprofloxacin on theophylline

clearance and steady-state concentrations in serum. Antimicrob Agents Chemother 1988;32:75–77.

116. Gregoire SL, Grasela TH Jr, Freer JP, et al. Inhibition of theophylline clearance by co-administered ofloxacin without alteration of theophylline effects. Antimicrob Agents Chemother 1987;31:375–378.

117. Ho G, Tierney MG, Dales RE. Evaluation of the effect of norfloxacin on the pharmacokinetics of theophylline. Clin Pharmacol Ther 1988;44:35–38.

118. Nix DE, Norman A, Schentag JJ. Effect of lomefloxacin on theophylline pharmacokinetics. Antimicrob Agents Chemother 1989;33:1006–1008.

119. Rogge MC, Solomon WR, Sedman AJ, et al. The theophylline–enoxacin interaction: I. effect of enoxacin dose size on theophylline disposition. Clin Pharmacol Ther 1988;44:579–587.

120. Sorgel F, Mahr G, Granneman R, Stephan U. Effects of two quinolone antibacterials, temafloxacin and enoxacin, on theophylline pharmacokinetics. Clin Pharmacokinet 1992;22(suppl 1):65–74.

121. Wijnands WJA, Vree TB, van Herwaarden CLA. Enoxacin decreases the clearance of theophylline in man. Br J Clin Pharmacol 1985;20:583–588.

122. Takagi K, Hasegawa T, Ogura Y, et al. Comparative studies on interaction between theophylline and quinolones. J Asthma 1988;25:63–71.

123. Wijnands WJA, Vree TB, van Herwaarden CLA. The influence of quinolone derivatives on theophylline clearance. Br J Clin Pharmacol 1986;22:677–683.

124. Sano M, Yamamoto I, Ueda J, et al. Comparative pharmacokinetics of theophylline following two fluoroquinolones co-administration. Eur J Clin Pharmacol 1987;32:431–432.

125. Kinzig-Schippers M, Fuhr U, Cesana M, et al. Absence of effect of rufloxacin on theophylline pharmacokinetics in steady-state. Antimicrob Agents Chemother 1998;42:2359–2364.

126. Takagi K, Yamaki K, Nadai M, Kuzuya T, Hasegawa T. Effect of a new quinolone, sparfloxacin, on the pharmacokinetics of theophylline in asthmatic patients. Antimicrob Agents Chemother 1991;35:1137–1141.

127. Sano M, Kawakatsu K, Ohkita C, et al. Effects of enoxacin, ofloxacin and norfloxacin on theophylline disposition in humans. Eur J Clin Pharmacol 1988;35:161–165.

128. Robson RA, Begg EJ, Atkinson HC, Saunders CA, Frampton CM. Comparative effects of ciprofloxacin and lomefloxacin on the oxidative metabolism of theophylline. Br J Clin Pharmacol 1990;29:491–493.

129. LeBel M, Vallee F, St. Laurent M. Influence of lomefloxacin on the pharmcokinetics of theophylline. Antimicrob Agents Chemother 1990;34:1254–1256.

130. Seelmann R, Mahr G, Gottschalk B, Stephan U, Sorgel F. Influence of fleroxacin on the pharmacokinetics of theophylline. Rev Infect Dis 1989;11 (suppl 5):S1100.

131. Soejima R, Niki Y, Sumi M. Effect of fleroxacin on serum concentrations of theophylline. Rev Infect Dis 1989;11 (suppl 5):S1099.

132. Beckman J, Elsasser W, Gundert-Remy U, Hertrampf R. Enoxacin—a potent inhibitor of theophylline metabolism. Eur J Clin Pharmacol 1987;33:227–230.

133. Wijnands WJA, Cornel JH, Martea M, Vree TB. The effect of multiple dose oral lomefloxacin on theophylline metabolism in man. Chest 1990;98:1440–1444.

134. Niki Y, Soejima R, Kawane H, et al. New synthetic quinolone antibacterial agents and serum concentration of theophylline. Chest 1987;92:663–669.

135. Wijnands WJA, van Herwaarden CLA, Vree TB. Enoxacin raises plasma theophylline concentrations [letter]. Lancet 1984;2:108–109.

136. Raoof S, Wollschlager C, Khan FA. Ciprofloxacin increases serum levels of theophylline. Am J Med 1987;82(suppl 4A):115–118.

137. Gisclon LG, Curtin CR, Fowler CL, Nayak RK. Absence of pharmacokinetic interaction between intravenous theophylline and orally administered levofloxacin. Proceedings of

the 35th Interscience Conference on Antimicrobial Agents and Chemotherapy, San Francisco, CA, September, 1995. Abstract A39.

138. Dickens GR, Wermeling D, Vincent J. Phase I pilot study of the effects of trovafloxacin (CP-99,219) on the pharmacokinetics of theophylline in healthy men. J Clin Pharmacol 1997;37:248–252.

139. Vincent J, Teng R, Dogolo L C, Willavize S A, Friedman H L. Effect of trovafloxacin, a new fluoroquinolone antibiotic, on the steady-state pharmacokinetics of theophylline in healthy volunteers. J Antimicrob Chemother 1997;39(suppl B):81–86.

140. Fourtillan J B, Granier J, Saint-Salvi B, et al. Pharmacokinetics of ofloxacin and theophylline alone and in combination. Infection 1986;14(suppl 1):S67–S69.

141. Batty KT, Davis TME, Ilett KF, Dusci LJ, Langton SR. The effect of ciprofloxacin on theophylline pharmacokinetics in healthy subjects. Br J Clin Pharmacol 1995;39:305–311.

142. Efthymiopoulos C, Bramer SL, Maroli A, Blum B. Theophylline and warfarin interaction studies with grapafloxacin. Clin Pharmacokinet 1997;33(suppl 1):39–46.

143. Niki Y, Hashiguchi K, Miyashita N, Nakajima M, Matsushima T, Soejima R. Effects of AM-1155 on serum concentration of theophylline. Proceedings of the 36th Interscience Conference on Antimicrobial Agents and Chemotherapy, New Orleans, LA, September, 1996. Abstract F73.

144. Stass HH, Kubitza D, Schweitert H, Wemer R. BAY 12-8039 does not interact with theophylline. Proceedings of the 20th International Congress of Chemotherapy, Sydney, Australia, June–July, 1997. Abstract 3356.

145. Stass H, Kubitza D. Lack of pharmacokinetic interaction between moxifloxacin, a novel 8-methoxyfluoroquinolone, and theophylline. Clin Pharmacokinet 2001;40(suppl 1):63–70.

146. Davy M, Allen A, Bird N, Rost KL, Fuder H. Lack of effect of gemifloxacin on the steady-state pharmacokinetics of theophylline in healthy volunteers. Chemotherapy 1999;45:478–484.

147. Kinzig-Schippers M, Fuhr U, Zaigler M, et al. Interaction of pefloxacin and enoxacin with the human cytochrome P450 enzyme CYP 1A2. Clin Pharmacol Ther 1999;65:262–274.

148. Carbo M, Segura J, de la Torre R, et al. Effect of quinolones on caffeine disposition. Clin Pharmacol Ther 1989;45:234–240.

149. Healy DP, Polk RE, Kanawati L, et al. Interaction between oral ciprofloxacin and caffeine in normal volunteers. Antimicrob Agents Chemother 1989;33:474–478.

150. Mahr G, Sorgel F, Granneman R, et al. Effects of temafloxacin and ciprofloxacin on the pharmacokinetics of caffeine. Clin Pharmacokinet 1992;22(suppl 1):90–97.

151. Harder S, Staib AH, Beer C, et al. 4-quinolones inhibit biotransformation of caffeine. Eur J Clin Pharmacol 1988;35:651–656.

152. Peloquin CA, Nix DE, Sedman AJ, et al. Pharmacokinetics and clinical effects of caffeine alone and in combination with oral enoxacin. Rev Infect Dis 1989;11(suppl 5):S1095.

153. Stille W, Harder S, Mieke S, et al. Decrease of caffeine elimination in man during co-administration of 4-quinolones. J Antimicrob Chemother 1987;20:729–734.

154. Janknegt R. Drug interactions with quinolones. J Antimicrob Chemother 1990;26(suppl D):7–29.

155. Healy DP, Schoenle JR, Stotka J, Polk RE. Lack of interaction between lomefloxacin and caffeine in normal volunteers. Antimicrob Agents Chemother 1991;35:660–664.

156. LeBel M, Teng R, Dogolo LC, Willavize S, Friedman HL, Vincent J. The effect of steady-state trovafloxacin on the steady-state pharmacokinetics of caffeine in healthy subjects. Proceedings of the 36th Interscience Conference on Antimicrobial Agents and Chemotherapy, New Orleans, LA, September, 1996. Abstract A1.

157. Stahlberg HJ, Gohler K, Guillaume M, Mignot A. Effects of gatifloxacin (GTX) on the pharmacokinetics of theophylline in healthy young volunteers. J Antimicrob Chemother 1999;44(suppl A):136. Abstract P435.

158. Manita S, Toriumi C, Kusajima H, Momo K. The influence of gatifloxacin (AM-1155) on pharmacokinetics and metabolism of theophylline in rats and humans. Proceedings of the 38th Interscience Conference on Antimicrobial Agents and Chemotherapy, San Diego, CA, September, 1998. Abstract A-16a.

159. Parent M, LeBel M. Meta-analysis of quinolone-theophylline interactions. DICP Ann Pharmacother 1991;25:191–194.

160. Barnett G, Segura J, de la Torre R, Carbo M. Pharmacokinetic determination of relative potency of quinolone inhibition of caffeine disposition. Eur J Clin Pharmcol 1990;39:63–69.

161. Toon S, Hopkins KJ, Garstang FM, et al. Enoxacin-warfarin interaction: pharmacokinetic and stereochemical aspects. Clin Pharmacol Ther 1987;42:33–41.

162. Millar E, Coles S, Wyld P, Nimmo W. Temafloxacin does not potentiate the anticoagulant effect of warfarin in healthy subjects. Clin Pharmacokinet 1992;22(suppl 1):102–106.

163. Rindone JP, Keuey CL, Jones WN, Garewal HS. Hypoprothrombinemic effect of warfarin is not influenced by ciprofloxacin. Clin Pharm 1991;10:136–138.

164. Rocci ML Jr, Vlasses PH, Dislerath LM, et al. Norfloxacin does not alter warfarin's disposition or anticoagulant effect. J Clin Pharmacol 1990;30:728–732.

165. Bianco TM, Bussey HI, Farnett LE, Linn WD, Roush MK, Wong YWJ. Potential warfarin–ciprofloxacin interaction in patients receiving long-term anticoagulation. Pharmacotherapy 1992;12:435–439.

166. Israel DS, Stotka JL, Rock W, et al. Effect of ciprofloxacin on the pharmacokinetics and pharmacodynamics of warfarin. Clin Infect Dis 1996;22:251–256.

167. Levofloxacin. Data on file (protocol LOFBO-PH10-098). Raritan, NJ: RW Johnson Pharmaceutical Research Institute.

168. Teng R, Apseloff G, Vincent J, Pelletier SM, Willavize AS, Friedman HL. Effect of trovafloxacin (CP-99,129) on the pharmacokinetics and pharmacodynamics of warfarin in healthy male subjects. Proceedings of the 36th Interscience Conference on Antimicrobial Agents and Chemotherapy, New Orleans, LA, September, 1996. Abstract A2.

169. Muller FO, Hundt HKL, Muir AR, et al. Study to investigate the influence of 400 mg BAY 12-8039 (M) given once daily to healthy volunteers on PK and PD of warfarin (W). Proceedings of the 38th Interscience Conference on Antimicrobial Agents and Chemotherapy, San Diego, CA, September, 1998. Abstract A-13.

170. Sparfloxacin (Zagam®) [package insert]. Research Triangle Park, NC: Bertek Pharmaceuticals, February 2003.

171. Davy M, Bird N, Rost KL, Fuder H. Lack of effect of gemifloxacin on the steady-state pharmacodynamics of warfarin in healthy volunteers. Chemotherapy 1999;45:491–495.

172. Jolson HM, Tanner LA, Green L, Grasela TH Jr. Adverse reaction reporting of interaction between warfarin and fluoroquinolones. Arch Intern Med 1991;151:1003–1004.

173. Kamada A. Possible interaction between ciprofloxacin and warfarin. DICP Ann Pharmacother 1990;24:27–28.

174. Leor J, Matetzki S. Ofloxacin and warfarin [letter]. Ann Intern Med 1988;109:761.

175. Linville D, Emory C, Graves L. Ciprofloxacin and warfarin interaction [letter]. Am J Med 1991;90:765.

176. Linnville T, Matanin D. Norfloxacin and warfarin [letter]. Ann Intern Med 1989;110; 751–752.

177. Mott FE, Murphy S, Hunt V. Ciprofloxacin and warfarin [letter]. Ann Intern Med 1989; 111:542–543

178. Dugoni-Kramer BM. Ciprofloxacin–warfarin interaction [letter]. DICP Ann Pharmacother 1991;25:1397.

179. Renzi R, Finkbeiner S. Ciprofloxacin interaction with sodium warfarin. Am J Emerg Med 1991;9:551–552.

180. Ravnan SL, Locke C. Levofloxacin and warfarin interaction. Pharmacotherapy 2001;21:884–885.

181. Ellis RJ, Mayo MS, Bodensteiner DM. Ciprofloxacin–warfarin coagulopathy: a case series. Am J Hematol 2000;63:28–31.

182. Jones CB, Fugate SE. Levofloxacin and warfarin interaction. Ann Pharmacother 2002;36:1554–1557.

183. Artymowicz RJ, Cino BJ, Rossi JG, Walker JL, Moore S. Possible interaction between gatifloxacin and warfarin [letter]. Am J Health-Sys Pharm 2002;59:1205–1206.

184a. Byrd DC, Gaskins SE, Parrish AM, Freeman LB. Warfarin and ciprofloxacin interaction: case report and controversy. J Am Board Fam Pract 1999;12:486–488.

184b. Anonymous. Fluoroquinolones and warfarin: suspected interactions. Can Fam Physician 2004;50:1417.

185. Mant T, Morrison P, Millar E. Absence of drug interaction between temafloxacin and low dose heparin. Clin Pharmacokinet 1992;22(suppl 1):98–101.

186. Avent CK, Krinsky D, Kirklin JK, et al. Synergistic nephrotoxicity due to ciprofloxacin and cyclosporine. Am J Med 1988;85:452–453.

187. Elston RA, Taylor J. Possible interaction of ciprofloxacin with cyclosporin A [letter]. J Antimicrob Chemother 1988;21:679–680.

188. Thomson DJ, Menkis AH, McKenzie FN. Norfloxacin–cyclosporine interaction. Transplantation 1988;46:312–313.

189. Nasir M, Rotellar C, Hand M, Kulczycki L, Alijani MR, Winchester JF. Interaction between ciclosporin and ciprofloxacin [letter]. Nephron 1991;57:245–246.

190. McLellan R, Drobitch RK, McLellan H, Acott PD, Crocker JFS, Renton KW. Norfloxacin interferes with cyclosporin disposition in pediatric patients undergoing renal transplantation. Clin Pharmacol Ther 1995;58:322–327.

191. Kruger HU, Schuler U, Proksch B, et al. Investigations of potential interaction between ciprofloxacin and cyclosporin A in patients with renal transplants. Antimicrob Agents Chemother 1990;34:1048–1052.

192. Lang J, de Villaine FJ, Guemi A, et al. Absence of pharmacokinetic interaction between pefloxacin and cyclosporin A in patients with renal transplants. Rev Infect Dis 1989;11(suppl 5):S1094.

193. Lang J, de Villaine F J, Garraffo R, Touraine J-L. Cyclosporine (cyclosporin A) pharmacokinetics in renal transplant patients receiving ciprofloxacin. Am J Med 1989;87(suppl 5A):82S–85S.

194. Pichard L, Fabre I, Fabre G, et al. Screening for inducers and inhibitors of cytochrome P-450 (cyclosporin A oxidase) in primary cultures of human hepatocytes and in liver microsomes. Drug Metab Dispos 1990;18:595–606.

195. Robinson JA, Venezio FR, Costanzo-Nordin MR, et al. Patients receiving quinolones and cyclosporin after heart transplantation. J Heart Transplant 1990;9:30–31.

196. Tan KKC, Trull AK, Shawket S. Co-administration of ciprofloxacin and cyclosporin: lack of evidence for a pharmacokinetic interaction. Br J Clin Pharmacol 1989;28:185–187.

197. Hooper TL, Gould FK, Swinburn CR, et al. Ciprofloxacin: a preferred treatment for legionella infections in patients receiving cyclosporin A [letter]. J Antimicrob Chemother 1988;22:952–953.

198. Van Buren DH, Koestner J, Adedoyin A, et al. Effect of ciprofloxacin on cyclosporine pharmacokinetics. Transplantation 1990;50:888–889.

199. Levofloxacin. Data on file (protocol N93-059). Raritan, NJ: RW Johnson Pharmaceutical Research Institute.

200. Capone D, Carrano R, Gentile A, et al. Pharmacokinetic interaction between tacrolimus and levofloxacin in kidney transplant recipients [abstract]. Nephrol Dial Transpl 2001;16:A207.

201. Olsen SJ, Uderman HD, Kaul S, Kollia GD, Birkhofer MJ, Grasela DM. Pharmacokinetics (PK) of concomitantly administered gatifloxacin and digoxin. Proceedings of the 39th Interscience Conference on Antimicrobial Agents and Chemotherapy, San Francisco, CA, September, 1999. Abstract 199.

202. Stass H, Kubitza D. Profile of moxifloxacin drug interactions. Clin Infect Dis 2001;32(suppl 1):S47–S50.

203. Vouden M, Allen A, Lewis A, Ehren N. Lack of pharmacokinetic interaction between gemifloxacin and digoxin in healthy elderly volunteers. Chemotherapy 1999;45:485–490.

204. Chien S-C, Rogge MC, Williams RR, Natarajan J, Wong F, Chow AT. Absence of a pharmacokinetic interaction between digoxin and levofloxacin. J Clin Pharm Ther 2002; 27:7–12.

205. Johnson RD, Dorr MB, Hunt TL, Conway S, Talbot GH. Pharmacokinetic interaction of sparfloxacin and digoxin. Clin Ther 1999;21:368–379.

206. Vincent J, Hunt T, Teng R, Robarge L, Willavize SA, Friedman HL. The pharmacokinetic effects of coadministration of morphine and trovafloxacin in healthy subjects. Am J Surg 1998;176(suppl 6A):32S–38S.

207. Morran C, McArdle C, Pettitt L, et al. Pharmacokinetics of orally administered ciprofloxacin in abdominal surgery. Am J Med 1989;87(suppl 5A):86S–88S.

208a. Grant EM, Zhong MK, Fitzgerald JF, Nicolau DP, Nightingale C, Quintiliani R. Lack of interaction between levofloxacin and oxycodone: pharmacokinetics and drug disposition. J Clin Pharmacol 2001;41:206–209.

208b. Labbe L, Robitaille NM, Lefez C et al. Effects of ciprofloxacin on the stereoselective disposition of mexiletine in man. Ther Drug Monit. 2004;26:492–498.

209. Kamali F, Thomas SHL, Edwards C. The influence of steady-state ciprofloxacin on the pharmacokinetics and pharmacodynamics of a single dose of diazepam in healthy volunteers. Eur J Clin Pharmacol 1993;44:365–367.

210. Wijnands WJA, Trooster JFG, Teunissen PC, et al. Ciprofloxacin does not impair the elimination of diazepam in humans. Drug Metab Dispos 1990;18:954–957.

211. Grasela DM, LaCreta FP, Kollia GD, Randall DM, Uderman HD. Open-label, nonrandomized study of the effects of gatifloxacin on the pharmacokinetics of midazolam in healthy male volunteers. Pharmacotherapy 2000;20:330–335.

212. Waite NM, Rybak MJ, Krakovsky DJ, et al. Influence of subject age on the inhibition of oxidative metabolism by ciprofloxacin. Antimicrob Agents Chemother 1991;35:130–134.

213. Loi C-M, Parker BM, Cusack BJ, Vestal RE. Aging and drug interactions. III. individual and combined effects of cimetidine and ciprofloxacin on theophylline metabolism in healthy male and female nonsmokers. J Pharmacol Exp Ther 1997;280:627–637.

214. Chandler MHH, Toler SM, Rapp RP, et al. Multiple-dose pharmacokinetics of concurrent oral ciprofloxacin and rifampin therapy in elderly patients. Antimicrob Agents Chemother 1990;34:442–447.

215. Bernard E, Garraffo R, Leclercq-Boscherel B, Garret C, Bidault R, Dellamonica P. Drug interaction between grepafloxacin (GFX) and rifampin (RIF) in healthy volunteers. Proceedings of the 39th Interscience Conference on Antimicrobial Agents and Chemotherapy, San Francisco, CA, September, 1999. Abstract 6.

216. Schrenzel J, Dayer P, Leemann T, Weidekamm E, Portmann R, Lew DP. Influence of rifampin on fleroxacin pharmacokinetics. Antimicrob Agents Chemother 1993;37: 2132–2138.

217a. Orisakwe OE, Agbasi PU, Afonne OJ, Ofeofule SI, Obi E, Orish CN. Rifampicin pharmacokinetics with and without ciprofloxacin. Am J Ther 2001;8:151–153.

217b. Orisakwe OE, Afonne OJ, Agbasi PU, Ofoefule SI. Urinary excretion of rifampicin in the presence of ciprofloxacin. Am J Ther 2004;11:171–174.

217c. Orisakwe OE, Akunyili DN, Agbasi PU, Ezejiofor NA. Some plasma and saliva pharmacokinetics parameters of rifampicin in the presence of pefloxacin. Am J Ther 2004; 11:283–287.

217d. Orisakwe OE, Agbasi PU, Ofoefule SI, et al. Effect of pefloxacin on the urinary excretion of rifampicin. Am J Ther 2004;11:13–16.

218. Markowitz JS, Gill HS, Devane CL, Mintzer JE. Fluoroquinolone inhibition of clozapine metabolism [letter]. Am J Psychiatry 1997;153:881.

219. Markowitz JS, DeVane CL. Suspected ciprofloxacin inhibition of olanzapine resulting in increased plasma concentration [letter]. J Clin Psychopharmacol 1999;19:289–291.

220. Herrlin K, Segerdahl M, Gustafsson LL, Kalso E. Methadone, ciprofloxacin, and adverse drug reactions [letter]. Lancet 2000;356:2069–2070.

221. Raaska K, Neuvonen PJ. Ciprofloxacin increases serum clozapine and N-desmethyl-clozapine: a study in patients with schizophrenia. Eur J Clin Pharmacol 2000;56: 585–589.

222. Dalle J-H, Auvrignon A, Vassal G, Leverger G. Interaction between methotrexate and ciprofloxacin. J Pediatr Hematol Oncol 2002;24:321–322.

223. Takahashi H, Higuchi H, Shimizu T. Severe lithium toxicity induced by combined levofloxacin administration [letter]. J Clin Psychiatry 2000;61:949–950.

224. Scholten PC, Droppert RM, Zwinkels MGJ, Moesker HL, Nauta JJP, Hoepelman IM. No interaction between ciprofloxacin and an oral contraceptive. Antimicrob Agents Chemother 1998;42:3266–3268.

225. Chien SC, Chow AT, Rogge MC, Williams RR, Hendrix CW. Pharmacokinetics and safety of oral levofloxacin in human immunodeficiency virus-infected individuals receiving concomitant zidovudine. Antimicrob Agents Chemother 1997;41:1765–1769.

226. Villani P, Viale P, Signorini L, et al. Pharmacokinetic evaluation of oral levofloxacin in human immmunodeficiency virus-infected subjects receiving concomitant antiretroviral therapy. Antimicrob Agents Chemother 2001;45:2160–2162.

227. Ofoefule SI, Obodo CE, Orisakwe OE, et al. Some plasma pharmacokinetic parameters of isoniazid in the presence of a fluoroquinolone antibacterial agent. Am J Ther 2001;8:243–246.

228. Ofoefule SI, Obodo CE, Orisakwe OE, et al. Salivary and urinary excretion and plasma-saliva concentration ratios of isoniazid in the presence of co-administered ciprofloxacin. Am J Ther 2002;9:15–18.

229. Kamali F. No influence of ciprofloxacin on ethanol disposition. Eur J Clin Pharmacol 1994;47:71–74.

230. Tillonen J, Homann N, Rautio M, Jousimies-Somer H, Salaspuro M. Ciprofloxacin decreases the rate of ethanol elimination in humans. Gut 1999;44:347–352.

231. Jokinen MJ, Olkkola KT, Ahonen J, Neuvonen PJ. Effect of ciprofloxacin on the pharmacokinetics of ropivacaine. Eur J Clin Pharmacol 2003;58:653–657.

232. Risk of serious seizures from concomitant use of ciprofloxacin and phenytoin in patients with epilepsy. CMAJ 1998;158:104–105.

233. Hull RL. Possible phenytoin–ciprofloxacin interaction [letter]. Ann Pharmacother 1993;27:1283.

234. Pollak PT, Slayter KL. Hazards of doubling phenytoin dose in the face of an unrecognized interaction with ciprofloxacin. Ann Pharmacother 1997;31:61–64.

235. Dillard ML, Fink RM, Parkerson R. Ciprofloxacin–phenytoin interaction [letter]. Ann Pharmacother 1992;26:263.

236. Brouwers PJ, DeBoer LE, Guchelaar H-J. Ciprofloxacin–phenytoin interaction [letter]. Ann Pharmacother 1997;31:498.

237. Otero M-J, Moran D, Valverde M-P, Dominguez-Gil A. Interaction between phenytoin and ciprofloxacin [letter]. Ann Pharmacother 1999;33:251–252.

238. Job ML, Arn SK, Strom JG, Jacobs NF, D'Souza MJ. Effect of ciprofloxacin on the pharmacokinetics of multiple-dose phenytoin serum concentrations. Ther Drug Monitor 1994;16:427–431.

239. Davis RL, Quenzer RW, Kelly HW, Powell JR. Effect of the addition of ciprofloxacin on theophylline pharmacokinetics in subjects inhibited by cimetidine. Ann Pharmcother 1992;26:11–13.

240. Gillum JG, Israel DS, Scott RB, Climo MW, Polk RE. Effect of combination therapy with ciprofloxacin and clarithromycin on theophylline pharmacokinetics in healthy volunteers. Antimicrob Agents Chemother 1996;40:1715–1716.

241. Loi C-M, Parker BM, Cusack BJ, Vestal RE. Individual and combined effects of cimetidine and ciprofloxacin on theophylline metabolism in male nonsmokers. Br J Clin Pharmacol 1993;36:195–200.

242. Hasegawa T, Nadai M, Kuzuya T, et al. The possible mechanism of interaction between xanthines and quinolone. J Pharm Pharmacol 1990;42:767–772.

243. Fuhr U, Strobl G, Manaut F, et al. Quinolone antibacterial agents: relationship between structure and in vitro inhibition of the human cytochrome P-450 isoform CYP1A2. Mol Pharmacol 1993;43:191–199.

244. Fuhr U, Anders E-M, Mahr G, Sorgel F, Staib AH. Inhibitory potency of quinolone antibacterial agents against cytochrome P-450 1A2 activity in vivo and in vitro. Antimicrob Agents Chemother 1992;36:942–948.

245. Sarkar M, Polk RE, Guzelian PS, Hunt C, Karnes HT. In vitro effect of fluoroquinolones on theophylline metabolism in human liver microsomes. Antimicrob Agents Chemother 1990;34:594–599.

246. Wingender W, Beerman D, Foerster D, et al. Mechanism of renal excretion of ciprofloxacin, a new quinolone carboxylic acid derivative in humans. Chemioterapia 1985;4 (suppl 2):403–404.

247. Levofloxacin. Data on file (protocol HR355/1/GB/101). Raritan, NJ: RW Johnson Pharmaceutical Research Institute.

248. Shimada J, Yamaji T, Ueda Y, Uchida H, Kusajima H, Irikura T. Mechanism of renal excretion of AM-715, a new quinolone carboxylic acid derivative, in rabbits, dogs, and humans. Antimicrob Agents Chemother 1983;23:1–7.

249. Jaehde U, Sorgel F, Reiter A, Sigl G, Naber KG, Schunack W. Effect of probenecid on the distribution and elimination of ciprofloxacin in humans. Clin Pharmacol Ther 1995;58:532–541.

250. Nakashima M, Uematsu T, Kosuge K, et al. Single- and multiple-dose pharmacokinetics of AM-1155, a new 6-fluoro-8-methoxy quinolone, in humans. Antimicrob Agents Chemother 1995;39:2635–2640.

251. Stass H, Sachse R. Effect of probenecid on the kinetics of a single oral 400 mg dose of moxifloxacin in healthy volunteers. Clin Pharmacokinet 2001;40(suppl 1):71–76.

252. Sudoh T, Fujimura A, Shiga T, et al. Renal clearance of lomefloxacin is decreased by furosemide. Eur J Clin Pharmacol 1994;46:267–269.

253. Sudoh T, Fujimura A, Harada K, Sunaga K, Ohmori M, Sakamoto K. Effect of ranitidine on renal clearance of lomefloxacin. Eur J Clin Pharmacol 1996;51:95–98.

254a. Martin DE, Shen J, Griener J, Raasch R, Patterson JH, Cascio W. Effects of ofloxacin on the pharmacokinetics and pharmacodynamics of procainamide. J Clin Pharmacol 1996; 36:85–91.

254b. Van Wart S, Phillips L, Ludwig EA, et al. Population pharmacokinetics and pharmacodynamics of garenoxacin in patients with community-acquired respiratory tract infections. Antimicrob Agents Chemother 2004;48:4766–4777.

255. Christ W. Central nervous system toxicity of quinolones: human and animal findings. J Antimicrob Chemother 1990;26(suppl B):219–225.

256. Anastasio GD, Menscer D, Little JM Jr. Norfloxacin and seizures [letter]. Ann Intern Med 1988;109:169–170.

257. Lucet J-C, Tilly H, Lerebours G, Gres J-J, Piguet H. Neurological toxicity related to pefloxacin [letter]. J Antimicrob Chemother 1988;21:811–812.

258. Rollof J, Vinge E. Neurologic adverse effects during concomitant treatment with ciprofloxacin, NSAIDs, and chloroquine: possible drug interaction. Ann Pharmacother 1993;27:1058–1059.

259. Slavich IL, Gleffe RF, Haas EJ. Grand mal epileptic seizures during ciprofloxacin therapy [letter]. JAMA 1989;261:558–559.

260. Simpson KJ, Brodie MJ. Convulsions related to enoxacin [letter]. Lancet 1985;2:161.

261. Rumsey S, Wilkinson TJ, Scott SD. Ciprofloxacin-induced seizures—the need for increased vigilance. Aust J Hosp Pharm 1995;25:145–147.

262. Yamamoto K, Naitoh Y, Inoue Y, et al. Seizure discharges induced by the combination of new quinolone carboxylic acid drugs and non-steroidal anti-inflammatory drugs. Chemotherapy 1988;36(suppl 2):300–324.

263. Matsuno K, Kunihiro E, Yamatoya O, et al. Surveillance of adverse reactions due to ciprofloxacin in Japan. Drugs 1995;49(suppl 2):495–496.

264. Naora K, Katagiri Y, Ichikawa N, Hayashibara M, Iwamoto K. Enhanced entry of ciprofloxacin into the rat central nervous system induced by fenbufen. J Pharmacol Exp Ther 1991;258:1033–1037.

265. Ichikawa N, Naora K, Hayashibara M, Katagiri Y, Iwamoto K. Effect of fenbufen on the entry of new quinolones, norfloxacin and ofloxacin, into the central nervous system in rats. J Pharm Pharmacol 1992;44:915–920.

266. Naora K, Katagiri Y, Iwamoto K, Tanaka K, Yamaguchi T, Sekine Y. Effect of fenbufen on the pharmacokinetics of sparfloxacin in rats. J Antimicrob Chemother 1992;30:673–683.

267. Naora K, Katagiri Y, Ichikawa N, Hayashibara M, Iwamoto K. A possible reduction in the renal clearance of ciprofloxacin by fenbufen in rats. J Pharm Pharmacol 1990;42:704–707.

268. Katagiri Y, Naora K, Ichikawa N, Hayashibara M, Iwamoto K. Absence of pharmacokinetic interaction between ofloxacin and fenbufen in rats. J Pharm Pharmacol 1989;41:717–719.

269. Naora K, Katagiri Y, Ichikawa N, Hayashibara M, Iwamoto K. A minor possibility of pharmacokinetic interaction between enoxacin and fenbufen in rats. J Pharmacobio-Dyn 1990;13:90–96.

270. Kamali F. Lack of a pharmacokinetic interaction between ciprofloxacin and fenbufen. J Clin Pharm Ther 1994;19:257–259.

271. Fillastre JP, Leroy A, Borsa-Lebas F, Etienne I, Gy C, Humbert G. Lack of effect of ketoprofen on the pharmacokinetics of pefloxacin and ofloxacin [letter]. J Antimicrob Chemother 1993;31:805–806.

272. Fillastre JP, Leroy A, Borsa-Lebas F, Etienne I, Gy C, Humbert G. Effects of ketoprofen (NSAID) on the pharmacokinetics of pefloxacin and ofloxacin in healthy volunteers. Drugs Exp Clin Res 1992;18:487–492.

273. Halliwell RF, Lambert JJ, Davey PG. Actions of quinolones and nonsteroidal antiinflammatory drugs on γ-aminobutyric acid currents of rat dorsal root ganglion neurons. Rev Infect Dis 1989;11(suppl 5):S1398–S1399.

274. Halliwell RF, Davey PG, Lambert JJ. The effects of quinolones and NSAIDs upon GABA-evoked currents recorded from rat dorsal root ganglion neurones. J Antimicrob Chemother 1991;27:209–218.

275. Akahane K, Sekiguchi M, Une T, Osada Y. Structure-epileptogenicity relationship of quinolones with special reference to their interaction with γ-aminobutyric acid receptor sites. Antimicrob Agents Chemother 1989;33:1704–1708.

276. Segev S, Rehavi M, Rubinstein E. Quinolones, theophylline, and diclofenac interactions with the γ-aminobutyric acid receptor. Antimicrob Agents Chemother 1988;32:1624–1626.

277. Hori S, Shimada J, Saito A, Matsuda M, Miyahara T. Comparison of the inhibitory effects of new quinolones on γ-aminobutyric acid receptor binding in the presence of antiinflammatory drugs. Rev Infect Dis 1989;11(suppl 5):S1397–S1398.

278. Motomura M, Kataoka Y, Takeo G, et al. Hippocampus and frontal cortex are the potential mediatory sites for convulsions induced by new quinolones and non-steroidal anti-inflammatory drugs. Int J Clin Pharmacol Ther Toxicol 1991;29:223–227.

279. Kawakami J, Shimokawa M, Yamamoto K, et al. Inhibition of $GABA_A$ receptor-mediated current responses by enoxacin (new quinolone) and felbinac (non-steroidal antiinflammatory drug) in *Xenopus* oocytes injected with mouse-brain messenger RNA. Biol Pharm Bull 1993;16:726–728.

280. Christ W, Gindler K, Gruene S, et al. Interactions of quinolones with opioids and fenbufen, a nonsteroidal antiinflammatory drug: involvement of dopaminergic neurotransmission. Rev Infect Dis 1989;11(suppl 5):S1393–S1394.

281. Kawakami J, Yamamoto K, Asanuma A, Yanagisawa K, Sawada Y, Iga T. Inhibitory effect of new quinolones on $GABA_A$ receptor-mediated response and its potentiation with felbinac in *Xenopus* oocytes injected with mouse-brain mRNA: correlation with convulsive potency in vivo. Toxicol Appl Pharmacol 1997;145:246–254.

282. Imanishi T, Akahane K, Akaike N. Attenuated inhibition by levofloxacin, l-isomer of ofloxacin, on GABA response in the dissociated rat hippocampal neurons. Neurosci Lett 1995;193:81–84.

283. Akahane K, Tsutomi Y, Kimura Y, Kitano Y. Levofloxacin, an optical isomer of ofloxacin, has attenuated epileptogenic activity in mice and inhibitory potency in GABA receptor binding. Chemotherapy 1994;40:412–417.

284. Yakushiji T, Shirasaki T, Akaike N. Non-competitive inhibition of $GABA_A$ responses by a new class of quinolones and non-steroidal anti-inflammatories in dissociated frog sensory neurones. Br J Pharmacol 1992;105:13–18.

285. Halliwell RF, Davey PG, Lambert JJ. A patch clamp study of the effects of ciprofloxacin and biphenyl acetic acid on rat hippocampal neurone $GABA_A$ and ionotropic glutamate receptors. Neuropharmacology 1995;34:1615–1624.

286. Tsuji A, Sato H, Okezaki E, Nagata O, Kato H. Effect of the anti-inflammatory agent fenbufen on the quinolone-induced inhibition of $\gamma$–aminobutyric acid binding to rat brain membranes in vitro. Biochem Pharmacol 1988;37:4408–4411.

287. Ito T, Miura Y, Kadokawa T, Hori S, Shimada J, Migahara T. Effects of enoxacin and its combination with 4-biphenylacetate, an active metabolite of fenbufen, on population spikes in rat hippocampal slices. Pharmacol Toxicol 1991;68:220–225.

288. Ito Y, Ishige K, Aizawa M, Fukuda H. Characterization of quinolone antibacterial-induced convulsions and increases in nuclear AP-1 DNA- and CRE-binding activities in mouse brain. Neuropharmacology 1999;38:717–723.

289. Marchand S, Pariat C, Bouquet S, Courtois P, Couet W. Pharmacokinetic-pharmacodynamic modelling of the convulsant interaction between norfloxacin and biphenyl acetic acid in rats. Br J Pharmacol 2000;129:1609–1616.

290. Marchand S, Pariat C, Boulanger A, Bouquet S, Couet W. A pharmacokinetic/pharmacodynamic approach to show that not all fluoroquinolones exhibit similar sensitivity toward the proconvulsant effect of biphenyl acetic acid in rats. J Antimicrob Chemother 2001;48:813–820.

291. Smolders I, Gousseau C, Marchand S, Couet W, Ebinger G, Michotte Y. Convulsant and subconvulsant doses of norfloxacin in the presence and absence of biphenylacetic acid alter extracellular hippocampal glutamate but not gamma-aminobutyric acid levels in conscious rats. Antimicrob Agents Chemother 2002;46:471–477.

292. Kohno K, Niwa M, Nozaki M, et al. Role of nitric oxide in the convulsive seizures induced by fluoroquinolones coadministered with 4-biphenylacetic acid. Gen Pharmacol 1997;29:767–770.

293. Masukawa T, Nakanishi K, Natsuki R, et al. Role of nitric oxide in the convulsions following the coadministration of enoxacin with fenbufen in mice. Jpn J Pharmacol 1998;76:425–429.

294. Jaillon P, Morganroth J, Brumpt I, Talbot G. Overview of electrocardiographic and cardiovascular safety for sparfloxacin. Sparfloxacin Safety Group. J Antimicrob Chemother 1996;37(suppl A):161–167.

295. Demolis JL, Charransol A, Funck-Bretano C, Jaillon P. Effects of a single oral dose of sparfloxacin on ventricular repolarization in healthy volunteers. Br J Clin Pharmacol 1996;41:499–503.

296. Morganroth J, Talbot GH, Dorr MB, Johnson RD, Geary W, Magner D. Effect of single ascending, supratherapeutic doses of sparfloxacin on cardiac repolarization (QTc interval). Clin Ther 1999;21:818–828.

297. Lipsky BA, Baker CA. Fluoroquinolone toxicity profiles: a review focusing on newer agents. Clin Infect Dis 1999;28:352–364.

298. Lode H, Vogel F, Elies W. Grepafloxacin: a review of its safety profile based on clinical trials and postmarketing surveillance. Clin Ther 1999;21:61–74.

299. Springsklee M, Reiter C, Meyer JM. Safety and tolerability profile of moxifloxacin. Proceedings of the 13th European Congress of Clinical Microbiology and Infectious Diseases, Berlin, Germany, March, 1999. Abstract P-0208.

300. Frothingham R. Rates of torsades de pointes associated with ciprofloxacin, ofloxacin, levofloxacin, gatifloxacin, and moxifloxacin. Pharmacotherapy 2001;21:1468–1472.

301. Samaha FF. QTC interval prolongation and polymorphic ventricular tachycardia in association with levofloxacin [letter]. Am J Med 1999;107:528–529.

302. Owens RC Jr, Ambrose PG. Torsades de pointes associated with fluoroquinolones. Pharmacotherapy 2002;22:663–672.

303a. Bertino JS Jr, Owens RC Jr, Carnes TD, Iannini PB. Gatifloxacin-associated corrected QT interval prolongation, torsades de pointes, and ventricular fibrillation in patients with known risk factors. Clin Infect Dis 2002;34:861–863.

303b. Amankwa K, Krishnan SC, Tisdale JE. Torsades de pointes associated with fluoroquinolones: importance of concomitant risk factors. Clin Pharmacol Ther 2004; 75:242–247.

304. Paltoo B, O'Donoghue S, Mousavi MS. Levofloxacin induced polymorphic ventricular tachycardia with normal QT interval. Pacing Clin Electrophysiol 2001;24:895–897.

305. Kang J, Wang L, Chen XL, Triggle DJ, Rampe D. Interactions of a series of fluoroquinolone antibacterial drugs with the human cardiac $K^+$ channel HERG. Mol Pharmacol 2001;59:122–126.

306. Anderson ME, Mazur A, Yang T, Roden DM. Potassium current antagonist properties and proarrhythmic consequences of quinolone antibiotics. J Pharmacol Exp Ther 2001;296:806–810.

307. Hagiwara T, Satoh S, Kasai Y, Takasuna K. A comparative study of the fluoroquinolone antibacterial agents on the action potential duration in guinea pig ventricular myocardia. Jpn J Pharmacol 2001;87:231–234.

308. Patmore L, Fraser S, Mair D, Templeton A. Effects of sparfloxacin, grepafloxacin, moxifloxacin, and ciprofloxacin on cardiac action potential duration. Eur J Pharmacol 2000;406:449–452.

309. Bischoff U, Schmidt C, Netzer R, Pongs O. Effects of fluoroquinolones on HERG currents. Eur J Pharmacol 2000;406:341–343.

310. Satoh Y, Sugiyama A, Chiba K, Tamura K, Hashimoto K. QT-prolonging effects of sparfloxacin, a fluoroquinolone antibiotic, assessed in the in vivo canine model with monophasic action potential monitoring. J Cardiovasc Pharmacol 2000;36:510–515.

311. Chiba K, Sugiyama A, Satoh Y, Shiina H, Hashimoto K. Proarrhythmic effects of fluoroquinolone antibacterial agents: in vivo effects as physiologic substrate for torsades. Toxicol Appl Pharmacol 2000;169:8–16.

312. Morganroth J, Hunt T, Dorr MB, Magner D, Talbot GH. The cardiac pharmacodynamics of therapeutic doses of sparfloxacin. Clin Ther 1999;21:1171–1181.

313. Morganroth J, Hunt T, Dorr MB, Magner D, Talbot GH. The effect of terfenadine on the cardiac pharmacodynamics of sparfloxacin. Clin Ther 1999;21:1514–1524.

314. Iannini PB, Doddamani S, Byazrova E, Curciumara I, Kramer H. Risk of torsades de pointes with non-cardiac drugs. prolongation of QT interval is probably a class effect of fluoroquinolones [letter]. BMJ 2001;322:46–47.

315a. Demolis JL, Kubitza D, Tenneze L, Funck-Brentano C. Effect of a single oral dose of moxifloxacin (400 mg and 800 mg) on ventricular repolarization in healthy subjects. Clin Pharmacol Ther 2000;68:658–666.

315b. Noel GJ, Goodman DB, Chien S, Solanki B, Padmanabhan M, Natarajan J. Measuring the effects of supratherapeutic doses of levofloxacin on healthy volunteers using four methods of QT correction and periodic and continuous ECG recordings. J Clin Pharmacol 2004;44:464–473.

316. Noel GJ, Natarajan J, Chien S, Hunt TL, Goodman DB, Abels R. Effects of three fluoroquinolones on QT interval in healthy adults after single doses. Clin Pharmacol Ther 2003;73:292–303.

317. Doig JC. Drug-induced cardiac arrhythmias: incidence, prevention and management. Drug Safety 1997;17:265–275.

318. Roden DM. A practical approach to torsades de pointes. Clin Cardiol 1997;20:285–290.

319. Janeira LF. Torsades de pointes and long QT syndromes. Clin Fam Phys 1995;52: 1447–1453.

320. Yu C-C, Kelly PA, Burckart GJ, Zeevi A. Sirolimus inhibition of lymphocyte proliferation is not antagonized by ciprofloxacin and other quinolone antibiotics. Transplant Proc 2001;33:2989–2991.

321. Kelly PA, Burckart GJ, Anderson D, Shapiro R, Zeevi A. Ciprofloxacin does not block the antiproliferative effect of tacrolimus [letter]. Transplantation 1997;63:172–173.

322a. Roberge RJ, Kaplan R, Frank R, Fore C. Glyburide–ciprofloxacin interaction with resistant hypoglycemia. Ann Emerg Med 2000;36:160–163.

322b. Lin G, Hays DP, Spillane L. Refractory hypoglycemia from ciprofloxacin and glyburide interaction. J Toxicol Clin Toxicol 2004;42:295–297.

323a. Menzies DJ, Dorsainvil PA, Cunha BA, Johnson DH. Severe and persistent hypoglycemia due to gatifloxacin interaction with oral hypoglycemic agents. Am J Med 2002;113:232–234.

323b. LeBlanc M, Belanger C, Cossette P. Severe and resistant hypoglycemia associated with concomitant gatifloxacin and glyburide therapy. Pharmacotherapy 2004;24:926–931.

323c. Khovidhunkit W, Sunthornyothin S. Hypoglycemia, hyperglycemia, and gatifloxacin. Ann Intern Med 2004;141:969.

323d. Happe MR, Mulhall BP, Maydonovitch CL, Holtzmuller KC. Gatifloxacin-induced hyperglycemia. Ann Intern Med. 2004;141:968–969.

324a. Gatifloxacin (Tequin®) [package insert]. Princeton, NJ: Bristol Myers-Squibb, October 2002.

324b. Frothingham R. Gatifloxacin associated with a 56-fold higher rate of glucose homeostasis abnormalities than comparator quinolones in the FDA spontaneous reporting database. Program and abstracts of the 44th Interscience Conference on Antimicrobial Agents and Chemotherapy, Washington, DC, October–November 2004; Abstract A-1092.

325. Grasela D, Lacreta F, Kollia G, Randall D, Stoltz R, Berger S. Lack of effect of multiple-dose gatifloxacin (GAT) on oral glucose tolerance (OGTT), glucose and insulin homeostasis, and glyburide pharmacokinetics (PK) in patients with type II non-insulin-dependent diabetes mellitus (NIDDM). Proceedings of the 39th Interscience Conference on Antimicrobial Agents and Chemotherapy, San Francisco, CA, September, 1999. Abstract 196.

326. Gajjar DA, LaCreta FP, Uderman HD, et al. A dose-escalation study of the safety, tolerability, and pharmacokinetics of intravenous gatifloxacin in healthy adult men. Pharmacotherapy 2000;20(6 pt 2):49S–58S.

327. Gajjar DA, LaCreta FP, Kollia GD, et al. Effect of multiple-dose gatifloxacin or ciprofloxacin on glucose homeostasis and insulin production in patients with noninsulin-

dependent diabetes mellitus maintained with diet and exercise. Pharmacotherapy 2000; 20(6 pt. 2):76S–86S.

328a.  Trissel LA. Handbook on Injectable Drugs. 12th ed. Bethesda, MD: American Society of Health-System Pharmacists, 2003.

328b.  Szentmary N, Kraszni M, Nagy ZZ. Interaction of indomethacin and ciprofloxacin in the cornea following phototherapeutic keratectomy. Graefes Arch Clin Exp Ophthalmol 2004;242:614–616.

# β-Lactam Antibiotics

## Melinda M. Neuhauser and Larry H. Danziger

## INTRODUCTION

The β-lactam antibiotics are a large class of diverse compounds used clinically in both the oral and parenteral forms. The β-lactam antibiotic agents have become the most widely used therapeutic class of antimicrobials because of their broad antibacterial spectrum and excellent safety profile. Reports of drug–drug interactions with the β-lactam antimicrobials are a relatively rare phenomenon, and when interactions do occur, they are generally minor. This chapter describes the drug–drug interactions of the β-lactam antibiotics: penicillins, cephalosporins, carbapenems, and monobactams.

As an overview, each β-lactam drug interaction has been categorized as major, moderate, or minor and is presented in Table 1. Interactions classified as major are considered well documented and have the potential to be life threatening or dangerous. Moderate interactions are those for which more documentation is needed or potential harm to the patient is less. Minor interactions are poorly documented, present minimal potential harm to the patient, or occur with a low incidence.

The clinical significance of drug–drug interactions associated with the β-lactam antibiotics and understanding of the management of these drug–drug interactions are presented.

## PENICILLIN DRUG INTERACTIONS

### Acid-Suppressive Agents

The combination of various penicillins (ampicillin, amoxicillin, bacampicillin, and amoxicillin/clavulanate) and $H_2$-receptor antagonists (cimetidine and ranitidine) or omeprazole has been evaluated for effects on the bioavailability of the specific penicillin investigated (1–5). With the exception of bacampicillin, the bioavailability of the penicillins was unaffected. The area under the curve (AUC) of bacampicillin was reduced in the presence of food, ranitidine, and sodium bicarbonate (5); however, another study did not demonstrate a difference in AUC with coadministration of omeprazole and bacampicillin (2). The concurrent administration of most penicillins and acid-suppressive agents poses no problems except possibly with bacampicillin.

From: *Infectious Disease: Drug Interactions in Infectious Diseases, Second Edition*
Edited by: S. C. Piscitelli and K. A. Rodvold © Humana Press Inc., Totowa, NJ

**Table 1**
**Significance of β-Lactam Drug Interactions**

| | Penicillins | Cephalosporins | Carbapenems | Monobactam |
|---|---|---|---|---|
| Major | In vitro aminoglycoside inactivation<br>Contraceptives, oral estrogen<br>Methotrexate | Contraceptives, oral estrogen<br>Methotrexate | | |
| Moderate | In vivo aminoglycoside inactivation<br>Aminoglycoside inactivation in sampling serum concentrations<br>Neomycin (oral)<br>Probenecid<br>Warfarin | Acid suppressive agents<br>Iron<br>Ethanol<br>Probenecid<br>Warfarin | Probenecid<br>Ganciclovir | Probenecid<br>Inducers of β-lactams |
| Minor | Acid-suppressive agents<br>Allopurinol<br>Aspirin<br>β-Adrenergic blockers<br>Calcium channel blockers<br>Chloramphenicol<br>Chloroquine<br>Ciprofloxacin<br>Cyclosporine<br>Heparin<br>Interferon-γ<br>Guar gum<br>Khat<br>Metformin<br>Phenytoin<br>Proguanil<br>Tetracyclines<br>Vecuronium | Aminoglycoside nephrotoxicity<br>Calcium channel blocker<br>Cholestyramine<br>Colistin<br>Furosemide<br>Metoclopramide<br>Nonsteroidal anti-inflammatory drugs<br>Phenytoin<br>Propantheline<br>Theophylline | Cyclosporine<br>Theophylline<br>Valproic acid | |

## Allopurinol

An increased incidence of skin rash has been reported in patients receiving either ampicillin or amoxicillin concomitantly with allopurinol. In an analysis of data collected in 4686 patients receiving ampicillin, 252 of which were also receiving allopurinol, rash was reported in 5.7% of the patients receiving ampicillin compared to 13.9% of patients receiving both ampicillin and allopurinol ($p = 0.0000001$) (6). There were no differences in age, sex, diagnosis, or admission laboratory value of serum urea nitrogen (BUN) that could be identified between the two groups. Similar results of an increased incidence of a rash have also been reported in patients receiving both amoxicillin and allopurinol (22%) vs amoxicillin alone (5.9%) (6).

Fessel attempted to determine the possible reasons for the higher incidence of rash in patients receiving allopurinol and ampicillin (7). Fessel compared the history of allergies to penicillin, allergies to other antibiotics, presence of hay fever, use of antihistamine medications, and the prevalence of asthma in 124 asymptomatic hyperuricemic individuals compared to 224 matched normouricemic controls. The following results were considered significant in asymptomatic hyperuricemic subjects vs the control subjects: history of penicillin allergy (14.1 vs 4.9%), hay fever (18.8 vs 8.0%), and use of antihistamine medications (9.9 vs 2.7%). The incidence of allergies to antibiotics excluding penicillin and prevalence of asthma were not significant between groups. The author hypothesized that hyperuricemic individuals tend to have a higher frequency of allergic reactions; therefore, this altered immunologic state may explain the increased incidence of ampicillin rashes rather than an ampicillin–allopurinol interaction.

The significance of this pharmacodynamic interaction tends to be minor. Clinicians may continue to prescribe these agents concomitantly. Patients should be monitored and counseled regarding this potential increased incidence of skin rashes when these two agents are prescribed concurrently.

## Aminoglycosides

Penicillins and aminoglycosides are commonly used in combination to treat a variety of infections. However, concomitant use of the extended-spectrum penicillin antimicrobials may result in inactivation of the aminoglycosides. Although the majority of interactions are reported in vitro, the potential for in vivo interactions are of concern, especially in those patients with end-stage renal failure (8–16).

### In Vivo Aminoglycoside Inactivation

McLaughlin and Reeves reported a case report of a patient undergoing hemodialysis and receiving gentamicin for 8 day for the treatment a soft tissue infection (9). Carbenicillin therapy was added on day 8. The authors reported that therapeutic serum concentrations for gentamicin could not be achieved despite administration of high doses following the addition of carbenicillin. Of note, the patient received more frequent dialysis sessions during this period, which may have also contributed to subtherapeutic gentamicin concentrations. Uber et al. noted similar pharmacokinetic findings when tobramycin and piperacillin were administered concomitantly in a chronic hemodialysis patient (10). McLauglin and Reeves also studied this interaction in an animal model (9). Rabbits that received only gentamicin were reported to have normal gentamicin concentrations ($n = 2$); rabbits receiving carbenicillin and gentamicin had undetectable levels at 30 hours ($n = 3$).

Other investigators have described a reduction in aminoglycoside concentration when coadministered with extended-spectrum penicillins, particularly in patients with end-stage renal failure *(11–16)*. Davies et al. evaluated gentamicin half-lives in the presence of therapeutic doses of ticarcillin or carbenicillin in eight patients with end-stage renal failure *(12)*. In patients receiving gentamicin concomitantly with ticarcillin, the gentamicin half-life was reduced from 31 to 22 hours, whereas gentamicin half-life was reduced from 50 to 8 hours in patients receiving carbenicillin and gentamicin.

Halstenson et al. assessed the effect of piperacillin administration on the disposition of netilmicin and tobramycin in 12 chronic hemodialysis patients *(11)*. The half-life of netilmicin was not significantly altered when netilmicin was given concurrently with piperacillin. In comparison, the half-life of tobramycin was considerably reduced in the presence of piperacillin ($59.62 \pm 25.18$ vs $24.71 \pm 5.41$ hours). Lau et al. were unable to document any such drug–drug interaction between piperacillin and tobramycin in subjects with normal renal function (defined as creatinine clearances of greater than or equal to 60 mL/minute) *(17)*. Hitt and colleagues reported no differences in pharmacokinetic parameters of once-daily gentamicin with the coadministration of several piperacillin/tazobactam regimens in subjects with normal renal function *(18)*. Similarly, Dowell et al. were unable to demonstrate differences in the pharmacokinetic parameters of tobramycin when administered alone or with piperacillin/tazobactam in subjects with moderate renal impairment (creatinine clearance between 40 and 59 mL/minute), mild renal impairment (creatinine clearance between 20 and 39 mL/minute), or normal renal function (creatinine clearance greater than 90 mL/minute) *(19)*.

It has been suggested that the extended-spectrum penicillins interact chemically with the aminoglycosides to form biologically inactive amides. The degree of inactivation is dependent on the specific aminoglycoside and β-lactam used *(12,20)*. In vivo inactivation of aminoglycosides occurs at such a slow rate that it appears to be clinically insignificant in patients with normal renal function *(17,20)*. Some investigators have stated that this interaction could possibly be relevant for patients with renal failure who have high serum concentrations of penicillins *(11,12,21)*; therefore, close therapeutic monitoring of aminoglycosides is warranted in this specific clinical situation.

### Neomycin

Concomitant administration of oral neomycin and penicillin V has been reported to reduce serum concentrations of penicillin *(22)*. In healthy volunteers, penicillin V concentrations decreased by over 50% following the administration of oral neomycin concomitantly with penicillin V *(22)*. Because of the significant decrease in penicillin exposure, oral neomycin should not be coadministered with penicillin V.

### In Vitro Aminoglycoside Inactivation

McLaughlin and Reeves described undetectable gentamicin concentrations and clinical failure in a patient who received an infusion of carbenicillin and gentamicin for *Pseudomonas* bacteremia *(9)*. In vitro inactivation of aminoglycosides can be significant when these agents are prepared in the same intravenous mixture for administration *(20)*. Within 2 hours of admixing at room temperature, an intravenous fluid mixture containing ampicillin (concentration equivalent to 12 g/day) and gentamicin resulted in a 50% decline in the gentamicin activity. After 24 hours, no measurable gentamicin activity was noted *(20)*. An intravenous fluid mixture containing gentamicin and carbenicillin demonstrated a 50% reduction in activity between 8 and 12 hours after admixing at room temperature. Aminoglycosides and penicillins should not be mixed together prior to infusion.

*In Vitro Inactivation Aminoglycoside in Sampling Serum Concentrations*

If high concentrations of penicillins are present in serum samples that are to be assayed for aminoglycoside concentrations, inactivation of the aminoglycosides by the penicillins can result in falsely decreased aminoglycoside concentrations *(8)*. Penicillin concentration, period of time prior to sampling, and storage temperature of the sample are factors that affect the extent of inactivation *(8)*. When measuring aminoglycoside serum concentrations through intravenous tubing, one should flush 5–10 mL of either normal saline or 5% dextrose in water (based on drug compatibilities) through the tubing before withdrawing blood to minimize the amount of β-lactam present in the intravenous tubing prior to sampling.

*Aminoglycosides—Synergy*

The concomitant use of β-lactam and aminoglycoside antimicrobials has been described as synergistic for several Gram-positive and Gram-negative organisms *(23–26)*. By inhibiting the cell wall synthesis, β-lactams increase the porosity of the bacterial cell wall, resulting in greater aminoglycoside penetration and access to target ribosomes *(27)*.

The use of penicillin or ampicillin in combination with an aminoglycoside has been documented to be advantageous in the treatment of enterococcal infections *(28)*. Moellering et al. also noted that whereas penicillin exhibits only bacteriostatic activity against enterococci, the combination of penicillin and streptomycin possesses bactericidal activity *(23)*. As a result, most severe enterococcal infections are routinely treated with penicillin or ampicillin plus an aminoglycoside.

Despite the well-documented in vitro synergy between β-lactams and aminoglycosides, limited clinical data are available supporting superior efficacy of synergistic vs nonsynergistic combinations for the treatment of Gram-negative infections. Anderson et al. retrospectively evaluated Gram-negative bacteremias to determine if the treatment with one or two antimicrobials effected outcome and whether in vitro synergy correlated with superior efficacy *(29)*. Of the 173 patients treated with two drugs, the clinical response rate was 83% in patients who received synergistic vs 64% with nonsynergistic antimicrobial regimens ($p < 0.05$). The use of synergistic antimicrobial combinations (aminoglycoside plus ampicillin or carbenicillin) was associated with better clinical response in patients with neutropenia ($p < 0.001$), shock ($p > 0.001$), *Pseudomonas aeruginosa* bacteremias ($p < 0.05$), and "rapidly or ultimately fatal" conditions ($p < 0.005$). In critically ill patients with Gram-negative bacteremia, the combination of an extended spectrum penicillin and aminoglycoside is a reasonable therapeutic approach.

## Anticoagulants

*Heparin*

A number of case reports have suggested that parenteral penicillins in combination with heparin have caused coagulopathies *(30–36)* and may predispose patients to clinically significant bleeding *(33–35,37)*. The exact mechanism of this interaction is unknown but may be a result of a direct effect on platelet function by penicillins, which may have an additive anticoagulant effect when combined with heparin *(31–32,37)*.

Wisloff et al. evaluated the bleeding time of patients receiving heparin and penicillins compared to heparin alone *(36)*. Fifty patients were placed on heparin (5000 IU sc for 7 days) following an elective vascular surgery procedure and were also randomly assigned to receive a combination of ampicillin and cloxacillin or no antibiotics. The patients who were receiving heparin along with the penicillins had a slightly longer bleeding time; however, this was still within an acceptable range in most cases.

Because patients receiving heparin are routinely monitored closely for coagulopathies and clinically significant bleeding, the potential interaction between these two drugs does not warrant further precautions.

### Warfarin

A decreased anticoagulant effect for warfarin has been documented when given concomitantly with nafcillin *(38–41)* or dicloxacillin *(38,42,43)*. Some clinicians have postulated that these antibiotics induce the cytochrome P450 system and may increase the metabolism of warfarin *(40,44,45)*. Another possible explanation may involve the ability of these highly protein-bound agents to displace warfarin. However, Qureshi et al. performed an in vitro study and demonstrated that nafcillin did not affect the protein binding of warfarin *(40)*.

Krstenansky et al. studied the effect of dicloxacillin in seven patients stabilized on warfarin therapy *(42)*. Prothrombin times (PTs) were obtained prior to treatment and on days 1, 3, 6, and 7 of dicloxacillin administration. A decrease in the PT was observed in all patients on day 6 or 7 compared to baseline PT values. The decrease in PT ranged from 0.3 to 5.6 seconds (mean $\pm$ SD of $-1.9 \pm 1.8$ seconds) and was statistically significant ($p < 0.05$).

Brown et al. presented a case report of a patient on 2.5 mg warfarin daily who developed an increased hypoprothrombinemic response after receiving high-dose intravenous penicillin (24 million units/day). On withdrawal of the penicillin, the patient's PT subsequently returned to his baseline *(46)*. Davydov et al. reported a case of a 58-year-old woman with an interaction of warfarin with amoxicillin/clavulanate, resulting in an elevated international normalized ratio (INR) and hematuria *(47)*. Although the exact mechanism of this interaction remains unknown, it has been proposed that broad-spectrum antibiotic use may lead to a decrease in vitamin K-producing bacteria within the gastrointestinal tract. This may then result in a vitamin K-deficient state (especially in patients with low dietary intake of vitamin K), potentially leading to an increased effect of warfarin. Clinicians should be aware of the potential interaction between penicillins and oral anticoagulants and monitor the PT and INR in patients receiving these agents concurrently.

### Aspirin

Large doses of aspirin may increase the serum concentrations and half-lives of penicillin, oxacillin, nafcillin, cloxacillin, and dicloxacillin when administered concurrently *(48,49)*. Eleven patients with arteriosclerotic disorders received penicillin G before and after high doses of aspirin (3 g/day) *(48)*. During aspirin administration, penicillin half-life increased from $44.5 \pm 15.8$ minutes to $72.4 \pm 35.9$ minutes ($p < 0.05$) *(48)*. The mechanism of this interaction remains unknown. Some have speculated that this interaction may occur as a result of aspirin displacing penicillin from protein-binding sites or of aspirin competing with penicillins for the renal tubular secretory proteins *(48–52)*. Avoidance of this combination is unnecessary.

### β-Adrenergic Blockers

Coadministration of ampicillin and atenolol may lead to a decrease in the serum concentration of atenolol. In a crossover study, six healthy subjects were orally administered 100 mg atenolol alone and with 1 g ampicillin. Atenolol pharmacokinetics were assessed after a single dose and after reaching steady state. These subjects previously received intravenous atenolol in another study, which was utilized to determine oral bioavailability in the present study. The bioavailability of atenolol was reduced from 60 (atenolol alone) to 36 (single-dose atenolol and ampicillin, $p < 0.01$) to 24% (steady-state concentrations of atenolol and ampicillin, $p < 0.01$) *(53)*. Other atenolol pharmacokinetic parameter values for AUC, $C_{max}$, and mean steady-state concentrations were also significantly reduced ($p < 0.01$). Despite the differences in atenolol serum concentration, blood pressure measurements did not differ between the groups over a 4-week treatment period.

McLean and colleagues also performed a crossover study administering oral atenolol and ampicillin to six volunteers *(54)*. Unlike the previous study, these investigators dosed ampicillin at clinically applicable doses of 250 mg four times a day as well as at higher doses of 1 g. The mean reduction of AUC was lower in the former dosing regimen compared to the latter one (18.2 vs 51.5%).

Although the clinical significance of this interaction is questionable, it would seem reasonable that patients should be monitored for this interaction when higher doses of ampicillin are used, especially in the presence of renal dysfunction; however, no empiric dosage alterations are recommended at this time.

### Calcium Channel Blockers

Nifedipine appears to increase the bioavailability of amoxicillin by facilitating its active transport mechanism within the gastrointestinal tract *(55)*. In a randomized crossover study conducted in eight healthy volunteers, each subject received 1 g oral amoxicillin with 20 mg nifedipine or placebo. The absolute bioavailability of amoxicillin was noted to increase from 65.25 to 79.2% with the addition of nifedipine ($p < 0.01$) *(55)*. The AUC also increased from 29.7 ± 5.3 mg · hours/L (amoxicillin alone) compared to 36.26 ± 6.9 mg · hours/L (amoxicillin and nifedipine) ($p < 0.01$). Because no adverse events were associated with the alterations of these pharmacokinetic parameters, no dosage adjustments are recommended.

Nafcillin has been postulated to enhance the elimination of agents metabolized through the cytochrome P450 system *(44,45)*. A crossover study was conducted to evaluate the induction potential of nafcillin on nifedipine, a substrate of the cytochrome P450 3A4 enzyme *(56)*. Healthy volunteers were randomly assigned to receive 5 days of oral nafcillin (500 mg four times daily) or placebo, which was followed by a single dose of nifedipine. The subjects who received nafcillin along with nifedipine were found to have a significant reduction in the nifedipine $AUC_{0-\infty}$ (80.9 ± 32.9 vs 216.4 ± 93.2 μg · hours/L; $p < 0.001$) and enhanced plasma clearance (138.5 ± 42.0 vs 56.5 ±

32.0 L/hour; $p < 0.002$) compared to the nifedipine-placebo group. Because of the limited available data, the clinical significance of this interaction is unknown.

## Chloramphenicol

The administration of a bacteriostatic agent such as chloramphenicol may antagonize the bactericidal activity of β-lactam antimicrobials (57,58). β-Lactam antimicrobials exhibit their bactericidal effect by binding to penicillin-binding proteins and inhibiting bacterial cell wall synthesis. For β-lactams to exert optimal bactericidal effects, bacteria should be actively growing and dividing. However, bacteriostatic agents such as chloramphenicol, which may inhibit protein synthesis, may interfere with the bactericidal activity of penicillins.

In vitro studies have demonstrated the concomitant use of penicillin and chloramphenicol to be antagonistic (57,59). However, human data do not support these findings (60,61). Patients with gonococcal infections who were treated with a combination of penicillin and chloramphenicol had better clinical outcomes than patients treated with penicillin alone (60). Superior outcomes were also reported among patients infected with typhoid fever who were treated with chloramphenicol plus ampicillin compared to chloramphenicol alone (61).

Relevant clinical information is limited for this drug–drug interaction. Because the in vivo and in vitro data concerning this interaction are contradictory, it is unnecessary to avoid the concurrent use of these antimicrobials.

## Chloroquine

Investigators conducted a study in healthy volunteers to evaluate the coadministration of chloroquine and ampicillin on the pharmacokinetics of ampicillin (62). Ampicillin pharmacokinetics alone or in the presence of chloroquine was determined by characterizing the drug's renal elimination. The mean percentage of dose excreted was 29% for ampicillin alone vs 19% for the ampicillin/chloroquine combination ($p < 0.005$). The coadministration of ampicillin and chloroquine resulted in a significant reduction in ampicillin bioavailability but not in time of maximal excretion (62). Based on limited data, coadministration of these agents may lead to a reduction in ampicillin concentrations. Although the clinical significance of this interaction remains unknown, concomitant administration of chloroquine and ampicillin should be avoided.

## Ciprofloxacin

Interactions between the penicillins and fluoroquinolones have been rarely documented (63,64). Barriere et al. assessed the effect of the concurrent administration of ciprofloxacin and azlocillin in a crossover trial (63). Six subjects were administered single doses of ciprofloxacin and azlocillin alone and in combination. Similar pharmacokinetic profiles were noted with azlocillin; however, when coadministered with azlocillin, a statistically significant reduction in total clearance and renal clearance of ciprofloxacin was noted. Based on limited data, coadministration of these agents need not be avoided.

## Contraceptives: Oral Estrogen

Several case reports of breakthrough bleeding and pregnancies have been reported in patients receiving oral contraceptives and antibiotics concomitantly (65–69). It has been postulated that antibiotics interfere with the enterohepatic circulation of oral estrogens, resulting in subtherapeutic estrogen concentrations (67–69). After oral estrogens are absorbed, they undergo hepatic metabolism to glucuronide and sulfate conjugates and are excreted into the bile. Bacteria residing in the gut hydrolyze the conjugates to active drug, which is then reabsorbed by the body (67). The proposed mechanism of this interaction involves the ability of antibiotics to destroy the gut bacteria required to hydrolyze the conjugated estrogen to their active form.

Studies in animal models assessing this interaction have shown mixed results (70,71). One investigation demonstrated no alterations in the pharmacokinetics of ethinylestradiol when administered with ampicillin (70). Another study found differences in both AUC and plasma clearance in the group that received antibiotics compared to those that received ethinylestradiol alone (71).

Several studies have been performed in humans to determine if the case reports and animal data represent significant findings (72–74). Freidman and colleagues prospectively evaluated the serum concentrations of gonadotropins and other hormones in 11 volunteers receiving Demulen® (50 µg ethinylestradiol and 1 mg ethynodiol diacetate) plus ampicillin or placebo during two consecutive menstrual cycles (73). Progesterone concentrations were similar between the Demulen-ampicillin and Demulen-placebo groups. Follicle-stimulating hormone and luteinizing hormone appeared to be similar between the two groups. None of the 11 patients underwent ovulation. Freidman and colleagues concluded that ampicillin should not reduce the effectiveness of Dumulen. Other researchers have criticized the results of this study because of its study design, which included a small number of subjects, a short duration of antimicrobial therapy, and a relatively high dose of estrogens (present in Demulin) (68).

Back and colleagues evaluated seven women receiving oral contraceptives (all containing $\geq$ 30 µg ethinyloestradiol) for at least 3 months who presented to their clinic with an infection that required the administration of ampicillin for 8 days (72). Blood samples were taken during concomitant oral estrogen and ampicillin therapy and during the next menstrual cycle without ampicillin. Six female volunteers receiving only oral contraceptives for at least 3 months were similarly evaluated for the potential drug interaction. Plasma concentrations of ethinyloestradiol, levonorgestrel, follicle-stimulating hormone, and progesterone were not significantly different between the two groups (oral contraceptive-ampicillin vs oral contraceptive alone). Despite the fact that a lower concentration of ethinyloestradiol was seen with two women on ampicillin, the authors concluded that alternative methods of protection are not necessary in most women (67).

Another study in volunteers analyzed the effect of administering ampicillin or metronidazole with an oral contraceptive preparation (74). This summary is limited to the group using ampicillin ($n = 6$). Subjects initially received a low-dose oral contraceptive (1 mg norethisterone acetate and 30 µg ethinyl estradiol). On days 6 and 7, plasma concentrations of ethinylestradiol and norethisterone were obtained. Subsequently, subjects were administered ampicillin (500 mg twice daily orally for 5–7 days) and the contraceptive steroid. Following antibiotic treatment, serum hormones, ampicillin, and progesterone concentrations were measured in the subjects. The concentrations of norethisterone and ethinylestradiol were not altered in the presence of ampicillin, and progesterone concentrations were in the appropriate range to suppress ovulation (74).

It is difficult to determine the clinical significance of this interaction because of the small number of clinical trials, small number of patients, minimal number of case reports, and the limited number of oral contraceptives studied. A review article suggested that the possibility of a clinically significant interaction between antibiotics and oral contraceptives is likely less than 1% (75). The author stated that women with a greater extent of enterohepatic circulation, previous breakthrough bleeding, or contraceptive failure may have a higher risk for this interaction (75). Because of the potential risk of contraceptive failure, clinicians should still counsel patients on this potential interaction and suggest alternative method(s) of contraception if antimicrobial therapy is necessary.

## Cyclosporine

Although nafcillin is not well established as an inducer of the cytochrome P450 system, the following case report suggests that nafcillin may reduce the serum concentrations of cyclosporine via induction of the cytochrome P450 system (76).

### CASE STUDY 1

On two separate occasions, a 34-year-old woman, status postrenal transplant, experienced a reduction in cyclosporine serum concentration following nafcillin administration (76). The patient received 2 g nafcillin intravenously every 6 hours for a positive culture of methicillin-susceptible *Staphylococcus aureus* from a perinephric abscess. On admission, the patient was receiving 400 mg cyclosporine daily with a corresponding trough serum concentration of 229 ng/mL. After initiation of nafcillin, her cyclosporine concentrations decreased to 119 ng/mL and 68 ng/mL on days 3 and 7 of nafcillin, respectively, despite stable daily doses of 400 mg cyclosporine. On discontinuation of nafcillin, trough serum concentrations of cyclosporine increased to 141 ng/mL and 205 ng/mL on days 2 and 4 without nafcillin therapy, respectively. No change in renal or hepatic function was noted throughout this entire treatment period. The second cyclosporine–nafcillin interaction occurred when the patient was later readmitted for drainage of retroperitoneal fluid collection. The patient experienced a similar decline in cyclosporine concentrations during concomitant therapy and subsequent increases in cyclosporine concentrations following discontinuation of nafcillin. Based on the findings of this case report, cyclosporine concentrations should be closely monitored during concomitant nafcillin administration.

## Erythromycin

The concurrent administration of erythromycin and penicillin may result in antagonism, synergy, or no effect (indifference) on the antibacterial activity of penicillin. β-Lactams exert their cidal effects on bacteria by binding to penicillin-binding proteins and inhibiting cell wall synthesis. For β-lactams to exercise their optimal bactericidal activity, bacteria should be actively growing and dividing; therefore, erythromycin can interfere with the bactericidal activity of penicillin by inhibiting protein synthesis.

In vitro studies have demonstrated the concomitant administration of penicillin and erythromycin to be synergistic, antagonistic, additive, or indifferent (77–84). These differences may be caused by such factors as the specific microorganism involved, susceptibility patterns to both agents, antibiotic concentrations, the inoculum effect, and time of incubation *(77,79,81,83–86)*. Similar to the disparate results demonstrated in vitro, case reports have shown penicillin and erythromycin antagonism in the treatment of scarlatina *(87)* and *Streptococcus bovis* septicemia *(88)*, whereas clinical improvement has been reported with the concurrent use of ampicillin and erythromycin in the treatment of pulmonary nocardiosis *(89)*.

Although there has been concern about the use of the combination of β-lactams and macrolides because of the possibility of antagonism, they have gained favor for the treatment of community-acquired pneumonia in the hospitalized patient. Several studies found that patients with bacteremic pneumococcal pneumonia treated with a β-lactam plus a macrolide had a lower mortality rate compared to those treated with a single agent *(90–92)*. As such, treatment guidelines for community-acquired pneumonia recommend a penicillin and macrolide as a preferred treatment option for hospitalized patients *(93)*. As evident from these clinical reports and in vitro testing, the antagonism risk between β-lactams and macrolides appears to be minimal.

### Guar Gum

Guar gum, which may be utilized as a food additive, has been reported to reduce serum concentrations of phenoxymethyl penicillin *(94)*. In a double-blind study, 10 healthy volunteers received guar gum or placebo granules along with 3 million units of phenoxymethyl penicillin. The peak penicillin concentration decreased significantly from $7560 \pm 1720$ to $5680 \pm 1390$ ng/mL ($p < 0.01$) when administered with placebo compared to guar gum. The $AUC_{0-6\ hours}$ of penicillin decreased significantly from $14,500 \pm 1860$ to $10,380 \pm 2720$ ng/mL · hour ($p < 0.001$) when administered with guar gum. The time to peak concentration was not altered significantly. As a result of the significant decrease in the peak serum concentrations and $AUC_{0-6\ h}$, phenoxymethyl penicillin should not be administered concomitantly with guar gum.

### Interferon-γ

Data suggested that penicillin may interact with a variety of cytokines by conjugating these biological proteins *(95,96)*. Benzylpenicillin has been shown to conjugate interferon (IFN)-γ, interleukin (IL)-1β, IL-2, IL-5, IL-13, and tumor necrosis factor (TNF)-α; however, based on a series of in vitro experiments, benzylpenicillin only appears to alter the biological activity of IFN-γ *(95)*. Using an in vitro bioassay, Brooks et al. noted that benzylpenicillin inhibited the ability of IFN-γ to induce CD54 expression on epithelial cells. Additional preclinical studies suggested that other regulatory functions of IFN-γ may also be modulated by benzylpenicillin *(96)*. Because IFN-γ promotes Th1 responses and inhibits Th2 and immunoglobulin E-mediated responses, disruption of IFN-γ activity by benzylpenicillin may result in clinically significant immunomodulatory effects, which promote allergy. Referred to Chapter 13 for additional information on drug–cytokine interactions.

### Khat

The chewing of khat (a natural substance obtained from shrubs grown in East Africa and Yemen) may reduce the bioavailability of ampicillin and amoxicillin *(97)*. In a crossover design, eight healthy adult male Yemeni subjects received ampicillin or amoxicillin under various conditions of khat chewing *(97)*. The urinary excretion method was utilized to determine the bioavailabilities of ampicillin and amoxicillin under the following conditions: antibiotic alone, 2 hours before khat chewing, immediately prior to khat chewing, immediately prior to khat chewing with a meal, midway through khat chewing, and 2 hours after khat chewing. The bioavailability of ampicillin (measured by percentage of ampicillin excreted unchanged in the urine, peak excretion, and time to peak excretion) was significantly decreased during all conditions except when administered 2 hours after khat chewing. In contrast, amoxicillin's bioavailability was only affected when amoxicillin was taken midway through khat chewing. Considering the limited use of khat in the developed countries, this should not be considered a clinically relevant drug–drug interaction. However, if ampicillin and amoxicillin are administered to an individual using khat, these agents should be taken at least 2 hours following khat chewing.

## Metformin

In a crossover study, healthy volunteers were randomly assigned to receive metformin alone or metformin along with cephalexin *(98)*. The coadministration of metformin and cephalexin led to an increase in $C_{max}$ and AUC of metformin by approx 30%. It appears that cephalexin interferes with renal clearance of metformin, which may be because of competition for renal transport proteins such as organic anion or cation transporter *(98,99)*. Limited data are available on the clinical significance of this interaction. Clinicians should exercise caution when using these two agents together.

## Methotrexate

Weak organic acids such as penicillins can compete with methotrexate (MTX) for renal tubular secretion *(100,101)* and reduce the renal elimination of MTX. Various studies in rabbits have demonstrated a reduction in the renal clearance of MTX and 7-hydroxymethotrexate *(100–103)*. One of the studies demonstrated nearly 50% reduction in MTX clearance when piperacillin was administered 10 minutes before and 4 hours after a single dose of MTX ($p \leq 0.05$) *(101)*. The AUC of MTX and its 7-hydroxymethotrexate metabolite also differed significantly from the control ($p \leq 0.05$).

Despite the rather significant results reported from animal studies, few case reports have documented this potential interaction *(104–109)*. Bloom and colleagues reported four cases in which the administration of various penicillins concomitantly with MTX resulted in the decreased clearance of MTX *(105)*. MTX clearance before and after the addition of the following antimicrobial agents was as follows: penicillin, 2.8 vs 1.8 L/hour; piperacillin, 11 vs 3.6 L/hour; ticarcillin, 5.8 vs 2.3 L/hour; and dicloxacillin/indomethacin, 6.4 vs 0.45 L/hour, respectively. Because of reduction in clearance, these patients required an extended leucovorin rescue. A case report described severe MTX toxicity following the concomitant administration of high-dose MTX and oxacillin, which led to a series of complications and ultimately the death of the patient *(109)*. In contrast, Herrick and colleagues reported no differences in renal clearance of MTX administered alone or with flucloxacillin in 10 patients *(110)*.

Avoiding the concomitant use of penicillins and MTX is justified to avoid potential toxicity. If the concomitant administration of penicillins and MTX is necessary, close monitoring of MTX concentrations and signs of toxicity is warranted.

## Oseltamivir

A pharmacokinetic study conducted in healthy volunteers evaluated the concurrent administration of oseltamivir (a prodrug) and amoxicillin *(111)*. No differences in the pharmacokinetic parameters of oseltamivir's active metabolite, Ro 64-0802, were noted when administered alone compared to coadministration with amoxicillin. Also, no pharmacokinetic differences were noted for amoxicillin with or without the administration of oseltamivir *(111)*. Based on these finding, oseltamivir may be prescribed with amoxicillin.

## Phenytoin

Highly protein-bound antibiotics such as nafcillin and oxacillin (both approx 90% bound to plasma proteins) *(112)* have the potential to interact with other highly protein-bound agents such as phenytoin *(113,114)*. Because of drug displacement from protein-binding sites, high doses of nafcillin or oxacillin may increase unbound concentrations of phenytoin in certain patient populations *(113,114)*.

Dasgupta et al. conducted an in vitro study to determine the potential drug interaction between oxacillin and phenytoin *(113)*. Serum was collected from three separate patient populations (A, B, and C). Serum for Group A was collected from healthy patients receiving phenytoin. Sera for Groups B and C were obtained from hypoalbuminemic and hyperuremic individuals, respectively. Subjects in these last two groups were not receiving phenytoin; therefore, the sera were supplemented with phenytoin. Each group was tested for total and unbound phenytoin concentrations with and without 15 or 50 µg/mL oxacillin, which represented estimated peak oxacillin concentrations following a 500-mg oral dose and a 1-g iv dose, respectively. Serum from Group A showed no statistical difference in unbound phenytoin concentrations with 15 µg/mL oxacillin; however, a significantly higher unbound phenytoin concentration with 50 µg/mL of oxacillin was observed when compared to serum not containing oxacillin (1.67 vs 1.47 µg/mL) ($p < 0.05$). Sera from subjects in Groups B and C also demonstrated a statistically significant increase in unbound phenytoin concentrations for both oxacillin concentrations compared to the group without oxacillin.

Dasgupta and colleagues performed another study to determine the potential effect of nafcillin on unbound phenytoin concentrations *(114)*. The study consisted of both in vitro and in vivo components. The authors observed both in vitro and in vivo displacement of phenytoin with the addition of nafcillin to serum. Although increases in unbound phenytoin appeared to be minor for the in vitro portion of the experiment, a significant increase in unbound phenytoin concentrations was noted in all groups compared to the control group ($p < 0.05$). Unbound phenytoin concentrations were also measured in four patients receiving phenytoin and nafcillin concurrently *(114)*. The investigators obtained unbound phenytoin concentrations during and after nafcillin therapy. Unbound phenytoin concentrations decreased following the discontinuation of nafcillin, although baseline phenytoin concentrations were not obtained.

Patients receiving antimicrobials with a high percentage of protein binding (90% or greater) and concomitant phenytoin should be monitored closely for signs of phenytoin toxicity. Furthermore, patients receiving high doses of any penicillin should have their unbound and total phenytoin concentrations monitored closely. Phenytoin dosage adjustments should be made according to extent of the interaction.

## Probenecid

The interaction of probenecid and penicillins (weak organic acids) occurs primarily as a result of the inhibition of the tubular secretion of penicillin, although other mechanisms may be possible as well *(115,116)*. The decrease in renal elimination results in increased penicillin serum concentrations. Studies have shown that the AUCs of amoxicillin, ampicillin, ticarcillin, and nafcillin may increase by approx 50 to 100% when coadministered with probenecid *(48,116–119)*. Other β-lactams such as penicillin and dicloxacillin have also demonstrated increased serum concentrations in the presence of probenecid *(48,120–123)*. Although probenecid significantly affects renal clearance of piperacillin/tazobactam, it does not significantly effect area under the curve or half-life of piperacillin/tazobactam *(124)*.

This drug–drug interaction may be clinically beneficial in certain situations in which higher penicillin serum concentrations are necessary (e.g., in the treatment of meningitis or endocarditis). However, careful monitoring or avoidance of this combination should be considered in certain patient populations in whom drug accumulation may occur (e.g., elderly patients or patients with impaired renal function).

## Proguanil

Babalola et al. conducted a study in healthy volunteers to evaluate the coadministration of proguanil and cloxacillin on the pharmacokinetics of cloxacillin *(125)*. Differences in pharmacokinetic parameter values for cloxacillin alone or in the presence of proguanil were determined by assaying urinary samples. Both the maximum excretion rate and total amount of excreted unchanged cloxacillin were reduced by approx 50% when taken with proguanil compared to proguanil alone ($p < 0.0001$). No differences were noted in cloxacillin half-life or $T_{max}$. The authors suggested that separating these two agents by 1–2 hours may avoid this potential interaction.

## Sulfonamides

The concurrent administration of penicillins and sulfonamides was evaluated in a pharmacokinetic study *(49)*. The unbound concentrations of penicillin G, penicillin V, nafcillin, and dicloxacillin were increased with the concurrent administration of several sulfonamides. The researcher postulated that this interaction occurred as a result of the displacement of penicillins from protein-binding sites *(49)*. In a separate study, Kunin reported that the coadministration of oral oxacillin and sulfonamides caused a decrease in oxacillin serum concentrations. The author postulated that perhaps the sulfonamides may cause reduced absorption of oral oxacillin; however, additional mechanisms cannot be ruled out *(49)*. Based on these limited clinical data, avoidance of penicillins and sulfonamides is not warranted.

## Tetracyclines

As stated in the Chloramphenicol section, the administration of a bacteriostatic agent, such as tetracycline or related compounds, may antagonize the bactericidal activity of β-lactams. Nonetheless, both antagonism and synergy between penicillins and tetracyclines has been documented in in vitro and in vivo studies *(126–130)*.

Lepper and Dowling reported the outcome of 57 patients diagnosed with pneumococcal meningitis who were treated with high-dose penicillin ($n = 43$) or high-dose penicillin along with the tetracycline antibiotic aureomycin (*n* = 14) *(131)*. Although the severity of illness appeared similar between the treatment groups, mortality rates were significantly higher in the patients who received combination therapy compared to penicillin alone (79 vs 30%). Olsson and colleagues also noted a trend toward increased mortality in patients with pneumococcal meningitis treated with penicillin in combination with a tetracycline derivative (85%; *n* = 7) vs penicillin alone (52%; *n* = 23) or erythromycin alone (50%; *n* = 6) *(132)*. Strom noted that treatment of hemolytic streptococci with penicillin in combination with chlortetracycline compared to penicillin alone had similar initial clinical response, but the penicillin/chlortetracycline group experienced a higher incidence of reinfection *(133)*.

Unlike the case studies involving meningitis, Ahern and Kirby reported similar clinical outcomes in patients treated with penicillin alone vs penicillin in combination with aureomycin for pneumococci pneumonia *(134)*. The authors suggested that the role of rapid, bactericidal activity of penicillin is of more clinical significance in treating meningitis compared to less-severe infections such as pneumonia. Adhern and Kirby stressed the importance of penicillin's role in treating meningitis because of the relatively limited phagocytic activity in the subarachnoid space compared to nonmeningeal infections such as pneumonia.

Avoiding the combination of penicillin and tetracycline derivatives appears appropriate in severe infections requiring rapid bactericidal activity such as meningitis. In less-severe infections, the use of these drugs in combination has not been documented to affect outcomes adversely.

### Vecuronium

The concurrent administration of vecuronium and acylaminopenicillins has been reported to prolong muscle paralysis in both humans and animals *(135–138)*. Condon et al. conducted a double-blind clinical trial to determine the ability of piperacillin or cefoxitin (control agent) to prolong the muscular blockade of vecuronium *(139)*. Patients were eligible for study enrollment if they were undergoing an elective operation with general anesthesia that required antibiotic prophylaxis. Patients were subsequently randomly assigned to receive piperacillin or cefoxitin as the prophylactic antibiotic prior to the operation. All patients received vecuronium for muscle relaxation. Prolongation of neuromuscular blockade was determined before and after the administration of the antibiotic by the electromyographic twitch response. Of the 27 evaluable patients enrolled in the study, 5 patients (2 on piperacillin and 3 on cefoxitin) exhibited a nonclinically significant prolongation of neuromuscular blockade. Otherwise, the rate and extent of neuromuscular blockade was similar between groups. It appears that this interaction is clinically insignificant, although knowledge of this potential prolongation may be useful in certain surgical settings.

### Miscellaneous Agents

The concomitant administration of penicillins and acidic drugs such as phenylbutazone, sulfinpyearazone, indomethacin, and sulfaphenazole may prolong the half-life of penicillin. This is postulated to occur as a result of competition between the acidic drugs and penicillin for renal tubular secretory proteins *(48)*. In this investigation, the half-life of penicillin was not noted to change significantly with concomitant administration of chlorothiazide, sulfamethizole, and sulfamethoxypyearidazine *(48)*.

Potential drug–drug interactions between the penicillins and theophylline have also been investigated. The coadministration of amoxicillin, ampicillin, ticarcillin/clavulanic acid, or ampicillin/sulbactam with theophylline was not noted to alter theophylline's properties *(140–144)*.

Deppermann et al. assessed the effect of the coadministration of pirenzepine, an antimuscarinic, with various antibiotics including amoxicillin in a double-blind, randomized crossover study *(4)*. Coadministration of pirenzepine with amoxicillin did not significantly alter the pharmacokinetics of amoxicillin.

## CEPHALOSPORIN DRUG INTERACTIONS

### Acid-Suppressive Agents

#### Ranitidine and Famotidine

Concomitant administration of the prodrugs cefpodoxime proxetil, cefuroxime axetil, and cefditoren pivoxil with agents that increase gastric pH, such as ranitidine, results in a reduction of the antibiotic serum concentrations *(5,145)*. The bioavailability of the cefpodoxime proxetil has been reported to decrease by approx 30–40% with concurrent administration of an $H_2$-receptor antagonist *(145,146)*. However, no impact on the bioavailability of cefpodoxime was noted when famotidine administration was separated from cefpodoxime by 2 hours. Similarly, the AUC of cefuroxime axetil was reduced by approx 40% with pretreatment of ranitidine and sodium bicarbonate *(5)*. The $C_{max}$ and AUC of cefditoren pivoxil were reduced by approx 25% with the concurrent administration of famotidine *(147)*. Other studies have found no significant effect on the bioavailability of cephalexin and cefaclor AF when administered concomitantly with $H_2$-receptor antagonists *(4,148)*. Based on the results from these studies, concurrent administration of $H_2$-receptor antagonists and cefuroxime axetil, cefpodoxime proxetil, and cefditoren pivoxil should be avoided. If these agents need to be administered concurrently, the cephalosporins should be given at least 2 hours after the $H_2$-receptor antagonist.

#### Antacids

The coadministration of antacids and certain cephalosporins, including Cefaclor CD®, cefdinir, cefpodoxime, and cefditoren may lead to decreased concentrations of the antibiotics *(145–149)*. A variety of studies have reported decreases in cephalosporin AUC and $C_{max}$ to be in the range of 20–40% for cefaclor, cefdinir, and cefpodoxime when administered with an antacid *(145,148,149)*. A minimal reduction in $C_{max}$ (14%) and AUC (11%) was noted with the concurrent administration of cefditoren with an antacid *(147)*. Other investigators have found no effect with cephalexin *(4)* or cefixime *(150)* when administered concomitantly with antacids. Certain cephalosporins, including Cefaclor CD, cefdinir, cefpodoxime, and cefditoren, should not be coadministered with antacids. If antacids are required during therapy, the cephalosporins should be separated from the antacid administration by at least 2 hours.

### Calcium Channel Blockers

Variable data exist regarding the effects of nifedipine on cephalosporin pharmacokinetics *(151,152)*. In a randomized crossover study, each healthy volunteer received cefixime with nifedipine or placebo *(152)*. The absolute bioavailability of cefixime was increased from 31 (cefixime alone) to 53% (cefixime and nifedipine) ($p < 0.01$). The $AUC_{0-\infty}$ also increased from 16.1 mg · (cefixime alone) compared to 25.4 mg · hours/L (cefixime and nifedipine) ($p < 0.01$) *(152)*. These investigators have also shown increased cephalexin concentrations with coadministration of nifedipine or diltiazem in an animal model *(153)*. The authors concluded that nifedipine can increase the absorption of these cephalosporins by enhancing the active transport mechanism in the intestine. In contrast, another study demonstrated that the pharmacokinetics of cefpodoxime did not change when coadministered with nifedipine *(151)*. Because of differences in specific antimicrobials and lack of adverse events seen with calcium channel blocker and cephalosporin combinations, no dosage changes are recommended when these agents are coadministered.

### Cholestyramine

The coadministration of cholestyramine with cefadroxil or cephalexin has been shown to cause a delay in absorption associated with a prolonged $T_{max}$ and reduction in $C_{max}$ *(154,155)*. Despite these pharmacokinetic alterations, other important parameters such as AUC or amount of drug excreted in the urine were minimally affected. Although data for this interaction are limited, the clinical significance is doubtful, particularly considering that cholestyramine does not appear to alter cephalosporin exposure.

### Contraceptives: Oral Estrogen

Refer to this topic in the discussion of penicillin.

### Ethanol: Disulfiramlike Reactions

Semisynthetic cephalosporins containing a methyltetrazolethiol (MTT) side chain, such as cefamandole, cefoperazone, cefmenoxime, cefotetan, and moxalactam, have been documented to cause disulfiramlike reactions in patients who consume ethanol during antibiotic treatment *(156–158)*. Cephalosporins with an MTT side chain inhibit acetaldehyde dehydrogenase, which results in the accumulation of acetaldehyde, a toxic metabolite of ethanol. Patients should be instructed not to consume alcohol during and for several days following antibiotic therapy. Refer to Chapter 12 regarding antimicrobials and food interactions for a more detailed review of this topic.

### Iron

Coadministration of ferrous sulfate appears to cause a chelation complex and reduce the absorption of cefdinir *(159)*. In a randomized three-way crossover study, six healthy male subjects received the following regimens: 200 mg cefdinir alone, 200 mg cefdinir plus 1050 mg ferrous sulfate sustained release, or 200 mg cefdinir followed by 1050 mg ferrous sulfate sustained release 3 hours later *(159)*. The $AUC_{0-12} \pm SD$ (µg · hours/mL) was significantly lower in the groups that received cefdinir concomitantly with ferrous sulfate ($0.78 \pm 0.25$ µg · hours/mL) or at 3 hours following the dose of cefdinir ($6.55 \pm 1.61$ µg · hours/mL) compared to cefdinir alone ($10.3 \pm 1.35$ µg · hours/mL) ($p < 0.05$). To avoid the potential for therapeutic failure of cefdinir, it should not be taken together with ferrous sulfate.

### Metoclopramide

A healthy volunteer, crossover study evaluated the effect of food, metoclopramide, propantheline, and probenecid on the pharmacokinetics of cefprozil *(160)*. In the metoclopramide arm of the study, volunteers received cefprozil alone or cefprozil given 0.5 hours after a dose of metoclopramide. Both isomers of cefprozil, *cis* and *trans*, were assayed in blood and urine. Cefprozil's isomers demonstrated a statistically significant reduction in mean residence time when administered after metoclopramide; however, there was no difference in $AUC_{0-\infty}$ or half-life of cefprozil among the treatment groups. Administration of metoclopramide prior to cefprozil did not affect its extent of absorption. Concurrent administration of these agents need not be avoided.

### Methotrexate

Rabbits receiving concomitant infusions of MTX and a cephalosporin (ceftriaxone, ceftazidime, ceftizoxime, or cefoperazone) have been demonstrated to have an increased renal elimination of MTX and 7-hydroxymethotrexate *(100,101)*.

In a case report, an 8-year-old boy receiving MTX for non-Hodgkin's lymphoma experienced a decrease in MTX clearance when MTX was coadministered with piperacillin *(104)*. The patient subsequently received MTX along with ceftazidime without any impact on MTX clearance. The differences seen in MTX renal elimination between cephalosporins and piperacillin may be because of the extent of tubular secretion (penicillins > cephalosporins) *(100,161)*.

Based on the limited data available, there have been no documented interactions resulting in decreased renal elimination of MTX with the concurrent administration of cephalosporins. However, because of the documented interaction between some penicillins and MTX, close monitoring of MTX concentrations and signs of toxicity (e.g., bone marrow suppression, nephrotoxicity, mucositis) is suggested during concurrent use of cephalosporins and MTX.

### Nonsteroidal Anti-Inflammatory Drugs

Diclofenac has been reported to cause an increase in the biliary excretion of ceftriaxone *(162)*. A study was conducted in patients in whom a cholecystectomy was performed and a drain was placed in the common bile duct *(162)*. The subjects who received ceftriaxone along with diclofenac demonstrated a 320% ($p < 0.05$) increase in the amount of ceftriaxone excreted in the bile and a 56% ($p < 0.05$) reduction in the amount excreted in the urine. Because of limited data, no therapeutic recommendations can be made.

### Phenytoin

Highly protein-bound antibiotics such as ceftriaxone (approx 90% bound to plasma proteins) *(112)* have the potential to interact with other highly protein-bound agents such as phenytoin *(114)*. Because of protein displacement, high doses of ceftriaxone may increase unbound concentrations of phenytoin in certain patient populations *(114)*. Dasgupta and colleagues performed an in vitro study to determine the effect of ceftriaxone in displacing phenytoin from protein-binding sites *(114)*. Estimated peak ceftriaxone concentrations (270 and 361 μmol/L) were added to pooled sera from patients receiving phenytoin. Three groups with varying albumin concentrations were evaluated. The greatest ceftriaxone-induced displacement effect was seen the group with the lowest albumin concentration (25 g/L). In this group, the unbound phenytoin concentrations (μmol/L) (SD) were 8.12 (0.28) for the control, 9.39 (0.12) for 270 μmol/L ceftriaxone, and 9.93 (0.36) for 361 μmol/L ceftriaxone. Although the increases appear minor, significant increases in unbound phenytoin concentrations were noted in all groups compared to the control group ($p < 0.05$). In patients receiving ceftriaxone concomitantly with phenytoin, monitoring of unbound and total serum concentrations of phenytoin in addition to watching for signs of phenytoin toxicity is warranted.

## Oral Anticoagulants

Semisynthetic cephalosporins containing an MTT substituent at the 3-position, such as cefamandole, cefoperazone, cefmenoxime, cefotetan, and moxalactam, have been associated with the development of a hypoprothrombinemia *(163)*. Several case reports have implicated these agents in prolonged PT or bleeding episodes in patients *(164– 170)*. Angaran and colleagues retrospectively assessed the effect of prophylactic administration of cefamandole or vancomycin on the warfarin anticoagulation response in 60 postsurgical patients *(171)*. Patients who received cefamandole had a higher proportion of elevated PTs compared with those who received vancomycin (14 vs 1, $p <$ 0.05). In another study, these same investigators characterized the effect of cefazolin, cefamandole, and vancomycin on warfarin anticoagulation in patients after cardiac valve replacement *(172)*. They noted that the greatest number of patients ($n = 6$) with elevated PTs received cefamandole compared to cefazolin ($n = 1$) and vancomycin ($n = 1$). In addition, cefamandole therapy was associated with a 15–20% greater change in PTs compared to the cefazolin and vancomycin ($p < 0.01$). Patients who are malnourished or who have renal insufficiency may be at higher risk for this interaction *(164)*. The exact mechanism of the hypoprothrombinemic phenomenon is unknown, although several mechanisms have been proposed *(97,173–176)*. Clinicians are cautioned to monitor for signs and symptoms of bleeding, PT, and activated partial thromboplastin time in patients receiving cephalosporins with an MTT side chain and concomitant therapy with oral anticoagulants.

## Probenecid

Probenecid can increase the serum concentrations of most renally eliminated cephalosporins *(148,160,177–191)*. Although other mechanisms may contribute, probenecid appears to inhibit tubular secretion of cephalosporins, resulting in their decreased renal elimination *(115,116)*. The AUCs of ceftizoxime, cefoxitin, cefaclor, and cefdinir have been reported to increase by approx 50–100% with the coadministration of probenecid *(115,179,180)*. Probenecid has been documented to prolong the half-life and increase the serum concentration of many other cephalosporins as well *(148,149,160,177–192)*. Certain cephalosporins, such as ceforanide, ceftazidime, ceftriaxone, and moxalactam, are eliminated through a different pathway, and their pharmacokinetics are not significantly altered by probenecid *(177,178,193–198)*.

Achieving high cephalosporin concentrations may be clinically beneficial in certain situations (e.g., in the treatment of meningitis or endocarditis); however, caution or avoidance of this combination should be considered in certain patient populations in which drug accumulation may occur (e.g., elderly patients or patients with impaired renal function).

### Propantheline

A healthy volunteer, crossover study evaluated the effect of food, metoclopramide, propantheline, and probenecid on the pharmacokinetics of cefprozil *(160)*. In the propantheline arm of the study, volunteers received cefprozil alone or cefprozil given 0.5 hours after a dose of propantheline. Both isomers of cefprozil, *cis* and *trans*, were assayed in blood and urine samples. There was no difference in cefprozil $AUC_{0-\infty}$ or half-life in either treatment group. The administration of propantheline prior to cefprozil does not affect the extent of cefprozil absorption. No special precautions seem necessary for this combination.

### Theophylline

The coadministration of cephalexin or cefaclor with theophylline has not been documented to significantly alter any pharmacokinetic parameters of theophylline *(199–201)*. However, Hammond and Abate reported a case of a possible interaction between theophylline and cefaclor, which resulted in theophylline toxicity *(202)*. It was unclear whether this was an actual drug–drug interaction or the effect of an acute viral illness on theophylline disposition. Based on these limited data, no dosage recommendations are necessary.

### Miscellaneous Agents

Older cephalosporins such as cephalothin and cephaloridine have been reported to cause nephrotoxicity *(203,204)*. The coadministration of these older cephalosporins with other potential nephrotoxic agents, including colistin *(204,205)*, various aminoglycosides *(203,206–212)*, and furosemide *(213–216)*, has been associated with an increased incidence of nephrotoxicity. The clinical impact of this interaction is limited because these cephalosporins are rarely used in current clinical practice; however, careful monitoring of renal function is warranted if such combinations are prescribed. These drug–drug interactions have not been documented as a clinically significant problem for any of the newer cephalosporins *(217–219)*.

## CARBAPENEMS

### Probenecid

Concomitant probenecid can increase the concentration of the carbapenems. It is proposed that probenecid inhibits tubular secretion of the carbapenems, resulting in their decreased renal elimination. Meropenem's half-life and AUC were increased by 33 and 55%, respectively, when coadministered with probenecid *(220)*. Probenecid has less impact on the renal elimination of ertapenem and imipenem. The combination of ertapenem and probenecid produced a 20% increase in half-life and a 25% increase in the AUC of ertapenem compared to ertapenem alone *(221)*. In contrast, imipenem's half-life and AUC only increased 6 and 13%, respectively, when coadministered with probenecid *(222)*.

Achieving high concentrations of carbapenems may be clinically beneficial in infections in which higher serum concentrations are necessary. However, caution or avoidance of this combination should be considered in patient populations in which drug accumulation may occur (such as elderly patients or patients with impaired renal function). The increased serum concentration noted as a result of this drug–drug interaction may increase the risk of central nervous system toxicity of these agents.

## Valproic Acid

Limited data suggest that the coadministration of carbapenems and valproic acid may lead to decreased concentrations of valproic acid. DeTurck and colleagues described two case reports in which valproic acid concentrations were decreased following the administration of meropenem and amikacin *(223)*. Both patients were receiving valproic acid for seizure prophylaxis. The first patient was receiving valproic acid as a continuous infusion following the placement of a ventricular drain to relieve obstructive hydrocephalus secondary to a subdural hemorrhage. Steady-state valproic acid concentrations were maintained between 50 and 100 mg/L; however, the addition of meropenem and amikacin therapy resulted in subtherapeutic valproic acid concentrations within 2 days. In the second case report, the authors described a female patient receiving valproic acid following clipping of multiple cerebral aneurysms. Similar to the previous case, valproic acid concentrations decreased suddenly with addition of meropenem. Other authors have reported data on three cases describing a potential interaction with valproic acid and panipenem/betamipron, a carbapenem *(224)*. Animal models have also found decreased valproic acid concentrations with the concurrent administration of imipenem *(225)*, meropenem *(226)*, or panipenem *(227)* and valproic acid. Monitoring for alteration in valproic acid concentrations during concurrent carbapenem therapy seems reasonable to avoid the possibility of subtherapeutic valproic acid serum concentrations.

## IMIPENEM/CILASTATIN

### Cyclosporine

Based on case reports, cyclosporine and imipenem/cilastatin may demonstrate additive central nervous system toxicity when administered concomitantly. Bösmuller and colleagues reported five transplant patients experiencing central nervous system toxicity during administration of cyclosporine and imipenem/cilastatin *(228)*. None of these patients reported a history of seizures. Four of the five patients experienced a seizure despite cyclosporine concentrations within normal therapeutic range. The fifth patient experienced myclonia; this was associated with an elevated cyclosporine concentration of 900 ng/mL. Symptoms of central nervous toxicity occurred within 1 day in four patients, and symptoms resolved in all patients with discontinuation of imipenem/cilastatin or dose reduction of cyclosporine.

Zazgornik and colleagues published a case report of a 62-year-old female receiving imipenem/cilastatin and cyclosporine who developed central nervous system toxicity *(229)*. The patient had recently received a renal transplant secondary to interstitial nephritis and was receiving imipenem/cilastatin for a urinary tract infection. Following the second dose of imipenem/cilastatin, the patient experienced confusion, agitation, and tremors, which resulted in the discontinuation of imipenem/cilastatin. The serum cyclosporine concentration, which was obtained 4 days after imipenem/cilastatin therapy, was elevated at 1000 ng/mL compared to a previous level of 400 ng/mL. In contrast, an investigation in a rat model demonstrated decreased cyclosporine serum concentrations when it was coadministered with imipenem/cilastatin *(230)*.

Because both imipenem and cyclosporine administered alone may have the potential to cause central nervous system side effects, it is difficult to determine what role the combination of these agents may have played in these reports. Based on these limited clinical data, avoidance of imipenem and cyclosporine is not warranted.

### *Theophylline*

Semel and Allen reported three cases of seizures occurring in patients receiving imipenem/cilastatin and theophylline *(231)*. None of the patients had a previous history of neurological or seizure disorder. The authors concluded that the seizures could be caused by both drugs' ability to inhibit γ-aminobutyric acid binding to receptors. It is difficult to differentiate the potential for seizures between the administration of imipenem/cilastatin alone and the combination of imipenem/cilastatin and theophylline. Avoiding coadministration of theophylline and imipenem/cilastatin is not warranted.

### *Ganciclovir*

Patients have experienced generalized seizures during concomitant imipenem/cilastatin and ganciclovir therapy *(232)*. No additional information is available on these patients. Because of these limited data, it is difficult to differentiate the potential for seizures of imipenem/cilastatin alone or the combination of imipenem/cilastatin and ganciclovir. The manufacturer does not recommend coadministration of imipenem/cilastatin and ganciclovir unless the benefits outweigh the risks.

## MONOBACTAMS

### *Inducers of β-Lactams*

Antimicrobials that can induce the production of β-lactamases, such as cefoxitin and imipenem, should not be used concurrently with aztreonam in the treatment of certain infections, depending on the causative microorganism *(233)*. This β-lactamase production by certain Gram-negative aerobes, such as *Enterobacter* and *Pseudomonas* species, may lead to the inactivation of aztreonam. Based on the organism isolated and susceptibility results, one should consider this potential interaction when choosing an antimicrobial regimen.

### *Probenecid*

Concomitant probenecid can increase aztreonam concentrations *(234)*. It is proposed that probenecid inhibits tubular secretion resulting in decreased aztreonam renal elimination. In a randomized crossover trial, six healthy men received aztreonam alone or aztreonam along with probenecid *(234)*. Coadministration of probenecid with aztreonam increased aztreonam concentrations from $81.7 \pm 3.4$ to $86.0 \pm 2.2$ μg/mL. This interaction seems to carry minimal clinical risk. No recommendation to avoid the concurrent administration of probenecid and aztreonam seems warranted.

### CASE STUDY 2

A 72-year-old male with a 10-year history of adult onset diabetes mellitus has been poorly controlled on rosiglitazone, with complications of diabetic retinopathy and multiple episodes of lower extremity infections. He also takes 5 mg warfarin daily status post-pulmonary embolism. Seven days ago, he presented to his local doctor with an infected left baby toe after "bumping it" on the leg of a chair. At that time, his doctor started him empirically on 500 mg dicloxacillin twice daily for 7 days. At his follow-up visit a week later, although his infection was better, it was noted that his INR had changed from 2.2 to less than 1.0.

A decreased anticoagulant effect for warfarin has been documented when given concomitantly with semisynthetic penicillins like nafcillin or dicloxacillin. It has been postulated that, because these antibiotics induce the P450 cytochrome system, this may lead to an increased warfarin metabolism.

Avoiding the concomitant use of dicloxacillin and warfarin is justified in this patient to avert this interaction. Selection of another antimicrobial that does not interfere with warfarin metabolism would be a more reasonable approach in this patient.

## CASE STUDY 3

A 45-year-old white male complaining of earache, pressure above his eyebrows, and cough producing thick, white purulent sputum for the last 2 weeks presented to the outpatient clinic for help. The patient also complained of inability to sleep because of feeling hot, having a constant pressure in his ears, and chest soreness. He stated that he has had a productive cough for several months at a time over the last 3 years. He routinely takes one 65-mg aspirin daily and one multivitamin supplemented with extra iron. The clinic doctor prescribed 300 mg cefdinir twice daily for 10 days. Despite taking the medication as directed, he returned to the clinic 5 days later with only minimal improvement of his symptoms and a temperature of 101.1°F. The clinic doctor discontinued the cefdinir and started another antibiotic.

The apparent clinical failure in this patient may have been caused by the coadministration of ferrous sulfate and cefdinir. This combination has been shown to result in a chelation complex that results in reduced absorption of cefdinir.

To avoid the potential for therapeutic failure with cefdinir therapy in this instance, the two drugs should not be taken together. Or, if the cefdinir therapy is considered essential, then the drug should be taken at least 2 hours before administration of the iron-containing product.

## REFERENCES

1. Rogers HJ, James CA, Morrison PJ. Effect of cimetidine on oral absorption of ampicillin and cotrimoxazole. J Antimicrob Chemother 1980;6:297–300.
2. Paulsen O, Hoglund P, Walder M. No effect of omeprazole-induced hypoacidity on the bioavailability of ampicillin and bacampicillin. Scand J Infect Dis 1989;21:219–223.
3. Stainforth DH, Clarke HL, Horton R, et al. Augmentin bioavailability following cimetidine, aluminum hydroxide and milk. Int J Clin Pharmacol Ther Toxicol 1985;23:154–157.
4. Deppermann KM, Lode H, Hoffken G, et al. Influence of ranitidine, pirenzepine, and aluminum magnesium hydroxide on the bioavailability of various antibiotics, including amoxicillin, cephalexin, doxycycline, and amoxicillin-clavulanic acid. Antimicrob Agents Chemother 1989;33:1901–1907.

5. Sommers DK, Van Wyk M, Moncrieff J. Influence of food and reduced gastric acidity on the bioavailability of bacampicillin and cefuroxime axetil. Br J Clin Pharm 1984:18: 535–539.

6. Jick H, Porter JB. Potentiation of ampicillin skin reactions by allopurinol or hyperuricemia. J Clin Pharmacol 1981;21:456–458.

7. Fessel WJ. Immunologic reactivity in hyperuricemia. N Engl J Med 1972;286:1218.

8. Townsend RS. In vitro inactivation of gentamicin by ampicillin. Am J Hosp Pharm 1989;46:2250–2251.

9. McLaughlin JE, Reeves DS. Clinical and laboratory evidence for inactivation of gentamicin by carbenicillin. Lancet 1971;1:261–264.

10. Uber WE, Brundage RC, White RL, et al. In vivo inactivation of tobramycin by piperacillin. DICP Ann Pharmacother 1991;25:357–359.

11. Halstenson CE, Hirata CA, Heim-Duthoy KL, et al. Effect of concomitant administration of piperacillin on the disposition of netilmicin and tobramycin in patients with end-stage renal disease. Antimicrob Agents Chemother 1990;34:128–133.

12. Davies M, Morgan JR, Anand C. Interactions of carbenicillin and ticarcillin with gentamicin. Antimicrob Agents Chemother 1975;7:431–434.

13. Weibert R, Keane W, Shapiro F. Carbenicillin inactivation of aminoglycosides in patients with severe renal failure. Trans Am Soc Artif Organs 1976;22:439.

14. Eykyn S, Philips I, Ridley M. Gentamicin plus carbenicillin. Lancet 1 1971;13:545,546.

15. Davies M, Morgan JR, Anand C. Interactions of carbenicillin and ticarcillin with gentamicin. Antimicrob Agents Chemother 1975:7:431–434.

16. Kradjian WA, Burger R. In vivo inactivation of gentamicin by carbenicillin and ticarcillin. Arch Intern Med 1980;140:1668–1670.

17. Lau A, Lee M, Flascha S, et al. Effect of piperacillin on tobramycin pharmacokinetics in patients with normal renal function. Antimicrob Agents Chemother 1983;24:533–537.

18. Hitt CM, Patel KB, Nicolau DP, Zhu Z, Nightingale CH. Influence of piperacillin-tazobactam on pharmacokinetics of gentamicin given once daily. Am J Health Syst Pharm 1997;1:2704–2708.

19. Dowell JA, Korth-Bradley J, Milisci M, et al. Evaluating possible pharmacokinetic interactions between tobramycin, piperacillin, and a combination of piperacillin and tazobactam in patients with various degrees of renal impairment. J Clin Pharmacol 2001;41:979–986.

20. Noone P, Pattison JR. Therapeutic implications of interaction of gentamicin and penicillins. Lancet 1971;2:575–578.

21. Ervin FR, Bullock WE, Nuttall CE. Inactivation of gentamicin by penicillins in patients with renal failure. Antimicrob Agents Chemother 1976;9:1009–1011.

22. Cheng SH, White A. Effect of orally administered neomycin on the absorption of penicillin V. N Engl J Med 1962;267:1296–1297.

23. Moellering RC, Wennersten C, Weinberg AN. Synergy of penicillin and gentamicin against enterococci. J Infect Dis 1971;S124:207.

24. Guenthner SH, Chao HP, Wenzel RP. Synergy between amikacin and ticarcillin or mezlocillin against nosocomial bloodstream isolates. J Antimicrob Chemother 1986;18:550–552.

25. Laverdiere M, Gallimore B, Restieri C, et al. In vitro synergism of ceftriaxone combined with aminoglycosides against *Pseudomonas aeruginosa*. Diagn Microbiol Infect Dis 1994;19:39–46.

26. Marks MI, Hammerberg S, Greenstone G, et al. Activity of newer aminoglycosides and carbenicillin, alone, and in combination against gentamicin-resistant *Pseudomonas aeruginosa*. Antimicrob Agents Chemother 1976;10:399–401.

27. Moellering RC, Wennersten, Weinberg AJ. Studies on antibiotic synergism against enterococci. I. Bacteriologic studies. J Lab Clin Med 1971;77:821–828.

28. Weinstein AJ, Moellering RC. Penicillin and gentamicin therapy for enterococcal infections. JAMA 1973;223:1030–1032.
29. Anderson ET, Young LS, Hewitt WL. Antimicrobial synergism in the therapy of Gram-negative rod bacteremia. Chemotherapy 1978;24:45–54.
30. Brown CH, Natelson EA, Bradshaw MW, et al. The hemostatic defect produced by carbenicillin. N Engl J Med 1974;291:265–270.
31. Brown CH, Natelson EA, Bradshaw MW, et al. Study of the effects of ticarcillin on blood coagulation and platelet function. Antimicrob Agents Chemother 1975;7:652–657.
32. Brown CH, Bradshaw MW, Natelson EA, et al. Defective platelet function following the administration of penicillin compounds. Blood 1976;6:949–956.
33. Andrassy K, Ritz E, Hasper B, et al. Penicillin-induced coagulation disorder. Lancet 1976;2:1039–1041.
34. Andrassy K, Weischedel E, Ritz E, et al. Bleeding in uremic patients after carbenicillin. Thrombos Haemost 1976;36:115–126.
35. Tabernero Romo JM, Corbacho L, Sanchez S, et al. Effects of carbenicillin on blood coagulation; a study in patients with chronic renal failure. Clin Nephrol 1979;11:31–34.
36. Wisloff F, Larsen JP, Dahle A, et al. Effect of prophylactic high-dose treatment with ampicillin and cloxacillin on bleeding time and bleeding in patients undergoing elective vascular surgery. Scand J Haematol 1983;31:97–101.
37. Lurie A, Ogilvie M, Gold CH, et al. Carbenicillin-induced coagulopathy. S Afr Med J 1974;48:457–461.
38. Taylor AT, Pritchard DC, Goldstein AO, et al. Continuation of warfarin-nafcillin interaction during dicloxacillin therapy. J Fam Pract 1994;39:182–185.
39. Heilker GM, Fowler JW, Self TH, et al. Possible nafcillin-warfarin interaction. Arch Intern Med 1994;154:822–824.
40. Qureshi GD, Reinders TP, Somori GJ, et al. Warfarin resistance with nafcillin therapy. Ann Intern Med 1984;100:527–529.
41. Shovick VA, Rihn TL. Decreased hypoprothrombinemic response to warfarin secondary to the warfarin-nafcillin interaction. Drug Intell Clin Pharm 1991;25:598–600.
42. Krstenansky PM, Jones WN, Garewal HS. Effect of dicloxacillin sodium on the hypoprothrombinemic response to warfarin sodium. Clin Pharm 1987;6:804–806.
43. Mailloux AT, Gidal BE, Sorkness CA. Potential interaction between warfarin and dicloxacillin. Ann Pharmacother 1996;30:1402–1407.
44. Davis RL, Berman W, Wernly JA, et al. Warfarin-nafcillin interaction. J Pediatr 1991;118:300–303.
45. Rolinson GN, Sutherland R. The binding of antibiotics to serum proteins. Br J Pharmacol 1965;25:638–650.
46. Brown MA, Korchinski ED, Miller DR. Interaction of penicillin-G and warfarin? Can J Hosp Pharm 1979;32:18,19.
47. Davydov L, Yermolnik M, Cuni LJ. Warfarin and amoxicillin/clavulanate drug interaction. Ann Pharmacother 2003;37:367–370.
48. Kampmann J, Molholm Hansen J, Siersbaek-Nielsen K, Laursen H. Effect of some drugs on penicillin half-life in blood. Clin Pharmacol Ther 1972;13:516–519.
49. Kunin CM. Clinical pharmacology of the new penicillins. II. Effect of drugs which interfere with binding to serum proteins. Clin Pharmacol Ther 1966;7:180–188.
50. Suffness M, Rose BS. Potential drug interactions and adverse effects related to aspirin. Drug Intell Clin Pharm 1974;8:694–699.
51. Moskowitz B, Somani SM, McDonald RH. Salicylate interaction with penicillin and secobarbital binding sites on human serum albumin. Clin Toxicol 1973;6:247–256.
52. Hayes AH. Therapeutic implications of drug interactions with acetaminophen and aspirin. Arch Intern Med 1981:141:301–304.
53. Schafer-Korting M, Kirch W, Axthelm T, et al. Atenolol interaction with aspirin, allopurinol, and ampicillin. Clin Pharmacol Ther 1983;33:283–288.

54. McLean AJ, Tonkin A, McCarthy P, et al. Dose-dependence of atenolol-ampicillin interaction. Br J Clin Pharmacol 1984;18:969–971.

55. Westphal JF, Trouvin JH, Deslandes A, et al. Nifedipine enhances amoxicillin absorption kinetics and bioavailability in humans. J Pharmacol Exp Ther 1990;255:312–317.

56. Lang CC, Jamal SK, Mohamed Z, et al. Evidence of an interaction between nifedipine and nafcillin in humans. Br J Clin Pharmacol 2003;55:588–590.

57. Jawetz E. Gunnison JB, Coleman VR. The combined action of penicillin with streptomycin or chloromycetin on enterococci in vitro. Science 1950;3:254–256.

58. Wallace JF, Smith H, Garcia M, et al. Studies on the pathogenesis of meningitis. VI Antagonism between penicillin and chloramphenicol in experimental pneumococcal meningitis. J Lab Clin Med 1967;70:408–418.

59. Yourassowsky E, Monsieur R. Antagonism limit of penicillin G and chloramphenicol against *Neisseria meningitidis*. Arzneimittel Forsch 1971;21:1385–1387.

60. Gjessing HC, Odegaard K. Oral chloramphenicol alone and with intramuscular procaine penicillin in the treatment of gonorrhoea. Br J Vener Dis 1967;43:133–136.

61. DeRitis F, Giammanco G, Manzillo G. Chloramphenicol combined with ampicillin in treatment of typhoid. Br Med J 1972;4:17,18.

62. Ali HM. Reduced ampicillin bioavailability following oral coadministration with chloroquine. J Antimicrob Chemother 1985;15:781–784.

63. Barriere SL, Catlin DH, Orlando PL, et al. Alteration in the pharmacokinetic disposition of ciprofloxacin by simultaneous administration of azlocillin. Antimicrob Agents Chemother 1990;34:823–826.

64. Peterson LR, Moody JA, Fasching CE, et al. In vivo and in vitro activity of ciprofloxacin plus azlocillin against 12 streptococcal isolates in a neutropenic site model. Diagn Microbiol Infect Dis 1987;7:127–136.

65. Dossetor J. Drug interaction with oral contraceptive steroids [editorial]. Br Med J 1980; 280:467,468.

66. DeSano EA, Hurley SC. Possible interaction of antihistamines and antibiotics with oral contraceptive effectiveness. Fertil Steril 1982;1:853,854.

67. Bainton R. Interaction between antibiotic therapy and contraceptive medication. Oral Surg Oral Med Oral Pathol 1986;61:453–455.

68. Silber TJ. Apparent oral contraceptive failure associated with antibiotic administration. J Adolesc Health Care 1983;4:287–289.

69. Miller DM, Helms SE, Brodell RT. A practical approach to antibiotic treatment in women taking oral contraceptives. J Am Acad Dermatol 1994;30:1008–1011.

70. Fernandez N, Sierra M, Diez MJ, et al. Study of the pharmacokinetic interaction between ethinylestradiol and amoxicillin in rabbits. Contraception 1997;55:47–52.

71. Back DJ, Brenckenridge AM, Cross KJ, et al. An antibiotic interaction with ethinyloestradiol in the rat and rabbit. J Steroid Biochem 1982;16:407–413.

72. Back DJ, Breckenridge AM, MacIver M, et al. The effects of ampicillin on oral contraceptive steroids in women. Br J Clin Pharmacol 1982;14:43–48.

73. Friedman CI, Huneke AL, Kim MH, et al. The effect of ampicillin on oral contraceptive effectiveness. Obstet Gynecol 1980;55:33–37.

74. Joshi JV, Joshi UM, Sankholi GM, et al. A study of interaction of low-dose combination oral contraceptive with ampicillin and metronidazole. Contraception 1980;22:643–652.

75. Weisberg E. Interactions between oral contraceptives and antifungals/antibacterials. Is contraceptive failure the result? Clin Pharmacokinet 1999;36:309–13.

76. Veremis SA, Maddux MS, Pollak R, et al. Subtherapeutic cyclosporine concentrations during nafcillin therapy. Transplantation 1987;43:913–915.

77. Finland M, Bach MC, Garner C, et al. Synergistic action of ampicillin and erythromycin against *Nocardia asteroides*: effect of time of incubation. Antimicrob Agents Chemother 1974;5:344–353.

78. Roberts CE, Rosenfeld LS, Kirby WM. Synergism of erythromycin and penicillin against resistant staphylococci: mechanism and relation to synthetic penicillins. Antimicrob Agents Chemother 1962:831–842.

79. Waterworth PM. Apparent synergy between penicillin and erythromycin or fusidic acid. Clin Med 1963:70:941–953.

80. Oswald EJ, Reedy RJ, Wright WW. Antibiotic combinations: an in vitro study of antistaphylococcal effects of erythromycin plus penicillin, streptomycin, or tetracycline. Antimicrob Agents Chemother 1961:904–910.

81. Herrell WE, Balows A, Becker J. Erythrocillin: a new approach to the problem of antibiotic-resistant staphylococci. Antibiot Med Clin Ther 1960;7:637–642.

82. Manten A. Synergism and antagonism between antibiotic mixtures containing erythromycin. Antibiot Chemother 1954;4:1228–1233.

83. Allen NE, Epp JK. Mechanism of penicillin-erythromycin synergy on antibiotic resistant *Staphylococcus aureus*. Antimicrob Agents Chemother 1978;13:849–853.

84. Manten A, Terra JI. The antagonism between penicillin and other antibiotics in relation to drug concentration. Chemotherapia 1964;8:21–29.

85. Chang TW, Weinstein L. Inhibitory effects of other antibiotics on bacterial morphologic changes induced by penicillin G. Nature 1966:211:763–765.

86. Garrod LP, Waterworth PM. Methods of testing combined antibiotic bactericidal action and the significance of the results. J Clin Pathol 1962;15:328–338.

87. Strom J. Penicillin and erythromycin singly and in combination in scarlatina therapy and the interference between them. Antibiot Chemother 1961;11:694–697.

88. Robinson L, Fonseca K. Value of the minimum bactericidal concentration of antibiotics in the management of a case of recurrent *Streptococcus bovis* septicaemia. J Clin Pathol 1982;35:879,880.

89. Bach MC, Monaco AP, Finland M. Pulmonary nocardiosis therapy with minocycline and with erythromycin plus ampicillin. JAMA 1973;224:1378–1381.

90. Martinez JA, Horcajada JP, Almela M, et al. Addition of a macrolide to a β-lactam-based empirical antibiotic regimen is associated with lower in-hospital mortality for patients with bacteremic pneumococcal pneumonia. Clin Infect Dis 2003;36:389–395.

91. Waterer GW, Somes GW, Wunderink RG. Monotherapy may be suboptimal for severe bacteremic pneumococcal pneumonia. Arch Intern Med 2001;161:1837–1842.

92. Mutson MA, Stanek. Bacteremic pneumococcal pneumonia in one American city: a 20-year longitudinal study, 1978–1997. Am J Med 1999;107:S34–S43.

93. Mandell LA, Bartlett JG, Dowell SF, et al. Update of practice guidelines for the management of community-acquired pneumonia in immunocompetent adults. Clin Infect Dis 2003;37:1405–1433.

94. Huupponen R, Seppala P, Iisalo E. Effect of guar gum, a fibre preparation on digoxin and penicillin absorption in man. Eur J Clin Pharmacol 1984;26:279–281.

95. Brooks BM, Thomas AL, Coleman JW. Benzylpenicillin differentially conjugates to IFN-γ, TNF-α, IL-1β, IL-4 and IL-13 but selectively reduces IFN-γ activity. Clin Exp Immunol 2003;131:268–274.

96. Brooks BM, Thomas AL, Coleman JW. Benzylpenicillin differentially conjugates to IFN-γ, TNF-α, IL-1β, IL-4 and IL-13 but selectively reduces IFN-γ activity. Clin Exp Immunol 2003;131:268–274.

97. Attef OA, Ali AA. Effect of khat chewing on the bioavailability of ampicillin and amoxycillin. J Antimicrob Chemother 1997;39:523–525.

98. Jayasagar G, Krishna Kumar M, Chandrasekhar K, et al. Effect of cephalexin on the pharmacokinetics of metformin in healthy human volunteers. Drug Metabol Drug Interact 2002;19:41–48.

99. Wang DS, Kusuhara H, Kato Y, et al. Involvement of organic cation transporter 1 in the lactic acidosis caused by metformin. Mol Pharmacol 2003;63:844–848.

100. Iven H, Brasch H. The effects of antibiotics and uricosuric drugs on the renal elimination of methotrexate and 7-hydroxymethotrexate in rabbits. Cancer Chemother Pharmacol 1988;21:337–342.

101. Iven H, Brasch H. Influence of the antibiotics piperacillin, doxycycline, and tobramycin on the pharmacokinetics of methotrexate in rabbits. Cancer Chemother Pharmacol 1986;17:218–222.

102. Najjar TA, Abou-Auda HS, Ghilzai NM. Influence of piperacillin on the pharmacokinetics of methotrexate and 7-hydroxymethotrexate. Cancer Chemother Pharmacol 1998:42:423–428.

103. Iven H, Brasch H. Cephalosporins increase the renal clearance of methotrexate and 7-hydroxymethotrexate in rabbits. Cancer Chemother Pharmacol 1990;26:139–143.

104. Yamamoto K, Sawada Y, Mutsashita Y, et al. Delayed elimination of methotrexate associated with piperacillin administration. Ann Pharmacother 1997;31:1261–1262.

105. Bloom NJ, Ignoffo RJ, Reis CA, et al. Delayed clearance (Cl) of methotrexate (MTX) associated with antibiotics and antiinflammatory agents [abstract]. Clin Res 1986;34:560A.

106. Nierenberg DW, Mamelok RD. Toxic reaction to methotrexate in a patient receiving penicillin and furosemide: a possible interaction [letter]. Arch Dermatol 1983;119:449,450.

107. Dean R, Nachman J, Lorenzana AN. Possible methotrexate-mezlocillin interaction. Am J Pediatr Hematol Oncol 1992;14:88–92.

108. Ronchera CL, Hernández T, Peris JE. Pharmacokinetic interaction between high-dose methotrexate and amoxycillin. Ther Drug Monit 1993;15:375–379.

109. Titier K, Lagrange F, Péhourcq, Moore N, et al. Pharmacokinetic interaction between high-dose methotrexate and oxacillin. Ther Drug Monit 2002;24:570–572.

110. Herrick AL, Grennan DM, Aarons L. Lack of interaction between methotrexate and penicillins. Rheumatology 1999;38:284–285.

111. Hill G, Cihlar T, Oo C, et al. The anti-influenza drug oseltamivir exhibits low potential to induce pharmacokinetic drug interactions via renal secretion-correlation of in vivo and in vitro studies. Drug Metab Dispos 2002;30:13–19.

112. Hardman JG, Limbird LE, Molinoff PB, Ruddon RW, Gilman AG, eds. Goodman and Gilman's The Pharmacological Basis of Therapeutics. New York: McGraw-Hill, 1996.

113. Dasgupta A, Sperelakis A, Mason A, et al. Phenytoin-oxacillin interactions in normal and uremic sera. Pharmacotherapy 1997;17:375–378.

114. Dasgupta A, Dennen DA, Dean R, et al. Displacement of phenytoin from serum protein carriers by antibiotics: studies with ceftriaxone, nafcillin, and sulfamethoxazole. Clin Chem 1991;37:98–100.

115. Welling PG, Selen SD, Kendall MJ, et al. Probenecid: an unexplained effect on cephalosporin pharmacology. Br J Clin Pharmacol 1979;8:491–495.

116. Gibaldi M, Schwartz MA. Apparent effect of probenecid on the distribution of penicillins in man. Clin Pharmacol Ther 1968;9:345–349.

117. Barbhaiya R, Thin RN, Turner P, et al. Clinical pharmacological studies of amoxycillin: effect of probenecid. Br J Vener Dis 1979;55:211–213.

118. Waller ES, Sharanevych MA, Yakatan GJ. The effect of probenecid on nafcillin disposition. J Clin Pharmacol 1982;22:482–489.

119. Corvaia L, Li SC, Ioannides-Demos LL, et al. A prospective study of the effects of oral probenecid on the pharmacokinetics of intravenous ticarcillin in patients with cystic fibrosis. J Antimicrob Chemother 1992;30:875–878.

120. Shanson DC, McNabb R, Hajipieris P. The effect of probenecid on serum amoxycillin concentrations up to 18 hours after a single 3 g oral dose of amoxycillin: possible implications for preventing endocarditis. J Antimicrob Chemother 1984;13:629–632.

121. Ziv G, Sulman FG. Effects of probenecid on the distribution, elimination, and passage into milk of benzylpenicillin, ampicillin, and cloxacillin. Arch Int Pharmacodyn Ther 1974;207:373–382.

122. Krogsgaard MR, Hansen BA, Slotsbjerg T, et al. Should probenecid be used to reduce the dicloxacillin dosage in orthopaedic infections? A study of the dicloxacillin-saving effect of probenecid. Pharmacol Toxicol 1994;74:181–184.

123. Hoffstedt B, Haidl S, Walder M. Influence of probenecid on serum and subcutaneous tissue fluid concentrations of benzylpenicillin and ceftazidime in human volunteers. Eur J Clin Microbiol 1983;2:604–606.

124. Ganes D, Batra A, Faulkner D, et al. Effect of probenecid on the pharmacokinetics of piperacillin and tazobactam in healthy volunteers. Pharm Res 1991;8:S299.

125. Babalola CP, Iwheye GB, Olaniyi AA. Effect of proguanil interaction on bioavailability of cloxacillin. J Clin Pharm Ther 2002;27:461–464.

126. Speck RS, Jawetz E, Gunnison JB. Studies on antibiotic synergism and antagonism. The interference of aureomycin or terramycin with the action of penicillin in infections in mice. Arch Intern Med 1951;88:168–174.

127. Gunnison JB, Coleman VR, Jawetz E. Interference of aureomycin and of terramycin with the action of penicillin in vitro. Proc Soc Exp Biol Med 1950;75:549–452.

128. Chuang YC, Liu JW, Ko WC, et al. In vitro synergism between cefotaxime and minocycline against *Vibrio vulnificus*. Antimicrob Agents Chemother 1997;41:2214–2217.

129. Chuang YC, Ko WC, Wang ST, et al. Minocycline and cefotaxime in the treatment of experimental murine *Vibrio vulnificus* infection. Antimicrob Agents Chemother 1998;42:1319–1322.

130. Ko WC, Lee HC, Chuang YC, et al. In vitro and in vivo combinations of cefotaxime and minocycline against *Aeromonas hydrophilia*. Antimicrob Agents Chemother 2001;45:1281–1283.

131. Lepper MH, Dowling HP. Treatment of pneumococcic meningitis with penicillin compared with penicillin plus aureomycin: studies including observations on an apparent antagonism between penicillin and aureomycin. Arch Intern Med 1951;88:489–494.

132. Olsson RA, Kirby JC, Romansky MJ. Pneumococcal meningitis in the adult. Clinical, therapeutic and prognostic aspects in 43 patients. Ann Intern Med 1961;55:545–549.

133. Strom J. The question of antagonism between penicillin and chlortetracycline, illustrated by therapeutical experiments in scarlatina. Antibiot Med 1955;1:6–12.

134. Ahern JJ, Kirby WMM. Lack of interference of aureomycin in treatment of pneumococcic pneumonia. Arch Intern Med 1953;91:197–203

135. Tryba M. Potentiation of non-depolarizing muscle relaxants of acetylaminopenicillin. Studies on the example of vecuronium [English abstract]. Anaethesist 1985;34:651–655.

136. Singh YN, Harvey AL, Marshall IG. Antibiotic-induced paralysis of the mouse phrenic nerve-hemidiaphragm preparation, and reversibility by calcium and by neostigmine. Anesthesiology 1978;48:418–424.

137. Harwood TN, Moorthy SS. Prolonged vecuronium-induced neuromuscular blockade in children. Anesth Analg 1989;68:534–536.

138. Mackie K, Pavlin EG. Recurrent paralysis following pipercillin administration. Anesthesiology 1990;72:561–563.

139. Condon RE, Munshi CA, Arfman RC. Interaction of vecuronium with pipercillin or cefoxitin evaluated in a prospective, randomized, double-blind clinical trial. Am Surg 1995;61:403–406.

140. Kadlec GJ, Ha LH, Jarboe CH, et al. Effect on ampicillin on theophylline half-life in infants and young children. South Med J 1978;71:1584.

141. Jonkman JH, Van der Boon WJ, Schoenmaker R, et al. Lack of effect of amoxicillin on theophylline pharmacokinetics. Br J Clin Pharmacol 1985;19:99–101.

142. Matera MG, Cazzola M, Lampa E, et al. Clinical pharmacokinetics of theophylline during co-treatment with ticarcillin plus clavulanic acid in patients suffering from acute exacerbation of chronic bronchitis. J Chemother 1993;5:233–236.

143. Cazzola M, Santangelo G, Guidetti E, et al. Influence of sulbactam plus ampicillin on theophylline clearance. Int J Clin Pharmacol Res 1991;11:11–15.

144. Jonkman JH, Van der Boon WJ, Schoenmaker R, et al. Clinical pharmacokinetics of amoxycillin and theophylline during cotreatment with both medicaments. Chemotherapy 1985;31:329–335.

145. Hughes GS, Heald DL, Barker KB, et al. The effects of gastric pH and food on the pharmacokinetics of a new oral cephalosporin, cefpodoxime proxetil. Clin Pharmacol Ther 1989;46:674–685.

146. Saathoff N, Lode H, Neider K, et al. Pharmacokinetics of cefpodoxime proxetil and interactions with an antacid and an $H_2$ receptor antagonist. Antimicrob Agents Chemother 1992;36:796–800.

147. Spectracef® [package insert]. Purdue Pharmaceutical Products, Stanford, CT, 2003.

148. Omnicef® [package insert]. Abbott Laboratories North Chicago, IL, 2001.

149. Satterwhite JH, Cerimele BJ, Coleman DL. Pharmacokinetics of cefaclor AF: effects of age, antacids, and $H_2$-receptor antagonists. Postgrad Med J 1992;68:S3–S9.

150. Healy DP, Sahia J, Sterling LP, et al. Influence of antacid containing aluminum and magnesium on the pharmacokinetics of cefixime. Antimicrob Agents Chemother 1989;33:1994–1997.

151. Deslandes A, Camus F, Lacroix C, et al. Effects of nifedipine and diltiazem on pharmacokinetics of cefpodoxime following its oral administration. Antimicrob Agents Chemother 1996;40:2879–2881.

152. Duverne C, Bouten A, Deslandes A, et al. Modification of cefixime bioavailability by nifedipine in humans: involvement of the dipeptide carrier system. Antimicrob Agents Chemother 1992;36:2462–2467.

153. Berlioz F, Julien S, Tsocas A, et al. Neural modulation of cephalexin intestinal absorption through the di- and tripeptide brush border transporter of rat jejunum in vivo. J Pharmacol Exp Ther 1999;288:1037–1044.

154. Marino EL, Vicente MT, Dominguez-Gil A. Influence of cholestyramine on the pharmacokinetic parameters of cefadroxil after simultaneous administration. Int J Pharmaceut 1983;16:23–30.

155. Parsons RL, Paddock GM, Hossack GM. Cholestyramine induced antibiotic malabsorption. Chemotherapy 4. In: Williams JD, Geddes AM, eds. Pharmacology of Antibiotics. New York: Plenum, 1975, pp. 191–198.

156. Kannangara DW, Gallagher K, Lefrock JL. Disulfiram-like reactions with newer cephalosporins: cefmenoxime. Am J Med Sci 1984;287:45–47.

157. Foster TS, Raehl CL, Wilson HD. Disulfiram-like reaction associated with a parenteral cephalosporin. Am J Hosp Pharm 1980;37:858,859.

158. Uri JV, Parks DB. Disulfiram-like reaction to certain cephalosporins. Ther Drug Monit 1983;5:219–224.

159. Ueno K, Tanaka K, Tsujimura K, et al. Impairment of cefdinir absorption by iron ion. Clin Pharmacol Ther 1993;54:473–475.

160. Shukla UA, Pittman KA, Barbhiaya RH. Pharmacokinetic interactions of cefprozil with food, propantheline, metoclopramide, and probenecid in healthy volunteers. J Clin Pharmacol 1992;32:725–731.

161. Neu HC. The in vitro activity, human pharmacology, and clinical effectiveness of new β-lactam antibiotics. Annu Rev Pharmacol Toxicol 1982;22:599–642.

162. Merle-Melet M, Bresler L, Lokiec F, et al. Effects of diclofenac on ceftriaxone pharmacokinetics in humans. Antimicrob Agents Chemother 1992;36:2331–2333.

163. Andrassy K, Bechtold H, Ritz E. Hypoprothrombinemia caused by cephalosporins. J Antimicrob Chemother 1985;15:133–136.

164. Freedy HR, Cetnarowski AB, Lumish RM, et al. Cefoperazone-induced coagulopathy. Drug Intell Clin Pharm 1986;20:281–283.

165. Rymer W, Greenlaw CW. Hypoprothrombinemia associated with cefamandole. Drug Intell Clin Pharm 1980;40;780–783.

166. Osborne JC. Hypoprothrombinemia and bleeding due to cefoperazone [letter]. Ann Intern Med 1985;102:721,722.
167. Cristiano P. Hypoprothrombinemia associated with cefoperazone treatment. Drug Intell Clin Pharm 1984;18:314–316.
168. Hooper CA, Haney BB, Stone HH. Gastrointestinal bleeding due to vitamin K deficiency in patients on parenteral cefamandole [letter]. Lancet 1980;1:39,40.
169. Pakter RL, Russell TR, Mielke CH, et al. Coagulopathy associated with the use of moxalactam. JAMA 1982;248:1100.
170. Marier RL, Faro S, Sanders CV, et al. Moxalactam in the therapy of serious infections. Antimicrob Agents Chemother 1982;21:650–654.
171. Angaran DM, Virgil MS, Dias VC. The comparative influence of prophylactic antibiotics on the prothrombin response to warfarin in the postoperative prosthetic cardiac valve patient. Ann Surg 1987;206:155–161.
172. Angaran DM, Dias VC, Arom KV, et al. The influence of prophylactic antibiotics on the warfarin anticoagulation response in the postoperative prosthetic cardiac valve patient. Cefamandole vs vancomycin. Ann Surg 1984;199:107–111.
173. Bechtold H, Andrassy K, Jahnchen E, et al. Evidence for impaired hepatic vitamin $K_1$ metabolism in patients treated with $N$-methyl-thiotetrazole cefalosporins. Thromb Haemost 1984;51:358–361.
174. Frick P, Riedler G, Brogli H. Dose response and minimal daily requirement for vitamin K in man. Applied Physiol 1967;23:387–389.
175. Lipsky J. $N$-Methyl-thio-tetrazole inhibition of the γ carboxylation of glutamic acid: possible mechanism for antibiotic associated hypothrombinemia. Lancet 1983;2:192,193.
176. Lipsky J, Lewis J, Novick W. Production of hypoprothrombinemia by moxalactam and 1-methyl-5-thiotetrazole in rats. Antimicrob Agents Chemother 1984;25:380,381.
177. Verhagen CA, Mattie H, Van Strijen E. The renal clearance of cefuroxime and ceftazidime and the effect of probenecid on their tubular excretion. Br J Clin Pharmacol 1994;37: 193–197.
178. Luthy R, Blaser J, Bonetti A, et al. Comparative multiple-dose pharmacokinetics of cefotaxime, moxalactam, and ceftazidime. Antimicrob Agents Chemother 1981;20: 567–575.
179. LeBel M, Paone RP, Lewis GP. Effect of probenecid on the pharmacokinetics of ceftizoxime. J Antimicrob Chemother 1983;12:147–155.
180. Reeves DS, Bullock DW, Bywater MJ, et al. The effect of probenecid on the pharmacokinetics and distribution of cefoxitin in healthy volunteers. Br J Clin Pharm 1981;11: 353–359.
181. Marino EL, Dominquez-Gil A. The pharmacokinetics of cefadroxil associated with probenecid. Int J Clin Pharmacol Ther Toxicol 1981;19:506–508.
182. Stoeckel K. Pharmacokinetics of Rocephin®, a highly active new cephalosporin with an exceptionally long biological half-life. Chemotherapy 1981;27:42–46.
183. Kaplan KS, Reisberg BE, Weinstein L. Cephaloridine: antimicrobial activity and pharmacologic behavior. Am J Med Sci 1967;253:667–674.
184. Duncan WC. Treatment of gonorrhoea with cefazolin plus probenecid. J Infect Dis 1974;130:398–401.
185. Mischler TW, Sugerman AA, Willard SA, Barmick L, Neiss ES. Influence of probenecid and food on the bioavailability of cephradine in normal male subjects. J Clin Pharmacol 1974;14:604–611.
186. Tuano SB, Brodie JL. Kirby WM. Cephaloridine vs cephalothin: relation of the kidney to blood level differences after parenteral administration. Antimicrob Agents Chemother 1966;6:101–106.
187. Griffith RS, Black HR, Brier GL, et al. Effect of probenecid on the blood levels and urinary excretion of cefamandole. Antimicrob Agents Chemother 1977;11:809–812.

188. Bint AJ, Reeves DS, Holt HA. Effect of probenecid on serum cefoxitin concentrations. J Antimicrob Chemother 1977;3:627,628.

189. Taylor WA, Holloway WJ. Cephalexin in the treatment of gonorrhea. Int J Clin Pharmacol 1972;6:7–9.

190. Ko H, Cathcart KS, Griffith DL, et al. Pharmacokinetics of intravenously administered cefmetazole and cefoxitin and effects of probenecid on cefmetazole elimination. Antimicrob Agents Chemother 1989;33:356–361.

191. Vlasses PH, Holbrook AM, Schrogie J, et al. Effect of orally administered probenecid on the pharmacokinetics of cefoxitin. Antimicrob Agents Chemother 1980;17:847–855.

192. Spina SP, Dillon EC Jr. Effect of chronic probenecid therapy on cefazolin serum concentrations. Ann Pharmacother 2003;37:621–624.

193. Stoeckel K, Trueb V, Dubach UC, et al. Effect of probenecid on the elimination and protein binding of ceftriaxone. Eur J Clin Pharmacol 1988;34:151–156.

194. O'Callaghan CH, Acred P, Harper PB, et al. GR 20263, a new broad-spectrum cephalosporin with antipseudomonal activity. Antimicrob Agents Chemother 1980;17:876–883.

195. DeSante KA, Israel KS, Brier GL, et al. Effect of probenecid on the pharmacokinetics of moxalactam. Antimicrob Agents Chemother 1982;21:58–61.

196. Patel IH, Soni PP, Carbone JJ, et al. Lack of probenecid effect on nonrenal excretion of ceftriaxone in anephric patients. J Clin Pharmacol 1990;30:449–453.

197. Kercsmar CM, Stern RC, Reed MD, et al. Ceftazidime in cystic fibrosis: pharmacokinetics and therapeutic response. J Antimicrob Chemother 1983;12:289–295.

198. Jovanovich JF, Saravolatz LD, Burch K, et al. Failure of probenecid to alter the pharmacokinetics of ceforanide. Antimicrob Agents Chemother 1981;20:530–532.

199. Pfeifer HJ, Greenblatt DJ, Friedman P. Effects of three antibiotics on theophylline kinetics. Clin Pharmacol Ther 1979;26:36–40.

200. Bachmann K, Schwartz J, Forney RB, et al. Impact of cefaclor on the pharmacokinetics of theophylline. Ther Drug Monitor 1986;8:151–154.

201. Jonkman JH, Van der Boon WJ, Schoenmaker R, et al. Clinical pharmacokinetics of theophylline during co-treatment with cefaclor. Int J Clin Pharmacol Ther Toxicol 1986;24:88–92.

202. Hammond D, Abate MA. Theophylline toxicity, acute illness, and cefaclor. Drug Intell Clin Pharm 1989;23:339,340.

203. Foord RD. Cephaloridine, cephalothin, and the kidney. J Antimicrob Chemother 1975;1(suppl):119–133.

204. Koch-Weser J, Sidel VW, Federman EB, et al. Adverse effects of sodium colistimethate. Manifestations and specific reaction rates during 317 courses of therapy. Ann Intern Med 1970;72:857–868.

205. Adler S, Segel DP. Nonoliguric renal failure secondary to sodium colistimethate: a report of four cases. Am J Med Sci 1971;262:109–114.

206. Plager JE. Association of renal injury with combined cephalothin-gentamicin therapy among patients severely ill with malignant disease. Cancer 1976;37:1937–1943.

207. Wade JC, Smith CR, Petty BG, et al. Cephalothin plus an aminoglycoside is more nephrotoxic than methicillin plus an aminoglycoside. Lancet 1978;2:604–606.

208. Gurwich EL, Sula J, Hoy RH. Gentamicin-cephalothin drug reaction. Am J Hosp Pharm 1978;35:1402,1403.

209. Hansen MM, Kaaber K. Nephrotoxicity in combined cephalothin-gentamicin therapy among patients severely ill with malignant disease. Cancer 1976;37:1937–1943.

210. Cabanillas F, Burgos RC, Rodriquez RC, et al. Nephrotoxicity of combined cephalothin-gentamicin regimen. Arch Intern Med 1975;135:850–852.

211. Fillastre JP, Laumonier R, Humbert G, et al. Acute renal failure associated with combined gentamicin and cephalothin therapy. Br Med J 1973;2:396,397.

212. Bobrow SL, Jaffe E, Young RC, et al. Anuria and acute tubular necrosis associated with gentamicin and cephalothin. JAMA 1972;222:1546,1547.

213. Kleinknecht D, Jungers P, Fillastre JP. Nephrotoxicity of cephaloridine. Ann Intern Med 1974;80:421,422.

214. Dodds MG, Foord RD. Enhancement by potent diuretics of renal tubular necrosis induced by cephaloridine. Br J Pharmacol 1970;40:227–236.

215. Norrby R, Stenqvist K, Elgefors B, et al. Interaction between cephaloridine and furosemide in man. Scand J Infect Dis 1976;8:209–212.

216. Simpson IJ. Nephrotoxicity and acute renal failure associated with cephalothin and cephaloridine. N Z Med J 1971;74:312–315.

217. Trollfors B, Norrby R, Kristianson K. Effects on renal function of treatment with cefoxitin sodium alone or in combination with furosemide. J Antimicrob Chemother 1978;4:S85–S89.

218. Korn A, Eichler HG, Gasic S. A drug interaction study of ceftriaxone and frusemide in healthy volunteers. Int J Clin Pharmacol Ther Toxicol 1986;24:262–264.

219. Walstad RA, Dahl K, Hellum KB, et al. The pharmacokinetics of ceftazidime in patients with impaired renal function and concurrent frusemide therapy. Eur J Clin Pharmacol 1988;35:273–279.

220. Bax RP, Bastain W, Featherstone A, et al. The pharmacokinetics of meropenem in volunteers. J Antimicrob Chemother 1989:24:311–320.

221. Invanz® [package insert]. Merck and Co., Whitehouse Station, NJ, 2003.

222. Norrby SR, Alestig K, Ferber F, et al. Pharmacokinetics and tolerance of *N*-formimidoyl thienamycin (MK0787) in humans. Antimicrob Agents Chemother 1983;23:293–299.

223. DeTurck BJ, Diltoer MW, Cornelis PJ, et al. Lowering of plasma valproic acid concentrations during concomitant therapy with meropenem and amikacin [letter]. J Antimicrob Chemother 1998;42:563,564.

224. Nagai K, Shimizu T, Togo A, et al. Decrease in serum levels of valproic acid during treatment with a new carbapenem, panipenem/βmipron. J Antimicrob Chemother 1997;39:295,296.

225. Torii M, Takiguchi Y, Saito F, et al. Inhibition by carbapenem antibiotic imipenem of intestinal absorption of valproic acid in rats. Pharm Pharmacol 2001;53:823–829.

226. Yokogawa K, Iwashita S, Kubota A, et al. Effect of meropenem on disposition kinetics of valproate and its metabolites in rabbits. Pharm Res 2001;18:1320–1326.

227. Yamamura N, Imura K, Naganuma H, et al. Panipenem, a carbapenem antibiotic, enhances the glucuronidation of intravenously administered valproic acid in rats. Drug Metab Dispos 1999;27:724–730.

228. Bösmuller C, Steurer W, Königsrainer A, et al. Increased risk of central nervous system toxicity in patients treated with cyclosporine and imipenem/cilastatin. Nephron 1991;58:362–364.

229. Zazgornik J, Schein W, Heimberger K, et al. Potentiation of neurotoxic side effects by coadministration of imipenem to cyclosporine therapy in a kidney transplant recipient—synergism of side effects or drug interaction. Clin Nephrol 1986;26:265,266.

230. Mraz W, Sido B, Knedel M, et al. Concomitant immunosuppressive and antibiotic therapy—reduction of cyclosporine A blood levels due to treatment with imipenem/cilastatin. Transplant Proc 1992;24:1704–1708.

231. Semel JD, Allen N. Seizures in patients simultaneously receiving theophylline and imipenem or ciprofloxacin or metronidazole. South Med J 1991;84:465–468.

232. Primaxin® [package insert]. Merck and Co., Whitehouse Station, NJ, 2003.

233. Azactam® [package insert]. Bristol-Myers Squibb, Princeton, NJ, 1999.

234. Swabb EA, Sugerman AA, Frantz M, et al. Renal handling of the monobactam aztreonam in healthy subjects. Clin Pharmacol Ther 1983;33:609–614.

# 10

# Antifungal Agents

## Paul O. Gubbins, Scott A. McConnell, and Jarrett R. Amsden

### INTRODUCTION

During the past several decades, fungi have become increasingly common pathogens, particularly among critically ill or immunosuppressed patients. Until recently, advances in antifungal therapy had not kept pace with this trend. Historically, antifungal development significantly lagged behind that of antibacterial therapy. For many years, there were few choices for the treatment of systemic mycoses. However, the recent past has seen the development of a new class of antifungal agents (the echinocandins); safer or more bioavailable formulations of marketed antifungal agents (itraconazole oral and iv solution, lipid formulations of amphotericin B); and a new addition to an existing class of agents (voriconazole). Today, antifungal agents differ sufficiently in terms of activity, toxicity, and drug interaction potential so that clinicians now have the luxury of considering these characteristics when tailoring therapy to treat a specific systemic fungal infection. Systemically acting antifungal agents can cause drug–drug interactions by a variety of mechanisms. Therefore, they have the potential to interact with a vast array of medicines. Given the patient populations in whom systemic mycoses typically occur, the increased use of antifungal therapy, and the growing but still relatively limited selection of antifungal agents, clinicians must understand the drug interaction profile of this small but increasingly important class of drugs.

### AMPHOTERICIN B BASIC PHARMACOLOGY

Amphotericin B, a polyene antifungal agent, has been the standard of therapy for systemic mycoses for many years. Pharmacologically, amphotericin B acts by binding to membrane-bound sterols, thereby disrupting biological membranes. Amphotericin B binds nonspecifically to ergosterol in fungal cells and to cholesterol in mammalian cells, which increases membrane permeability. In addition, amphotericin B stimulates cytokine release and causes arteriolar vasoconstriction, especially in the renal vasculature (1,2). These pharmacological effects of amphotericin B lead to either infusion-related toxicities, including hypotension, fever, rigors, and chills, or dose-dependent

From: *Infectious Disease: Drug Interactions in Infectious Diseases, Second Edition*
Edited by: S. C. Piscitelli and K. A. Rodvold © Humana Press Inc., Totowa, NJ

adverse effects, such as renal dysfunction, azotemia, renal tubular acidosis, electrolyte imbalance, cardiac arrhythmias, and anemia.

Infusion-related adverse effects, although noxious to the patient, rarely affect the ability to use amphotericin B or other agents. In contrast to the infusion-related adverse effects, dose-dependent adverse effects often limit the use of amphotericin B and interfere with ability to use other agents. Amphotericin B drug–drug interactions are primarily a consequence of its dose-dependent adverse effects.

*Distribution*

Following iv administration, amphotericin B is widely distributed. The liver is the primary repository of amphotericin B in humans, but amphotericin B also distributes to the spleen, kidneys, and heart *(1)*. Amphotericin B deoxycholate is highly protein bound (>95%), primarily to albumin and $\alpha_1$-acid glycoprotein *(3)*. This binding is nonlinear and concentration dependent. That is, the percentage of bound drug increases as the amphotericin B deoxycholate concentration increases. This unique binding may be caused by the low solubility of unbound amphotericin B deoxycholate in human plasma (<1 µg/mL), relative to the large binding capacity of plasma proteins *(3)*. Amphotericin B deoxycholate has a very large apparent volume of distribution (2–4 L/kg), suggesting that it distributes to tissues *(3,4)*. The formulation of amphotericin B in a lipid vehicle alters its distribution and reduces its renal toxicity *(3–5)*.

*Elimination*

Historically, amphotericin B deoxycholate pharmacokinetics have been poorly understood. However, investigators using sensitive analytical methods and sampling for an extensive time period vastly improved our understanding of how the human body handles amphotericin B deoxycholate. One week after the administration of 0.6 mg/kg amphotericin B deoxycholate to healthy volunteers, investigators were able to account for over 90% of the administered dose *(4)*. Amphotericin B deoxycholate is mostly excreted as unchanged drug in the urine and feces. In fact, approximately two-thirds of amphotericin B deoxycholate was recovered in the urine (20.6%) and feces (42.5%) *(4)*. Urinary and fecal clearances of unchanged drug accounted for 75% of amphotericin B deoxycholate total clearance. Amphotericin B deoxycholate is apparently cleared from its distribution sites very slowly and the terminal half-life $(t_{1/2}\beta)$ of amphotericin B deoxycholate is approx 127 hours *(4)*. The formulation of amphotericin B in a lipid vehicle significantly alters its distribution and elimination *(4)*.

*Scope of Problem*

Amphotericin B drug–drug interactions are primarily a result of its nephrotoxicity. Amphotericin B causes nephrotoxicity through several mechanisms, including reducing glomerular filtration and renal blood flow. In addition, it causes direct cellular damage to the proximal and distal tubules, which interferes with reabsorption of electrolytes. Amphotericin B-induced nephrotoxicity can cause the accumulation of toxic concentrations of renally eliminated drugs (i.e., 5-fluorocytosine [5-FC]), resulting in secondary nonrenal adverse effects. More important, amphotericin B-induced nephrotoxicity can be additive to that of other commonly administered nephrotoxins (i.e., aminoglycosides, cyclosporine, cisplatin, foscarnet, and tacrolimus). These additive toxicities can further complicate drug therapy regimens and increase the risk of severe renal failure, which may necessitate hemodialysis.

Certain amphotericin B-associated electrolyte disturbances, such as hypokalemia, can be compounded by other medications that share this toxicity. The subtle nature of this interaction can be easily overlooked; however, it may lead to direct cardiac or skeletal muscle toxicity, increase the risk of digoxin toxicity, or exacerbate the risk of cardiotoxicity (i.e., torsades de pointes) from medications such as quinidine.

## 5-FC Basic Pharmacology

5-Fluorocytosine (5-FC) is a fluorinated pyrimidine related to 5-fluorouracil (5-FU). Absorption of 5-FC is rapid and complete. In the fasting state, 5-FC bioavailability is approx 90% *(6)*. The apparent volume of distribution of 5-FC approximates total body water *(6)*. Moreover, 5-FC is minimally bound to plasma proteins. Approximately 90% of a 5-FC dose is excreted renally as unchanged drug, and renal clearance is highly correlated with creatinine clearance (CrCL) *(6)*. As CrCL declines and serum creatinine concentrations (Scr) increase, $t_{1/2}$ of 5-FC becomes prolonged. 5-FC undergoes virtually no metabolism *(6)*. Once thought improbable, the deamination of 5-FC to 5-FU occurs routinely in humans and is thought to contribute to the primary toxicity of 5-FC, myelosuppression *(6)*.

### Scope of Problem

Because there are few indications for 5-FC use, very few significant drug interactions with 5-FC have been identified. Renal dysfunction produced by nephrotoxic drugs such as amphotericin B or aminoglycosides prolong 5-FC elimination and increase its serum concentrations. Therefore, these drug interactions may predispose patients to 5-FC toxicity.

## Azoles Basic Pharmacology

The systemic azoles ketoconazole, itraconazole, fluconazole, and voriconazole exert a fungistatic effect by inhibiting cytochrome P450 (CYP)-dependent C-14 α-demethylase, the enzyme necessary for the conversion of lanosterol to ergosterol. This leads to the depletion of ergosterol, the essential sterol of the fungal cell membrane, and ultimately compromises cell membrane integrity *(7)*. Chemically, the azoles are all weak bases. Ketoconazole and itraconazole are very lipophilic and generally water insoluble. Voriconazole is lipophilic and has limited water solubility. In contrast, fluconazole is only slightly lipophilic and very water soluble. These physicochemical properties are the basis for the drug–drug interactions involving this class.

The systemic azoles are substrates and inhibitors of CYP isoforms to varying degrees. In addition, certain azoles are substrates and inhibitors of the multidrug resistance 1 (MDR1) gene product, P-glycoprotein (P-gp) *(8,9)*. As described in Chapter 3, P-gp is a large transmembrane efflux protein that shares substrate specificity and is extensively co-localized with CYP3A in the intestine, liver, and kidney *(9,10)*. In general, P-gp may limit exposure of a variety of tissues to xenobiotics.

### Absorption

When administered orally, ketoconazole exhibits pH-dependent dissolution and absorption. Food does not consistently alter the absorption and systemic availability of ketoconazole *(7)*. The relative bioavailability of the ketoconazole tablet is approx 80% *(7)*.

Itraconazole is marketed as a capsule containing itraconazole-coated sugar pellets and solubilized in a 40% hydroxpropyl-β-cyclodextrin solution for oral and iv use. The absorption of itraconazole is incomplete, and the drug is subjected to significant first-pass metabolism. Absorption from the capsule form is slow, variable, and optimal under acidic gastric conditions or in the fed state *(11)*. In contrast to the capsule, itraconazole in the oral solution form requires no dissolution, so its absorption is not influenced by gastric pH *(12)*. In addition, the absorption of itraconazole from the oral solution is optimal in the fasted state *(13)*. Under fasting conditions, absorption from the oral solution is rapid and less variable than from the capsule under fed conditions. However, even in the presence of food, higher serum concentrations are achieved with the oral solution compared to the capsule. The absolute bioavailability of the oral solution is 55%, approx 30% higher than that of the capsule formulation *(11,14)*. However, the two formulations are bioequivalent *(14)*.

Because fluconazole is water soluble and more polar than the other systemic azoles, it can be formulated as an iv form without the use of a solubilizing agent. This chemical property also allows fluconazole to circumvent much of the hepatic metabolism required by the other azoles for elimination. Oral fluconazole formulations are rapidly and nearly completely absorbed, with a bioavailability in excess of 93% *(15)*. Fluconazole absorption is not dependent on acidic gastric conditions or the presence of food *(15)*.

Voriconazole is available in both iv and oral formulations. Intravenous voriconazole is formulated with the solubilizing agent sulfobutyl ether β-cyclodextrin. Following oral dosing, voriconazole absorption is rapid and nearly complete, with a relative bioavailability of approx 90% *(16)*. The dissolution of voriconazole is not affected by increases in gastric pH, but fatty foods decrease its bioavailability to approx 80% *(17)*.

## Distribution

Following oral administration, ketoconazole and itraconazole are highly protein bound (99%) and widely distributed in the body *(7,11)*. Therefore, in body fluids the unbound concentrations of these compounds are much lower compared to their plasma concentrations. Voriconazole is moderately bound (58%) to plasma proteins and is widely distributed throughout the body *(12)*. In contrast to these azoles, fluconazole minimally binds proteins (11%) and thus circulates mostly as free drug *(15)*. Fluconazole also distributes extensively into a variety of body fluids and hepatic and renal tissues *(15)*. Notably, unlike ketoconazole and itraconazole, both fluconazole and voriconazole distribute into the cerebrospinal fluid and central nervous system tissues *(15–18)*.

## Metabolism/Elimination

Ketoconazole exhibits dose-dependent elimination and is hepatically metabolized to inactive metabolites by CYP isoforms. Less than 5% of an administered dose of ketoconazole is eliminated unchanged in the urine *(7)*.

Itraconazole also exhibits dose-dependent elimination and is extensively metabolized to many metabolites by CYP3A4. The complete metabolic pathway of itraconazole is not fully elucidated, and it may be acted on by additional isoforms. The drug is somewhat extracted by the liver (hepatic extraction ratio [He] = 0.5) *(19)*. The principle metabolite, hydroxyitraconazole, is bioactive and is primarily formed via enteric CYP3A4 *(11)*.

Fluconazole is distinct among systemic azoles in that approx 91% of an orally administered dose is excreted in the urine. Most (80%) is excreted as unchanged drug; two inactive metabolites account for the remaining 11% *(20)*.

Voriconazole undergoes extensive hepatic metabolism by CYP enzymes to eight metabolites that are inactive *(21)*. Less than 2% of an administered dose is excreted in the urine unchanged *(16,22)*. The hepatic metabolism of voriconazole is more complex than other azoles and involves several different CYP enzymes: CYP2C19, CYP3A4, and CYP2C9 *(16,17,22)*. Voriconazole is primarily metabolized to its principle N-oxide metabolite by CYP2C19, CYP3A4, and to a lesser extent CYP2C9 *(22)*. Nonetheless, CYP2C19 metabolism is the primary pathway, and this isoform exhibits genetic polymorphism. This polymorphism has eight known variant alleles, which if expressed, result in deficient or absent enzyme activity and manifest as a poor-metabolizing phenotype. This phenotype is an inherited autosomal recessive trait that is present in 2 to 5% of Caucasians, 12 to 23% of Asian populations, and 38 to 79% of Polynesians and Micronesians *(22,23)*. Populations exhibiting the homozygous poor-metabolizing phenotype will have nearly a fourfold increase in drug exposure compared to those exhibiting the homozygous efficient-metabolizing phenotype. Furthermore, populations exhibiting the heterozygous efficient-metabolizing phenotype will have nearly a twofold increase in drug exposure compared to the homozygous efficient-metabolizing phenotype *(16)*.

Voriconazole is also metabolized by CYP2C9, which also exhibits polymorphisms. This polymorphism has six known variant alleles, of which two are associated with reduced enzyme activity. The variant alleles are expressed among Caucasians and less frequently among African Americans, but they are not expressed in Asian populations *(23,24)*. Last, CYP3A4 is also involved in voriconazole metabolism; however, to date significant polymorphisms have not been identified with this enzyme. Nonetheless, variability in CYP3A4 expression is widely documented and may contribute somewhat to interindividual variability in voriconazole pharmacokinetics.

In healthy volunteers, the CYP2C19 genotype is the most important covariate determining plasma voriconazole concentrations. However, voriconazole exposure varies greatly across the genotypes and is confounded by drug–drug and perhaps drug–disease interactions *(22)*. Therefore, genotyping or genotypic specific dose adjustments are not clinically indicated. Nonetheless, clinicians should be aware of the complexities of voriconazole metabolism.

### Scope of Problem

As reviewed in Chapter 2, drug interactions occur primarily in the gastrointestinal (GI) tract, liver, and kidneys by a variety of mechanisms. Drug interactions in the GI tract can occur as a result of alterations in pH, complexation with ions, or interference with transport proteins and enzymatic processes involved in enteric (i.e., presystemic) drug metabolism. Drug interactions in the liver can occur as a result of interference with transport proteins and Phase I or II drug metabolism. In the kidney, drug interactions can occur through interference with glomerular filtration, active tubular excretion, or other mechanisms. The azoles are one of the few drug classes that can cause or be involved in drug interactions at all of these sites by one or more of the above mechanisms. Many of the drug–drug interactions involving the azoles occur classwide. Therefore, when using the azoles, clinicians must be aware of the many real and potential drug–drug interactions associated with this class.

In contrast to the treatment of bacterial infections, treatment alternatives for systemic mycoses are more limited. The azoles are the largest and one of the safest class of systemic antifungals available. Thus, given the few antifungal agents from which to choose, clinicians must also be able to discern the potential interactions of clinical significance from those of theoretical significance, so that this therapeutic drug class can be used optimally.

### Echinocandins Basic Pharmacology

The echinocandin class of antifungal agents is the first new systemic antifungal class introduced in nearly two decades. This class is fungicidal and disrupts cell wall synthesis by inhibiting a novel target, 1,3,-β-D-glucan synthase. This enzyme is present in most fungal pathogens but is not present in mammalian cells *(25)*. The echinocandins are large molecular weight semisynthetic lipopeptides and thus cannot be formulated for oral dosing. Caspofungin, the lone available agent in the United States, is a complex, large (MW = 1093 Da), water-soluble (log $p$ -1.2), cyclic hexapeptide *(26)*. Within several years, other echinocandins (e.g., micafungin and anidulafungin) will likely be added to the list of available agents in this class.

### Distribution

The distribution of caspofungin in humans has not been adequately studied. However, animal data reveal that the primary repositories of caspofungin in a murine tissue penetration model were the liver, kidneys, and large intestines *(27)*. This model also showed that caspofungin does not readily distribute into the central nervous system. Caspofungin is apparently highly protein bound (≈96%) *(28)*.

### Elimination

Caspofungin exhibits predictable linear pharmacokinetics, and with a half-life of 8–11 hours it can be dosed once daily *(29)*. In healthy male adults, following iv administration caspofungin undergoes hydrolysis or *N*-acetylation to form several inactive metabolites. Caspofungin also undergoes spontaneous chemical degradation to an open-ring compound. Caspofungin and its metabolites are then slowly excreted, primarily in the urine and to a lesser extent in the feces *(26)*. Approximately 1.4% of an administered caspofungin dose is excreted in the urine as unchanged drug *(29)*. In healthy elderly subjects, advances in age produced a modest effect on pharmacokinetics when compared to pooled data from younger healthy volunteers *(30)*. However, these differences were not deemed significant enough to warrant dosage adjustments in the elderly. Similarly, little or no differences in caspofungin pharmacokinetics were observed with gender or race *(25,31)*. In addition, dosage adjustment is not required in patients with impaired renal function; however, the dose should be reduced by 50% in patients with significant hepatic impairment *(25)*.

### Scope of Problem

Because the echinocandins are a new class of compounds, their propensity to interact with other compounds is still being elucidated. Although early in vitro evidence indicated agents in this class were poor substrates for CYP enzymes, several human studies involving tacrolimus and cyclosporine suggested that the class may potentially

**Table 1**
**Drug Interactions Caused by Amphotericin B Formulations**

| Interaction | Drugs | Comments |
|---|---|---|
| Additive/synergistic effects | | |
| • Direct or indirect nephrotoxicity | Cyclosporine Tacrolimus Aminoglycosides | Monitor Scr, BUN, electrolytes, consider renal-sparing amphotericin B formulations or other antifungal agents |
| • Fluid and electrolyte disturbance (i.e., water retention, hypokalemia, hypomagnesemia) | Thiazide and loop diuretics, aminoglycosides, corticosteroids | Monitor Scr, BUN, electrolytes; supplement electrolytes as needed |
| Enhanced pharmacological effect | | |
| • Increase cardiac automaticity and inhibition of $Na^+$-$K^+$ ATPase (adenosine triphosphatase) pump | Digoxin | Effects secondary to amphotericin B-induced hypokalemia |
| • Myelosuppression | 5-Fluorocytosine (5-FC) | Effect caused by diminished renal clearance of 5-FC secondary to amphotericin B-associated nephrotoxicity |

interact with other drugs, and that these interactions may involve CYP. Nonetheless, to date it appears that, compared to other antifungal classes, these compounds are relatively devoid of significant drug interactions. Further study of the drug interaction potential of this class is likely as agents such as caspofungin gain wider use and additional agents are introduced into clinical practice.

## IMPORTANT DRUG INTERACTIONS

### *Amphotericin B Formulations*

#### *Synergistic/Additive Nephrotoxicity*

Amphotericin B-induced nephrotoxicity can be additive to that caused by other agents that damage the kidneys by similar mechanisms (i.e., cyclosporine, tacrolimus, aminoglycosides), or it can lead to the accumulation of toxic serum concentrations of renally eliminated drugs such as 5-FC. Electrolyte disturbances resulting from amphotericin B-induced nephrotoxicity can be additive to those of other medications (i.e., thiazide and loop diuretics), or they may augment the pharmacological effects of drugs such as digoxin, with potentially deleteriously results. Drug interactions caused by amphotericin B formulations are summarized in Table 1.

MECHANISM

Amphotericin B causes nephrotoxicity via direct toxicity to the proximal and distal tubule and indirectly via reduced renal blood flow. Directly, it causes renal tubular acidosis and impairs proximal and distal reabsorption of electrolytes. Indirectly, amphotericin B produces afferent arteriolar vasoconstriction, which causes ischemic damage and reduces glomerular filtration *(1)*. Amphotericin B shares these several mechanisms of renal injury with cyclosporine, tacrolimus, or aminoglycosides. Therefore, using amphotericin B in combination with these agents may produce additive or synergistic renal toxicity.

CLINICAL IMPORTANCE

Amphotericin B is commonly used in critically ill patients at high risk for renal dysfunction and electrolyte disturbances as a consequence of their underlying illness or concomitant nephrotoxic medications. Amphotericin B-associated nephrotoxicity can make the use of concomitant medications difficult.

MANAGEMENT

When amphotericin B interactions occur, they may be somewhat unavoidable. Therefore, clinicians should focus on limiting the risk or severity of these interactions. In patients receiving aminoglycosides, cyclosporine, or tacrolimus who need amphotericin B, the lipid formulations of amphotericin B should be substituted for amphotericin B deoxycholate. Increases in Scr and nephrotoxicity may still occur when these formulations are used with cyclosporine, tacrolimus, or the aminoglycosides, but the increases are generally not clinically significant, or incidence of such toxicity is markedly reduced *(32,33)*. Depending on the suspected pathogen and the severity of the patient's underlying illness, other iv antifungal agents that can be safely dosed in patients with diminished renal function (i.e., caspofungin, fluconazole) should also be considered. Although voriconazole and itraconazole are formulated as an iv dosage form, the potential accumulation of their solubilizing agents in patients with diminished renal function is a concern.

Although individually amphotericin B deoxycholate and cyclosporine cause hypomagnesemia, this electrolyte disturbance is not additive when the two drugs are given in combination *(34)*. Nonetheless, judicious laboratory monitoring of renal function (i.e., Scr, serum urea nitrogen [BUN]), and electrolytes (i.e., $K^+$, Mg, $PO_4$) should be a standard of care. More important, blood or serum concentrations of the aminoglycosides, cyclosporine, or tacrolimus should be closely monitored. Because amphotericin B may produce renal vascular effects in the absence of glomerular damage, changes in the blood or serum concentrations of these agents may precede alterations in Scr and provide early evidence of impending acute renal damage. Another measure that should be employed is the use of hydration with normal saline, especially if amphotericin B deoxycholate is used.

*Secondary Nonrenal Toxicities*

Amphotericin B can interact with concomitantly administered drugs that are primarily eliminated renally. This interaction leads to the accumulation of the renally eliminated drug and results in elevated serum concentrations and secondary nonrenal toxicities associated with the agent.

MECHANISM

Flucytosine toxicities such as bone marrow suppression, hepatic necrosis, and diarrhea have been associated with elevated plasma 5-FC concentrations and often occur in the presence of renal dysfunction *(6)*. 5-FC is primarily excreted renally as unchanged drug, and very little of the parent drug is deaminated to 5-FU *(6)*. However, 5-FU serum concentrations similar to those that produce hematological toxicity in patients receiving it as cancer chemotherapy have been observed in noncancer patients following 5-FC administration *(6)*. Therefore, amphotericin B-associated renal dysfunction prolongs 5-FC elimination, which results in accumulation and elevated serum 5-FC concentrations. The 5-FC is then deaminated, resulting in elevated concentrations of 5-FU, which can cause bone marrow and GI mucosa toxicity *(6)*.

EFFECT ON PHARMACOKINETICS/DYNAMICS

The incidence of 5-FC toxicity in patients receiving amphotericin B is approx 20 to 40% *(35,36)*. The effects of amphotericin B on the pharmacokinetics of 5-FC have not been rigorously studied. Rather, most of the effects of amphotericin B on the pharmacokinetics of 5-FC have been extrapolated from studies of 5-FC in patients with varying degrees of renal function. Because renal clearance of 5-FC correlates well with CrCL, renal dysfunction significantly prolongs $t_{1/2}$ and decreases plasma clearance. In one study of the effect of amphotericin B-induced nephrotoxicity, peak 5-FC concentrations $C_{max}$ increased 14 to 142% *(37)*.

Because 5-FC is administered only in combination with amphotericin B, there are few direct comparisons of 5-FC toxicity in the presence and absence of amphotericin B therapy. In a large study of amphotericin B and 5-FC toxicity in patients with cryptococcal meningitis, evidence of myelosuppression occurred in 22% *(35)*. Toxicity was predominantly observed in patients treated with ≥3 mg/kg normalized for CrCL (mL/minute) for 2 or more weeks. These doses were not more frequently administered to patients with renal dysfunction. In fact, no correlation between 5-FC-induced blood dyscrasias (leukopenia and thrombocytopenia), underlying disease, or concomitant drug therapy was observed *(35)*.

CLINICAL IMPORTANCE

The importance of this interaction is outweighed by the efficacy of this combination for the treatment of cryptococcal meningitis. Nonetheless, clinicians should be aware of this interaction so that this combination can be used optimally.

MANAGEMENT

Because the use of this combination often cannot be avoided, Scr and 5-FC blood concentrations should be monitored. The benefits of therapeutic drug monitoring for 5-FC have been demonstrated *(38)*. Ideally, concentrations should be maintained between 25 and 100 µg/mL to minimize 5-FC toxicity and avoid the emergence of 5-FC resistance *(38)*. Several nomograms for dosing 5-FC based on CrCL in patients with renal dysfunction have been published. However, these methods are based on Scr; therefore, they should not be used unless the renal dysfunction is chronic, and they should be used cautiously in elderly patients. Furthermore, these methods should be used only to make initial estimates. Thereafter, plasma concentrations should be monitored and the results used to make any necessary adjustments. The use of lower doses (100 mg/kg/day) of 5-FC has been recommended *(38)*. Although likely, whether lower doses of 5-FC actually improve the safety of this combination needs to be further evaluated.

*Miscellaneous Electrolyte Disturbances*

Amphotericin B-associated electrolyte disturbances may represent an often-overlooked source of drug–drug interactions. These electrolyte disturbances can be additive to those of other medications, or they may augment the pharmacological effects of drugs such as nondepolarizing skeletal muscle relaxants and digoxin *(6)*.

MECHANISM

Hypokalemia secondary to persistent wasting of urinary potassium is perhaps the most significant amphotericin B-associated electrolyte disturbance. This adverse effect can lead to hypokalemic cardiopathy, which can be compounded by concomitant medications. Amphotericin B-induced hypokalemia can increase cardiac automaticity and facilitate inhibition of the $Na^+$-$K^+$ ATPase (adenosine triphosphatase) pump by digoxin. The combination of amphotericin B and drugs that cause hypokalemia and salt and water retention (i.e., corticosteroids) can further compound the hypokalemic cardiopathy.

LITERATURE

Corticosteroids potentiate amphotericin B-induced hypokalemia and have contributed to reversible cardiomegaly and congestive heart failure in several patients treated with amphotericin B and hydrocortisone. In a series of cases, patients received 25–40 mg/day of hydrocortisone for 13–44 days *(39)*. Laboratory data and clinical findings suggested the cardiomegaly and congestive heart failure were caused by urinary wasting and salt and water retention, which led to circulatory overload. The authors stated that the salt and water retention caused by the hydrocortisone was augmented by the hypokalemia, which was caused primarily by amphotericin B *(39)*. Amphotericin B-induced hypokalemia reportedly also potentiates digoxin toxicity *(6)*.

CLINICAL IMPORTANCE

Based on few and conflicting data, and often with little concern, hydrocortisone is frequently added to the amphotericin B admixture to prevent infusion-related toxicity. These cases illustrate that these medications should be used only after careful consideration of the patient's clinical condition.

MANAGEMENT

When hydrocortisone or other medications that effect the fluid and electrolyte status of the patient are used with amphotericin B, fluid status, electrolytes, and cardiac function should be closely monitored.

### 5-Fluorocytosine

*Secondary Nonrenal Toxicities*

As described previously, concomitantly administered drugs (i.e., amphotericin B, aminoglycosides) that reduce glomerular filtration will prolong 5-FC elimination. Without 5-FC dosage adjustment, accumulation of toxic concentrations will likely occur. Although this same potential exists when 5-FC is administered to patients receiving either cyclosporine or tacrolimus, there are no reports describing such an interaction between these drugs *(40)*.

*Synergistic/Additive Myelosuppression and Cytotoxicity*

5-FC may interact with drugs that are myelosuppressive or cytotoxic, such as zidovudine and ganciclovir, and increase the risk of blood dyscrasias.

MECHANISM

Approximately 25% of administered 5-FC is deaminated to 5-FU, which contributes directly to 5-FC-associated myelosuppression. In addition, 5-FU can be further acted on to form 5-fluordeoxyuridylic acid, which can inhibit thymidylate synthetase and interfere with deoxyribonucleic acid (DNA) synthesis. This may also contribute to 5-FC-associated myelosuppression. Zidovudine is acted on intracellularly by thymidine kinase and converted to zidovudine monophosphate. The hematological toxicity associated with zidovudine has been attributed to intracellular accumulation of zidovudine monophosphate *(41)*.

LITERATURE

Because of the concern over the potential myelotoxicity, clinicians have been hesitant to use 5-FC in patients with acquired immunodeficiency syndrome (AIDS). There have been several studies using 5-FC in combination with amphotericin B or the azoles for the treatment of cryptococcosis in AIDS patients. Although the 5-FC-containing regimens have demonstrated efficacy in AIDS patients, these reports shed little light on the safety of this agent in this population *(38)*.

## Systemic Azoles
### Mechanisms of Interactions

As a result of their physicochemical properties, primarily their lack of aqueous solubility, the systemic azoles, particularly itraconazole and ketoconazole, are prone to many drug–drug interactions. The systemic azoles can interact, by different mechanisms, with a variety of medications at several sites within the body. These interactions primarily affect the pharmacokinetic processes of the systemic azoles as well as those of the interacting drug.

The systemic azoles itraconazole, ketoconazole, and voriconazole are lipophilic. Therefore, they cannot be formulated as an iv dosage form without the use of a solubilizing agent, or their administration is limited to the oral route. Thus, they may be prone to interactions within the GI tract that may interfere with absorption. As discussed below, fluconazole differs physicochemically from other azoles and is therefore less prone to drug interactions, particularly within the GI tract. As a consequence of their nonpolar chemical nature, to some extent all systemic azoles undergo oxidative Phase I metabolism in the liver and perhaps in the intestine via CYP. Enteric metabolism is quite extensive for itraconazole and ketoconazole.

### Interactions Affecting Solubility and Absorption
pH INTERACTIONS

Drug dissolution rate determines the intestinal lumen concentration of drug in solution available for absorption *(42)*. Therefore, intralumen pH can indirectly affect absorption. Weakly basic drugs such as itraconazole and ketoconazole dissolve more slowly at higher pH, whereas weakly acidic drugs dissolve faster at higher pH. Itraconazole and ketoconazole are weak bases with high p$K_a$ (3.7 and 2.94–6.51, respectively), and their dissolution and subsequent absorption in large fluid volumes (i.e., >50 mL) is optimal at pH 1.0–4.0 *(43)*. The absorption of itraconazole and ketoconazole is impaired above these pH values. Fluconazole and voriconazole are also weak bases, with lower p$K_a$ values ($\approx$2.0 and 1.63, respectively), and thus their dissolution is not affected by increases in gastric pH.

BINDING INTERACTIONS

Binding interactions (i.e., complexation and chelating interactions) between ketoconazole, or potentially itraconazole, and metal ion-containing drugs, vitamin supplements, and antacids can also diminish dissolution and subsequent absorption. Interactions between the azole and metal ions can be a simple interaction by which the azole may be soluble but, as a result of the ionic binding, unavailable for transport across the GI epithelium. Conversely, the interactions can be complex. The interacting drug may also influence the intralumen pH and thereby affect azole dissolution and absorption. These electrostatic binding interactions can occur between the protonated species of ketoconazole (ketoconazole$^{2+}$ or ketoconazole$^{+}$) and the polyanion of sucralfate *(44)*. This interaction between either ketoconazole$^{2+}$ or ketoconazole$^{+}$ and the sucralfate polyanion renders ketoconazole unavailable for transport across the GI epithelium *(44)*. Thus, even though reducing GI pH increases ketoconazole solubility, the interaction with sucralfate still decreases ketoconazole absorption under acidic conditions *(44)*. Although there is no reported interaction between itraconazole and sucralfate, given its chemical similarity to ketoconazole, such an interaction may occur.

### Interactions Affecting CYP-Mediated Biotransformation

Ketoconazole, itraconazole, and voriconazole are lipophilic and cannot be excreted into the urine by the kidney without extensive conversion to hydrophilic metabolites. In contrast, fluconazole is much less lipophilic and requires less biotransformation. The azoles are all inhibitors and substrates of CYP, although the affinities of itraconazole and ketoconazole for specific isoforms differ from that of fluconazole and voriconazole.

As inhibitors of CYP isoforms, the systemic azoles exhibit rapidly reversible binding *(45)*. As reviewed in Chapter 2, this type of binding to CYP by an inhibitor or its metabolite results in either competitive or noncompetitive inhibition *(45)*. The extent of inhibition by a noncompetitive inhibitor is dependent only on the concentration of the inhibitor relative to its $K_i$ value. Conversely, the extent of inhibition by a competitive inhibitor is dependent on the substrate concentration relative to its $K_m$ *(46)*. The azoles are potent reversible inhibitors that generally exert competitive inhibition *(45)*. However, ketoconazole and fluconazole have also demonstrated noncompetitive or mixed-type inhibition, indicating a direct interaction with the heme moiety of CYP *(45,46)*. There are no published data describing whether voriconazole also exhibits noncompetitive or mixed-type inhibition. The pharmacokinetic properties of the azoles also influence azole-drug interactions *(41)*.

The systemic azoles predominantly inhibit CYP3A4, which is extensively expressed in the liver and GI tract. As a result, at both of these sites the systemic azoles, particularly itraconazole, ketoconazole, and voriconazole, are prone to CYP-mediated interactions, which can affect either their biotransformation or that of many compounds. In vitro, the inhibitory potential of azoles on other CYP isoforms varies. Ketoconazole interacts extensively with the heme moiety of CYP3A (i.e., Type 2 binding), resulting in noncompetitive inhibition of oxidative metabolism of many CYP3A substrates *(45)*. In addition to being a potent inhibitor of CYP3A4, ketoconazole inhibits other isoforms, albeit to a lesser extent *(41)*. These isoforms include CYP1A2, CYP2E1, CYP2D6, and the CYP2C subfamily. Thus, ketoconazole may interact with a wide range of drugs *(41)*. Unlike ketoconazole, to date itraconazole is only known to inhibit CYP3A4.

Although fluconazole undergoes minimal CYP-mediated metabolism, like the other azoles, in vitro it inhibits CYP3A4, but much more weakly than other agents in this class *(47)*. However, unlike itraconazole and ketoconazole, in vitro fluconazole is a comparatively stronger inhibitor of several other isoforms (i.e., CYP2C9 and perhaps

CYP2C19) *(47)*. When evaluating in vitro studies of the inhibitory potential, it is important to note fluconazole binds noncompetitively to CYP, and in vivo it circulates largely as free drug. Therefore, determination of the ability of fluconazole to inhibit CYP in vitro may not accurately predict its potential to inhibit CYP in vivo. Fluconazole also interacts with phase II enzymes involved in glucuronidation *(15)*. Voriconazole and perhaps some of its metabolites are inhibitors of CYP2C9, CYP2C19, and to a lesser extent CYP3A4. Therefore, it has the potential to interact with a wide array of other medicines *(48)*.

### Interactions Affecting P-gp-Mediated Efflux and Other Transporters

Drug transporters are increasingly recognized as key determinants of drug disposition. These transport proteins are expressed in a variety of tissues and allow for the efficient directional movement (i.e., uptake or efflux) of many drugs. Although there are likely many transport proteins involved in drug disposition, most research has focused on the role of the efflux transporter MDR1 (P-gp). The MDR1 gene product P-gp is expressed in a variety of tissues and functions as a transmembrane efflux pump/transport system on a broad range of substrates. P-gp is extensively expressed in the apices of mature enterocytes in the GI tract, bile canicular membrane of hepatocytes in the liver, cells of the blood–brain barrier, glomerular mesangium and apical membrane of the proximal tubule epithelia *(9)*. In these tissues, P-gp serves several different functions, all of which limit systemic exposure to many drugs. In the GI tract, P-gp reduces drug absorption, whereas in the liver and proximal tubules of the kidney, it is involved in the elimination of endogenous and exogenous compounds from the systemic circulation. In the blood–brain barrier, P-gp limits distribution *(45)*.

Growing evidence suggests that uptake transporters, specifically the members of the organic anion transporting polypeptide (OATP) family of transport proteins may also be important to drug disposition. Like the efflux transporter P-gp, members of the OATP family of transporters are expressed in the GI tract, liver, kidney, and at the blood–brain barrier. Moreover, these uptakes have been found capable of transporting a large array of structurally diverse compounds *(49)*.

P-gp is extensively co-localized with CYP3A, and the two proteins exhibit significant overlap in substrate specificity *(9)*. Even though many P-gp inhibitors are substrates or inhibitors of CYP3A4, the inhibitory potency of a compound toward the two proteins can be mutually exclusive. CYP3A4 inhibition is not an intrinsic characteristic of P-gp inhibitor *(50)*.

The systemic azoles vary in their interactions with P-gp. Itraconazole and ketoconazole, and perhaps fluconazole, are P-gp substrates *(9,51,52)*. However, itraconazole and ketoconazole inhibit P-gp, whereas fluconazole apparently does not *(8)*. There are no published data characterizing the interaction between voriconazole and P-gp. Nonetheless, it is likely that voriconazole is neither a substrate nor an inhibitor *(53)*. Therefore, interactions between itraconazole or ketoconazole and another CYP3A substrate can result from the inhibition of CYP-mediated metabolism, reduced P-gp-mediated efflux, or a combination of the two. Consequently, separating the effect of P-gp from that of CYP3A4 can be difficult. Interactions between itraconazole and digoxin or quinidine demonstrate this complexity.

To date, the interaction between the azoles and OATP transporters has not been elucidated. Nonetheless, as our understanding of the role of OATP transporters in drug disposition evolves, so too will our understanding of the factors governing the absorption, elimination, and tissue penetration of the azoles and other drugs.

### Ketoconazole

#### Literature

Itraconazole, fluconazole, and voriconazole have largely supplanted ketoconazole for the treatment of systemic mycoses. Ketoconazole can interact with other medications through pH and binding mechanisms or by interacting with CYP or P-gp.

#### pH and Binding Interactions

CLINICAL IMPORTANCE

Given the limited role of ketoconazole in the treatment of superficial or systemic mycosis, pH and binding interactions involving this azole are generally not important. However, in patients who, for lack of an alternative, require ketoconazole therapy, these interactions could compromise therapy and lead to clinical failure.

MANAGEMENT OF pH AND BINDING INTERACTIONS

Clearly, concomitant administration of agents that elevate gastric pH (i.e., antacids, $H_2$-antagonists, proton pump inhibitors) should be avoided in patients requiring ketoconazole therapy. If sucralfate or antacids are prescribed with ketoconazole, their administration should be separated by at least 2 hours *(54)*.

#### Interactions Affecting CYP-Mediated Biotransformation of Other Drugs

EFFECT ON PHARMACOKINETICS/DYNAMICS

Ketoconazole is a potent inhibitor of CYP3A4 in vitro, and in vivo studies established that it can inhibit the enteric or hepatic metabolism of many CYP3A4 substrates *(41,54,55)*. Most studies of ketoconazole interactions with CYP3A4 substrates attributed pharmacokinetic changes of the substrate (i.e., increased $C_{max}$, area under the curve [AUC], and $t_{1/2}$, or a corresponding decrease in its metabolite:parent drug ratios) to ketoconazole inhibition of CYP3A4. However, ketoconazole can also inhibit P-gp, so it is difficult to attribute ketoconazole drug interactions solely to CYP3A4 inhibition *(55)*. Most data concerning ketoconazole interactions with other CYP3A4 substrates were gathered before the importance of P-gp, particularly intestinal P-gp, in determining systemic availability was realized. Therefore, it is possible that P-gp inhibition, especially in the GI tract, contributes somewhat to ketoconazole drug interactions that were previously attributed to CYP3A4 inhibition.

#### Interactions Affecting P-gp-Mediated Efflux

EFFECT ON PHARMACOKINETICS/DYNAMICS

When ketoconazole was administered with oral and iv cyclosporine, investigators attributed pharmacokinetic changes in cyclosporine (i.e., decreased systemic clearance $CL_{iv}$ and a significant increase in oral bioavailability) to inhibition of intestinal CYP3A4 by ketoconazole *(56)*. However, it is now recognized that oral cyclosporine availability is determined primarily by intestinal P-gp rather than CYP3A4 *(55)*.

CLINICAL IMPORTANCE OF CYP AND P-GP-MEDIATED EFFLUX INTERACTIONS

Because the role of ketoconazole in the treatment of systemic mycoses has diminished, reports describing drug interactions with this agent have lessened. The clinical importance of these drug interactions lies in the mechanism behind them (i.e., ketoconazole inhibition of CYP3A4 and P-gp). Although CYP3A and P-gp substrates overlap substantially, it is likely that the substrates vary in their dependency on either CYP3A or P-gp for oral availability and systemic clearance. Thus, inhibiting CYP3A or P-gp may be an important clinical means for improving the oral absorption of drugs with poor oral availability or reducing the interpatient variability in pharmacokinetic behavior of certain drugs *(55)*.

MANAGEMENT OF CYP AND P-GP-MEDIATED EFFLUX INTERACTIONS

By exploiting the ketoconazole-cyclosporine interaction, several investigators demonstrated that ketoconazole can be utilized safely in transplant patients to lower the daily dose of cyclosporine and thereby lower the drug costs associated with transplantation. The use of ketoconazole enabled cyclosporine dosage reductions of approx 80% and reduced drug costs associated with transplantation 50–75% within the first year posttransplantation *(57,58)*. The use of ketoconazole may produce added benefits, including reduced rates of rejection and opportunistic fungal infections and a delay in the first rejection episode *(57,58)*. Ketoconazole also significantly increases methylprednisolone and prednisolone concentrations *(54)*. Although data suggest the ketoconazole-prednisolone interaction is not clinically significant, there is disagreement regarding the significance and the management of this interaction *(54,58)*.

## Itraconazole

### Literature

Drug interactions with itraconazole are summarized in Tables 2 and 3.

### Gastric pH Interactions

Itraconazole is an extremely weak base that is highly lipophilic ($P = 460,000$), virtually water insoluble (<5 μg/mL), and ionized at low pH *(19)*. Consequently, dissolution and subsequent absorption of itraconazole capsules are optimal in acidic intragastric conditions. However, the dissolution and subsequent absorption of itraconazole capsules are not dependent solely on a low intragastric pH; a long gastric retention time and a meal high in fat content are also critical for absorption of the capsules *(59)*. The potential for changes in gastric pH to affect the absorption of the itraconazole capsule has been demonstrated by studies of its administration with drugs that increase pH and data demonstrating the effects of food on its absorption. However, changes in pH do not affect the absorption of the oral solution *(12)*.

Drugs that increase gastric pH, such as $H_2$-receptor antagonists and proton pump inhibitors, reduce the absorption and oral availability of the itraconazole capsule approx 30–60% following a single dose or multiple doses *(60–62)*. Studies assessing the impact of pH on the itraconazole capsule are difficult to perform because, in addition to intragastric pH, many other conditions, including gastric emptying time, dietary caloric and fat content, and compounds that affect enteric CYP, must be controlled. Often, studies that demonstrate an effect have not taken into account these conditions *(63)*.

To protect against acid-induced hydrolysis, didanosine (ddI), a nucleoside reverse transcriptase inhibitor, was previously marketed as several buffered oral formulations. In a loosely controlled trial, simultaneous administration of the itraconazole capsule and the ddI buffered oral tablet significantly reduced itraconazole absorption *(63)*. However, ddI has since been reformulated as nonbuffered enteric-coated encapsulated beads, and there is no appreciable affect on itraconazole or hydroxyitraconazole pharmacokinetics when this formulation is administered with the itraconazole capsule *(64)*.

**Table 2**
**Itraconazole Interactions Effecting Pharmacokinetics/Dynamics of Other Drugs**

| Drug | Effect on drug | Suggested mechanism | Reference |
|---|---|---|---|
| **HMG-CoA reductase inhibitors** | | | |
| • Lovastatin | ↑ $C_{max}$, $AUC_{0-24}$, and $t_{1/2} \geq$ 15–20× | Inhibition of hepatic CYP3A; perhaps intestine | 69, 74 |
| • Simvastatin | ↑ $C_{max}$, $AUC_{0-\infty} \geq$ 10×; ↑ $t_{1/2}$ | Inhibition of hepatic CYP3A; perhaps intestine | 70, 73 |
| • Atorvastatin | ↔ $C_{max}$, ↑ $AUC_{0-72}$, $t_{1/2} \approx$ 3× | Inhibition of hepatic CYP3A; perhaps intestine | 71, 72 |
| • Fluvastatin | No effect on $C_{max}$, AUC, $t_{1/2}$ | | 74 |
| • Pravastatin | No effect on $C_{max}$, AUC, $t_{1/2}$ | | 70, 72 |
| • Rosuvastatin | No effect on $C_{max}$, AUC, $t_{1/2}$ | | 75 |
| **Benzodiazepines** | | | |
| • Midazolam | ↑ $C_{max}$, $AUC_{0-\infty}$, $t_{1/2}$, $F \approx$ 2×; ↓ $CL \approx$ 67% | Inhibition of hepatic CYP3A; perhaps intestine | 76, 79 |
| • Triazolam | ↑ $C_{max}$, $T_{max} \approx$ 2×; ↑ $AUC_{0-\infty}$, $t_{1/2} \approx$ 20× | Inhibition of hepatic CYP3A; perhaps intestine | 77, 78 |
| • Diazepam | ↑ $AUC_{0-\infty}$, $t_{1/2} \approx$ 35% | Inhibition of hepatic CYP3A | 80 |
| • Estazolam | No clinically significant effect | | 81 |
| • Bromazepam | No clinically significant effect | | 82 |
| • Temazepam | No clinically significant effect | | 83 |
| • Oxazepam | No clinically significant effect | | 83 |
| **Other anxiolytics, sedatives, and hypnotics** | | | |
| • Buspirone | ↑ $C_{max}$ 13×, $AUC_{0-\infty}$ 19× | Inhibition of hepatic and enteric CYP3A4 | 84 |
| • Zolpidem | No clinically significant effect | | 85 |
| **Antipsychotic agents** | | | |
| • Haloperidol | ↑ Concentrations 30% | Inhibition of hepatic CYP3A | 87 |
| • Clozapine | No clinically significant effect | | 88 |
| **Cyclosporine and tacrolimus** | | | |
| • Cyclosporine | ↑ $C_{min}$ 50% | Inhibition of hepatic CYP3A, P-gp in intestine? | 89, 90 |
| • Tacrolimus | ↑ $C_{min} \approx$ 5× | Inhibition of hepatic CYP3A, P-gp in intestine? | 91 |

| Drug | Effect | Suggested mechanism | Reference |
|---|---|---|---|
| Corticosteroids | | | |
| • Methylprednisolone | ↑ $C_{max}$, $T_{max}$, ↑ $AUC_{0-\infty}$, $t_{1/2} \approx 4\times$ | Inhibition of hepatic and enteric CYP3A4 | 92–94 |
| • Dexamethasone | ↑ $AUC_{0-\infty}$ three- to fourfold | Inhibition of hepatic and enteric CYP3A4 may involve P-gp | 95 |
| • Prednisolone | ↑ $AUC_{0-\infty}$, $t_{1/2}$ 13–30% | Inhibition of hepatic and enteric CYP3A4? | 93, 96 |
| • Budesonide | ↑ $C_{max}$, $AUC_{0-\infty}$, and $t_{1/2}$ 1.5- to 4-fold | Inhibition of hepatic and enteric CYP3A4 | 97 |
| Calcium channel blockers | | | |
| • Felodipine | ↑ $C_{min}$, $AUC_{0-\infty}$ 5-7×, $t_{1/2}$ 71% | Inhibition of hepatic and enteric CYP3A4 | 98 |
| Miscellaneous drugs inhibited by itraconazole | | | |
| • Oxybutynin | ↑ $C_{min}$, $AUC_{0-\infty}$, ≈ 2× | Inhibition of hepatic and enteric CYP3A4 | 99 |
| • Fentanyl | No significant effect | | 100 |
| • Selegiline | No significant effect | | 101 |
| • Busulfan | ↑ $C_{ss}$ 25%; ↑ CL/F 20% | Inhibition of hepatic CYP3A; perhaps intestine | 19 |
| • Digoxin | ↑ $t_{1/2}$ 38%; $AUC_{0-\infty}$ 68%, ↓ $CL_R$ 20% | Inhibition of renal P-gp | 107 |
| • Quinidine | ↑ $C_{max}$, $t_{1/2}$; $AUC_{0-\infty}$ 1.6-2.4×, ↓ $Cl_R$ 49-60%, partial clearance 3-hydroxyquinidine 84% and quinidine N-oxide 73% | Inhibition of hepatic CYP3A; renal P-gp | 108, 109 |
| • Cimetidine | ↑ $AUC_{0-24}$, ↓ CL 25% | Inhibition of P-gp-mediated renal tubular secretion | 112 |

## Table 3
### Pharmacokinetic Drug Interactions That Affect Itraconazole Plasma Concentrations

| Drug | Effect | Suggested mechanism | Reference |
|---|---|---|---|
| Famotidine | ↓ $C_{max}$, $C_{min}$, and AUC 30–53% | ↑ Gastric pH and ↓ absorption | 60, 61 |
| Omeprazole | ↓ $C_{max}$ 66% and $AUC_{0-24}$ 64% (itraconazole capsules) | ↑ Gastric pH and ↓ absorption | 62 |
| Didanosine (buffered formulation) | ↓ Concentrations 100% | ↑ Gastric pH and ↓ absorption | 63 |
| Phenytoin | ↓ $C_{max}$, AUC, $t_{1/2}$ 80–90%; ↑ CL/F 14× | Induction of CYP3A in liver; perhaps intestine | 104 |
| Phenobarbital | ↓ Concentrations to 30 ng/mL | Induction of CYP3A | 103 |
| Carbamazepine | ↓ Concentrations to undetectable | Induction of CYP3A | 103 |

EFFECT OF GASTRIC pH INTERACTIONS ON ITRACONAZOLE PHARMACOKINETICS/DYNAMICS

Generally, pH interactions with itraconazole manifest as a reduction in its $C_{max}$, AUC, and $T_{max}$. The coadministration of drugs that increase gastric pH with oral itraconazole will also likely lower serum concentrations of hydroxyitraconazole. However, pH interactions may change the metabolic ratio (i.e., metabolite: parent compound). Hydroxyitraconazole is formed primarily by the enteric CYP metabolism of itraconazole; thus, if there is an effect, it would likely manifest as a reduction in the metabolic ratio.

CLINICAL IMPORTANCE OF GASTRIC pH INTERACTIONS

Drug interactions with the itraconazole capsule resulting from elevated gastric pH may be unavoidable in patients who require high-dose corticosteroid therapy (i.e., transplant recipients).

MANAGEMENT OF GASTRIC pH INTERACTIONS

In patients receiving drugs that elevate gastric pH and who require itraconazole therapy, the oral solution rather than the capsule dosage form should be used. However, the marketed oral solution is somewhat dilute and may not be practical in certain patients, who will require either itraconazole or drugs that elevate gastric pH for a prolonged period of time. Consequently, there is still a need for the capsule dosage form. Therefore, clinicians should understand that the itraconazole capsule form can be absorbed in patients receiving drugs that elevate gastric pH. However, this absorption will be reduced and variable. For that reason, itraconazole trough serum concentrations ($C_{min}$) should be monitored periodically to document adequate oral availability. Several studies have tried to establish a threshold concentration in·humans that is predictive of response. The results of these studies varied, but in general, for optimal effectiveness investigators advocate itraconazole plasma trough concentration of at least 0.25 µg/mL (measured by high-performance liquid chromatography) *(19)*. However, evidence suggests that 0.5 µg/mL is the minimal desirable target concentration for the prevention and treatment of invasive fungal infections, especially in neutropenic hosts *(65)*. Nonetheless, given the variability of serum itraconazole concentrations observed with the capsule or oral solution, clinical response should guide judgments on the adequacy of the concentrations achieved.

*Interactions Affecting CYP-Mediated Biotransformation of Other Drugs*

EFFECT ON PHARMACOKINETICS/DYNAMICS

Itraconazole is a substrate and potent inhibitor of CYP3A4. Therefore, it can inhibit the intestinal or hepatic biotransformation of other CYP3A4 substrates. Likewise, because itraconazole is itself a CYP3A4 substrate, inducers of this isoform may augment its metabolism.

*Inhibitory Effects on Pharmacokinetics/Dynamics of Other Drugs*

HMG-CoA REDUCTASE INHIBITORS

The 3-hydroxy-3 methylglutaryl coenzyme A (HMG-CoA) reductase inhibitors are primarily CYP or P-gp substrates, and one, pravastatin, is a substrate of hepatic OATP-C *(49,66)*. Itraconazole is an inhibitor of P-gp and CYP3A4, so it may be difficult to attribute itraconazole drug interactions solely to CYP3A4 inhibition. Coadministration of the HMG-CoA reductase inhibitors with itraconazole can produce elevated systemic concentrations of these agents, which may result in rare, but severe, life-threatening toxicities *(19)*. Although the contribution of P-gp inhibition to this interaction is unclear, CYP3A inhibition is likely involved. All but one of the HMG-CoA reductase inhibitors undergo significant CYP-mediated metabolism. Lovastatin, simvastatin, and atorvastatin are all CYP3A substrates, whereas fluvastatin and rosuvastatin are metabolized by CYP2C9 *(66,67)*. In contrast, pravastatin is metabolized via several different CYP- and non-CYP-mediated reactions. CYP-dependent metabolism, specifically CYP3A4 and CYP3A5, is involved only in the formation of two of its minor metabolites *(68)*. Thus, compared to other HMG-CoA reductase inhibitors, like lovastatin, the CYP-dependent metabolism of pravastatin is quantitatively negligible *(68)*.

The inhibitory effects of itraconazole on the metabolism of these agents varies. Itraconazole significantly increases the $C_{max}$ and $AUC_{0-\infty}$ of lovastatin or simvastatin, whereas it affects atorvastatin pharmacokinetics considerably less *(69–72)*. The effect of this interaction on the exposure of certain HMG-CoA reductase inhibitors is dramatic. Itraconazole competitively inhibits CYP3A4-mediated metabolism of simvistatin, and coadministration of these two agents may increase simvastatin exposure up to 100 times that observed after a single dose of simvastatin administered alone *(73)*. The predicted maximum effect of the interaction on lovastatin exposure is approx 2.5 times that observed with simvastatin *(73)*. In contrast, this azole has no significant CYP-mediated effect on the pharmacokinetics of the HMG-CoA reductase inhibitors that are not metabolized by CYP3A4 (fluvastatin, pravastatin, and rosuvastatin) *(70,72–75)*.

### BENZODIAZEPINES

Coadministration of itraconazole with triazolam, midazolam, or diazepam can result in significant pharmacokinetic interactions and subsequently alter the pharmacodynamics of these agents. The most dramatic effects have been observed with triazolam and midazolam, which are exclusively metabolized by CYP3A4 in the intestine and liver *(55,76,77)*. The oral administration of either agent with itraconazole increases their oral availability and apparently decreases their clearance. This interaction manifests as significant changes in triazolam or midazolam $C_{max}$, $t_{max}$, $t_{1/2}$, and $AUC_{0-\infty}$ *(76,77)*. The effect of itraconazole on the clearance of triazolam cannot be fully determined without an intravenous formulation. However, following intravenous midazolam, itraconazole substantially reduces plasma clearance but does not affect the steady-state volume of distribution $V_{ss}$ of midazolam, which is reflected by a prolongation in its $t_{1/2}$ *(77)*.

Midazolam ($F = 30\%$) and triazolam ($F \approx 50\%$) undergo significant first-pass metabolism *(55,77)*. In addition, the significant interaction between itraconazole and triazolam occurs even when triazolam is administered up to 24 hours after itraconazole *(78)*. The interaction between itraconazole and midazolam is evident 4 days after the end of a 4-day course of itraconazole *(79)*. Furthermore, itraconazole significantly reduces the metabolic ratio of midazolam *(79)*. These data indicate the interaction between either of these agents and itraconazole likely results from inhibition of enteric and hepatic CYP3A4 by itraconazole.

More important, administration of itraconazole with either agent results in long-lasting pharmacodynamic effects, including prolonged amnesia, significantly reduced psychomotor performance tests, and severe sedation *(76,77)*. The effects of itraconazole on the pharmacodynamics of iv midazolam were also notable but less marked than after oral midazolam *(76)*. These effects can occur with a single 200-mg dose of itraconazole. Itraconazole concentrations at steady state are disproportionately higher than those following a single dose. Therefore, with repeated itraconazole dosing or increased doses, the affect on the pharmacokinetics and pharmacodynamics of these agents will likely be greater *(76)*. In addition, given the prolonged elimination of itraconazole, these effects will likely persist for at least several days *(76,78)*.

In contrast to midazolam and triazolam, diazepam does not undergo significant first-pass metabolism, and it is acted on by an additional isoform, CYP2C19 *(80)*. Concomitant itraconazole produces a small, yet statistically significant, increase in diazepam $AUC_{0-\infty}$, and slightly prolongs its $t_{1/2}$. However, it does not alter the pharmacodynamic effects of diazepam *(80)*. Estazolam is a short-acting benzodiazepine that is chemically similar to midazolam and triazolam. Although the CYP-dependent metabolism of estazolam has not been rigorously studied, it undergoes extensive oxidative metabolism, presumably by CYP3A4/5. However, surprisingly, 100 mg itraconazole capsules daily for 3 days does not alter plasma concentrations, other pharmacokinetic measures, or the pharmacodynamic effect of a single dose of estazolam *(81)*. Similarly, itraconazole coadministration did not affect the pharmacokinetics or pharmacodynamics of bromazepam, which suggests CYP3A4 is not significantly involved in the oxidative metabolism of this benzodiazepine *(82)*. Temazepam is a pharmacologically active metabolite of diazepam that possesses excellent oral availability *(F > 95%)* and is metabolized primarily via Phase II metabolism to temazepam glucuronide. CYP-mediated conversion to oxazepam represents a minor metabolic pathway for temazepam *(83)*. Therefore, not surprisingly, temazepam demonstrates no pharmacokinetic or pharmacodynamic interaction with itraconazole *(83)*.

OTHER ANXIOLYTICS, SEDATIVES, AND HYPNOTICS

Buspirone is a nonbenzodiazepine anxiolytic agent that, like oral midazolam and triazolam, undergoes extensive first-pass metabolism *(F ≈ 5%) (84)*. Administration of itraconazole with oral buspirone produces a pharmacokinetic interaction similar in magnitude (i.e., significant increase in $AUC_{0-\infty}$ and $C_{max}$) to that of oral triazolam and midazolam *(84)*. However, itraconazole does not effect the $t_{1/2}$ of buspirone. This suggests that the interaction likely results from inhibition of intestinal CYP3A4 by itraconazole. Changes in buspirone pharmacokinetics produced by itraconazole also manifest pharmacodynamically as moderate reductions in several psychomotor performance tests *(84)*. In addition, noxious adverse effects may be more common, but they disappear rapidly.

Zolpidem, a short-acting imidazopyridine hypnotic, is a substrate of CYP3A4 and, to a lesser extent, CYP1A2. Unlike midazolam, triazolam, and buspirone, it undergoes minimal first-pass metabolism and possesses good oral availability. Itraconazole minimally affects (i.e., slight increase in $AUC_{0-\infty}$) the pharmacokinetics and pharmacodynamics of this agent *(85)*.

ANTIPSYCHOTIC AGENTS

Haloperidol, a butyrophenone-derivative antipsychotic agent, is well absorbed from the GI tract but undergoes first-pass metabolism. The oral availability is approx 60%. Although the exact metabolic fate of haloperidol is unknown, it is acted on by CYP2D6 and perhaps CYP3A4 *(86)*. Itraconazole significantly increases plasma concentrations of haloperidol and its metabolite (reduced haloperidol) *(87)*. Although concomitant itraconazole does not produce any changes in haloperidol pharmacodynamics, this combination may significantly increase the incidence of haloperidol-associated neurological side effects *(88)*. The atypical antipsychotic agent clozapine is primarily metabolized by CYP1A2, but CYP3A4 and CYP2D6 catalyze secondary metabolic pathways *(86)*. Because CYP3A4 catalyzes a minor pathway in clozapine metabolism, itraconazole does not affect the pharmacokinetics or pharmacodynamics of this agent *(88)*.

CYCLOSPORINE AND TACROLIMUS

Pharmacokinetic interactions between tacrolimus or cyclosporine and the azoles are well known. Itraconazole inhibits intestinal and hepatic CYP-mediated metabolism of cyclosporine and tacrolimus *(40,41,57)*. The impact of itraconazole on cyclosporine pharmacokinetics varies among individuals, so elevated cyclosporine concentrations may not occur in all patients *(57)*. Generally, itraconazole causes a doubling of cyclosporine $C_{min}$, with a subsequent increase in serum creatinine *(57,89)*. Furthermore, itraconazole causes a 50% reduction in the relationship between cyclosporine oral dose rate and steady-state $C_{min}$ (dose rate-$C_{ss-min}$), compared with cyclosporine alone *(90)*. Generally, a change in this ratio can be attributed to a change in apparent clearance and perhaps in distribution *(19)*.

Similar to cyclosporine, tacrolimus is metabolized by intestinal and hepatic CYP3A4, and therefore it likely possesses a similar drug interaction profile. In one case report, a hepatopulmonary patient was initially started on 4 mg/kg of tacrolimus, but shortly thereafter trough concentrations of tacrolimus rose nearly fivefold after high-dose itraconazole (i.e., 600 mg twice daily) was started *(91)*. This necessitated a 50% reduction in the daily tacrolimus dose. On discontinuation of itraconazole after nearly 2 months of therapy, a 3.5-fold increase in the daily tacrolimus dose was necessary to maintain adequate target concentrations.

CORTICOSTEROIDS

Corticosteroids are widely used for their anti-inflammatory and immunosuppressive properties. As a result of their immunosuppressive effects, patients, particularly solid organ, bone marrow, or peripheral stem cell transplant recipients, are at risk for opportunistic systemic mycoses such as invasive aspergillosis. Two separate studies have demonstrated that itraconazole inhibits the metabolism of oral methylprednisolone (i.e., two- to threefold increases in $C_{max}$, $AUC_{0-\infty}$, and $t_{1/2}$) *(92,93)*. In addition, in both studies itraconazole coadministration reduced morning plasma cortisol concentration by approx 80% *(92,93)*. The effects of itraconazole on the pharmacokinetics and pharmacodynamics of iv methylprednisolone were similar. Itraconazole increased the systemic exposure ($AUC_{0-\infty}$) nearly threefold and more than doubled the $t_{1/2}$ of methylprednisolone *(94)*. In addition, the systemic clearance of methylprednisolone was reduced 40%, and morning plasma cortisol concentration was reduced approx 90% *(94)*. The metabolism of methylprenisolone has not been fully elucidated, but collectively these data suggest CYP3A4 is likely involved.

Dexamethasone is a CYP3A4 substrate, and similar to methylprednisolone, itraconazole increased the systemic exposure ($AUC_{0-\infty}$) of iv and oral dexamethasone approximately three- and fourfold, respectively *(95)*. Moreover, morning plasma cortisol concentrations were also significantly reduced. Dexamethasone is also a P-gp substrate, and thus this efflux protein could be involved in this reaction. In contrast to methylprednisolone and dexamethasone, coadministration of itraconazole affects the pharmacokinetics and pharmacodynamics of prednisolone to a lesser extent. Itraconazole coadministration increases prednisolone $AUC_{0-24}$ and $t_{1/2}$ 13 to 30%, but produces only minimal changes in prednisolone $C_{max}$ or pharmacodynamics *(93,96)*.

Inhaled corticosteroids are not immune to systemic drug interactions. Depending on the inhalation device and the skill of the patient, only about one-third of an inhaled corticosteroid dose is delivered directly to the lungs; the rest is inadvertently swallowed *(97)*. Drug that is delivered to the lungs is absorbed into the systemic circulation. In contrast, if the inhaled corticosteroid is a CYP3A4 substrate, prior to reaching the systemic circulation the fraction of a dose that is swallowed undergoes extensive metabolism by enteric and hepatic CYP3A4 to active or inactive metabolites. Budesonide, an inhaled glucocorticoid, reaches the systemic circulation directly by pulmonary absorption and indirectly through GI absorption. Oral itraconazole significantly inhibited the metabolism of inhaled budesonide (i.e., 1.5- to 4-fold increases in $C_{max}$, $AUC_{0-\infty}$, and $t_{1/2}$) in a crossover study of 10 healthy adults *(97)*. The extent of this interaction was quite variable between subjects. However, this study included men and women; thus, this observation may be a reflection of sex-related differences in the expression or activity of CYP3A4. Similar to the interaction with oral and iv corticosteroids, the interaction enhanced the adrenal suppressive effects of budesonide, as reflected by a significant reduction in morning plasma cortisol concentrations *(97)*.

In all of the above studies, coadministration of itraconazole with iv, oral, or inhaled corticosteroids enhanced their adrenal-suppressant effects, as reflected by reductions in morning plasma cortisol concentrations. Even though itraconazole can directly inhibit cortisol synthesis, this effect is associated with high doses administered for a prolonged period. All these studies were placebo-controlled trials, and subjects received 200 mg itraconazole daily for only 4 days. In addition, there was no difference in morning plasma cortisol concentrations between the itraconazole and placebo phases prior to corticosteroid administration *(92–97)*. Therefore, the enhanced adrenal-suppressant effects were attributed to feedback inhibition caused by the increased systemic exposure of the corticosteroids *(92–97)*.

CALCIUM CHANNEL BLOCKERS

Felodipine, a dihydropyridine calcium channel blocker, is a CYP3A4 substrate. Following oral administration, felodipine undergoes extensive first-pass metabolism, which results in low oral availability $(F = 15\%)$ *(98)*. Itraconazole coadministration results in a significant pharmacokinetic interaction and substantially increases the pharmacodynamic effects of felodipine. Itraconazole increases felodipine $C_{max}$ eightfold, $AUC_{0-\infty}$ approximately sixfold, and $t_{1/2}$ approximately twofold *(98)*. In one crossover study, the inhibition in felodipine metabolism was so marked that in most subject's felodipine $C_{min}$ with itraconazole 32 hours after dosing was higher than felodipine $C_{max}$ without itraconazole.

More important, the changes in felodipine pharmacokinetics reduced systolic and diastolic blood pressure significantly and were associated with a significant increase in heart rate *(98)*. Although systemic clearance was not assessed, the observed changes suggest that the interaction results from inhibition of intestinal and hepatic CYP3A4 by itraconazole. These interactions likely occur with other dihydropyridine calcium channel blockers *(41)*.

Miscellaneous Drugs

Itraconazole increases the $C_{max}$ and $AUC_{0-\infty}$ of oxybutynin *(99)*. However, oral itraconazole has no significant effect on the pharmacokinetics or pharmacodynamics of iv fentanyl administered to healthy volunteers in doses similar to that used during the induction of general anesthesia (3 μg/kg) *(100)*. Itraconazole also has no effect on the pharmacokinetics of selegiline *(101)*. In bone marrow transplant recipients, itraconazole increased steady-state busulfan concentrations and lowered plasma clearance. These changes were associated with an increased incidence of toxicity *(19)*. A case report noted a substantial potentiation of warfarin's effect with concomitant itraconazole therapy. This observation is intriguing because the metabolism of the pharmacologically active S-enantiomer of warfarin is carried out almost exclusively by CYP2C9, and there is no evidence that itraconazole inhibits the activity of this CYP isoform. A well-controlled, rigorous pharmacokinetic evaluation of these two drugs administered in combination has not been reported but is certainly needed *(102)*.

Clinical Importance of Itraconazole Interactions Affecting CYP Metabolism

Itraconazole has a very broad and extensive drug interaction profile, and many of these interactions are clinically important. Myopathy (skeletal muscle toxicity), which is manifested by myalgia and markedly elevated creatinine phosphokinase levels, is a rare, but potentially severe, side effect of elevated HMG-CoA reductase inhibitor concentrations *(70)*. This adverse effect could ultimately progress to rhabdomyolysis and renal failure *(70)*. In patients treated with lovastatin monotherapy, the incidence of skeletal muscle toxicity is 0.1 to 0.2% *(68)*. This risk dramatically increases to approx 30% within 1 year when lovastatin is combined with potent CYP3A4 inhibitors like cyclosporine *(68)*. This toxicity has been reported in a patient receiving lovastatin in combination with itraconazole and can likely occur with simvastatin and perhaps atorvastatin *(70–72)*. In addition, concomitant itraconazole therapy with these HMG-CoA reductase inhibitors may increase the risk of their associated dose-dependent adverse effects (i.e., hepatotoxicity) *(67)*.

The interaction between itraconazole and midazolam, triazolam, and buspirone produces significant changes in the pharmacodynamic effects of these drugs. Because of the potency of these agents, the changes in pharmacodynamics are severe and can be long-lasting. Patients receiving even low doses of these agents (particularly midazolam and triazolam) may have an impaired capacity to perform intellectual or motor skills for prolonged periods of time. The interaction with iv midazolam is less significant. Because the interaction does not change $V_{ss}$ when small bolus doses are used, the effect should not be increased. However, a high-dose bolus injection or a prolonged infusion may produce a significant interaction.

The clinical significance of the interaction between itraconazole and cyclosporine is unclear. The effect of itraconazole on cyclosporine concentrations is less than that produced by ketoconazole, so nephrotoxicity associated with this interaction is rare *(41)*. In contrast, the significance of the interaction between itraconazole and tacrolimus is unknown; nonetheless, the risk of this interaction and subsequent tacrolimus toxicity is likely high.

Itraconazole interacts significantly with oral, iv, or inhaled corticosteroids that are apparently metabolized to a significant extent by CYP3A4. This interaction increases the systemic exposure of these corticosteroids, which results in prolonged suppression of endogenous cortisol production. The studies to date have involved healthy volunteers administered a 4-day regimen of placebo or itraconazole followed by a single dose of corticosteroid. Therefore, the clinical significance of this interaction has not been fully determined. Nonetheless, given the extent and duration of the pharmacodynamic effect of this interaction in healthy patients, it is likely that the interaction could be even more problematic in patients administered prolonged courses of these agents together.

Given the extent of the increase in felodipine pharmacodynamic effects when given with itraconazole, this interaction is very significant clinically. Despite no evidence that itraconazole inhibits CYP2C9, and even though the coadministration of itraconazole and warfarin has not been rigorously evaluated in a controlled fashion, given the danger of excessive anticoagulation, the itraconazole-warfarin interaction should be considered clinically significant.

## MANAGEMENT OF INTERACTIONS AFFECTING CYP-MEDIATED METABOLISM OF OTHER DRUGS

Patients receiving lovastatin, simvastatin, or atorvastatin in combination with itraconazole should be monitored closely for clinical and laboratory signs of skeletal muscle toxicity (myalgia, arthralgia, creatinine phosphokinase elevations) and hepatotoxicity (transaminase elevations). The empiric administration of lower doses of these agents in the presence of itraconazole may be prudent. However, because pravastatin, fluvastatin, and rosuvastatin do not interact with itraconazole, they are the preferred HMG-CoA reductase inhibitors for use in patients receiving concurrent therapy with itraconazole.

Because of the prolonged elimination of itraconazole, the interaction with triazolam, and likely midazolam, cannot be avoided *(79)*. The benzodiazepines temazepam, oxazepam, and lorazepam undergo Phase II metabolism, so they should also be considered alternatives to triazolam and midazolam. Other alternatives include diazepam, estazolam, and the short-acting imidazopyridine zolpidem. Although all are CYP3A4 substrates, none is significantly affected by itraconazole.

In patients receiving itraconazole and either cyclosporine or tacrolimus, the dose of their immunosuppressive agent should be reduced by at least 50% *(19)*. In addition, their renal function and serum immunosuppressive concentrations should be closely monitored.

Patients requiring concomitant itraconazole and oral or iv corticosteroid therapy should receive prednisolone because of a lack significant pharmacokinetic interaction or pharmacodynamic effect with this agent. If patients are receiving dexamethasone or methylprednisolone (dosed chronically or as pulse therapy), corticosteroid dose reduction and careful follow-up are needed during concomitant itraconazole therapy.

Given the considerable clinical significance of the interaction between itraconazole and felodipine, this combination should be avoided. Similarly, calcium channel blockers that are chemically related to felodipine (i.e., amlodipine, isradepine, nifedipine) should also be avoided. If these combinations cannot be avoided, then the dose of felodipine or related agents should be reduced, and the patient's heart rate and blood pressure should be closely monitored until the patient's condition is stable. Termination of the interaction between itraconazole and warfarin requires discontinuation of itraconazole and perhaps infusion of fresh-frozen plasma and packed red blood cells to reverse excessive anticoagulation *(102)*. The combination of itraconazole and warfarin should be avoided. If antifungal therapy is needed, an amphotericin B formulation or caspofungin should be used.

*Interactions With Other Drugs That Accelerate CYP-Mediated Metabolism of Itraconazole*

EFFECT ON ITRACONAZOLE PHARMACOKINETICS/DYNAMICS

Phenytoin, phenobarbital, carbamazepine, and rifampin are well-known inducers of CYP3A4. Coadministration of itraconazole with any of these agents results in a pharmacokinetic interaction that markedly reduces its serum concentrations *(103–105)*. The onset of induction varies with each anticonvulsant, so changes in itraconazole serum concentrations may not be detectable for approximately several days to 2 weeks *(103)*. Clinically, the effects of induction may not be apparent for several days. After discontinuation of these anticonvulsants, induction can persist for approximately several days to 2 weeks *(103)*.

Changes in itraconazole pharmacokinetics produced by enzyme induction can be striking. Phenytoin reduces the AUC and $t_{1/2}$ of itraconazole and hydroxyitraconazole approx 90%. Similarly, phenytoin reduces their $C_{max}$ approx 20% and their $C_{min}$ approx 50- to 100-fold *(104)*. Rifampin also induces metabolism and lowers serum concentrations of itraconazole *(105)*.

CLINICAL SIGNIFICANCE OF INTERACTIONS THAT ACCELERATE
CYP-MEDIATED METABOLISM OF ITRACONAZOLE

The coadministration of CYP3A inducers with itraconazole produces clinically significant interactions. Often, induction of itraconazole metabolism leads to undetectable or subtherapeutic serum itraconazole concentrations. Therefore, the magnitude of this interaction is sufficient to compromise therapy in patients with fungal infections who are being treated with itraconazole.

MANAGEMENT OF INTERACTIONS THAT ACCELERATE
CYP-MEDIATED METABOLISM OF ITRACONAZOLE

The magnitude of induction and the dose-dependent pharmacokinetics make it unlikely that increasing the dose of itraconazole and monitoring serum concentrations can circumvent this interaction. Generally, these combinations should be avoided if possible. However, this is often not possible, especially in patients with human immunodeficiency virus (HIV) receiving rifampin or rifabutin. In these cases, if alternative antifungal therapy (i.e., amphotericin B, caspofungin) cannot be used, then itraconazole serum concentrations should be closely monitored, and the patient's clinical condition should be used as a guide in assessing the adequacy of the achieved concentrations. Alternative antimycobacterial regimens that do not contain rifampin or rifabutin should only be considered if alternative antifungal agents cannot be used. In patients receiving anticonvulsant therapy, gabapentin or levetiracetam may represent an alternative that is devoid of CYP3A-inducing properties.

*Interactions Affecting P-gp-Mediated Efflux*

EFFECT ON PHARMACOKINETICS/DYNAMICS OF OTHER DRUGS

As discussed earlier in the chapter, because of the substrate overlap and co-localization of CYP3A and P-gp, it is difficult to distinguish the contribution of each to interactions involving itraconazole and other CYP3A4 substrates. This complexity is best illustrated by the interaction between quinidine and itraconazole, which apparently involves both mechanisms. *(106–110)*. On the other hand, in some cases the distinction can be made. Digoxin represents one of the few drugs that interact with P-gp but not CYP3A.

## DIGOXIN

When first reported, the interaction between itraconazole was somewhat enigmatic, digoxin was not known to be significantly metabolized, and itraconazole was not known to have effects on renal transport systems. In the initial case reports, itraconazole elevated serum digoxin concentrations, which resulted in symptomatic digoxin toxicity and necessitated 60 to 75% reductions in digoxin doses to achieve safe and effective concentrations *(111)*. A rigorous pharmacokinetic analysis revealed that itraconazole significantly increased digoxin $AUC_{0-72}$ approx 50% and reduced renal clearance approx 20%. Although $C_{max}$ and $t_{1/2}$ were also increased, these changes were not significant *(107)*. Although itraconazole increases serum digoxin concentrations, the hepatic metabolism of digoxin is minimal ($\approx$10%), so this interaction cannot be attributed to inhibition of CYP-mediated metabolism *(41)*. Thus, these changes were attributed to a reduction in clearance or competition for tissue-binding sites with a subsequent reduction in volume of distribution *(111)*. Digoxin is primarily eliminated renally as unchanged drug, predominantly through P-gp-mediated renal tubular secretion *(106)*. Therefore, the interaction between itraconazole and digoxin can be attributed to inhibition of P-gp-mediated renal secretion of digoxin by itraconazole. The reduced P-gp-mediated efflux causes decreased renal clearance and increases serum concentrations of digoxin *(107)*.

## QUINIDINE

In contrast, the role of P-gp in the interaction between itraconazole and quinidine is less clear. Orally administered quinidine undergoes first-pass metabolism ($F$ = 70–90%), and approx 80% is metabolized via CYP isoforms to form 3-hydroxyquinidine and quinidine N-oxide *(108)*. Quinidine is also actively secreted by the renal tubules, which most likely involves P-gp. The formation of the 3-hydroxy metabolite is apparently dependent primarily on CYP3A4, whereas formation of the N-oxide depends on CYP2C9 and perhaps CYP3A4 *(109)*. The coadministration of itraconazole can significantly increase quinidine $C_{max}$ and exposure (AUC) nearly 2- and 2.5-fold, respectively, and the metabolic ratio (the metabolite/parent AUC) decreased 20% *(108)*. These findings suggest that itraconazole decreases first-pass and hepatic CYP3A4 metabolism of quinidine. However, coadministration of itraconazole also prolongs the quinidine elimination $t_{1/2}$ and significantly decreases the renal clearance of quinidine 49 to 60% *(108,109)*. In addition, coadministration of itraconazole significantly reduces the partial clearances by the 3-hydroxylation and N-oxidation 84 and 73%, respectively *(109)*. Interestingly peak serum quinidine metabolite concentrations are diminished, but not significantly, by itraconazole administration. Certainly, the interaction involves the inhibition of enteric and hepatic CYP3A4 to some degree. Nonetheless, the reductions observed in renal and partial clearances provide strong evidence that inhibition of renal P-gp also contributes to the interaction *(109)*. Thus, the changes in quinidine pharmacokinetics produced by concomitant itraconazole administration may be attributed to inhibition of enteric and hepatic CYP3A4 metabolism and P-gp-mediated tubular secretion of quinidine by itraconazole *(108–110)*.

MISCELLANEOUS DRUGS

As our understanding of the role of efflux proteins on the disposition of the azoles improves, the number of drugs that interact with itraconazole involving this mechanism will likely grow. Because of the overlapping tissue tropisms of CYP and P-gp, in vitro and in vivo studies of the renal clearance of P-gp substrates will likely best identify the contribution of P-gp in drug–drug interactions. This was illustrated using cimetidine, a P-gp substrate capable of interacting with itraconazole through a variety of mechanisms. Investigators used a renal cell monolayer expressing P-gp (MDR1-Madin-Darby canine kidney [MDCK] cells) to establish a model that demonstrated itraconazole significantly reduced transcellular efflux of cimetidine and then confirmed these findings in vivo *(111,112)*. In healthy volunteers, systemic cimetidine exposure $AUC_{0-240}$ increased 25%, and clearance was reduced to a similar degree following coadministration with itracona-zole *(112)*.

CLINICAL IMPORTANCE OF INTERACTIONS INVOLVING P-GP-MEDIATED EFFLUX

Because of the narrow therapeutic index of digoxin, the itraconazole-digoxin interaction is of considerable clinical significance. Case reports have documented patients experiencing symptomatic evidence of digoxin toxicity while receiving this combination *(113)*. Like digoxin, quinidine also has a relatively narrow therapeutic index, and elevated concentrations can produce life-threatening toxicity. Therefore, the clinical significance of the interaction is considerable *(107)*.

MANAGEMENT OF INTERACTIONS AFFECTING P-GP-MEDIATED EFFLUX OF OTHER DRUGS

In patients receiving itraconazole and digoxin, it is recommended that serum digoxin concentrations be closely monitored and that patients be questioned about nonspecific symptoms of digoxin toxicity *(113)*. Similarly, plasma quinidine concentrations should be closely monitored in patients receiving itraconazole and quinidine *(107)*.

## Fluconazole

### Mechanisms of Interactions

Fluconazole differs markedly from ketoconazole and itraconazole in terms of its physicochemical properties. Therefore, it does not share the drug interaction profiles of itraconazole and ketoconazole.

### Interactions Affecting Solubility and Absorption

PH AND BINDING INTERACTIONS

Fluconazole is water soluble and slightly lipophilic and has a low $pK_a$ (2.03), so it dissolves readily even at elevated pH. The disposition of fluconazole is unaffected by concomitant therapy with drugs that increase gastric pH, such as $H_2$-receptor antagonists and proton pump inhibitors. In addition, fluconazole absorption is unaffected by aluminum and magnesium hydroxide *(15)*.

### Interactions Affecting CYP-Mediated Biotransformation

Fluconazole exerts noncompetitive or mixed-type inhibition of CYP by interacting directly with the heme moiety of CYP2C9, CYP3A4, and CYP2C19 *(42,46)*. In vitro fluconazole is a much less potent inhibitor of CYP than ketoconazole *(47)*. Because fluconazole is a noncompetitive inhibitor, the extent of enzyme inhibition depends only on its concentration relative to its $K_i$ value *(47)*. In general, inhibition of 10 to 90% occurs in the range of noncompetitive inhibitor concentration 0.1–10 $K_i$ *(47)*. The extent of inhibition by fluconazole in vivo may be difficult to predict from in vitro studies *(47)*. For example, in vitro fluconazole demonstrates less-potent CYP3A4 inhibition than equivocal concentrations of itraconazole; in vivo, however, serum concentrations are approx 30 times higher than itraconazole *(76)*. This demonstrates the limited value of in vitro studies for predicting in fluconazole drug interactions in vivo. In addition, fluconazole circulates largely as unbound drug and exhibits predictable renal clearance and linear pharmacokinetics, so greater inhibition may occur with more elevated concentrations achieved with higher doses.

### Literature

Drug interactions with fluconazole are summarized in Table 4.

### Interactions Affecting CYP-Mediated Biotransformation of Other Drugs
#### EFFECT ON PHARMACOKINETICS/DYNAMICS

Fluconazole undergoes CYP-mediated metabolism, and compared to other azoles, it is a weak CYP3A4 inhibitor. However, it interacts with CYP2C9 and perhaps CYP2C19, and it circulates largely as free drug. Therefore, it may inhibit the hepatic biotransformation of CYP2C9 substrates. In addition, with sufficiently high doses, fluconazole may also inhibit the hepatic biotransformation of certain CYP3A4 substrates. Even though only a small percentage of fluconazole undergoes CYP-mediated metabolism, this percentage may greatly increase in the presence of a potent CYP inducer.

### Inhibitory Effects on Pharmacokinetics/Dynamics of Other Drugs
#### BENZODIAZEPINES

Coadministration of fluconazole with triazolam or midazolam results in significant pharmacokinetic interactions that subsequently alter the pharmacodynamics of these agents. The oral administration of either agent with fluconazole increases its oral availability and apparently decreases its Cl (i.e., increases $C_{max}$, $t_{1/2}$, and $AUC_{0-\infty}$) *(76, 114–116)*. Following iv midazolam, fluconazole substantially reduces plasma clearance but does not affect the steady-state volume of distribution $V_{ss}$ of midazolam, which is reflected by a prolongation in its $t_{1/2}$ *(76)*. Fluconazole also significantly reduces the metabolic ratio of midazolam *(114)*. Although the interaction between these agents likely results from inhibition of intestinal and hepatic CYP3A4, the data suggest that the interaction occurs primarily in the liver *(76,114–116)*. This interaction results in significant increases in pharmacodynamic effects that are long-lasting *(76,114–116)*. The effects of fluconazole on the pharmacodynamics of iv midazolam were also notable but less marked than after oral midazolam *(76,114)*. Fluconazole exhibits linear pharmacokinetics, so its effects did not increase with repeated dosing *(76)*. However, with increasing doses, the extent of the interaction between fluconazole and triazolam increased accordingly *(116)*.

#### CYCLOSPORINE AND TACROLIMUS

In vitro evidence predicts that fluconazole serum concentrations approximate the $K_i$ value for inhibition of cyclosporine metabolism, so the extent of cyclosporine inhibition will be closely correlated to the dose of fluconazole *(47)*. Indeed, this relationship has been seen in vivo. The initial study of concomitant 100 mg fluconazole daily with cyclosporine failed to demonstrate a significant interaction *(117)*. However, subse-

**Table 4**
**Fluconazole Drug–Drug Interactions**

| Drug | Effect on drug | Suggested mechanism | Reference |
|---|---|---|---|
| Benzodiazepines | | | |
| • Midazolam | ↑ $C_{max}$, $AUC_{0-\infty}$, $t_{1/2}$, $F \approx 2\times$; ↓ CL $\approx 51\%$ | Inhibition of hepatic and enteric CYP3A | 76, 114 |
| • Triazolam | ↑ $C_{max}$, $AUC_{0-\infty}$; $t_{1/2} \approx 1.25\text{-}2.5\times$ | Inhibition of hepatic CYP3A; perhaps intestine | 115, 116 |
| Cyclosporine and tacrolimus | | | |
| • Cyclosporine | ↑ $C_{min}$, $C_{ss}$, AUC $\approx 50\%$, ↓ CL $\approx 55\%$ | Inhibition of hepatic CYP3A; P-gp in intestine? | 118, 121 |
| • Tacrolimus | No significant effect | | 121 |
| Anticonvulsants | | | |
| • Phenytoin | ↑ $C_{min} \approx 1.25\times$, $AUC_{0-24}$ 75% | Dose-dependent Inhibition of hepatic CYP3A4 | 122 |
| Anticoagulants | | | |
| • Warfarin | Inhibits primary metabolic pathway $\approx 70\%$ | Inhibition of hepatic CYP2C9 | 42 |
| Miscellaneous drugs inhibited by fluconazole | | | |
| • Losartan | No significant effect | | 123 |
| • Alfentanil | ↑$AUC_{0-10}$, $t_{1/2} \approx 2\times$,↓CL $\approx 50\%$, $V_{ss} \approx 20\%$ | Inhibition of hepatic CYP3A4 | 124 |
| • Glyburide | ↑ Serum concentrations | Dose-dependent inhibition of hepatic CYP3A4 | 41 |
| • Saquinavir HGC | ↑ $C_{max}$ 56%, AUC 50%, ↓ CL/F 50% | Inhibition of hepatic CYP3A4 | 125 |
| • Ritonavir | No significant effect | | 125 |
| • Cyclophosphamide | ↓ CL; ↑ $t_{1/2}$ | Inhibition of hepatic CYP2C9 and CYP3A4 | 126 |
| Effects of other drugs on fluconazole pharmacokinetics/dynamics | | | |
| • Rifampin | ↓ $AUC_{0-\infty}$, $t_{1/2} \approx 20\%$;↑ $K_{el} \approx 20\%$ | Induction of hepatic CYP | 128 |
| Effect of fluconazole on drugs metabolized by Phase II reactions | | | |
| • Zidovudine | ↓ CL/F 43%; ↑ AUC 74%; ↑ $C_{max}$ 84%; $t_{1/2} \approx 1.2\times$ | Inhibition of GZDV formation by UDPGT | 129 |

quent reports using higher doses of fluconazole demonstrated that it causes slow increases in cyclosporine serum concentrations, although the incidence of subsequent nephrotoxicity was variable *(118,119)*.

A dose-dependent interaction has also been reported between fluconazole and tacrolimus *(120)*. However, the potential for fluconazole to interact with either cyclosporine or tacrolimus may also depend on the route of administration. A study of iv fluconazole (400 mg) and iv cyclosporine demonstrated statistically significant increases in steady-state cyclosporine concentrations and a significant reduction in steady-state cyclosporine clearance *(121)*. These differences were not thought to be clinically significant. In this same study, there was no significant effect of iv fluconazole on iv tacrolimus *(121)*. The investigators suggested that the lack of observed significant interaction with iv cyclosporine may reflect fluconazole's inhibition of gut metabolism. Whether this is true for tacrolimus is unknown. However, the oral availability of cyclosporine is determined primarily by intestinal P-gp rather than by CYP3A4, and fluconazole is not an inhibitor of P-gp *(9,10,55)*.

PHENYTOIN

Coadministration of fluconazole with phenytoin results in a significant increase in phenytoin $AUC_{0-24}$ and $C_{min}$ *(122)*. Given that fluconazole minimally binds to protein, this interaction likely results from CYP2C9 inhibition. Oddly, in one study phenytoin did not affect the pharmacokinetics of fluconazole. The unidirectional nature of this interaction is unclear; however, in this healthy volunteer study, for safety concerns the phenytoin dose was limited, and phenytoin exposure may have been inadequate to induce CYP *(122)*.

WARFARIN

Warfarin is administered as a racemic mixture, and the S-enantiomer is primary responsible for pharmacological activity. The metabolic pathways of racemic warfarin are complex and involve several CYP isoforms. However, metabolism of the S-enantiomer is carried out almost exclusively by CYP2C9. An interaction between fluconazole and warfarin can be predicted from in vitro studies *(42)*. Therapeutic plasma concentrations of fluconazole exceed its in vitro $K_i$ for inhibition of CYP2C9-mediated warfarin metabolism by at least twofold *(42)*. Fluconazole inhibits this pathway approx 70% and produces a 38% increase in international normalized ratio in patients previously stabilized on warfarin therapy *(42,102)*.

MISCELLANEOUS DRUGS

Fluconazole decreases the metabolism of the angiotensin II receptor antagonist losartan. Although fluconazole significantly reduced the active metabolite's $C_{max}$ and $AUC_{0-\infty}$, there was no significant change in these parameters for the parent compound *(123)*. Intravenous and oral fluconazole reduce the clearance of alfentanil more than 50% and cause doubling of its $t_{1/2}$ *(124)*. Pharmacodynamic changes were noted as a result of the increased alfentanil concentrations. The route of fluconazole administration does not influence the extent of this interaction *(124)*. Increased concentrations of the oral hypoglycemic glyburide and hypoglycemic episodes have been reported when this agent is administered with fluconazole *(41)*. Fluconazole significantly increased the $C_{max}$ and AUC of the hard gel saquinavir capsule (56 and 50%, respectively) and reduced apparent saquinavir clearance 50%, but it had no effect on ritonavir pharmacokinetics *(125)*.

Cyclophosphamide is a prodrug that is metabolized by CYP to produce the active moieties responsible for its cytotoxic effects in treating cancer in children *(126)*. Cyclophosphamide undergoes extensive metabolism and must first be hydroxylated to eventually produce the cytotoxic alkylating agent. This hydroxylation is catalyzed by several CYP isoforms; however, CYP2C9, and CYP3A4 are the two most important principal isoforms in this reaction *(127)*. Fluconazole reduces the clearance and increases the $t_{1/2}$ of cyclophosphamide in children *(126)*. Moreover, human liver microsomal studies reveal that peak free-plasma fluconazole concentrations achieved with routine dosing are sufficient to cause significant inhibition of cyclophosphamide metabolism in vivo *(126)*.

CLINICAL IMPORTANCE OF FLUCONAZOLE INTERACTIONS AFFECTING CYP METABOLISM

The interaction between fluconazole and midazolam or triazolam produces significant changes in the pharmacodynamic effects of these drugs. Because of the potency of these agents, the changes in pharmacodynamics are severe and can be long-lasting. Patients receiving even low doses of these agents (particularly midazolam and triazolam) may have an impaired capacity to perform intellectual or motor skills for prolonged periods of time. The interaction with iv midazolam is less significant. Because the interaction does not change $V_{ss}$ when small bolus doses are used, the effect should not be increased. However, a high-dose bolus injection or a prolonged infusion may produce a significant interaction.

Because of the dose dependency of the fluconazole interaction with cyclosporine and the variable effects on renal function, the clinical significance of this interaction is unclear. With daily fluconazole doses of 400 mg or more, this interaction will be more significant.

Because phenytoin exhibits Michaelis-Menten pharmacokinetics and the interaction with fluconazole likely increases $K_m$, patients receiving this combination may be predisposed to phenytoin toxicity.

Given the danger of excessive anticoagulation, clinically the fluconazole-warfarin interaction is considerably significant. Similarly, because of the consequences of excessive hypoglycemia, the fluconazole-glyburide interaction is also clinically significant. The interaction between saquinavir and fluconazole, although notable, is likely not clinically significant. The increase in saquinavir concentrations generally is less than the intrinsic interindividual variability normally observed in its pharmacokinetic variables.

The interaction between fluconazole and cyclophosphamide is potentially clinically significant in that it may reduce the therapeutic efficacy of cyclophosphamide. Further study to determine whether fluconazole reduces the formation of 4-hydroxycyclophosphamide in vivo is needed. If there is a reduction, such studies will also need to determine whether the reduction translates into a diminished therapeutic effect of cyclophosphamide before the significance of this interaction can be fully appreciated.

MANAGEMENT OF INTERACTIONS AFFECTING
CYP-MEDIATED METABOLISM OF OTHER DRUGS

Because the interaction between triazolam, and likely midazolam, occurs even with low doses of fluconazole, these combinations should generally be avoided. The benzodiazepines temazepam, oxazepam, and lorazepam undergo Phase II metabolism, so they may be alternatives to triazolam and midazolam. However, fluconazole also inhibits certain phase II enzymes, so until the interaction potential of agents with fluconazole is known, they should be used cautiously. Other alternatives such as diazepam and the short-acting imidazopyridine zolpidem also require further study to determine their potential to interact with fluconazole.

When fluconazole is used with cyclosporine, the lowest effective dose of fluconazole should be used to minimize the risk of this interaction occurring. Cyclosporine blood concentrations and serum creatinine monitoring should be performed routinely to detect any deterioration in renal function.

Phenytoin serum concentrations should be monitored prospectively with the addition of fluconazole therapy. If the two are used together for prolonged times, the patient should be monitored for breakthrough fungal infections.

The therapeutic concentrations of fluconazole are generally more than twofold its $K_i$; therefore, it is unlikely that lowering the dose of fluconazole 50% will be beneficial in patients receiving warfarin. Termination of the interaction between fluconazole and warfarin requires discontinuation of fluconazole and perhaps infusion of fresh-frozen plasma and packed red blood cells to reverse excessive anticoagulation *(102)*.

When fluconazole is used with glyburide, the lowest effective dose of fluconazole should be used to minimize the risk of this interaction occurring. Blood glucose concentrations should be monitored, and the patient should be aware of signs and symptoms of hypoglycemia.

### Interactions With Other Drugs That Accelerate CYP-Mediated Metabolism of Fluconazole

#### EFFECT ON FLUCONAZOLE PHARMACOKINETICS/DYNAMICS

Even though fluconazole is minimally metabolized, drugs such as rifampin and its derivatives can accelerate its biotransformation. Coadministration of rifampin with fluconazole significantly induces the CYP-mediated metabolism of fluconazole, thereby significantly reducing $AUC_{0-\infty}$ and causing a significant increase in its elimination rate constant *(128)*.

#### CLINICAL SIGNIFICANCE OF INTERACTIONS THAT ACCELERATE CYP-MEDIATED METABOLISM OF FLUCONAZOLE

The coadministration of rifampin with fluconazole produces a clinically significant interaction. Without a dosage adjustment in fluconazole, the resulting induction of fluconazole metabolism leads to undetectable or subtherapeutic serum fluconazole concentrations. Therefore, the magnitude of this interaction is sufficient to compromise therapy in patients with fungal infections who are being treated with fluconazole.

#### MANAGEMENT OF INTERACTIONS THAT ACCELERATE CYP-MEDIATED METABOLISM OF FLUCONAZOLE

In many instances, the induction of fluconazole CYP-mediated metabolism cannot be overcome by increasing the fluconazole dose. However, in patients receiving rifampin, the dose of fluconazole should be doubled.

### Effect of Fluconazole on Drugs Metabolized by Phase II Reactions

Fluconazole lowers concentrations of the Phase II enzyme, uridine diphosphate-glucuronosyl transferase (UDPGT) in rats *(15)*. In humans, this enzyme is responsible for catalyzing the biotransformation of zidovudine (ZDV) to its major metabolite, GZDV *(129)*. Coadministration of fluconazole (400 mg daily) significantly decreased

ZDV oral clearance and formation of GZDV, which subsequently led to increases in $AUC_{0-\infty}$, $C_{max}$, and $t_{1/2}$ of ZDV *(129)*. Urinary recovery of GZDV was also significantly reduced *(129)*.

CLINICAL SIGNIFICANCE OF FLUCONAZOLE INTERACTIONS INVOLVING PHASE II REACTIONS

Although fluconazole's effect on UDPGT is implicated in this reaction, the exact mechanism of ZDV metabolic inhibition by fluconazole is unknown. The clinical significance of this interaction is undetermined.

MANAGEMENT OF FLUCONAZOLE INTERACTIONS INVOLVING PHASE II REACTIONS

Patients receiving this combination should be monitored closely for the development of ZDV toxicity.

## Voriconazole

### Mechanism of Interaction

Chemically, voriconazole is a derivative of fluconazole. The chemical modifications not only broadened and improved the spectrum of activity of the molecule, but also changed the way it is eliminated from the body. As discussed previously, unlike fluconazole, voriconazole is extensively metabolized by CYP to its principle N-oxide metabolite by CYP2C19, CYP3A4, and to a lesser extent CYP2C9 *(22)*. Because CYP2C19 and CYP2C9 exhibit genetic polymorphisms, when assessing the effect of voriconazole on other drugs and vice-versa, genotype status for CYP2C19 and perhaps CYP2C9, the coadministration of other substrates or inhibitors of CYP2C19, CYP3A4, or CYP2C9, and voriconazole's inhibitory effects on these isoforms all must be considered. Therefore, the potential for voriconazole to interact with other medicines is greater than that of fluconazole. Voriconazole is likely neither a substrate nor an inhibitor of P-gp; thus, induction or inhibition of CYP-mediated drug metabolism are the primary mechanisms by which voriconazole participates in drug–drug interactions *(53)*.

### Interactions Affecting Solubility and Absorption
PH AND BINDING INTERACTIONS

Voriconazole is soluble in dilute acid and has a low $pK_a$ (1.63); it dissolves readily even at elevated pH. Voriconazole's disposition is unaffected by concomitant therapy with drugs that increase gastric pH, such as $H_2$-receptor antagonists and proton pump inhibitors.

### Literature

Drug interactions with voriconazole are summarized in Tables 5 and 6.

### Interactions Affecting CYP-Mediated Biotransformation of Other Drugs
VORICONAZOLE INHIBITORY EFFECTS ON PHARMACOKINETICS/DYNAMICS OF OTHER DRUGS
WARFARIN

The pharmacologically active S-enantiomer of warfarin is primarily metabolized by CYP2C9. Although CYP2C9 is only minimally involved in the CYP-mediated metabolism of voriconazole, the azole apparently inhibits it to an extent similar to that of fluconazole. In the only study to date, 300 mg voriconazole administered twice daily by mouth significantly potentiated warfarin-induced prolongation of prothrombin time *(130)*. Voriconazole increased the pharmacodynamic effect of warfarin 41%, which resulted in a 100% increase from the baseline prothrombin time. The effects of the interaction lasted

## Table 5
## Voriconazole Interactions Affecting Pharmacokinetics/Dynamics of Other Drugs[a]

| Drug | Effect on drug | Suggested mechanism | Reference |
|---|---|---|---|
| Warfarin | Inhibits primary metabolic pathway; increases warfarin pharmacodynamic effect 41%; ↑ partial thromboplastin time 100% | Inhibition of hepatic CYP2C9 | 130 |
| Cyclosporine and tacrolimus | | | |
| • Cyclosporine | ↑ $C_{min}$ 248%, $AUC_{0-12}$ 70% | Inhibition of hepatic CYP3A4 | 131 |
| • Tacrolimus | ↑ $C_{min}$ | Inhibition of hepatic CYP3A4 | 132, 133 |
| Miscellaneous drugs | | | |
| • Phenytoin | ↑ $C_{max}$ 70%, AUC 80% | Inhibition of hepatic CYP2C9 and CYP3A4 | 134 |
| • Omeprazole | ↑ $C_{max}$ 2.4-fold, $AUC_{0-24}$ 3.8-fold, ↑ $t_{1/2}$ 1.15 hour | Inhibition of hepatic CYP2C19 and CYP3A4 | 136 |
| • Prednisolone | ↑ $AUC_{0-\infty}$ 13–30% | Inhibition of hepatic CYP3A4? | 137 |
| • Rifabutin | ↑ $C_{max}$, AUC twofold | Inhibition of hepatic CYP | 17, 48 |
| • Digoxin | No significant effect | | 53 |
| • Indinavir | No significant effect | | 138 |
| • Mycophenolic acid | No significant effect | | 139 |

[a] Voriconazole may also increase the plasma concentrations of several drugs, including benzodiazepines, calcium channel blockers, HMG-CoA reductase inhibitors, vinca alkaloids, sulfonylureas, nonnucleoside reverse transcriptase inhibitors, protease inhibitors, sirolimus, quinidine, and pimozide. However, published data describing these possible interactions are lacking.

**Table 6**
**Drug Interactions That Affect Voriconazole Plasma Concentrations**[a]

| Drug | Effect | Suggested Mechanism | Reference |
|---|---|---|---|
| Drugs that accelerate voriconazole metabolism | | | |
| • Phenytoin | ↓ $C_{max}$ 53%, AUC 72% | Induction of hepatic CYP | *134* |
| • Rifampin | ↓ $C_{max}$, AUC 95% | Induction of hepatic CYP | *140* |
| • Rifabutin | ↓ $C_{max}$, AUC 60–80% | Induction of hepatic CYP | *140* |
| H₂-receptor antagonists | | | |
| • Cimetidine | No significant effect | | *141* |
| • Ranitidine | No significant effect | | *141* |
| Macrolide antibiotics | | | |
| • Erythromycin | No significant effect | | *142* |
| • Azithromycin | No significant effect | | *142* |
| Miscellaneous drugs | | | |
| • Omeprazole | No significant effect | | *143* |
| • Indinavir | No significant effect | | *138* |

[a] Other agents such as saquinavir, amprenavir, and nelfinavir, delavirdine, or efavirenz may inhibit voriconazole metabolism, however, published data describing these possible interactions are lacking.

6 days *(130)*. Therapeutic doses of warfarin normally exhibit large intersubject variability, which may be partly because of the genotype status for CYP2C19 and CYP2C9 *(130)*. However, in this study the incidence of homozygous poor metabolizer CYP2C19 phenotype was approx 6% (1 of 17 healthy volunteers), which is consistent with general population estimates. The subject who exhibited this phenotype had the highest voriconazole concentrations, but the maximum increase in prothrombin time was comparable to others.

CYCLOSPORINE/TACROLIMUS

In a controlled study, voriconazole significantly increased cyclosporine exposure ($AUC_{0-12}$) and trough concentrations ($C_{min}$) (70 and 248%, respectively) in renal transplant recipients *(131)*. A corresponding increase in nonserious cyclosporine-associated toxicities was observed. The magnitude of this interaction is greater than that seen with either ketoconazole or fluconazole. Similarly, tacrolimus trough concentrations following single or repeated dosing are significantly increased with repeated voriconazole coadministration *(132,133)*. Human liver microsomal studies qualitatively predicted the in vivo interaction. However, the magnitude of inhibition observed in vivo was much greater. Moreover, the in vitro studies suggested that voriconazole inhibits tacrolimus metabolism (presumably via CYP3A4 inhibition) by competitive and noncompetitive means *(132)*.

PHENYTOIN

Steady-state plasma phenytoin concentrations increase dramatically following repeated oral administration of 400 mg voriconazole twice daily for 10 days *(134)*. Steady-state phenytoin $C_{max}$ and AUC increased approx 70 and 80%, respectively, with coadministration of voriconazole *(134)*.

OMEPRAZOLE

Omeprazole, a proton pump inhibitor, is completely metabolized by CYP2C19 and CYP3A4 to 5-hydroxy-omeprazole and omeprazole-sulfone, respectively *(135)*. The latter metabolite is ultimately metabolized to the 5-hydroxy metabolite *(135)*. Steady-state omeprazole concentrations increased dramatically following repeated oral administration of 400 mg voriconazole twice daily for 1 day followed by 200 mg twice daily for 6 days *(136)*. Steady-state omeprazole $C_{max}$ and $AUC_{0-24}$ increased approx 2.2-fold and 3.8-fold, respectively, with coadministration of voriconazole. In addition, omeprazole $t_{1/2}$ increased by approx 1.15 hours with voriconazole administration *(136)*.

MISCELLANEOUS DRUGS

Oral prednisolone exposure is increased 13 and 30% by steady-state voriconazole dosing of 250 mg daily or 200 mg twice daily, respectively. These changes are similar in magnitude to those observed with itraconazole coadministration *(137)*. Voriconazole may also increase the plasma concentrations of several drugs, including benzodiazepines, calcium channel blockers, HMG-COA reductase inhibitors, vinca alkaloids, sulfonylureas, nonnucleoside reverse transcriptase inhibitors, protease inhibitors, sirolimus, quinidine, and pimozide, but no data from large, well-controlled studies describing these interactions are available *(16,17,48)*. In addition, voriconazole increases steady-state plasma rifabutin $C_{max}$ and AUC approximately twofold *(17,48)*. Voriconazole may also inhibit the metabolism of select protease inhibitors and nonnucleoside reverse transcriptase inhibitors *(16)*.

DRUGS THAT ARE NOT INHIBITED BY VORICONAZOLE

Voriconazole produces no clinically significant effects on the pharmacokinetics and pharmacodynamics of digoxin, indinavir, or mycophenolic acid *(16,48,53,138,139)*. The lack of interaction with digoxin is consistent with the belief that voriconazole interacts very little, if at all, with P-gp.

CLINICAL IMPORTANCE OF VORICONAZOLE INTERACTIONS AFFECTING CYP METABOLISM

Given the danger of prolonged and excessive anticoagulation, the voriconazole-warfarin interaction is clinically significant. In the lone study of this interaction, subjects were withdrawn from the study when the investigators deemed it was no longer in their best interest to continue. As a result, two (12%) of enrolled subjects were withdrawn because of increased prothrombin time during the drug coadministration phase and were excluded from analysis. Thus, the actual magnitude of this interaction could have been underestimated.

The magnitude of the interaction between cyclosporine and voriconazole is greater than that observed with other azoles. Although no serious adverse events occurred in the study of this interaction, patients receiving this combination had a high rate of nonserious adverse events, particularly during voriconazole administration. These adverse events were likely caused by elevated cyclosporine blood concentrations. Similarly, clinically achievable concentrations of voriconazole significantly inhibit tacrolimus metabolism by up to 50%. In doing so, tacrolimus trough concentrations rise rapidly in the presence of voriconazole.

As described below, phenytoin can significantly lower voriconazole concentrations. This induction can be overcome by doubling the voriconazole dose (i.e., from 200 to 400 mg). However, increasing the voriconazole dose too much can in turn lead to inhibition of phenytoin CYP-mediated metabolism and an increased risk of phenytoin toxicity.

Given the magnitude of the interaction between voriconazole and omeprazole, patients receiving this combination can be predisposed to an increase risk of experiencing omeprazole-related adverse effects. Although there are few published data, interactions between voriconazole and sirolimus (significant increase in sirolimus concentrations); quinidine (potential QT prolongation and possible occurrence of torsade de pointes); or ergot alkaloids (ergotism) are so significant that these combinations are contraindicated.

## MANAGEMENT OF INTERACTIONS AFFECTING CYP-MEDIATED METABOLISM OF OTHER DRUGS

In patients receiving warfarin who require voriconazole therapy, the dose of warfarin should be reduced according to international normalized ratio and prothrombin time values. In addition, these markers should be monitored closely if this combination is used.

When voriconazole is initiated in patients receiving cyclosporine, the cyclosporine dose should be halved. In addition, cyclosporine blood concentrations should be carefully monitored and the cyclosporine dose adjusted accordingly. Furthermore, on discontinuation of voriconazole, cyclosporine blood concentrations should continue to be monitored carefully and the cyclosporine dose adjusted accordingly. Similar to cyclosporine, tacrolimus blood concentrations should be closely monitored and the dose adjusted accordingly.

Using higher voriconazole doses in patients also receiving phenytoin can overcome the induction of CYP by phenytoin. However, because of the increased risk of phenytoin toxicity in patients receiving high-dose voriconazole (400 mg twice daily) plasma phenytoin concentrations should be closely monitored. The dose of omeprazole should be reduced 50% in patients receiving or starting on voriconazole therapy. Sirolimus, quinidine, and ergot alkaloids should be avoided in patients receiving or starting on voriconazole therapy.

### Interactions With Other Drugs That Accelerate CYP-Mediated Metabolism of Voriconazole

Coadministration of voriconazole with drugs that are well-known inducers of CYP (i.e., phenytoin, phenobarbital, carbamazepine, and rifampin) can result in a pharmacokinetic interaction that markedly reduces its serum concentrations (17,18,48). In some cases, the reduction in voriconazole concentrations can be overcome by adjusting its dose.

#### PHENYTOIN

Voriconazole 200 mg per day for 7 days produced plasma concentrations similar to control values. However, steady-state voriconazole plasma concentrations following coadministration of phenytoin (300 mg/day) for 2 weeks were significantly reduced for up to 12 hours postdose. Peak ($C_{max}$) steady-state plasma voriconazole concentrations and systemic exposure were reduced approx 53 and 72%, respectively. Increasing the dose of voriconazole from 200 mg twice daily to 400 mg twice daily compensated for the effect of phenytoin on plasma voriconazole concentrations (134). As described above, increasing dosages of voriconazole subsequently led to inhibition of CYP-mediated metabolism of phenytoin.

MISCELLANEOUS DRUGS

Voriconazole serum concentrations are significantly reduced by rifampin and rifabutin. Both of these known CYP inducers reduce the $C_{max}$ and exposure of voriconazole *(140)*. Rifampin reduced these values approx 95%, whereas rifabutin reduced these values approx 60–80% *(140)*. Doubling the voriconazole dose up to 400 mg twice daily partially overcame the induction of rifampin, and increasing the voriconazole dose 1.75 times fully compensated for the induction caused by rifabutin *(140)*. However, similar to phenytoin, the interaction between voriconazole and rifabutin is bidirectional. Voriconazole significantly increased steady-state rifabutin concentrations ($C_{max}$ and AUC) to toxic concentrations *(48)*. Although there are no published studies, the nonnucleoside reverse transcriptase inhibitors efavirenz and nevirapine may also induce the metabolism of voriconazole *(16)*.

CLINICAL SIGNIFICANCE OF INTERACTIONS THAT
ACCELERATE CYP-MEDIATED METABOLISM OF VORICONAZOLE

Clinically, interactions that reduce voriconazole serum concentrations are significant. Reductions in voriconazole serum concentrations can lead to therapeutic failure. Voriconazole possesses a broad spectrum of activity, including resistant strains of *Candida* species; therefore, if it fails there is a choice of only a few suitable alternative therapeutic agents (i.e., caspofungin, lipid amphotericin B).

MANAGEMENT OF INTERACTIONS THAT ACCELERATE
CYP-MEDIATED METABOLISM OF VORICONAZOLE

Generally, given the magnitude of the interaction, induction of voriconazole cannot be completely overcome by increasing the dose of voriconazole; therefore some of these combinations (rifabutin, rifampin, phenobarbital, and carbamazepine) are contraindicated. In contrast, the induction effects of phenytoin on voriconazole can be overcome by doubling the voriconazole dose. However, this dosage adjustment should be done cautiously because high-dose voriconazole (i.e., 400 mg twice daily) can inhibit phenytoin and predispose the patient to phenytoin toxicity. Therefore, if this combination is used, phenytoin concentrations should be strictly monitored.

*Interactions With Other Drugs That Inhibit CYP-Mediated Metabolism of Voriconazole*

Few drugs have demonstrated the capability to inhibit the metabolism of voriconazole. Protease inhibitors such as saquinavir, amprenavir, and nelfinavir may inhibit voriconazole metabolism *(16)*. Moreover, selected nonnucleoside reverse transcriptase inhibitors such as delavirdine or efavirenz may also inhibit voriconazole metabolism *(16)*.

*Drugs That Do Not Interact With Voriconazole*

Little or no clinically relevant effects on the steady-state pharmacokinetics of voriconazole have been observed when it has been coadministered with indinavir, $H_2$-receptor antagonists (cimetidine or ranitidine), macrolide antibiotics (erythromycin or azithromycin), or omeprazole *(138,141–143)*.

---

### CASE STUDY:
### AZOLE DRUG INTERACTIONS *(144)*

C. B. was an 8-year-old boy with a history of seizure disorder managed with valproic acid and primidone. Primidone therapy had been started approx 1 month before his illness, and he was on an escalating dose schedule. Three weeks before presentation, C. B. developed a cough and an intermittent fever (40.0°C). He was treated for community-acquired pneumonia but continued to be febrile, with a productive cough, daily chills that were not responsive to antipyretics, and anorexia. He was referred to a children's hospital in April 1995, where an extensive workup established the diagnosis of presumed blastomycosis. Itraconazole, 100 mg capsules once daily (3.3 mg/kg/day), was started. After 4 days of therapy, the patient's condition had worsened. At this time, an exploratory right thoracotomy and open lung biopsy revealed multiple necrotic areas of the lung, and examination of the tissue produced findings consistent with *Blastomyces dermatitidis*. Therapy with oral itraconazole capsules was continued at an increased dosage, 100 mg twice daily (6.6 mg/kg/day). After 10 days, his cough had become more productive, and he had remained febrile (40.0°C). Serum itraconazole and hydroxyitraconazole concentrations were measured by high-performance liquid chromatography and found to be undetectable (lower limit of quantitation [LLQ] = 25 ng/mL). Intravenous amphotericin B, 1 mg/kg/day, was initiated. After 9 days, C. B.'s condition had begun to improve. The patient received a total of 35 mg/kg of amphotericin B. A desire to shorten the course of amphotericin B therapy prompted a second attempt at therapy with itraconazole in conjunction with amphotericin B 1 month after discharge. After 9 days of oral itraconazole capsules, 100 mg twice daily (6.6 mg/kg/day), serum itraconazole and hydroxyitraconazole concentrations were again undetectable despite directly observed itraconazole administration. Throughout therapy, the patient remained on valproic acid and primidone, and antiepileptic drug concentrations were within normal limits. Six months following the end of amphotericin B therapy, C. B.'s pneumonia was cured and without relapse.

## Echinocandins

### Mechanisms of Interactions

Caspofungin undergoes spontaneous chemical degradation and metabolism via hydrolysis and *N*-acetylation *(26)*. These metabolic pathways are not thought to involve CYP. However, whether CYP is involved in caspofungin metabolism has not been fully determined. Nonetheless, to date there is no published evidence that caspofungin is either a substrate or inhibitor of CYP or P-gp. Thus, some believe that the potential of caspofungin to interact with other drugs through these mechanisms is very low *(31)*. However, interaction studies suggest that caspofungin does mildly inhibit the metabolism of CYP substrates, and that its concentrations are reduced by concomitant administration of CYP inducers.

### Caspofungin Inhibitory Effects on Pharmacokinetics/Dynamics of Other Drugs
#### CYCLOSPORINE AND TACROLIMUS

In a Phase I study, caspofungin produced no significant change in cyclosporine pharmacokinetics *(145,146)*. However, in this study coadministration with cyclosporine produced transient elevations (two to three times upper limit of normal) in alanine transaminase in 5 of 12 health subjects. Subjects had received 35 or 70 mg of caspofungin for 3 or 10 days, respectively, and experienced the elevations within a day of the concomitant cyclosporine *(145)*. Similar, albeit smaller, increases in aspartate transaminase were also seen in these 5 subjects *(145)*. Interestingly, in a Phase I study evaluating the potential for drug interactions between caspofungin and tacrolimus, caspofungin produced a modest reduction (approx 20%) in tacrolimus exposure ($AUC_{0-12}$) and $C_{max}$ *(147)*.

DRUGS THAT ARE NOT INHIBITED BY CASPOFUNGIN

In addition to cyclosporine, clinical studies have shown that caspofungin produces no significant change in the pharmacokinetics of amphotericin B, itraconazole, mycophenolate, or rifampin *(31,145,146,148)*.

CLINICAL IMPORTANCE OF CASPOFUNGIN INTERACTIONS
THAT AFFECT BIOTRANSFORMATION OF OTHER DRUGS

Although the mechanism(s) involved with the pharmacodynamic interaction between caspofungin and cyclosporine are unknown, the increases in transaminases that occurred fueled product labeling that recommends the coadministration of these agents only when the benefit of the combination outweighs the risk. The mechanism underlying the interaction between caspofungin and tacrolimus is unknown; nonetheless, clinically the interaction is moderately significant.

MANAGEMENT OF INTERACTIONS THAT AFFECT
THE BIOTRANSFORMATION OF OTHER DRUGS

Until there is additional study of the mechanism responsible for the interaction between caspofungin and cyclosporine, the concomitant administration of these agents is contraindicated. When caspofungin is administered with tacrolimus, standard monitoring of tacrolimus blood concentrations and appropriate tacrolimus dosage adjustment is recommended *(147)*.

*Interactions With Other Drugs That Affect Biotransformation of Caspofungin*

DRUGS THAT INCREASE CASPOFUNGIN EXPOSURE:

*Cyclosporine*

In the Phase I study just described previously, concomitant cyclosporine administration elevated caspofungin plasma concentrations and increased caspofungin exposure approx 35% *(146)*. The exact mechanism of this apparent inhibition is unknown. Moreover, whether cyclosporine affects the caspofungin distribution, or elimination, or both is also unknown. Given the slow metabolism and excretion of caspofungin and the uncertainty surrounding its interaction with CYP, this interaction may reflect an alteration in the distribution of caspofungin to tissues. Clearly, more study of this interaction is needed to fully elucidate the mechanism.

CLINICAL IMPORTANCE OF INTERACTIONS
THAT INCREASE CASPOFUNGIN EXPOSURE

Although the mechanism(s) involved with the pharmacokinetic interaction between cyclosporine and caspofungin are unknown, increases in transaminases were noted in this study. Whether the increase in caspofungin exposure was primarily or partially responsible for the changes is unknown. Nonetheless, until there are additional data regarding this interaction, coadministration of these agents should only occur when the benefit of the combination outweighs the risk.

DRUGS THAT DECREASE CASPOFUNGIN EXPOSURE:

### Rifampin and Other CYP Inducers

Although there is no evidence that caspofungin interacts significantly with CYP, data suggest that coadministration of caspofungin with drugs that are known to induce CYP results in reduced caspofungin concentrations. These drugs include efavirenz, nevirapine, phenytoin, and carbamazepine *(145)*. In addition, coadministration of dexamethasone may also decrease caspofungin concentrations *(145)*. On the other hand, nelfinavir has no clinically significant effect on caspofungin concentrations *(148)*.

Two placebo-controlled studies demonstrated that rifampin both inhibits and induces caspofungin disposition, with the net effect resulting in a slight induction at steady-state. Both studies assessed the effect of 600 mg rifampin per day on caspofungin 50 mg iv daily. In the first study, both drugs were started on the same day and continued for 14 days. Surprisingly, in patients who received caspofungin and rifampin, caspofungin exposure and trough concentrations were nearly double those of subjects who received only caspofungin. This apparent inhibition occurred in the initial days of concomitant administration, and by day 14, the pharmacokinetics of caspofungin in patients receiving the combination were similar to those of subjects who received only caspofungin. In the second study, in patients randomly assigned to receive the combination, rifampin was administered for 14 days, and then caspofungin was coadministered for the final 14 days. Caspofungin pharmacokinetics in these patients were compared to a group of subjects who received caspofungin alone for 14 days. In this study, pretreatment with 14 days of rifampin produced no significant change in caspofungin exposure. However, rifampin pretreatment reduced caspofungin trough concentrations approx 30% *(148)*. The investigators surmised that initially rifampin may inhibit uptake of caspofungin into its tissue compartment, and then with continued administration, rifampin induces the disposition of caspofungin *(148)*.

CLINICAL SIGNIFICANCE OF INTERACTIONS THAT REDUCE CASPOFUNGIN EXPOSURE

Interactions that reduce caspofungin serum concentrations may be clinically significant. Reductions in caspofungin serum concentrations could lead to therapeutic failure. Caspofungin possesses activity against *Aspergillus* species and *Candida* species, including species with reduced susceptibility to other antifungal agents (i.e., *Candida glabrata* and *Candida krusei*); therefore, if it fails there is a choice of only a few suitable alternative therapeutic agents (i.e., voriconazole, lipid amphotericin B).

MANAGEMENT OF INTERACTIONS THAT REDUCE CASPOFUNGIN EXPOSURE

If patients receiving caspofungin require rifampin therapy, a caspofungin dose of at least 70 mg daily should be considered *(148)*. There are no data to guide dosing should patients receiving caspofungin require therapy with other drugs known to induce CYP. In these cases, alternatives to those agents should be considered; caspofungin could be switched to an amphotericin B formulation; or the caspofungin dose should be increased based on clinical response and patient tolerance.

## SUMMARY

Antifungal drug–drug interactions occur through a variety of mechanisms with a wide array of agents. Interactions involving amphotericin B occur predictably as a result of its toxicities. In contrast, interactions involving the azoles result as a consequence of their physiochemical properties. Itraconazole is subject to pH-based and metabolic interactions. Drugs that will likely interact with itraconazole include agents that increase gastric pH or lipophilic CYP3A4 substrates with poor oral availability. Because itraconazole also interacts with P-gp, identifying the principal cause of itraconazole drug interactions is complicated. In addition, because of itraconazole's complex pharmacokinetic properties, predicting the extent or duration of effects of the interaction is difficult. Fluconazole is not affected by agents that increase gastric pH, but its potential to cause CYP-mediated interactions is more than that suggested by in vitro studies. CYP-mediated interactions involving fluconazole are often dose dependent. Because of its linear and predictable pharmacokinetic properties, these interactions may sometimes be avoided or managed by using the lowest effective fluconazole dosage. Fluconazole is not affected by agents that interact with P-gp.

Like fluconazole, voriconazole is not affected by drugs that increase gastric pH interactions or by those that interact with P-gp. However, unlike fluconazole, voriconazole is extensively metabolized by multiple CYP pathways. Moreover, voriconazole exhibits unpredictable nonlinear pharmacokinetics, and it inhibits multiple CYP isoforms. In addition, the CYP pathways that affect voriconazole exhibit genetic polymorphisms. Therefore, the propensity for voriconazole to be involved in CYP-mediated drug interactions is greater than that of fluconazole. Furthermore, in addition to whether a compound is a CYP substrate or inhibitor, a person's CYP phenotype may also be important when evaluating the risk of a drug interaction involving voriconazole.

The echinocandin class is the newest among the antifungals. Clinical experience with this class is growing, yet to date this class is relatively devoid of significant drug–drug interactions. However, more study is needed to elucidate the mechanisms of the modest interactions noted to date.

## REFERENCES

1. Gallis HA, Drew RH, Pickard WW. Amphotericin B: 30 years of clinical experience. Rev Infect Dis 1990;12:308–329.
2. Yamaguchi H, Abe S, Tokuda Y. Immunomodulating activity of antifungal drugs. Ann NY Acad Sci 1993;685:447–457.
3. Bekersky I, Fielding RH, Dressler DE, Lee JW, Buell DN, Walsh TJ. Plasma protein binding of amphotericin B and pharmacokinetics of bound versus unbound amphotericin B after administration of intravenous liposomal amphotericin B (AmBisome) and amphotericin B deoxycholate. Antimicrob Agents Chemother 2002;46:834–840.
4. Bekersky I, Fielding RH, Dressler DE, Lee JW, Buell DN, Walsh TJ. Pharmacokinetics, excretion, and mass balance of liposomal amphotericin B (AmBisome) and amphotericin B deoxycholate in humans. Antimicrob Agents Chemother 2002;46:828–833.
5. Wong-Beringer A, Jacobs RA, Guglielmo BJ. Lipid formulations of amphotericin B: clinical efficacy and toxicities. Clin Infect Dis 1998;27:603–618.
6. Daneshmend TK, Warnock DW. Clinical pharmacokinetics of systemic antifungal drugs. Clin Pharmacokinet 1983;8:17–42.
7. Como JA, Dismukes WE. Oral azole drugs as systemic antifungal therapy. N Engl J Med 1994;330:263–272.
8. Wang EJ, Lew K, Casciano CN, Clement RP, Johnson WW. Interaction of common azole antifungals with p-glycoprotein. Antimicrob Agents Chemother 2002;46:160–165.
9. Wacher VJ, Wu CY, Benet LZ. Overlapping substrate specificities and tissue distribution of cytochrome P450 3A and P-glycoprotein: implications for drug delivery and activity in cancer chemotherapy. Mol Carcinogen 1995;13:129–134.

10. Wacher VJ, Silverman JA, Zhang Y, Benet LZ. Role of P-glycoprotein and cytochrome P450 in limiting oral absorption of peptides and peptidomimetics. J Pharm Sci 1998;87: 1322–1330.

11. Heykants J, Van Peer A, Van de Velde V, et al. The clinical pharmacokinetics of itraconazole: an overview. Mycoses 1989;32(Suppl 1):67–87.

12. Johnson MD, Hamilton CD, Drew RH, Sanders LL, Pennick GJ, Perfect JR. A randomized comparative study to determine the effect of omeprazole on the peak serum concentration of itraconazole oral solution. J Antimicrob Chemother 2003;51:453–457.

13. Van de Velde VJ, Van Peer A, Heykants JJP, et al. Effect of food on the pharmacokinetics of a new hydroxypropyl-β-cyclodextrin formulation of itraconazole. Pharmacotherapy 1996;16:424–428.

14. Barone JA, Moskovitz BL, Guarnieri J, et al. Enhanced bioavailability of itraconazole in hydroxypropyl-β-cyclodextrin solution versus capsules in healthy volunteers. Antimicrob Agents Chemother 1998;42:1862–1865.

15. Debruyne D, Ryckelynk JP. Clinical Pharmacokinetics of fluconazole. Clin Pharmacokinet 1993;24:10–27.

16. Pearson MM, Rogers PD, Cleary JD, Chapman SW. Voriconazole: A new triazole antifungal. Ann Pharmacotherapy 2003;37:420–432.

17. Johnson LB, Kauffman CA. Voriconazole: A new triazole antifungal agent. Clin Infect Dis 2003;36:630-637.

18. Schwartz S, Milatovic D, Thiel E. Successful treatment of cerebral aspergillosis with a novel triazole (voriconazole) in a patient with acute leukemia. Brit J Haematol 1997;97: 663–665.

19. Poirier JM, Cheymol G. Optimization of itraconazole therapy using target drug concentrations. Clin Pharmacokinet 1998;35:461–473.

20. Brammer KW, Coakley AJ, Jezequel SG, Tarbit MH. The disposition and metabolism of [$^{14}$C] fluconazole in humans. Drug Metab Disp 1991;19:764–767.

21. Sabo JA, Abdel-Rahman SM. Voriconazole: A new triazole antifungal. Ann Pharmacotherapy 2000;34:1032–1043.

22. Hyland R, Jones BC, Smith DA. Identification of the cytochrome P450 enzymes involved in the *N*-oxidation of voriconazole. Drug Metab Disp 2003;31:540–547.

23. Goldstein JA. Clinical relevance of genetic polymorphisms in the human CYP2C subfamily. Br J Clin Pharmacol 2001;52:349–355.

24. Lee CR. Goldstein JA. Pieper JA. Cytochrome P450 2C9 polymorphisms: a comprehensive review of the in-vitro and human data. Pharmacogenetics 2002;12:251–263.

25. Denning DW. Echinocandins: A new class of antifungal. J Antimicrob Chemother 2002; 49:889–891.

26. Balani SK, Xu X, Arison BH, et al. Metabolites of caspofungin acetate, a potent antifungal agent, in human plasma and urine. Drug Metab Disp 2000;28:1274–1278.

27. Hajdu R, Thompson R, Sundelof JG, et al. Preliminary animal pharmacokinetics of the parenteral antifungal agent MK-0991 (L-743,872). Antimcrob Agents Chemother 1997; 41:2339–2344.

28. Chiller T, Farrokhshad K, Brummer E, Stevens DA. The influence of human sera on the in vitro activity of MK-0991 against *Aspergillus fumigatus*. Program and Abstracts 39th Interscience Conference on Antimicrobial Agents and Chemotherapy. San Francisco, CA, September 26–29 1999, Abstract 153.

29. Stone JA, Holland SD, Wickersham PJ, et al. Single- and multiple-dose pharmacokinetics of caspofungin in healthy men. Antimicrob Agents Chemother 2002;46:739–745.

30. Stone JA, Ballow CH, Holland SD, et al. Single dose caspofungin pharmacokinetics in healthy elderly subjects. Program and Abstracts 40th Interscience Conference on Antimicrobial Agents and Chemotherapy. Toronto, Ontario, September 17–20, 2000, Abstract 853.

31. Stone JA, McCrea JB, Wickersham PJ, et al. A phase I study of caspofungin evaluating the potential for drug interactions with itraconazole, the effect of gender and the use of a loading dose regimen. Program and Abstracts 40<sup>th</sup> Interscience Conference on Antimicrobial Agents and Chemotherapy. Toronto, Ontario, September 17–20 2000, Abstract 854.

32. White MH, Bowden RA, Sandler ES, et al. Randomized, double-blind clinical trial of amphotericin B colloidal dispersion vs. amphotericin B in the empirical treatment of fever and neutropenia. Clin Infect Dis 1998;27:296–302.

33. Ringdén O, Andström E, Remberger M, Svahn BM, Tollemar J. Safety of liposomal amphotericin B (AmBisome) in 187 transplant recipients treated with cyclosporine. Bone Marrow Transplant 1994;14(Suppl 5):S10–S14.

34. June CH, Thompson CB, Kennedy MS, Nims J, Thomas ED. Profound hypomagnesemia associated with the use of cyclosporine for marrow transplantation. Transplantation 1985; 39:620–624.

35. Stamm AM, Diaso RB, Dismukes WE, et al. Toxicity of amphotericin B plus flucytosine in 194 patients with cryptococcal meningitis. Am J Med 1987;83:236–242.

36. Bennett JE, Dismukes WE, Duma RJ, et al. A comparison of amphotericin B alone and combined with flucytosine in the treatment of cryptococcal meningitis. N Engl J Med 1979;301:126–131.

37. Block ER, Bennett JE. Pharmacological studies with 5-fluorocytosine. Antimicrob Agents Chemother 1972;1:476–482.

38. Viviani MA. Flucytosine-what is its future? J Antimicrob Chemother 1995;35:241–244.

39. Chung DK, Koenig MG. Reversible cardiac enlargement during treatment with amphotericin B and hydrocortisone. Am Rev Respir Dis 1971;103:831–841.

40. Paterson DL, Singh N. Interactions between tacrolimus and antimicrobial agents. Clin Infect Dis 1997;25:1430–1440.

41. Albengres E, Le Louët H, Tillement JP. Systemic antifungal agents: drug interactions of clinical significance. Drug Safety 1998;18:83–97.

42. Fleisher D, Li C, Zhou Y, Pao LH, Karim A. Drug, meal and formulation interactions influencing drug absorption after oral administration: clinical implications. Clin Pharmacokinet 1999;36:233–254.

43. Lange D, Pavao JH, Wu J, Klausner M. Effect of a cola beverage on the bioavailability of itraconazole in the presence of H2 blockers. J Clin Pharmacol 1997;37:535–540.

44. Hoeschele JD, Roy AK, Pecoraro VL, Carver PL. In vitro analysis of the interaction between sucralfate and ketoconazole. Antimicrob Agents Chemother 1994;38:319–325.

45. Thummel KE, Wilkinson GR. In vitro and in vivo drug interactions involving human CYP3A. Annu Rev Pharmacol Toxicol 1998;38:389–430.

46. Omar G, Whiting PH, Hawksworth GM, Humphrey MJ, Burke MD. Ketoconazole and fluconazole inhibition of the metabolism of cyclosporin A by human liver in vitro. Ther Drug Monit 1997;19:436–445.

47. Black DJ, Kunze KL, Wienkers LC, et al. Warfarin-fluconazole II. A metabolically based drug interaction: in vivo studies. Drug Metab Disp 1996;24:422–428.

48. Muijser RBR, Goa KL, Scott LJ. Voriconazole in the treatment of invasive aspergillosis. Drugs 2002;62:2655–2664.

49. Kim RB. Organic anion-transporting polypeptide (OATP) transporter family and drug disposition. Eur J Clin Invest 2003;33(Suppl. 2):1–5.

50. Wandel C, Kim RB, Kajiji S, Guengerich P, Wilkinson GR, Wood AJ. P-glycoprotein and cytochrome P-450 3A inhibition: dissociation of inhibitory potencies. Cancer Res 1999;59:3944–3948.

51. Eytan GD, Regev R, Oren G, Assaraf YG. The role of passive transbilayer drug movement in multidrug resistance and its modulation. J. Biol Chem 1996;271:12,897–12,902.

52. Ferte J. Analysis of tangled relationships between P-glycoprotein-mediated multidrug resistance and the lipid phase of the cell membrane. Eur J Biochem 2000;267;277–294.

53. Purkins L, Wood N, Kleinermans D, Nichols D. Voriconazole does not affect the steady-state pharmacokinetics of digoxin. Br J Clin Pharmacol 2003;56(Suppl 1):45–50.

54. Baciewicz AM, Baciewicz FA. Ketoconazole and fluconazole drug interactions. Arch Intern Med 1993;153:1970–1976.

55. Hall SD, Thummel KE, Watkins PB, et al. Molecular and physical mechanisms of first-pass extraction. Drug Metab Disp 1999;27:161–166.

56. Gomez DY, Wacher VJ, Tomlanovich SJ, Hebert MF, Benet LZ. The effects of ketoconazole on intestinal metabolism and bioavailability of cyclosporine. Clin Pharmacol Ther 1995;58:15–19.

57. Campana C, Regazzi MB, Buggia I, Molinaro M. Clinically significant drug interactions with cyclosporin: an update. cyclosporine with antimicrobial agents. Clin Pharmacokinet 1996;30:141–179.

58. Keogh A, Spratt P, McCosker C, Macdonald P, Mundy J, Kaan A. Ketoconazole to reduce the need for cyclosporine after cardiac surgery. N Engl J Med 1995;333:628–633.

59. Zimmermann T, Yeates RA, Laufen H, Pfaff G, Wildfeuer A. Influence of concomitant food intake on the oral absorption of two triazole antifungal agents, itraconazole and fluconazole. Eur J Clin Pharmacol 1994;46:147–150.

60. Kanda Y, Kami M, Matsuyama T, et al. Plasma concentrations of itraconazole in patients receiving chemotherapy for hematological malignancies: the effect of famotidine on the absorption of itraconazole. Hematol Oncol 1998;16:33–37.

61. Lim SG, Sawyerr AM, Hudson M, Sercombe J, Pounder RE. Short report: the absorption of fluconazole and itraconazole under conditions of low intragastric acidity. Aliment Pharmacol Ther 1993;7:317–321.

62. Jaruratanasirikul S, Sriwiriyajan S. Effect of omeprazole on the pharmacokinetics of itraconazole. Eur J Clin Pharmacol 1998;54:159–161.

63. May DB, Drew RH, Yedinak KC, Bartlett JA. Effect of simultaneous didanosine administration on itraconazole absorption in healthy volunteers. Pharmacotherapy 1994;14:509–513.

64. Damle B, Hess H, Kaul S, Knupp C. Absence of clinically relevant drug interactions following simultaneous administration of didanosine-encapsulated, enteric-coated bead formulation with either itraconazole or fluconazole. Biopharm Drug Disp 2002;23:59-66.

65. Glasmacher A, Hahn C, Molitor E, Sauerbruch T, Marklein G, Schmidt-Wolf IG. Definition of a minimal effective trough concentration of itraconazole for antifungal prophylaxis in severely neutropenic patients with hematologic malignancies. 39th Interscience Conference on Antimicrobial Agents and Chemotherapy, San Francisco, CA, September 26–29, 1999, Abstract 1417.

66. Christians U, Jacobsen W, Floren LC. Metabolism and drug interactions of 3-hydroxy-3-methylglutaryl coenzyme A reductase inhibitors in transplant patients: are the statins mechanistically similar? Pharmacol Ther 1998;80:1–34.

67. McCormick AD, McKillop D, Butters CJ, et al. ZD4522- An HMG-CoA reductase inhibitor free of metabolically mediated drug interactions: Metabolic studies in human in vitro systems [abstract]. J Clin Pharmacol 2000;40:1055.

68. Jacobsen W, Kirchner G, Hallensleben K, et al. Comparison of cytochrome P-450-dependent metabolism and drug interactions of the 3-hydroxy-3-methylglutaryl-COA-reductase inhibitors lovastatin and pravastatin in the liver. Drug Metab Disp 1999;27:173–179.

69. Neuvonen PJ, Jalava KM. Itraconazole drastically increases plasma concentrations of lovastatin and lovastatin acid. Clin Pharmacol Ther 1996;60:54–61.

70. Neuvonen PJ, Kantola T, Kivistö KT. Simvastatin but not pravastatin is very susceptible to interaction with the CYP3A4 inhibitor itraconazole. Clin Pharmacol Ther 1998;63:332–341.

71. Kantola T, Kivistö KT, Neuvonen PJ. Effect of itraconazole on the pharmacokinetics of atorvastatin. Clin Pharmacol Ther 1998;64:58–65.

72. Mazzu AL, Lasseter KC, Shamblin EC, Agarwal V, Lettieri J, Sundaresen P. Itraconazole alters the pharmacokinetics of atorvastatin to a greater extent than either cerivastatin or pravastatin. Clin Pharmacol Ther 2000;68:391–400.

73. Ishigam M, Uchiyama M, Kondo T, et al. Inhibition of in vitro metabolism of simvastatin by itraconazole in humans and predictions of in vivo drug-drug interactions. Pharm Res 2001;18:622–631.

74. Kivistö KT, Kantola T, Neuvonen PJ. Different effects of itraconazole on the pharmaco-kinetics of fluvastatin and lovastatin. Br J Clin Pharmacol 1998;46:49–53.

75. Cooper KJ, Martin PD, Dane AL, Warwick MJ, Schneck DW, Cantarini MV. Effect of itraconazole on the pharmacokinetics of rosuvastatin. Clin Pharmacol Ther 2003;73:322–329.

76. Olkkola KT, Ahonen J, Neuvonen PJ. The effect of the systemic antimycotics, itraconazole and fluconazole, on the pharmacokinetics and pharmacodynamics of intra-venous and oral midazolam. Anesth Analg 1996;82:511–516.

77. Varhe A, Olkkola KT, Neuvonen PJ. Oral triazolam is potentially hazardous to patients receiving systemic antimycotics ketoconazole or itraconazole. Clin Pharmacol Ther 1994; 56:601–607.

78. Neuvonen PJ, Varhe A, Olkkola KT. The effect of ingestion time interval on the interac-tion between itraconazole and triazolam. Clin Pharmacol Ther 1996;60:326–331.

79. Backman JT, Kivistö KT, Olkkola KT, Neuvonen PJ. The area under the plasma concen-tration-time curve for oral midazolam is 400-fold larger during treatment with itraconazole than with rifampicin. Eur J Clin Pharmacol 1998;54:53–58.

80. Ahonen J, Olkkola KT, Neuvonen PJ. The effect of the antimycotic itraconazole on the pharmacokinetics and pharmacodynamics of diazepam. Fundam Clin Pharmacol 1996;10: 314–318.

81. Otsuji Y, Okuyama N, Aoshima T, et al. No effect of itraconazole on the single oral dose pharmacokinetics and pharmacodynamics of estazolam. Ther Drug Monit 2002;24:375–378.

82. Oda M, Kotegawa T, Tsutsumi K, Ohtani Y, Kuwatani K, Nakano S. The effect of itra-conazole on the pharmacokinetics and pharmacodynamics of bromazepam in healthy volunteers. Eur J Clin Pharmacol 2003;59:615–619.

83. Ahonen J, Olkkola KT, Neuvonen PJ. Lack of effect of the antimycotic itraconazole on the pharmacokinetics or pharmacodynamics of temazepam. Ther Drug Monit 1996;18: 124–127.

84. Kivistö KT, Lamberg TS, Kantola T, Neuvonen PJ. Plasma buspirone concentrations are greatly increased by erythromycin and itraconazole. Clin Pharmacol Ther 1997;62:348–354.

85. Luurila H, Kivistö KT, Neuvonen PJ. Effect of itraconazole on the pharmacokinetics and pharmacodynamics of zolpidem. Eur J Clin Pharmacol 1998;54:163–166.

86. Bertz RJ, Granneman GR. Use of in vitro and in vivo data to estimate the likelihood of metabolic pharmacokinetic interactions. Clin Pharmacokinet 1997;32:210–258.

87. Yasui N, Kondo T, Otani K, et al. Effects of itraconazole on the steady-state plasma concentrations of haloperidol and its reduced metabolite in schizophrenic patients: in vivo evidence of the involvement of CYP3A4 for haloperidol metabolism. J Clin Psycho-pharmacol 1999;19:149–154.

88. Raaska K, Neuvonen PJ. Serum concentrations of clozapine and N-desmethylclozapine are unaffected by the potent CYP3A4 inhibitor itraconazole. Eur J Clin Pharmacol 1998; 54:167–170.

89. Kramer MR, Marshall SE, Denning DW, et al. Cyclosporine and itraconazole in heart and lung transplant recipients. Ann Intern Med 1990;113:327–329.

90. McLachlan AJ, Tett SE. Effect of metabolic inhibitors on cyclosporine pharmacokinetics using a population approach. Ther Drug Monit 1998;20:390–395.

91. Billaud EM, Guillemain R, Tacco F, Chevalier P. Evidence for a pharmacokinetic interaction between itraconazole and tacrolimus in organ transplant patients. Br J Clin Pharmacol 1998;46:271–272.

92. Varis T, Kaukonen KM, Kivistö KT, Neuvonen PJ. Plasma concentrations and effects of oral methylprednisolone are considerably increased by itraconazole. Clin Pharmacol Ther 1998;64:363–368.

93. Lebrun-Vignes B, Archer VC, Diquet B, et al. Effect of itraconazole on the pharmacokinetics of prednisolone and methylprednisolone and cortisol secretion in healthy subjects. Br J Clin Pharmacol 2001;51:443–450.

94. Varis T, Kivistö KT, Backman JT, Neuvonen PJ. Itraconazole decreases the clearance and enhances the effects of intravenously administered methylprednisolone in healthy volunteers. Pharmacol Toxicol 1999;85:29–32.

95. Varis T, Kivistö KT, Backman JT, Neuvonen PJ. The cytochrome P450 3A4 inhibitor itraconazole markedly increases the plasma concentrations of dexamethasone and enhances its adrenal-suppressant effect. Clin Pharmacol Ther 2000;68:487–494.

96. Varis T, Kivistö KT, Neuvonen PJ. The effect of itraconazole on the pharmacokinetics and pharmacodynamics of oral prednisolone. Eur J Clin Pharmacol 2000;56:57–60.

97. Raaska K, Niemi M, Neuvonen M, Neuvonen PJ, Kivistö KT. Plasma concentrations of inhaled budesonide and its effects on plasma cortisol are increased by the cytochrome P4503A4 inhibitor itraconazole. Clin Pharmacol Ther 2002;72:362–369.

98. Jalava KM, Olkkola KT, Neuvonen PJ. Itraconazole greatly increases plasma concentrations and effects of felodipine. Clin Pharmacol Ther 1997;61:410–415.

99. Lukkari E, Juhakoski A, Aranko K, Neuvonen PJ. Itraconazole moderately increases serum concentrations of oxybutynin but does not affect those of the active metabolite. Eur J Clin Pharmacol 1997;52:403–406.

100. Palkama VJ, Neuvonen PJ, Olkkola KT. The CYP3A4 inhibitor itraconazole has no effect on the pharmacokinetics of i.v. fentanyl. Br J Anaesth 1998;81:598–600.

101. Kivistö KT, Wang JS, Backman JT, et al. Selegiline pharmacokinetics are unaffected by the CYP3A4 inhibitor itraconazole. Eur J Clin Pharmacol 2001;57:37–42.

102. Lomaestro BM, Piatek MA. Update on drug interactions with azole antifungal agents. Ann Pharmacotherapy 1998;32:915–928.

103. Bonay M, Jonville-Bera AP, Diot P, Lemarie E, Lavandier M, Autret E. Possible interaction between phenobarbital, carbamazepine and itraconazole. Drug Safety 1993;9: 309–311.

104. Ducharme MP, Slaughter RL, Warbasse LH, et al. Itraconazole and hydroxyitraconazole serum concentrations are reduced more than tenfold by phenytoin. Clin Pharmacol Ther 1995;58:617–624.

105. Jaruratanasirikul S, Sriwiriyajan S. Effect of rifampicin on the pharmacokinetics of itraconazole in normal volunteers and AIDS patients. Eur J Clin Pharmacol 1998;54: 155–158.

106. de Lannoy IA, Silverman M. The mdr-1 gene product P-glycoprotein mediates transport of the cardiac glycoside, digoxin. Biochem Biophys Res Comm 1992; 189:551–557.

107. Jalava KM, Partanen J, Neuvonen PJ. Itraconazole decreases renal clearance of digoxin. Ther Drug Monit 1997;19:609–613.

108. Kaukonen KM, Olkkola KT, Neuvonen PJ. Itraconazole increases plasma concentrations of quinidine. Clin Pharmacol Ther 1997;62:510–517.

109. Damkier P, Hansen LL, Brøsen K. Effect of diclofenac, disulfram, itraconazole, grapefruit juice and erythromycin on the pharmacokinetics of quinidine. Br J Clin Pharmacol 1999;48:829–838.

110. de Lannoy IA, Koren G, Klein J, Charuk J, Silverman M. Cyclosporin and quinidine inhibition of renal digoxin excretion: evidence for luminal secretion of digoxin. Am J Physiol 1992;263:F613–F622.

111. Karyekar CS, Eddington ND, Garimella TS, Gubbins PO, Dowling TC. Evaluation of P-glycoprotein mediated renal drug interactions in an MDR1-MDCK model. Pharmacotherapy 2003;23:436–442.

112. Karyekar CS, Eddington ND, Briglia A, Gubbins PO, Dowling TC. Renal interaction between itraconazole and cimetidine. J Clin Pharmacol 2004;44:919–927.

113. Sachs MK, Blanchard LM, Green PJ. Interaction of itraconazole and digoxin. Clin Infect Dis 1993;16:400–403.

114. Ahonen J, Olkkola KT, Neuvonen PJ. Effect of route of administration of fluconazole on the interaction between fluconazole and midazolam. Eur J Clin Pharmacol 1997;51:415–419.

115. Varhe A, Olkkola KT, Neuvonen PJ. Fluconazole, but not terbinafine, enhances the effects of triazolam by inhibiting its metabolism. Br J Clin Pharmacol 1996;41:319–323.

116. Varhe A, Olkkola KT, Neuvonen PJ. Effect of fluconazole dose on the extent of fluconazole-triazolam interaction. Br J Clin Pharmacol 1996;42:465–470.

117. Krüger HU, Schuler U, Zimmermann R, Ehninger G. Absence of significant interaction of fluconazole with cyclosporin. J Antimicrob Chemother 1989;24:781–786.

118. Canafax DM, Graves NM, Hilligoss DM, Carleton BC, Gardner MJ, Matas AJ. Interaction between cyclosporine and fluconazole in renal allograft recipients. Transplantation 1991;51:1014–1018.

119. Lopez-Gil JA. Fluconazole-cyclosporine interaction: a dose-dependent effect? Ann Pharmacotherapy 1993;27:427–430.

120. Manez R, Martin M, Raman D, et al. Fluconazole therapy in transplant recipients receiving FK506. Transplantation 1994;57:1521–1523.

121. Osowski CL, Dix SP, Lin LS, Mullins RE, Geller RB, Wingard JR. Evaluation of the drug interaction between intravenous high-dose fluconazole and cyclosporine or tacrolimus in bone marrow transplant recipients. Transplantation 1996;61:1268–1272.

122. Blum RA, Wilton JH, Hilligoss DM, et al. Effect of fluconazole on disposition of phenytoin. Clin Pharmacol Ther 1991;49:420–425.

123. Kaukonen KM, Olkkola KT, Neuvonen PJ. Fluconazole but not itraconazole decreases the metabolism of losartan to E-3174. Eur J Clin Pharmacol 1998;53:445–449.

124. Palkama VJ, Isohanni MH, Neuvonen PJ, Olkkola KT. The effect of intravenous and oral fluconazole on the pharmacokinetics and pharmacodynamics of intravenous alfentanil. Anesth Analg 1998;87:190–194.

125. Koks CHW, Crommentuyn KML, Hoetelmans RMW, et al. The effect of fluconazole on ritonavir and saquinavir pharmacokinetics in HIV-1 infected adults. Br J Clin Pharmacol 2001;51:631–635.

126. Yule SM, Walker D, Cole M, et al. The effect of fluconazole on cyclophosphamide metabolism in children. Drug Metab Disp 1999;27:417–421.

127. Ren S, Yang JS, Kalhorn TF, Slattery JT. Oxidation of cyclophosphamide to 4-hydroxycyclophosphamide and deschloroethylcyclophosphamide in human liver microsomes. Cancer Res 1997;57:4229–4235.

128. Apseloff G, Hilligoss DM, Gardner MJ, et al. Induction of fluconazole metabolism by rifampin: in vivo study in humans. J Clin Pharmacol 1991;31:358–361.

129. Sahai J, Gallicano K, Pakuts A, Cameron DW. Effect of fluconazole on zidovudine pharmacokinetics in patients infected with Human Immunodeficiency Virus. J Infect Dis 1994;169:1103–1107.

130. Purkins L, Wood N, Kleinermans D, Nichols D. Voriconazole potentiates warfarin-induced prothrombin time prolongation. Br J Clin Pharmacol 2003;56(Suppl 1):24–29.

131. Romero AJ, Pogamp PL, Nilsson LG, Wood N. Effect of voriconazole on the pharmacokinetics of cyclosporine in renal transplant recipients. Clin Pharmacol Ther 2002;71:226–234.

132. Venkataramanan R, Zang S, Gayowski T, Singh N. Voriconazole inhibition of the metabolism of tacrolimus in a liver transplant recipient and in human liver microsomes. Antimicrob Agents Chemother 2002;46:3091–3093.

133. Wood N, Tan K, Allan R, Fielding A, Nichols DJ. Effect of voriconazole on the pharmacokinetics of tacrolimus. Program and Abstracts 41st Interscience Conference on Antimicrobial Agents and Chemotherapy. Chicago, IL, December 16–19, 2001, Abstract 20.

134. Purkins L, Wood N Ghahramani P, Love ER, Eve MD, Fielding A. Coadministration of voriconazole and phenytoin: pharmacokinetic interaction, safety, and toleration. Br J Clin Pharmacol 2003;56(Suppl 1):37–44.

135. Andersson T, Miners JO, Veronese ME, Birkett DJ. Identification of human liver cytochrome P450 isoforms mediating secondary omeprazole metabolism. Br J Clin Pharmacol 1994;597–604.

136. Wood N, Tan K, Allan R, Fielding A, Nichols DJ. Effect of voriconazole on the pharmacokinetics of omeprazole. Program and Abstracts 41st Interscience Conference on Antimicrobial Agents and Chemotherapy. Chicago, IL, December 16–19, 2001, Abstract 19.

137. Ghahramani P, Purkins L, Klienermans D, Nichols DJ. The pharmacokinetics of voriconazole and its effect on prednisolone disposition. Program and Abstracts 40th Interscience Conference on Antimicrobial Agents and Chemotherapy. Toronto, Ontario, September 17–20, 2000, Abstract 842.

138. Purkins L, Wood N, Klienermans, Love ER.. No clinically significant pharmacokinetic interaction between voriconazole and indinavir in healthy volunteers. Br J Clin Pharmacol 2003;56(Suppl 1):62–68.

139. Wood N, Abel S, Fielding A, Nichols DJ, Bygrave E. Voriconazole does not affect the pharmacokinetics of mycophenolic acid. Program and Abstracts 41st Interscience Conference on Antimicrobial Agents and Chemotherapy. Chicago, IL, December 16–19, 2001, Abstract 24.

140. Ghahramani P, Purkins L, Klienermans D, Nichols DJ. Effects of rifampicin and rifabutin on the pharmacokinetics of voriconazole. Program and Abstracts 40th Interscience Conference on Antimicrobial Agents and Chemotherapy. Toronto, Ontario, September 17–20, 2000, Abstract 844.

141. Purkins L, Wood N, Klienermans, Nichols D. Histamine H2-receptor antagonists have no clinically significant effect on the steady-state pharmacokinetics of voriconazole. Br J Clin Pharmacol 2003;56(Suppl 1):51–55.

142. Purkins L, Wood N, Ghahramani P, Kleinermans D, Layton G, Nichols D. No clinically significant effect of erythromycin or azithromycin on the pharmacokinetics of voriconazole in healthy male volunteers. Br J Clin Pharmacol 2003;56(Suppl 1):30–36.

143. Wood N, Tan K, Purkins L, et al. Effect of omeprazole on the steady-state pharmacokinetics of voriconazole. Br J Clin Pharmacol 2003;56(Suppl 1):56–61.

144. Schutze GE, Hickerson SL, Fortin E, et al. Blastomycosis in children, Clin Infect Dis 1996;22:496–502.

145. Ullman AJ. Review of the safety, tolerability, and drug interactions of the new antifungal agents caspofungin and voriconazole. Curr Med Res Opinion 2003;19:263–271.

146. Letscher-Bru V, Herbrecht R. Caspofungin: the first representative of a new antifungal class. J Antimicrob Chemother 2003;51:513–521.

147. Stone J, Holland S, Wickersham P, et al. Drug interactions between caspofungin and tacrolimus. Program and Abstracts 41st Interscience Conference on Antimicrobial Agents and Chemotherapy. Chicago, IL, December 16–19, 2001, Abstract 13.

148. Stone J, Migoya E, Hickey L, et al. Drug interactions between caspofungin and nelfinavir or rifampin. Program and Abstracts 43rd Interscience Conference on Antimicrobial Agents and Chemotherapy. Chicago, IL; September 14–17, 2003, Abstract 1605.

# 11

# Miscellaneous Antibiotics

## Gregory M. Susla

## INTRODUCTION

This chapter discusses the interactions of antibiotics that may be the only available agents from a class of antibiotics that is used clinically today. Chloramphenicol and tetracycline are older agents that are less frequently prescribed; so many clinicians may not be familiar with their interactions with other medications. Many of the interacting agents also are less frequently prescribed, such as first-generation oral hypoglycemic agents. Because many of the interactions in this chapter are based on single case reports, it is difficult to determine the mechanism of the interaction and if a true interaction exists. The existence of some interactions may be questioned because of other potential causes that may have been present when the interaction was discovered.

The interactions described in this chapter are summarized in Table 1.

## CHLORAMPHENICOL

Chloramphenicol is a broad-spectrum antibiotic that has been shown to interact with a number of medications, including analgesics-antipyretics, other antibiotics, oral hypoglycemic agents, anticoagulants, and anticonvulsants. Most of these interactions are limited to case reports with small numbers of patients. The mechanism of the interaction for several of the interactions is unknown or is limited to speculation.

### Acetaminophen

Chloramphenicol has been reported to increase, decrease, and have no effect on the half-life of acetaminophen. Spika and colleagues evaluated the effect of multiple doses of acetaminophen on chloramphenicol metabolism in patients with bacterial meningitis (1). Significant differences in chloramphenicol peak serum concentration, volume of distribution, half-life, and clearance occurred between samples obtained before and during treatment with acetaminophen. Peak serum concentrations fell, volume of distribution and clearance increased, and half-life shortened. The greatest change was in clearance, which increased by more than 300% from baseline values. During treatment with acetaminophen, the percentage of chloramphenicol excreted unchanged in the urine decreased; its succinate metabolite remained unchanged; the glucuronide metabolite increased by approx 300%.

From: *Infectious Disease: Drug Interactions in Infectious Diseases, Second Edition*
Edited by: S. C. Piscitelli and K. A. Rodvold © Humana Press Inc., Totowa, NJ

**Table 1**
**Antibiotics Interactions**

| Primary drug | Interacting drug | Mechanism | Effects | Comments/management |
|---|---|---|---|---|
| Chloramphenicol | Acetaminophen | Increased chloramphenicol clearance | Reduced chloramphenicol concentrations<br>Potential for therapeutic failure | Monitor chloramphenicol concentrations and adjust dose as needed<br>Use alternative agent for antipyresis or analgesia |
| | Anticonvulsants | Increased chloramphenicol clearance | Reduced chloramphenicol concentrations<br>Potential for therapeutic failure | Monitor chloramphenicol concentrations and adjust dose as needed<br>Patients should be monitored for clinical and microbiological response to therapy |
| | Anticonvulsants | Decreased metabolism of phenytoin and phenobarbital | Increased serum concentrations of these anticonvulsants with increased CNS toxicity | Monitor phenytoin and phenobarbital concentrations and adjust dose as needed |
| | Oral hypoglycemic agents | Decreased metabolism of tolbutamide and excretion of chlorpropamide | Increased half-life of tolbutamide and chlorpropamide with increased risk of hypoglycemia | Monitor blood glucose and adjust dose of oral hypoglycemic agents as needed<br>Monitor for clinical signs and symptoms of hypoglycemia |
| | Penicillins | Antagonism of bacteriocidal agents | Potential risk of therapeutic failure when both agents are administered concurrently | Monitor clinical and microbiological response to therapy<br>Monitor MIC and MBC of antibiotic combination and each antibiotic alone<br>Use alternative class of antibiotic |
| | Rifampin | Increased chloramphenicol clearance | Reduced chloramphenicol concentrations<br>Potential for therapeutic failure | Monitor chloramphenicol concentrations and adjust dose as needed<br>Patients should be monitored for clinical and microbiological response to therapy |
| | Oral anticoagulants | Enhanced metabolism of warfarin<br>Decreased gut production of vitamin K<br>Altered production of prothrombin by hepatic cells | Increased risk of major and minor bleeding | Monitor PT/INR when beginning or discontinuing chloramphenicol therapy<br>Monitor for clinical signs of bleeding |

| Drug | Interacting agent | Mechanism | Effect | Recommendation |
|---|---|---|---|---|
| | Immunosuppressive agents | Decreased cyclosporine and tacrolimus clearance | Increased cyclosporine and tacrolimus concentrations / Potential for cyclosporine and tacrolimus toxicity | Monitor cyclosporine and tacrolimus concentrations and adjust dose as needed |
| Clindamycin | Nondepolarizing neuromuscular blocking agents | Local anesthetic effect on myelinated muscle / Stimulates nerve terminal and blocks postsynaptic cholinergic receptor / Direct depressant action on muscle | Prolonged duration of neuromuscular blockade | Patients receiving this combination of medications should have their neuromuscular function monitored with peripheral nerve stimulation to access the degree of paralysis induced by these agents / Patients should be monitored for the potential development of respiratory failure |
| | Aminoglycosides | No clear evidence to support the hypothesis that clindamycin leads to an increased risk of nephrotoxicity when prescribed concurrently with aminoglycoside antibiotics | | |
| Vancomycin | Indomethacin | Nonsteroidal antiinflammatory agents may cause renal failure | Increased concentrations of renally eliminated medications | Serum concentrations of medications should be monitored when possible and dosage regimens adjusted to maintain serum concentrations within the accepted therapeutic ranges |
| | Nondepolarizing neuromuscular blocking agents | It is unclear regarding the exact mechanism of this interaction | High vancomycin concentrations may be associated with prolonged paralysis following a dose of nondepolarizing blocking agent | Vancomycin dose should be adjusted for body weight and infused over recommended times to prevent excessively high peak concentrations |
| | Heparin | Inactivation of vancomycin | Reduced vancomycin activity | Infuse the two drugs through the same intravenous line serially, with a 0.9% sodium chloride solution flushing the line between the two drugs to prevent mixing at high concentrations |

*Continued on next page*

**Table 1 (*Continued*)**
**Antibiotics Interactions**

| Primary drug | Interacting drug | Mechanism | Effects | Comments/management |
|---|---|---|---|---|
| Sulfonamides | Oral anticoagulants | Some sulfonamides appear to impair the hepatic metabolism of oral anticoagulants<br>Competition for plasma protein-binding sites may play an additional role | An enhanced hypoprothrombinemic response to warfarin with an increased risk of minor and major bleeding | Monitor PT/INR when beginning or discontinuing sulfonamide therapy<br>Monitor for clinical signs of bleeding |
| Tetracycline | Heavy metals, trivalent cations | Chelate tetracycline products in the gastrointestinal tract | Impair their absorption and decrease bioavailability<br>Potential for therapeutic failure | Tetracycline products should be administered 2 hours before or 6 hours after an antacid<br>$H_2$-receptor antagonists and proton pump inhibitors may be prescribed in place of antacids<br>Alternative antibiotics may be prescribed in place of a tetracycline<br>Patients should be monitored for clinical and microbiological response to therapy |
| | Colestipol | Bind tetracycline products in the gastrointestinal tract | Impair their absorption and decrease bioavailability<br>Potential for therapeutic failure | Tetracycline products should be administered 2 hours before or 3 hours after colestipol<br>Alternative antibiotics may be prescribed in place of a tetracycline<br>Patients should be monitored for clinical and microbiological response to therapy |
| | Digoxin | Tetracycline can suppress the gut flora responsible for metabolizing digoxin in the gastrointestinal tract | Increased digoxin absorption and bioavailability may result in toxicity | Serum digoxin concentrations should be monitored and the dose adjusted with initiating or discontinuing antibiotic therapy |
| | Anticonvulsants | Anticonvulsants increase the hepatic metabolism of doxycycline, reducing its serum concentration | Increased potential for therapeutic failure | Patients should be monitored for clinical and microbiological response to therapy<br>Renally eliminated tetracycline or other classes of antibiotics should be prescribed to avoid this interaction |

| Drug | Mechanism | Significance | Recommendations |
| --- | --- | --- | --- |
| | | | Doxycycline should be administered twice a day in patients on chronic anticonvulsant therapy |
| Warfarin | Doxycycline enhances the anticoagulation response to oral anticoagulants | An enhanced hypoprothrombinemic response to warfarin with an increase risk of minor and major bleeding | Patients should be monitored for clinical signs and symptoms of bleeding when these drugs are used concurrently; PT and/or INR should be monitored when these drugs are used concurrently; Alternative antibiotics should be prescribed for patients on oral anticoagulants |
| Lithium | It is unclear if there is a direct interaction between lithium and tetracycline | Potential for increased serum lithium concentrations and lithium toxicity | Patients should be monitored for signs and symptoms of lithium toxicity when receiving lithium and tetracycline concurrently; Monitor serum lithium concentrations when receiving lithium and tetracycline |
| Theophylline | A reduction in theophylline metabolism | The reduction in clearance appears to be quite variable so that it may be difficult to predict how much the theophylline concentration will increase following the addition of tetracycline to the medication regimen | Patients should be monitored clinically for signs and symptoms of theophylline toxicity; Serum theophylline concentration should be closely monitored in patients at high risk for developing theophylline toxicity |
| Oral contraceptives | Prospective trials have failed to documented a consistent effect | Unexpected pregnancies | It is not known if noncompliance played a role in some of these unplanned pregnancies; Women should be counseled to use other methods of birth control during tetracycline therapy |
| Psychotropic agents | In is unclear as to the exact mechanism of the interaction | Possible potential for acute psychotic behavior | Monitor for signs and symptoms of acute psychotic behavior; Use alternative class of antibiotic |

*Continued on next page*

**Table 1 (*Continued*)**
**Antibiotics Interactions**

| Primary drug | Interacting drug | Mechanism | Effects | Comments/management |
|---|---|---|---|---|
| Tetracycline (*Continued*) | Methotrexate | Decreased methotrexate clearance | Increased methotrexate concentration<br>Potential for methotrexate toxicity | Monitor methotrexate concentrations<br>Maintain leucovorin rescue until methotrexate concentrations are below the desired range |
| | Rifampin | Increased doxycycline clearance | Increased potential for therapeutic failures in patients with *Brucellosis* infections | Monitor clinical and microbiological response to therapy<br>Use alternative class of antibiotic |
| Aminoglycosides | Amphotericin B | Additive direct nephrotoxicity effects on kidney | The concurrent administration of aminoglycoside antibiotics and amphotericin B may increase the risk of developing renal failure | Aminoglycoside concentrations should be monitored and the dosage regimen adjusted to maintain serum concentrations within the desired therapeutic range<br>Attempts should be made to avoid other conditions that increase the risk for developing nephrotoxicity (i.e., hypotension, intravenous contrast media)<br>Avoid prescribing other agents that cause nephrotoxicity |
| | Neuromuscular blocking agents | Aminoglycosides have been shown to interfere with acetylcholine release and exert a postsynaptic curare-like action<br>These agents have membrane-stabilizing properties and exert their effect on acetylcholine release by interfering with calcium ion fluxes at the nerve terminal, an action similar to magnesium ions | These drugs may cause postoperative respiratory depression when administered before or during operations and may also cause a transient deterioration in patents with myasthenia gravis | Patient should be monitored for prolonged postoperative paralysis if they received neuromuscular blocking agents and aminoglycoside antibiotics during the perioperative or immediate postoperative period |

344

| | | |
|---|---|---|
| | Aminoglycosides also possess a smaller but significant decrease in postjunctional receptor sensitivity and spontaneous release | Serum concentrations of medications should be monitored when possible and dosage regimens adjusted to maintain serum concentrations within the accepted therapeutic ranges |
| Indomethacin | Nonsteroidal anti-inflammatory agents may cause renal failure | Increased concentrations of renally eliminated medications |
| Cyclosporine | Additive direct nephrotoxicity effects on kidney | Concurrent administration of aminoglycoside antibiotics and cyclosporine may increase the risk of developing renal failure | Aminoglycoside and cyclosporine concentrations should be monitored and the dosage regimen adjusted to maintain serum concentrations within the desired therapeutic range<br><br>Attempts should be made to avoid other conditions that increase the risk for developing nephrotoxicity (i.e., hypotension, intravenous contrast media)<br><br>Avoid prescribing other agents that cause nephrotoxicity |
| Cisplatin | Additive direct nephrotoxicity effects on kidney | Concurrent administration of aminoglycoside antibiotics and cisplatin-based chemotherapy regimens may increase the risk of developing renal failure | Aminoglycoside concentrations should be monitored and the dosage regimen adjusted to maintain serum concentrations within the desired therapeutic range<br><br>Attempts should be made to avoid other conditions that increase the risk for developing nephrotoxicity (i.e., hypotension, intravenous contrast media)<br><br>Avoid prescribing other agents that cause nephrotoxicity |

*Continued on next page*

345

**Table 1 (*Continued*)**
**Antibiotics Interactions**

| Primary drug | Interacting drug | Mechanism | Effects | Comments/management |
|---|---|---|---|---|
| Aminoglycosides (*Continued*) | Loop diuretics | Ethacrynic acid may cause direct additive ototoxic effects on the ear | When ethacrynic acid is used alone or in combination with aminoglycosides, it should be used in low doses and titrated to maintain adequate urine output or fluid balance<br><br>It is unclear whether furosemide directly increases the nephrotoxicity and ototoxicity of aminoglycosides | Aminoglycoside concentrations should be monitored and the dosage regimens adjusted to maintain concentrations within the therapeutic range<br><br>Furosemide should be used with caution in patients receiving aminoglycoside antibiotics; careful attention should be paid to the patient's weight, urine output, fluid balance, and indices of renal function |
| | Vancomycin | Unclear if vancomycin increases the nephrotoxicity of aminoglycosides | The development of nephrotoxicity | Aminoglycoside and vancomycin concentrations should be monitored and the dosage regimen adjusted to maintain serum concentrations within the desired therapeutic range<br><br>Attempts should be made to avoid other conditions that increase the risk for developing nephrotoxicity (i.e., hypotension, intravenous contrast media)<br><br>Avoid prescribing other agents that cause nephrotoxicity |
| | Anti-*Pseudomonas* penicillins | Penicillins combine with aminoglycoside antibiotics in equal molar concentrations at a rate dependent on the concentration, temperature, and medium composition<br><br>The greater the concentration of the penicillin, the greater the inactivation of the aminoglycoside | Unexpected low serum aminoglycoside concentrations for a given dose | Blood samples for aminoglycosides concentrations should be sent to the laboratory within 1–2 hours so that the sample can be spun down and frozen if not assayed immediately<br><br>The two antibiotics should never to be given at the same time; schedule administration time of the antibiotic so that the administration of the aminoglycoside occurs toward the end of the penicillin dosing interval |

| Antibiotic | Interacting drug | Mechanism | Effect | Recommendation |
|---|---|---|---|---|
| | | The inactivation is thought to occur by way of a nucleophilic opening of the β-lactam ring, which then combines with an amino group of the aminoglycoside, leading to the formation of a microbiologically inactive amide | | If a patient is receiving this antibiotic combination and unusually low aminoglycoside concentrations occur, the above factors should be checked |
| Linezolid | Selective serotonin reuptake inhibitors | Decreased serotonin metabolism by inhibition of monoamine oxidase | Development of the serotonin syndrome | Review patient profile before prescribing linezolid<br>Use alternative class of antibiotic<br>If necessary, treat serotonin syndrome with serotonin antagonist cyproheptadine |
| | Systemic decongestants | Decreased metabolism by inhibition of monoamine oxidase | Increased blood pressure | Review patient profile before prescribing linezolid<br>Use alternative class of antibiotic<br>Consider using topical nasal decongestants |
| Quinupristin-dalfopristin | Medications metabolized by cytochrome P450 3A4 enzyme | Decreased metabolism of medications by cytochrome P450 3A4 enzyme | Prolonged therapeutic effects or increased adverse reactions | Review patient profile before prescribing quinupristin-dalfopristin<br>Use alternative class of antibiotic<br>Monitor patients closely for signs of adverse effects |
| Telithromycin | Azole antifungal agents | Decreased telithromycin metabolism | Increased telithromycin concentrations | Use alternative class of antibiotic |
| | Cisapride | Decreased cisapride metabolism | Increased cisapride concentrations resulting in QTc interval prolongation | Avoid concomitant use of telithromycin and cisapride<br>Use alternative class of antibiotic |
| | Simvastatin | Decreased simvastatin metabolism | Increased simvastatin and metabolite concentrations<br>Increased the risk of developing myopathy | Similar interaction possible with atorvastatin and lovastatin<br>Use alternative class of antibiotic |

Continued on next page

**Table 1 (*Continued*)**
**Antibiotics Interactions**

| Primary drug | Interacting drug | Mechanism | Effects | Comments/management |
|---|---|---|---|---|
| | Midazolam | Decreased midazolam metabolism | Increased midazolam concentrations<br>Increased risk for CNS and respiratory depression | Reduce midazolam dose<br>Monitor patient's level of consciousness and respiratory status |
| | Warfarin | Enhanced metabolism of warfarin<br>Decreased gut production of vitamin K<br>Altered production of prothrombin by hepatic cell | Increased risk of major and minor bleeding | Monitor PT/INR when beginning or discontinuing telithromycin therapy<br>Monitor for clinical signs of bleeding<br>Alternative antibiotics should be prescribed in patients on oral anticoagulants |
| | Verapamil | Decreased metabolism of verapamil | Increased risk of cardiac decompensation, heart block, or bradycardia | Monitor cardiac function and ECG<br>Use alternative class of antibiotic |
| | Rifampin | Increased telithromycin clearance | Reduced telithromycin concentrations<br>Potential for therapeutic failure | Patients should be monitored for clinical and microbiologic response to therapy |
| | Anticonvulsants | Increased telithromycin clearance | Reduced telithromycin concentrations<br>Potential for therapeutic failure | Patients should be monitored for clinical and microbiologic response to therapy |
| | Metoprolol | Decreased metoprolol metabolism | Increase metoprolol concentrations potentially precipitating acute decompensated heart failure | Monitor patient's cardiac status<br>Use alternative class of antibiotic |
| | Digoxin | Unknown | Increased digoxin absorption and bioavailability may result in toxicity | Serum digoxin concentrations should be monitored and the dose adjusted with initiating or discontinuing antibiotic therapy |

348

| Theophylline | A reduction in theophylline metabolism | The reduction in clearance appears to be quite variable so that it may be difficult to predict how much the theophylline concentration will increase following the addition of tetracycline to the medication regimen | Patients should be monitored clinically for signs and symptoms of theophylline toxicity<br>Serum theophylline concentration should be closely monitored in patients at high risk for developing theophylline toxicity<br>Alternative antibiotics should be prescribed in patients on theophylline |
| Sotalol | Decreased sotalol absorption | Decreased sotalol concentration<br>Loss of antiarrhythmic effects | Monitor patient's ECG<br>Use alternative class of antibiotic |
| Oral contraceptives | Prospective trials have failed to documented a consistent effect | Unexpected pregnancies | It is not know if noncompliance played a role in some of these unplanned pregnancies<br>Women should be counseled to use other methods of birth control during tetracycline therapy |

MBC, minimum bactericidal concentration; MIC, minimum inhibitory concentration.

Kearns et al. evaluated the effect of acetaminophen in acutely ill pediatric patients *(2)*. Chloramphenicol pharmacokinetic parameters were compared between a group of patients receiving acetaminophen and a group not receiving acetaminophen. There was no statistical difference in the chloramphenicol pharmacokinetic parameters between the two groups. However, there was a clinically significant increase in chloramphenicol clearance and decrease in half-life between the initial dose and final dose in the patients receiving acetaminophen. Following acetaminophen therapy, the chloramphenicol half-life decreased by approx 33%, from 3.4 to 2.2 hours, and its clearance increased by more than 50%, from 5.5 to 8.9 mL/minute/kg. The peak chloramphenicol serum concentrations were lower after the final dose than at steady state, 15.7 vs 22.7 mg/L, respectively.

Stein et al. were unable to document any effect of acetaminophen on chloramphenicol metabolism in hospitalized adult patients *(3)*. In a randomized crossover design, patients received either chloramphenicol or chloramphenicol with acetaminophen for 48 hours. There was no significant difference in peak and trough chloramphenicol concentrations, half-life, or area under the concentration–time curve (AUC) between the two treatment periods.

Although the mechanism of this interaction is unclear, it appears to be an alteration in clearance. This interaction may take several days to manifest its full effect, and in some studies patients may not have been studied for a long enough period of time to evaluate fully the effects of acetaminophen on chloramphenicol pharmacokinetic parameters. Although Spika et al. *(1)* suggested that the increase in chloramphenicol clearance was caused by an increased in glucuronidation, this has not been confirmed by other investigators.

This interaction may be important in patients receiving chloramphenicol for the treatment of central nervous system (CNS) infections or infections caused by organisms resistant to more traditional antibiotics. Reduced peak concentrations or increases in clearance without appropriate adjustments in dosage regimens to account for these changes may result in therapeutic failures. Patients receiving chloramphenicol and acetaminophen should have chloramphenicol serum concentrations monitored every 2–3 days during a course of therapy, especially during the later part of therapy when it appears that chloramphenicol levels may begin to decline. Dosage regimens should be adjusted to maintain chloramphenicol concentrations within the desired therapeutic range. Other agents such as aspirin or ibuprofen may be used as alternatives to acetaminophen for antipyresis and analgesia.

### Anticonvulsants

Anticonvulsants have been shown to increase the metabolism of chloramphenicol by increasing its hepatic metabolism. Phenobarbital has been shown to stimulate the metabolism of chloramphenicol in several case reports *(4,5)*. In addition, chloramphenicol has been shown to reduce the metabolism of phenytoin and phenobarbital when both agents are administered concurrently *(6–10)*. The onset of these interactions appears to be rapid and may persist for several days after chloramphenicol is discontinued.

The reduction in phenytoin and phenobarbital metabolism is mostly likely because of a competition for metabolic enzymes. The clinical significance of the interaction is the potential for patients to develop phenytoin or phenobarbital toxicity after beginning chloramphenicol therapy. Patients may show signs of lethargy, excessive sedation, nystagmus, hallucinations, or other mental status changes. Because phenytoin undergoes nonlinear metabolism, toxic serum concentrations may not occur for several days after starting chloramphenicol. After the maximum rate of phenytoin metabolism is exceeded, serum concentrations will rise rapidly and may remain elevated for a period of time after the chloramphenicol is discontinued. Because of phenobarbital's long half-life, its sedative effects can be expected to resolve slowly as the serum concentration falls.

Patients receiving chloramphenicol with either phenytoin or phenobarbital must have their anticonvulsant serum concentrations monitored frequently, preferably every 3–5 days if possible, to detect increases in the concentrations. Patients also should be monitored clinically for the development of signs and symptoms of phenytoin or phenobarbital toxicity.

Phenobarbital has been shown to increase the metabolism of chloramphenicol, resulting in a reduction in its peak serum concentrations. Bloxham reported two patients who received chloramphenicol and phenobarbital for the treatment of meningitis *(4)*. In one patient, peak chloramphenicol serum concentrations fell from 31 mg/L on days 2 and 3 to less than 5 mg/L on day 5. Patients receiving concurrent therapy with chloramphenicol and phenobarbital should have chloramphenicol concentrations monitored daily for reductions in the serum concentration. The chloramphenicol dosage regimen needs to be adjusted to maintain therapeutic concentrations and prevent therapeutic failures.

## Oral Hypoglycemic Agents

Several investigators have documented chloramphenicol's ability to decrease the hepatic metabolism of tolbutamide, resulting in increases in its half-life and serum concentrations *(10,11)*. Patients receiving tolbutamide and chloramphenicol concurrently may experience greater reductions in their serum glucose values and hypoglycemia with its associated complications. However, frank hypoglycemia has not been reported when this combination has been given together.

Petitpierre and Fabre reported the ability of chloramphenicol to inhibit the renal excretion of chlorpropamide *(12)*. They reported that five patients taking these agents together experienced an increase in their chlorpropamide half-lives from 30–36 hours to up to 40–146 hours. Hypoglycemia was not documented in these patients.

Patients taking oral hypoglycemic agents should monitor their blood glucose frequently when taking chloramphenicol. The oral hypoglycemic dosage regimen may need to be adjusted to maintain the blood glucose within a desirable range. Patients should also be instructed to monitor for signs of hypoglycemia and to carry glucose-containing products to reverse any episodes of hypoglycemia that may develop. If possible, alternative antibiotics should be selected to avoid this interaction. Because a patient's blood glucose may be controlled on a stable oral hypoglycemic dose, switching oral hypoglycemic agents to avoid this interaction is not recommended.

## Antibiotics

### Penicillins

Chloramphenicol has been reported to antagonize the effect of β-lactam antibiotics. A number of reports have been published suggesting that bacteriostatic and bactericidal antibiotics may antagonize each other in vitro *(13,14)* and in vivo *(15,16)*.

Despite this information, many authorities do not believe that this is a clinically significant interaction and have used this combination of antibiotics as a standard of practice for many years for the treatment of bacterial meningitis.

French and colleagues described a case in which chloramphenicol and ceftazidime were used together to treat an infant with *Salmonella* meningitis *(16)*. The combination failed to eradicate the infection, but subsequent treatment with ceftazidime alone was successful. In vitro tests of serum and cerebrospinal fluid taken at that time showed that the serum could inhibit the growth of an inoculum of the salmonella at a dilution of 1:2 and the cerebrospinal fluid at a dilution of 1:16, but neither fluid could kill the organism at any dilution. A specimen of cerebrospinal fluid taken during treatment with ceftazidime alone inhibited and killed the standard inoculum of salmonella in vitro at a dilution of 1:32.

Minor degrees of antagonism have been demonstrated in occasional laboratory experiments between almost any pair of drugs, but generally the most consistent interfering drugs are bacteriostatic agents such as chloramphenicol, tetracyclines, and macrolides *(14)*. All these agents appear to act predominantly as inhibitors of protein synthesis in microorganisms. They actively antagonize agents such as the penicillins, which primarily block the synthesis of cell wall mucopeptides. It is believed that protein synthesis must proceed actively to permit active mucopeptide synthesis; therefore, inhibitors of protein synthesis can antagonize inhibitors of cell wall synthesis.

### Rifampin

Prober *(17)* and Kelly et al. *(18)* each reported two cases in which the coadministration of rifampin and chloramphenicol resulted in significantly lower chloramphenicol serum concentrations. Two patients were treated with chloramphenicol for *Haemophilus influenzae*. During the last 4 days of treatment, the patients received 20 mg/kg/day of rifampin. After 12 doses of chloramphenicol, the peak serum concentrations of chloramphenicol in these two patients were 21.5 and 38.5 mg/L, respectively, and trough concentrations were 13.7 and 28.8 mg/L. After the administration of rifampin, peak chloramphenicol concentrations progressively declined. By day 3 of rifampin coadministration, the peak concentration of chloramphenicol was reduced by 85.5% to 3.1 mg/L in one patient and by 63.8% to 8 mg/L in the second patient. Serum concentrations increased back into the therapeutic range after the daily dose of chloramphenicol was increased to 125 mg/kg/day. The reduction in serum concentrations was most likely caused by rifampin stimulating the hepatic metabolism of chloramphenicol, increasing its clearance and decreasing its serum concentrations.

Patients should have chloramphenicol concentrations monitored daily while they are receiving rifampin. The chloramphenicol dosage regimen may need to be adjusted to maintain concentrations within the therapeutic range because subtherapeutic concentrations may result in therapeutic failure. Patients also should be monitored clinically for their response to therapy.

### Anticoagulants

Chloramphenicol may enhance the hypoprothrombinemic response to oral anticoagulants. Christensen and Skovsted documented a two- to fourfold increase in dicumarol half-life when coadministered with chloramphenicol *(10)*.

Several potential mechanisms may be responsible for this interaction. Chloramphenicol has been shown to inhibit the metabolism of dicumarol, probably by inhibiting hepatic microsomal enzymes *(10)*. Some investigators have proposed that chloramphenicol decreases vitamin K production by gastrointestinal bacteria *(19,20)*; however, bacterial production of vitamin K appears to be less important than dietary intake. Moreover, chloramphenicol does not usually have much effect on bowel flora *(21)*. Vitamin K depletion by chloramphenicol may affect the production of vitamin K-dependent clotting factors in the hepatocyte *(22)*.

The clinical consequences of an increased prothrombin time (PT) or international normalized ratio (INR) would be increased risk of bleeding. This includes not only minor bleeding such as nosebleeds and bleeding from the gums, but also major bleeding into the gastrointestinal tract, CNS, or retroperitoneal space. The PT/INR should be monitored daily when chloramphenicol is started or discontinued in patients taking oral anticoagulants. There may be an increase in clot formation and thromboembolic complications if the warfarin dose is not increased after the chloramphenicol is stopped.

### Immunosuppressive Agents Cyclosporine and Tacrolimus

Several reports have appeared in the literature describing an interaction between chloramphenicol and immunosuppressive agents, specifically cyclosporine and tacrolimus. Bui and Huang reported the interaction in a renal transplant patient receiving cyclosporine *(23)*. The patient required cyclosporine 50–75 mg twice daily to maintain trough concentrations in the 100–150 mg/L prior to hospital admission. The patient's cyclosporine dose required increasing to 300 mg twice daily during her hospital admission to maintain similar trough concentrations because of rifampin therapy for the treatment of line sepsis. Ten days after the rifampin was stopped, 875 mg chloramphenicol every 6 hours was started for the treatment of an *Enterococcus* sinusitis. The trough cyclosporine concentration on the following day increased to 280 mg/L. Despite stepwise lowering of the cyclosporine dose to 50–100 mg daily, the concentrations continued to rise for the next 2 weeks, reaching a plateau of 600 mg/L. After stopping the chloramphenicol, the cyclosporine concentration stabilized between 100 and 150 mg/L on a dose of 50 mg twice daily. Steinfort and McConachy reported a similar experience in a heart transplant patient receiving chloramphenicol and cyclosporine *(24)*.

Two reports have documented a similar interaction between chloramphenicol and tacrolimus in transplant patients *(25,26)*. Schulman and colleagues reported a 7.5-fold increase in tacrolimus dose-adjusted AUC, 22.7 vs 171 mg·h/L and an increased in tacrolimus half-life from 9.1 to 14.7 hours following the addition of chloramphenicol to a stable tacrolimus regimen *(25)*. Taber and colleagues documented the chloramphenicol–tacrolimus interaction in a liver transplant patient. The patient was stabilized on an outpatient tacrolimus dose of 5 mg twice daily with trough concentrations ranging between 9 and 11 ng/mL. The tacrolimus 12-hour trough concentration increased to more than 60 ng/mL after 3 days of 1850 mg chloramphenicol every 6 hours. The patient complained of lethargy, fatigue, headaches, and tremors. The tacrolimus concentration decreased to 8.2 ng/mL 7 days after the chloramphenicol was stopped. The tacrolimus regimen was restarted at 5 mg twice daily, resulting in stable trough concentrations between 6.7 and 11.0 ng/mL *(26)*.

The mechanism of the interaction is most likely caused by chloramphenicol's inhibition of the cyctochrome P450 3A4 enzyme, which is responsible for the metabolism of cyclosporine and tacrolimus. If chloramphenicol has to be used in a patient receiving cyclosporine or tacrolimus, a prospective decrease in dose may be warranted. Cyclosporine and tacrolimus concentrations should be closely monitored with appropriate dose adjustments while patients are receiving chloramphenicol. Cyclosporine and tacrolimus administration should be stopped in patients with elevated trough concentrations, especially in patients slowing signs of cyclosporine or tacrolimus toxicity until the concentrations returned to the normal therapeutic range. The agents may be restarted at appropriately adjusted doses to maintain the trough concentrations within the therapeutic range.

## CLINDAMYCIN

### Nondepolarizing Neuromuscular Blocking Agents

Clindamycin has been shown to interact with nondepolarizing neuromuscular blocking agents and aminoglycoside antibiotics. Becker and Miller investigated the neuromuscular blockade induced by clindamycin alone and when mixed with *d*-tubocurarine or pancuronium in an in vitro guinea pig lumbrical nerve-muscle preparation *(27)*. Clindamycin initially increased twitch tension, but with higher concentrations twitch tensions subsequently decreased. With 15–20% twitch depression induced by clindamycin, neostigmine or calcium slightly but not completely antagonized the blockade. Clindamycin at a dose that did not depress twitch tension potentiated *d*-tubocurarine- and pancuronium-induced neuromuscular blockade.

Several clinical reports documented clindamycin's ability to prolong neuromuscular blockade following depolarizing and nondepolarizing neuromuscular blocking agents *(28–30)*. Best and colleagues reported on a patient who received 300 mg clindamycin intravenously 30 minutes before surgery to repair a nasal fracture *(28)*. To facilitate intubation, 120 mg succinylcholine was administered, with no additional nondepolarizing neuromuscular blocking agents administered during the surgery. Approximately 5 hours after surgery and 20 minutes after receiving 600 mg clindamycin intravenously, the patient complained of profound overall body weakness and was noted to have bilateral ptosis, difficulty speaking, and rapid shallow respirations. After several minutes, her weakness rapidly became more profound, with one-fifth muscle strength noted in all extremities. Nerve stimulation showed marked neuromuscular blockade with the train-of-four (TOF) stimulation noted to be 0/4. The patient was treated with 4 mg neostigmine iv and 0.8 mg glycopyrrolate iv, enabling the patient to move all extremities and develop a more normal respiratory pattern. Follow-up nerve stimulation showed a TOF of 4/4, and within 20 minutes of the reversal agent, the patient returned to baseline muscle strength (5/5) in all extremities.

Clindamycin-induced neuromuscular blockade is difficult to reverse. No reversal could be obtained by using either calcium or neostigmine *(31)*. The mode of action of clindamycin on neuromuscular function is complex. Although it has a local anesthetic effect on myelinated nerves, it also stimulates the nerve terminal and simultaneously blocks the postsynaptic cholinergic receptor. It appears that its major neuromuscular blocking effect is a direct depressant action on the muscle by the un-ionized form of clindamycin *(32)*. Clindamycin also has been shown to decrease the quantal content of acetylcholine released with presynaptic stimulation in vitro *(33)*, possibly the result of effects on presynaptic voltage-gated $Ca^{2+}$ channels *(34)*.

This pharmacodynamic interaction may be of clinical significance in patients receiving clindamycin and depolarizing or nondepolarizing neuromuscular blocking agent during the perioperative period or in an intensive care unit. This interaction may result in a prolonged period of neuromuscular blockade, resulting in recurarization with respiratory failure and an extended period of mechanical ventilation.

Patients receiving this combination of agents should be monitored clinically with peripheral nerve stimulation using TOF or other mode of nerve stimulation to assess neuromuscular function and degree of neuromuscular blockade.

## Aminoglycosides

One report suggested that clindamycin may increase the risk of nephrotoxicity when administered concurrently with aminoglycoside antibiotics. Butkus and colleagues reported three patients who developed acute renal failure when gentamicin and clindamycin were administered concurrently *(35)*. The evidence for combined nephrotoxicity consisted of the temporal relationship between administration of the antibiotics and the development of acute renal failure with rapid recovery after the antibiotics were stopped.

This interaction is supported by circumstantial evidence. Although both agents were administered concurrently, none of the patients had gentamicin concentrations monitored during therapy. The reversible renal failure is consistent with that seen with aminoglycosides. It occurs during the course of therapy and resolves rapidly once the aminoglycoside antibiotic is stopped. There is no evidence to suggest that the administration of clindamycin in the setting of appropriately dosed aminoglycoside antibiotics leads to an increased risk of nephrotoxicity.

## VANCOMYCIN

### Nonsteroidal Anti-Inflammatory Agents

Spivey and Gal compared the vancomycin pharmacokinetic parameters in six neonates with patent ductus arteriosus treated with indomethacin and vancomycin to five patients receiving vancomycin alone *(36)*. The vancomycin half-life (24.6 vs 7.0 hours) and volume of distribution (0.71 vs 0.48 L/kg) increased, and the clearance decreased (23 vs 54 mL/kg/hour) in the indomethacin-treated group compared to the control group. This may have been because of the ability of nonsteroidal anti-inflammatory agents to cause reversible renal failure, impairing the elimination of all renally eliminated medications.

Renal function should be closely monitored in patients receiving nonsteroidal anti-inflammatory agents. If renal failure develops, the doses of all renally eliminated medications should be adjusted to the level of residual renal function. Serum concentrations of medications should be monitored and dosage regimens adjusted to maintain serum concentrations within the accepted therapeutic ranges.

### Vecuronium

Huang and colleagues described the depression of neuromuscular function that developed after the intravenous administration of vancomycin *(37)*. Tracheal intubation was facilitated with vecuronium. Twenty minutes after induction of anesthesia, T1 had returned to 35% of the preinduction baseline, but T4 was barely perceptible. An infusion of 1 g vancomycin was administered, and the T1 decreased immediately after the start of the infusion to less than 10% of the preinduction level; T4 was totally absent. The infusion lasted 35 minutes. A blood sample was drawn 25 minutes after stopping the infusion to determine the vancomycin concentration; it was 70 mg/L. Within 3 minutes after stopping the vancomycin infusion, the electromyogram (EMG) began to recover. Twenty minutes later, the operation was completed, and the vecuronium was reversed with atropine and edrophonium. Initially, the EMG response demonstrated the recovery of the neuromuscular function to near-preinduction levels, but the responses decreased approx 5 minutes later to the same level they were before the edrophonium was given. The patient was awake and breathing spontaneously but was unable to sustain a headlift. Twenty minutes after the injection of edrophonium, the patient's muscle tone was judged to be adequate by both clinical assessment and EMG.

The exact mechanism of this pharmacodynamic interaction is unclear. The patient was administered a rather large dose of vancomycin for her body size, and the infusion was infused over 35 minutes rather than the usual recommended infusion time of 60 minutes. Both of these factors resulted in the high postinfusion peak serum concentration. The neuromuscular depression seen in this patient may have been because of the high serum concentration of vancomycin, but this level can occur during treatment of patients with vancomycin.

Vancomycin should be administered cautiously to patients undergoing surgery with neuromuscular blocking agents and patients in the intensive care unit receiving chemical paralysis. The doses should be adjusted for body weight and infused over recommended times.

## Heparin

Barg and colleagues described the inactivation of vancomycin by heparin when the substances were infused simultaneously through the same intravenous line, resulting in a reduction in vancomycin activity (38). Mixtures of heparin and vancomycin in various concentrations were made and tested against a clinical isolate of methicillin-resistant *Staphylococcus aureus*. A precipitate formed at the concentrations achieved in the intravenous line, and when the vancomycin concentrations were measured by bioassay, a 50–60% reduction in vancomycin activity was noted. When these two solutions were prepared and mixed at microgram concentrations, concentrations typically seen in patients, a precipitate was no longer observed, and vancomycin activity was not reduced. Heparin appeared to inactivate vancomycin at the concentrations typically achieved when these two agents are administered simultaneously though the same intravenous catheter. The authors concluded that infusions of the two drugs through the same intravenous line could be done serially, with a 0.9% sodium chloride solution flushing the line between the two drugs to prevent mixing at high concentrations.

The interaction between vancomycin and aminoglycosides is discussed in the section Aminoglycosides. Angaran and colleagues determined that vancomycin had no effect on the PT response to warfarin in patients undergoing prosthetic value surgery (39).

## SULFONAMIDES

### Warfarin

Several reports have described an enhanced hypoprothrombinemic response to warfarin when sulfamethoxazole (SMX), usually in combination with trimethoprim (TMP), was added to a patient's therapy *(40–43)*. Two pharmacokinetic studies in healthy adults confirmed that SMX enhances the hypoprothrombinemic response to warfarin in most people *(43,44)*. Although the SMX seems more likely to have been responsible than the TMP, a TMP effect cannot be ruled out.

O'Reilly conducted two studies evaluating the stereoselective interaction between TMP-SMX and warfarin. In one study, patients received 1.5 mg/kg of racemic warfarin with and without 320 mg TMP-1600 mg SMX beginning 7 days before warfarin and continuing daily throughout the period of hypoprothrombinemia *(44)*. There was a significant increase in the areas of the one-stage PT, from 53 to 83 units, during the administration of TMP-SMX. In a follow-up study, O'Reilly studied the effects of TMP-SMX on each of the warfarin enantiomers *(45)*. Subjects received each enantiomer alone and in combination with 80 mg TMP-400 mg SMX. TMP-SMX had no effect on the *R*-isomer. The areas of the one-stage PT increased by approx 70%, from 40 to 67 units, when the *S*-isomer and TMP-SMX were given together. Additional case reports described the prolongation in PT following the addition of TMP-SMX to medication regimens containing warfarin *(40–43)*.

Some sulfonamides appear to impair the hepatic metabolism of oral anticoagulants. Competition for plasma protein-binding sites may play an additional role. Although sulfonamides reportedly decrease vitamin K production by the gastrointestinal bacteria, evidence for such an effect is lacking.

Patients should be monitored closely for an increase in PT/INR when SMX-containing products are coadministered with warfarin. Patients should be monitored clinically for signs of bleeding with initiating and decreased effects on discontinuing TMP-SMX. Other antibiotics may be prescribed to avoid this interaction, or other forms of anticoagulation such as unfractionated or low molecular weight heparin may be used as alternatives to warfarin.

## TETRACYCLINES

Tetracyclines have been documented to interact with a number of medications. The most common interaction is with heavy metals, which chelate tetracyclines and impair their absorption from the gastrointestinal tract. More important interactions may occur with oral contraceptives, for which tetracycline may reduce effectiveness and increase the risk of pregnancy.

### Heavy Metals

Numerous studies have documented the ability of heavy metals to chelate tetracycline products and impair their absorption *(46–48)*. These products contain divalent and trivalent cations such as aluminum, magnesium, and calcium. Antacids also may impair the dissolution of tetracyclines. Bismuth subsalicylate, a common ingredient in antidiarrheal medications, also has been shown to impair the absorption of tetracyclines through a similar chelation mechanism *(49,50)*.

This is a pharmacokinetic interaction because it impairs absorption and reduces oral bioavailability. The clinical consequences of this interaction could be potential therapeutic failure because of inadequate tetracycline serum and tissue concentrations.

Oral tetracycline products should be taken 2 hours before or 6 hours after antacids. This may not completely avoid the interaction but should minimize it. Because this interaction is not based on an alteration in pH, $H_2$-receptor antagonists and proton pump inhibitors may be alternative medications. In addition, other antibiotics may be prescribed to avoid the interaction.

Bismuth can reduce the bioavailability of tetracycline, similar to heavy metals. Ericsson and colleagues evaluated the influence of a 60-mL dose of bismuth subsalicylate on the absorption of doxycycline (49). Doxycycline bioavailability was reduced by 37 and 51% when given simultaneously and as a multiple-dose regimen, respectively, before doxycycline. Peak serum concentrations of doxycycline were significantly decreased when bismuth subsalicylate was given 2 hours before doxycycline but not when given 2 hours after doxycycline. Albert and coworkers documented a 34% reduction in doxycycline bioavailability when the two products were administered simultaneously (50). A further discussion on the effect of various foods containing divalent cations is given in Chapter 12.

## Colestipol

Colestipol reduces the bioavailability of tetracycline by impairing its absorption in the gastrointestinal tract. Friedman et al. showed that when colestipol and tetracycline were given together, there was a 50% reduction in tetracycline bioavailability (51). In a single dose, three-way crossover study, subjects ingested 500 mg tetracycline with 180 mL water, 180 mL water and 30 g colestipol, and 180 mL orange juice and 30 g colestipol. There were significant differences in the 48-hour urinary excretion of tetracycline. More than 50% of the dose was recovered in the urine when the tetracycline was administered with water. Only 23–24% was recovered in the urine when it was administered with colestipol. There was no significant difference among the three groups in the mean value excretion half-life.

This is a pharmacokinetic interaction because it impairs absorption and reduces oral bioavailability as a result of tetracycline adsorbing onto colestipol-binding sites. The clinical consequences of this interaction could be potential therapeutic failure because of inadequate tetracycline serum and tissue concentrations.

Oral tetracycline should be taken 2 hours before or at least 3 hours after a dose of colestipol. In addition, other antibiotics may be prescribed to avoid the interaction.

## Digoxin

Tetracycline can reduce the gastrointestinal bacterial flora responsible for metabolizing digoxin in the gastrointestinal tract and increase digoxin absorption and bioavailability in some patients. Lindenbaum and colleagues administered digoxin to healthy volunteers for 22–29 days. After 10 days, 500 mg tetracycline every 6 hours for 5 days was started (52). During the period of antibiotic administration, digoxin reduction products fell, urine digoxin output rose, and digoxin steady-state serum concentrations increased by as much as twofold in some subjects. Preantibiotic serum digoxin serum concentrations ranged between 0.37 and 0.76 µg/L and increased to 0.8–1.33 µg/L following antibiotic therapy. It also was noted that these effects persisted for several months after the antibiotics were stopped. There were no reports of digoxin toxicity in the patients who experienced an increase in their digoxin concentrations.

The mechanism of this pharmacokinetic interaction appears to be the inhibition of digoxin metabolism by suppression of gut bacteria. The clinical implications of this interaction are the possibility that therapy with antibiotics in subjects producing large amounts of digoxin reduction products may precipitate toxicity. Unrecognized changes in gut flora might result in variability in digoxin response in the direction of either drug toxicity or therapeutic failure.

### Anticonvulsants

Phenobarbital and phenytoin have been shown to reduce the serum concentrations of doxycycline *(53–55)*. Penttilla and colleagues conducted three trials to evaluate the effect of anticonvulsants on doxycycline metabolism *(53)*. In one study, they compared the half-life of doxycycline in patients taking long-term phenytoin or carbamazepine therapy to a control group of patients not receiving anticonvulsants. The doxycycline half-life in the patients receiving chronic anticonvulsants ranged between 7 and 7.5 hours compared to 15 hours in the control subjects. In a second crossover trial, they determined the half-life of doxycycline in five patients after 10 days of phenobarbital therapy and in another five patients taking phenobarbital chronically *(54)*. The half-life of doxycycline was 15 hours in the control patients before phenobarbital therapy began. After 10 days of therapy, the half-life was reduced to 11 hours. The doxycycline half-life was 7 hours in the patients taking phenobarbital chronically. In a third trial, they evaluated the effect of chronic anticonvulsant therapy on a variety of tetracycline products and compared this to results in control patients *(55)*. The doxycycline half-life averaged 7 hours, and the peak concentrations were lower in the patients on chronic anticonvulsant therapy compared to the control group. There was no difference in the half-lives of oxytetracycline, methacycline, chlortetracycline, and demethylchlortetracycline between the patients on anticonvulsants and control patients.

The enhanced hepatic metabolism of doxycycline is the mechanism of this pharmacokinetic interaction. The clinical consequences of this interaction could be a reduction in serum doxycycline concentrations and the potential for therapeutic failure. An alternative class of antibiotics should be selected for these patients because they may be receiving anticonvulsants for the control of a seizure disorder, and it would not be wise to switch anticonvulsants to avoid this interaction.

### Warfarin

Tetracyclines may be associated with an increased hypoprothrombinemic response in patients taking oral anticoagulants. Several case reports described patients stabilized on chronic warfarin therapy who experienced increases in PT after the addition of doxycycline to their medication regimens *(56,57)*. Westfall and coworkers described a patient maintained on warfarin therapy with stable PT values approximately two times the control value *(56)*. After the initiation of 100 mg doxycycline twice a day, the patient's PT increased to 51 s and was associated with unusually heavy menstrual flow. On medical evaluation, her hemoglobin and hematocrit had dropped to 5.7 g/dL and 18.9%, respectively.

Caraco and Rubinow described two patients taking chronic oral anticoagulation who presented with severe hemorrhage and disturbed anticoagulation tests after the addition of doxycycline to their medication regimens *(57)*. In the first patient, the PT ratio increased from 1.49 to 3.82 following the addition of 100 mg doxycycline daily. In the second patient, the PT ratio increased from between 1.5 and 2.5–4.09 following the addition of 100 mg doxycycline twice daily.

The mechanism of this pharmacodynamic interaction is unclear but may involve a reduction in the plasma prothrombin activity by impairing prothrombin utilization or decreasing vitamin K production by the gastrointestinal tract.

The clinical significance of this interaction is the increased anticoagulant effect, which may result in an increased risk of bleeding. Patients should be closely monitored for clinical signs of bleeding, such as nosebleeds or bleeding from the gums, and the PT monitored and warfarin dose adjusted to maintain the PT/INR in the therapeutic range. Other antibiotics may be prescribed to avoid this interaction, or other forms of anticoagulation such as unfractionated or low molecular weight heparin may be used as alternatives to warfarin.

### Lithium

One case report described the increase in lithium concentrations following a course of tetracycline *(58)*. However, a prospective trial documented small decreases in the serum lithium concentration when both agents were administered concurrently *(59)*.

McGennis reported a patient taking lithium chronically for a history of manic depression *(58)*. Two days after starting tetracycline, it was noted that her serum lithium level increased from 0.81 to 1.7 mmol/L. The patient exhibited slight drowsiness, slurred speech, and a fine tremor of both hands consistent with lithium toxicity. At the time lithium and tetracycline were stopped, the serum lithium concentration was 2.74 mmol/L. The concentration declined to within the therapeutic range 5 days after stopping both agents.

Fankhauser and coworkers evaluated the effect of tetracycline on steady-state serum lithium concentrations in healthy volunteers and compared the frequency and severity of adverse effects in the lithium and lithium-tetracycline treatment phases *(59)*. There was a significant decrease in the serum lithium concentration between the control and treatment phases (0.51 vs 0.47 mEq/L, $p = 0.01$). It is unclear whether this is a clinically significant decrease in the serum lithium concentration. There was no difference in adverse effects between the control and treatment phases of the trial.

The mechanism of this interaction is not known. One possibility may be that tetracycline-induced renal failure may reduce urinary lithium excretion. Although it is unlikely that a significant interaction exists, patients should be monitored for signs of lithium toxicity when this combination is prescribed. Renal function should also be monitored to prevent increases in the serum lithium concentrations secondary to reductions in renal function. Another class of antibiotics should be prescribed to avoid this interaction.

### Psychotropic Agents

Steele and Couturier reported the possible interaction between tetracycline and respiradone and/or sertraline in a 15-year-old male with Asperger's disorder, Tourette's disorder, and obsessive-compulsive disorder *(60)*. Tetracycline was added to a respiradone-sertraline treatment regimen, resulting in an acute exacerbation of motor and vocal tics. The authors postulated that the increase in tics may have resulted from a tetracycline-respiradone interaction leading to a reduction in respiradone levels, a tetracycline-sertraline interaction leading to increased levels of sertraline, or the natural course of Tourette's disorder. The sertraline dose was increased with no concomitant increase in tics, and subsequent discontinuation of tetracycline resulted in an improvement in tics, which suggests the possibility of an interaction between tetracycline and respiradone. The mechanism of this potential interaction is unknown, but the authors recommended that the addition of antibiotics to psychotropic medications requires close monitoring because of the potential for the interaction.

### Theophylline

Several case reports described increases in theophylline serum concentrations during a course of tetracycline administration *(61,62)*. However, prospective trials have failed to document a consistent effect *(63–66)*.

Four prospective studies have evaluated the interaction between theophylline and tetracycline. Pfeifer et al. gave nine patients tetracycline for 48 hours and did not observe a statistically significant interaction *(63)*. However, six subjects had a decrease in theophylline clearance during the combined tetracycline-theophylline period, and in four of the subjects, the decrease was greater than 15%. Mathis and colleagues studied eight healthy volunteers by giving them a single intravenous injection of aminophylline before and after 7 days of tetracycline *(64)*. Theophylline clearance decreased by an average of 9%, but four patients had greater than 15% decrease in clearance; one patient had a 32% decrease in clearance. Gotz and Ryerson evaluated the interaction between tetracycline and theophylline in five patients with chronic obstructive airways disease *(65)*. Theophylline clearance decreased by an average of 11% following the 5-day course of tetracycline. Jonkman et al. evaluated the effects of doxycycline on theophylline pharmacokinetic parameters in healthy volunteers during a 9-day course of theophylline alone and with the coadministration of doxycycline *(66)*. There was no influence of doxycycline on absorption, elimination, and volume of distribution of theophylline. Mean steady-state plasma concentrations were not significantly different between the two treatment periods.

The mechanism for the interaction is unknown but appears to be a reduction in the hepatic metabolism of theophylline. The reduction in metabolism appears to be quite variable. It may take several days for the interaction to occur, so increases in serum theophylline may not be clinically significant after short courses of tetracycline. Patients taking longer courses of tetracycline may be at risk for developing theophylline toxicity.

Patients should be closely monitored when tetracycline is added to a medication regimen containing theophylline. Although short courses may not result in clinically significant increases in the serum theophylline concentration, patients maintained in the upper end of the therapeutic range may be at risk of developing theophylline toxicity even with modest increases in the serum theophylline concentration. Also, the reduction in clearance appears to be quite variable, so it may be difficult to predict how much the theophylline will increase following the addition of tetracycline to the medication regimen. All patients should be monitored clinically for signs and symptoms of theophylline toxicity. Serum theophylline concentration should be monitored every 2–3 days in patients at high risk for developing theophylline toxicity.

### Oral Contraceptives

Several case reports suggest that tetracycline can reduce the effectiveness of oral contraceptives *(67,68)*. One retrospective study showed that the oral contraceptive failure rate was within the expected range associated with the typical pattern of use *(69)*. However, prospective trials have failed to document a consistent effect *(70,71)*. These case reports of unintended pregnancies have occurred following the concurrent administration of tetracycline and other antibiotics with oral contraceptives. Two small controlled studies evaluated the effect of tetracycline on the serum levels of ingredients contained in commonly prescribed oral contraceptives. Neely et al. compared the serum concentrations of ethinyl estradiol, norethindrone, and endogenous progesterone during a control period and after a 7-day course of doxycycline starting on day 14 of their cycle *(70)*. There were no statistically significant differences in serum concentrations of ethinyl estradiol, norethindrone, and endogenous progesterone between the control and treatment phases. Murphy et al. studied the effect of tetracycline on ethinyl estradiol and norethindrone after 24 hours and 5–10 days of therapy with tetracycline *(71)*. There was no significant decrease in ethinyl estradiol or norethindrone concentrations after 24 hours or after 5–10 days of therapy.

The mechanism for the interaction is unknown but may be because of interference with the enterohepatic circulation of estrogens in the intestines, making this a pharmacokinetic interaction. Other antibiotics have also been reported to reduce the effectiveness of oral contraceptives when administered concurrently. It is not known if noncompliance played a role in some of these unplanned pregnancies.

Although the evidence of the interaction between tetracycline and oral contraceptives is limited to case reports, women should be counseled to use other methods of birth control during tetracycline therapy.

### Methotrexate

Tortajada-Ituren and colleagues reported an interaction between doxycycline and high-dose methotrexate *(72)*. A 17-year-old female was receiving high-dose methotrexate as part of a chemotherapy regimen. The patient had undergone 10 cycles of the regimen without complications. Her mean methotrexate pharmacokinetic parameters following the 10 cycles were a methotrexate clearance of 2.95 L/hour; 2.96-hours half-life; 4.27-hour mean residence time; and 12.53-L volume of distribution. On admission to the hospital for the 11th cycle of chemotherapy, the patient was noted to have a palprebal abscess in her left eye, which was treated with 100 mg doxycycline twice daily. The high-dose (18 g) methotrexate was administered according to her usual protocol. During the first 24 hours after the methotrexate infusion, the patient developed facial erythema, malaise, and vomiting, which had not occurred during the first 10 cycles. The doxycycline was stopped 48 hours after chemotherapy. The pharmacokinetic monitoring was prolonged for 168 hours, revealing a significant decrease in methotrexate clearance (1.29 L/hour) and significant increase in half-life (6.26 hours) and mean residence time (9.03 hours) compared to the values obtained during the first 10 cycles. Her hospital stay was prolonged to 11 days compared to an average of 7.7 days during the first 10 cycles.

Although the mechanism of the interaction is unknown, one proposed theory suggests that tetracyclines may displace methotrexate from plasma protein-binding sites *(73)*. In an attempt to validate this mechanism in their patient, the authors determined the degree of methotrexate plasma protein binding in two plasma samples with similar methotrexate concentrations from the 7th and 11th cycles. The unbound methotrexate concentrations were determined with an ultrafiltration process. The unbound methotrexate fractions during the 7th and 11th cycles were 53 and 41%, respectively.

Although case reports of a tetracycline–methotrexate interaction are limited, tetracyclines should be avoided in patients receiving high-dose methotrexate therapy. If therapy with a tetracycline is required, pharmacokinetic monitoring should be continued until the methotrexate concentrations are below the desired range, and the leucovorin rescue should be continued, if necessary, until all signs and symptoms of methotrexate toxicity disappear.

### Rifampin

Colmenero and colleagues studied the possible interaction between rifampin and doxycycline in 20 patients with brucellosis *(74)*. Patients were treated with either doxycyline and streptomycin or doxycyline and rifampin. The doxycycline levels in the patients treated with rifampin were significantly lower than in those patients treated with doxycycline and streptomycin. The doxycycline clearance in patients treated with rifampin was significantly higher than in the patients treated with doxycycline and streptomycin, 3.59 and 1.55 L/hours, respectively. The elimination half-life (4.32 vs 10.59 hours) and AUC were significantly lower in patients in the rifampin-treated patients (30.4 vs 72.6 mg*hours/mL). In addition, there were lower doxycycline levels in the rifampin treatment group, which had rapid acetylaters. There were no treatment failures in the patients receiving doxycyline and streptomycin; there were two treatment failures in the doxycyline-rifampin group.

Rifampin is a potent inducer of hepatic microsomal enzymes. Although doxycyline is only partially metabolized, the effect of rifampin may be significant enough to lower doxycyline concentrations to subtherapeutic levels. Caution should be used when treating patients with combined rifampin and doxycycline therapy. If possible, an alternative antibiotic should be prescribed to avoid potential treatment failures.

## AMINOGLYCOSIDES

Aminoglycoside antibiotics are involved in a number of drug interactions, many of which result in an increased risk of nephrotoxicity.

### Amphotericin B

The concurrent use of aminoglycoside antibiotics Amphotericin B may lead to an increased risk of developing nephrotoxicity. Churchill and Seely reported four patients who developed nephrotoxicity when both agents were administered together *(75)*. All of the patients received amphotericin B at an approximate dose of 0.5 mg/kg/day. Two of the four patients had documented gentamicin trough concentrations of 5 mg/L. All patients developed progressive renal failure during the first several days of combined therapy. In the patients who survived, renal function returned to baseline values after both agents were discontinued.

The mechanism of this is the potential of additive nephrotoxicity from both agents. Amphotericin B is associated with a predictable rise in creatinine within the first several days of therapy. Aminoglycoside antibiotics are associated with acute tubular necrosis, especially in the setting of elevated serum concentrations. In the case report, three patients had documented gentamicin concentrations significantly higher than the desired 2 mg/L. This mostly likely contributed to the development of nephrotoxicity in these patients.

Patients receiving aminoglycoside antibiotics and amphotericin B should be closely monitored for the development of renal failure. The aminoglycoside serum concentrations should be monitored every 2–3 days and the dosage regimen adjusted to maintain peak and trough concentrations within the desired therapeutic range. Every attempt should be made to avoid other conditions (i.e., hypotension) that might increase the risk of developing renal failure and to avoid administering other medications (i.e., intravenous contrast media, loop diuretics) that might increase the risk of developing renal failure.

### Neuromuscular Blocking Agents

Aminoglycoside agents are known to potentiate paralysis from neuromuscular blocking agents *(76–79)*. Often, this has occurred in the setting of the instillation of aminoglycoside-containing irrigation solutions into the intra-abdominal cavity during surgery. Dupuis et al. evaluated prospectively the interaction between aminoglycosides and atracurium and vecuronium in 44 patients *(80)*. Twenty-two patients had therapeutic concentrations of gentamicin or tobramycin, and 22 patients served as controls. Onset time, clinical duration, and time to spontaneous recovery $T_1/T_4$ ratio of 0.7 after atracurium or vecuronium injection were measured. Although no statistically significant differences were found in onset time, clinical duration was longer in patients receiving tobramycin or gentamicin and paralyzed with vecuronium than in controls. The neuromuscular blockade produced by atracurium was not significantly influenced by the presence of therapeutic serum concentrations of tobramycin or gentamicin. The clinical duration of patients receiving atracurium alone or in the presence of an aminoglycoside was approx 40 minutes in each group, and the time to recovery of a $T_1/T_4$ ratio >0.7 approx 60–70 minutes. The clinical duration was significantly longer in the vecuronium patients receiving aminoglycosides than in the vecuronium control patients, 30 vs 55 minutes, respectively. The time to recovery of a $T_1/T_4$ ratio >0.7 in the patients receiving vecuronium with aminoglycosides also was longer in the patients receiving an aminoglycoside, 55 vs 105 minutes, respectively.

Aminoglycosides have been shown to interfere with acetylcholine release and exert a postsynaptic curare-like action *(81)*. These agents have membrane-stabilizing properties and exert their effect on acetylcholine release by interfering with calcium ion fluxes at the nerve terminal, an action similar to magnesium ions. Aminoglycosides also possess a smaller but significant decrease in postjunctional receptor sensitivity and spontaneous release.

These drugs may cause postoperative respiratory depression when administered before or during operations and may also cause a transient deterioration in patients with myasthenia gravis. Patients should be monitored for prolonged postoperative paralysis if they received neuromuscular blocking agents and aminoglycoside antibiotics during the perioperative or immediate postoperative period.

### Indomethacin

Zarfin et al. evaluated the effect of indomethacin on gentamicin and amikacin serum concentration in 22 neonates with patent ductus arteriosus treated with indomethacin and aminoglycosides *(82)*. The aminoglycoside doses were held stable before the initiation of indomethacin therapy. After the addition of indomethacin, there was a significant rise in aminoglycoside trough and peak concentrations, a reduction in urine output, and a significant rise in serum creatinine. This may have been because of the ability of nonsteroidal anti-inflammatory agents to cause reversible renal failure. In this setting, the elimination of all renally eliminated medications would be expected to be reduced with elevation in serum concentrations.

Renal function should be closely monitored in patients receiving nonsteroidal anti-inflammatory agents. If renal failure develops, the doses of all renally eliminated medications should be adjusted to the level of remaining renal function. Serum concentrations of medications should be monitored when possible and dosage regimens adjusted to maintain serum concentrations within the accepted therapeutic ranges.

### Cyclosporine

Cyclosporine and aminoglycosides are both nephrotoxic and produce additive renal damage when administered together. Termeer et al. reported that the combined use of gentamicin and cyclosporine in renal transplant patients increased the incidence of acute tubular necrosis to 67%, compared with 5–10% when gentamicin was used alone or when cyclosporine was used with other, nonnephrotoxic antibiotics *(83)*. Animal studies have also documented the additive nephrotoxicity of aminoglycosides when administered with cyclosporine.

The mechanism appears to be additive injury to the renal tubule. Aminoglycosides induce renal failure by inhibiting the intracellular phospholipases in lysosomes of tubular cells in the proximal tubule. Cyclosporine-induced acute renal failure is related primarily to its effects on the renal blood vessels. Cyclosporine acutely reduces renal blood flow, with a corresponding increase in renal vascular resistance and a reduction in glomerular filtration rate.

Patients receiving aminoglycoside antibiotics and cyclosporine should be closely monitored for the development of renal failure. The aminoglycoside and cyclosporine serum concentrations should be monitored every 2–3 days and the dosage regimen adjusted to maintain peak and trough concentrations within the desired therapeutic range. Every attempt should be made to avoid other conditions (i.e., hypotension) that might increase the risk of developing renal failure and to avoid administering other medications (i.e., intravenous contrast media, loop diuretics) that might increase the risk of developing renal failure.

### Chemotherapeutic Agents

Numerous reports have documented the additive nephrotoxicity when aminoglycosides are administered to patients receiving cisplatin-type chemotherapeutic agents *(84–90)*. Cisplatin-type chemotherapeutic agents have been associated with a reduction in renal function. Patients who received aminoglycoside antibiotics during or after a course of cisplatin-based chemotherapy regimens have demonstrated additional reductions in renal function.

The mechanism appears to be direct injury to the renal tubule. Aminoglycosides induce renal failure by inhibiting the intracellular phospholipases in lysosomes of tubular cells in the proximal tubule. Cisplatin-induced renal failure is mediated by a toxic effect on the renal tubular cells, resulting in acute tubular necrosis.

Prior administration of cisplatin is not an absolute contraindication to the use of aminoglycoside antibiotics. When clinically indicated, patients who have previously received cisplatin and have apparently normal renal function should be treated cautiously with standard doses of aminoglycoside antibiotics, and pharmacokinetic monitoring should be performed routinely, with the dosage regimens adjusted to maintain serum concentrations within the normal therapeutic range.

### Loop Diuretics

Several reports described the increased risk of nephro- and ototoxicity when aminoglycosides and loop diuretics are administered together *(91,92)*. Some case reports suggested there is increased ototoxicity when ethacrynic acid is given in combination with aminoglycosides *(92)*. The data supporting the association between furosemide and aminoglycosides are controversial *(93)*.

### Ethacrynic Acid

High doses of ethacrynic given alone have been shown to produce hearing loss in patients with renal failure *(94,95)*. Hearing loss can range between partial and full deafness and is usually irreversible. When patients receiving ethacrynic acid have been given an aminoglycoside such as kanamycin or streptomycin, hearing loss has been reported to occur within 15 minutes after an injection of the diuretic and to last for several hours. Some patients had reduced hearing loss; others remained deaf *(94)*.

The mechanism of this pharmacodynamic interaction is not known. Ethacrynic is thought to produce hearing loss by an alteration in the formation of perilymph in the cochlea. This may be disputed because not all patients experience vertigo or nausea. Other possible causes of deafness may be the cysteine adduct of ethacrynic acid, a substance known to be ototoxic, or a direct toxicity to the auditory nerves by ethacrynic acid. Aminoglycosides produce ototoxicity by destroying the sensory hair cells in the cochlea and vestibular labyrinth.

Ethacrynic acid and the older-generation aminoglycosides are rarely used in clinical practice. However, some patients may be unable to take loop diuretics such as furosemide or bumetanide, so ethacrynic acid may be their only available option. When ethacrynic acid is used alone or in combination with aminoglycosides, it should be used in the lowest dose that maintains adequate urine output or fluid balance. Aminoglycoside concentrations should be monitored and the dosage regimens adjusted to maintain concentrations within the therapeutic range. Patients should be monitored with audiograms if therapy is to be continued for an extended duration, and audiograms should be performed in patients who complain of hearing loss.

## Furosemide

Kaka et al. reported a suspected case of furosemide increasing the peak and trough concentrations of tobramycin in a 72-year-old woman *(91)*. The patient received intermittent doses of furosemide for the management of congestive heart failure. The patient developed a Gram-negative aspiration pneumonia. Tobramycin was started, with serum concentrations drawn after the loading dose followed by a maintenance dose of 180 mg iv every 8 hours. Twelve hours after an intravenous dose of 120 mg furosemide, the tobramycin trough and peak concentrations around the fourth dose were 5.3 and 16.2 mg/L, respectively. The authors concluded that moderate doses of furosemide can increase tobramycin concentrations, thus increasing the risk of ototoxicity and nephrotoxicity in some patients.

It is unclear whether furosemide was the cause of the increased tobramycin concentrations in this patient. Although furosemide has been reported to both increase and decrease the clearance of gentamicin, there are other possible explanations for the elevated tobramycin concentrations in this patients. The authors determined the patient's tobramycin pharmacokinetic parameters after the initial dose and used these parameters to determine the patient's maintenance dosage regimen. The maintenance regimen may have been overly aggressive for the patient's age, weight, and underlying renal function. There was extreme variability in the tobramycin pharmacokinetic parameters between the first and fourth doses, suggesting errors in drug administration or sampling technique rather than changes in the patient's clinical status or the administration of furosemide.

Smith and Lietman analyzed the data from three prospective, controlled, randomized, double-blind clinical trials to determine whether furosemide increased the nephrotoxicity and ototoxicity of aminoglycosides. There was no difference in the incidence of nephrotoxicity or ototoxicity between the groups receiving aminoglycosides alone and the group receiving aminoglycosides and furosemide *(93)*.

It is unclear whether furosemide directly increases the nephrotoxicity and ototoxicity of aminoglycosides. Furosemide may increase the risk of developing nephrotoxicity by causing excessive diuresis, hypovolemia, and a reduction in renal blood flow. Furosemide should be used with caution in patients receiving aminoglycoside antibiotics. Careful attention should be paid to the patient's weight, urine output, fluid balance, and indices of renal function. Aminoglycoside concentrations should be monitored and the dosage regimen adjusted to maintain concentrations within the therapeutic range.

## Vancomycin

Several reports have been published evaluating the potential of vancomycin to increase the nephrotoxicity of aminoglycoside antibiotics. Two studies were retrospective reviews and two studies were prospective evaluations. Cimino et al. retrospectively evaluated 229 courses of therapy in 229 oncology patients *(96)*. Forty patients received vancomycin alone, 148 patients received aminoglycosides alone, and 40 patients received vancomycin and an aminoglycoside antibiotic. The incidence of nephrotoxicity in patients administered an aminoglycoside was 18%; for vancomycin, it was 15%, and for an aminoglycoside and vancomycin, 15%. They could not show that the concurrent administration of vancomycin had an additive effect on the incidence of nephrotoxicity.

Pauly et al. retrospectively evaluated the incidence of nephrotoxicity in 105 patients who received at least 5 days of combined therapy *(97)*. Twenty-eight (27%) patients developed nephrotoxicity during combined vancomycin-aminoglycoside therapy. However, 22 patients had other insults, such as amphotericin B, sepsis, or liver disease that could account for the increase in nephrotoxicity. There were no control groups of patients receiving vancomycin or aminoglycosides alone to provide a comparative incidence of nephrotoxicity between these groups. The results of these two studies are limited by their retrospective design, the small number of patients who received vanco-mycin and an aminoglycoside, and the patients who had other potential causes for developing nephrotoxicity.

Mellor et al. prospectively evaluated 39 courses of vancomycin therapy in 34 patients *(98)*. Twenty-seven courses were associated with aminoglycoside administration either concurrently or within 2 weeks of the first dose of vancomycin. A reduction in renal function was seen during (7%) and after (9%) vancomycin therapy. There was no evidence of synergistic toxicity between vancomycin and aminoglycosides. One feature of the patients with renal dysfunction was the severity of their underlying disease. Each case of nephrotoxicity occurred in association with either sepsis or gastrointestinal hemorrhage.

Ryback and colleagues prospectively evaluated the incidence of nephrotoxicity in patients receiving vancomycin alone or in combination with an aminoglycoside, following 224 patients receiving 231 courses of therapy *(99)*. One hundred and sixty-eight patients received vancomycin alone, 63 patients received vancomycin with an aminoglycoside, and 103 patients received an aminoglycoside alone. Eight patients (5%) receiving vancomycin alone, 14 patients (22%) receiving vancomycin with an aminoglycoside, and 11 patients (11%) receiving an aminoglycoside alone were found to have nephrotoxicity. Factors thought to be associated with an increased risk of neph-rotoxicity in patients receiving vancomycin were concurrent therapy with an aminogly-coside, length of treatment with vancomycin (>21 days), and vancomycin trough concentrations (>10 mg/L).

Both of these studies were small prospective studies. Although they had control groups, it is unclear how well matched the control groups were to the group of patients receiving vancomycin and an aminoglycoside for underlying disease states and renal function. The increased risk of nephrotoxicity when vancomycin is administered with an aminoglycoside antibiotic is controversial. The clinical studies published to date did not show a clear association between the combination use of these agents and an increased risk of nephrotoxicity. Patients receiving vancomycin and aminoglycoside antibiotics should be closely monitored for the development of renal failure. The aminogly-coside and vancomycin serum concentrations should be monitored and the dosage regi-men adjusted to maintain peak and trough concentrations within the desired therapeutic range. Every attempt should be made to avoid other conditions (i.e., hypotension) that might increase the risk of developing renal failure and to avoid administering other medications (i.e., intravenous contrast media, loop diuretics) that might increase the risk of developing renal failure.

## LINEZOLID

Linezolid is a synthetic oxazolidinone antibiotic that selectively inhibits bacterial protein synthesis. As a class, oxazolidinones are known to inhibit monoamine oxidase (MAO). Two forms of MAO exit in humans: Type A and Type B. MAO-A preferentially deaminates noradrenaline, adrenaline, and seratonin, and Type B deaminates dopamine. Linezolid has been shown to be a weak, competitive inhibitor of MAO-A.

### Selective Serotonin Reuptake Inhibitors

Several reports have been published describing the development of the serotonin syndrome in patients who were prescribed linezolid while they were taking selective serotonin reuptake inhibitors (SSRIs). Wigen and Goetz described the serotonin syndrome developing in a patient who was prescribed linezolid shortly after discontinuing therapy with paroxetine *(100)*. The patient developed delirium, hypertension, hostility, anger, and tremors 24 hours after starting on linezolid. The patient returned to her baseline mental status within 48 hours after stopping linezolid. Hachem et al. described two patients taking SSRIs who developed the seratonin syndrome following the initiation of linezolid therapy *(101)*. Both patients developed hypertension requiring medical therapy and an altered mental status manifested by confusion, delirium, tremors, and fatigue. One patient developed cardiac palpitations. One patient's symptoms abated within 1 day after stopping linezolid and sertraline; the second patient required 9 days for the normalization of blood pressure after discontinuing linezolid and citalopram. Lavery described the development of the seratonin syndrome after linezolid was prescribed in a patient taking sertraline, bupropion, and trazodone *(102)*. The patient's symptoms began to improve within an hour after starting cyproheptadine, a seratonin antagonist, and normalized completely after 48 hours of cyproheptadine therapy. Two reports suggested that mirtazapine *(103)* and venlafaxine *(104)* may be safe to administer in patients receiving linezolid.

Serotonin is removed from the nerve synapse by reuptake into the nerve terminal or degradation by MAO. Linezolid's ability to inhibit MAO degradation of serotonin results in increased serotonin levels and the development of the serotonin syndrome. Patient medication profiles should be reviewed for medications that are metabolized by MAO before linezolid is prescribed. When possible, alternative antibiotics should be prescribed to avoid the risk of the development of the serotonin syndrome in susceptible individuals. Because of the long half-lives of some of the SSRIs, the serotonin syndrome may develop in patients whose SSRI was discontinued several days before initiating linezolid therapy. Management of the serotonin syndrome is primarily supportive, with removal of the offending agent, with symptoms resolving within 24–36 hours. If necessary, cyproheptadine appears to be an effective antiserotonin agent. It usually relieves symptoms after the first dose but may be administered every 1–4 hours until a therapeutic response is obtained.

### Cough and Cold Preparations

Many over-the-counter cough and cold preparations contain ingredients that are metabolized by MAO or are SSRIs. Decongestants such as pseudoephedrine and phenylpropanolamine are metabolized by MAO. The cough suppressant dextromethorphan has been shown to block serotonin reuptake and has been implicated in precipitating the serotonin syndrome when coingested with MAO inhibitors.

Hendershot and colleagues reviewed the data from three linezolid clinical trials to evaluate the pharmacokinetic and pharmacodynamic responses to the coadministration of linezolid with pseudoephedrine, phenylpropanolamine, and dextromethorphan *(105)*. Significant increases in systolic blood pressure (SBP) were observed following the coadministration of linezolid with either pseudoephedrine or phenylpropanolamine. The mean maximum increase from baseline in SBP was 32 and 38 mmHg with the coadministration with pseudoephedrine and phenylpropanolamine, respectively. Treatment emergent SBP greater than 160 mmHg was observed following the coadministration of linezolid with pseudoephedrine in five subjects and in two patients in the linezolid-phenylpropanolamine-treated group. Dizziness was the most frequent adverse event when linezolid and pseudoephedrine were given concomitantly, and headache was the most frequent adverse event when linezolid and phenylpropanolamine were given together. There were no statistically or clinically significant effects on heart rate in either treatment group. There were no statistically or clinically significant changes in blood pressure, heart rate, or temperature and no abnormal neurological examination results in the dextromethorphan-linezolid treatment group.

Linezolid's ability to inhibit the MAO degradation of pseudoephedrine and phenylpropanolamine resulted in the significant increases in blood pressure that was seen when linezolid was coadministered with the decongestants. Patients should be counseled to consult with their pharmacist or physician before taking systemic decongestants while taking linezolid. Topical nasal decongestants such as sodium chloride or oxymetazoline may be alternative agents for patients requiring decongestants while receiving linezolid.

## DAPTOMYCIN

### Aminoglycosides

Daptomycin is a recently approved lipopeptide with activity limited to Gram-positive bacteria. Daptomycin is renally excreted, with approx 50–60% of a dose appearing in the urine of healthy volunteers. Woodworth and colleagues evaluated the disposition of daptomycin and tobramycin on each other because both drugs have the potential to induce nephrotoxicity *(106)* Neither drug affected the disposition of the other agent. There were no changes in the pharmacokinetic parameters when daptomycin and tobramycin were given alone or when they were given in combination. The mean baseline renal tubular enzyme excretion values were 12.2 U/day for alanine aminopeptidase and 2.6 U/day for $N$-acetyl-$\beta$-glucosaminidase. Excretion of alanine aminopeptidase increased to 16.9, 18.8, and 17.8 U/day after daptomycin, tobramycin, and the combination, respectively. $N$-Acetyl-$\beta$-glucosaminidase excretion increased to 4.4, 4.2, and 3.9 U/day after the same respective treatments. The results suggest that there is no need to alter either aminoglycoside or daptomycin dosages if the agents are coadministered, and the two drugs can be administered together without additional precautions. Although minor renal damage may occur following the coadministration of the antibiotics, the nephrotoxicity sustained should be no more than from the aminoglycoside itself.

## QUINUPRISTIN-DALFOPRISTIN

### *Cytochrome P450 3A4-Metabolized Drugs*

In vitro drug interaction studies have demonstrated that quinupristin-dalfopristin significantly inhibits cyctochrome P450 3A4 metabolism. There are no published drug interaction studies in normal volunteers and only limited reports of interactions in patients receiving quinupristin-dalfopristin for therapeutic indications. The manufacturer's package insert indicates that it is reasonable to expect that the concomitant administration of quinupristin-dalfopristin and other drugs primarily metabolized by the cytochrome P450 3A4 enzyme system may likely result in increased plasma concentrations of these drugs, which could increase or prolong their therapeutic effect or increase adverse reactions *(107)*.

In healthy volunteers, the coadministration of quinupristin-dalfopristin with midazolam increased midazolam $C_{max}$ and AUC by 14 and 33%, respectively. Also, in healthy volunteers the $C_{max}$ and AUC of nifedipine were increased by 18 and 44%, respectively, when the two agents were coadministered. Additional studies in transplant patients indicated that quinupristin-dalfopristin can inhibit the metabolism of cyclosporine and tacrolimus. Stamatakis and Richards reported an interaction between cyclosporine and quinupristin-dalfopristin in a renal transplant patient *(108)*. The patient's baseline cyclosporine levels ranged from 80 to 105 ng/mL. At 2 and 3 days after the initiation of quinupristin-dalfopristin therapy, trough cyclosporine concentrations increased to 261 and 291 ng/mL, respectively. Following the discontinuation of quinupristin-dalfopristin, the cyclosporine blood concentrations decreased, and the dosage was increased to the previous regimen.

Medications known to be metabolized through the cytochrome P450 3A4 pathway, especially those with a narrow therapeutic index, should be administered with caution and closely monitored for adverse effects.

## ANTI-PSEUDOMONAS PENICILLINS

Aminoglycosides and penicillins are often administered in combination for their additive or synergistic effects in the treatment of serious Gram-negative infections. Numerous reports have been published documenting the ability of commonly used antipseudomonal penicillins to inactivate aminoglycoside antibiotics in vivo *(109–116)* and in vitro *(117–123)*. These have usually documented unusually low aminoglycoside concentrations in patients receiving this combination, despite high doses of aminoglycosides. Carbenicillin inactivates all aminoglycosides at faster rates and to a greater extent than ticarcillin, mezlocillin, and piperacillin. Tobramycin is the least stable, and amikacin is the most stable aminoglycoside. Gentamicin has intermediate stability.

Pickering and Gearhart evaluated the effect of time on the in vitro interaction between mixtures of four aminoglycosides at two concentrations with carbenicillin, piperacillin, mezlocillin, azlocillin, and mecillinam at three concentrations *(119)*. The inactivation of the aminoglycoside was shown to be directly proportional to the concentration of the penicillin. Aminoglycoside inactivation was greater at 72 hours of incubation with the penicillins than after 24 hours of incubation. Inactivation by each penicillin was greater for tobramycin and gentamicin than for netilmicin and amikacin, especially at higher penicillin concentrations. At concentrations of 500 µg/mL, significantly less inactivation of amikacin occurred compared to netilmicin. No significant change in aminoglycoside activity occurred when the aminoglycosides were stored with the penicillins at –70°C for 30 days.

There are several reports of in vivo inactivation of aminoglycosides by ticarcillin and carbenicillin. These have occurred in patients with renal failure, for whom the penicillin concentrations would be expected to be high. Thompson and colleagues studied the inactivation of gentamicin by piperacillin and carbenicillin in patients with end-stage renal disease *(115)*. Patients received a single dose of gentamicin, 4 g piperacillin every 12 hours for four doses, or 2 g carbenicillin every 8 hours for six doses and gentamicin plus piperacillin or carbenicillin. Subjects were studied on off-dialysis days. Gentamicin was inactivated to a greater extent by carbenicillin than by piperacillin. In the subjects in the carbenicillin group, the terminal elimination half-life of gentamicin was 61.6 hours when gentamicin was administered alone and 19.4 hours when gentamicin was administered with carbenicillin. In the subjects in the piperacillin group, the mean gentamicin half-life when gentamicin was given alone was 53.9 hours, and it was 37.7 hours when it was administered with piperacillin. Control samples verified that no in vitro inactivation occurred.

Penicillins combine with aminoglycoside antibiotics in equal molar concentrations at a rate dependent on the concentration, temperature, and medium composition. The greater the concentration of the penicillin, the greater is the inactivation of the aminoglycoside. The inactivation is thought to occur by way of a nucleophilic opening of the β-lactam ring, which then combines with an amino group of the aminoglycoside, leading to the formation of a microbiologically inactive amide. The inactivation occurs less in pooled human sera than in other media, including whole blood. Spinning down whole blood can help slow the inactivation. Significant serum inactivation occurs at room temperature and under refrigeration. Only when the blood sample is centrifuged and frozen is the inactivation arrested.

Rich reviewed the procedure for handling aminoglycoside concentrations in patients receiving this combination of antibiotics *(124)*. Blood samples for aminoglycoside concentrations drawn from patients receiving the combination should be sent on ice to the laboratory within 1–2 hours so that the sample can be spun down and frozen to arrest any inactivation. Samples left exposed at room temperature will decay 10% in 1 hour. The two antibiotics should not be given at the same time. The administration times should be scheduled so that the administration of the aminoglycoside occurs at the end of the penicillin dosing interval, when its concentrations are the lowest. If a patient is receiving this antibiotic combination and unusually low aminoglycoside concentrations occur, the above factors should be checked. Inactivation with β-lactam antibiotics is further described in Chapter 9.

## TELITHROMYCIN

Telithromycin is a semisynthetic antibacterial in the ketolide class of antibiotics that selectively inhibits bacterial protein synthesis. Telithromycin is known to inhibit medications metabolized Cytochrome (CYP) P450 isoenzymes 3A4 and 2D6, as well as other concomitantly prescribed medications. The information on telithromycin drug interactions is limited to information published in the manufacturer's package insert *(125)*.

## CYP 3A4 Inhibitors

Azole antifungal agents inhibit the metabolism of telithromycin. Itraconazole increased the $C_{max}$ and AUC of telithromycin by 22 and 54%, respectively, while ketoconazole increased these parameters by 51 and 95%, respectively. Other classes of antibiotics should be considered in patients these agents.

Grapefruit juice had no affect on the pharmacokinetic parameters of telithromycin in healthy subjects.

## CYP 3A4 Substrates

Telithromycin is a potent inhibitor of the CYP P450 3A4 system. Co-administration of telithromycin with drugs metabolized by the CYP 3A4 system may result in increased concentrations of the substrate drug resulting in increased or prolonged therapeutic or adverse effects.

### Cisapride

Telithromycin increased the steady-state peak plasma concentrations of cisapride by 95% resulting in significant prolongation of the QTc interval. Cisapride is a restricted drug with limited clinical use. Other classes of antibiotics should be considered to avoid this potentially fatal interaction.

### Statins

There appears to be a time dependent effect on the magnitude of the interaction between telithromycin and simvastatin. There were a 5.3- and 8.9-fold increase in the simvastatin $C_{max}$ and AUC, respectively, accompanied by a 15- and 12-fold increase in the $C_{max}$ and AUC of the simvastatin metabolite when the two agents were co-administered. However, there only was a 3.4- and 4.0-fold increase in the simvastatin $C_{max}$ and AUC and a 3.2- and 4.3-fold increase in the $C_{max}$ and AUC of the simvastatin metabolite when the two agents are administered 12 hours apart. A similar interaction is possible with atorvastatin and lovastatin. Increased statin concentrations resulting from this interaction may increase the risk of myopathy. Patients being treated chronically with these statins and requiring antibiotic therapy should be treated with antibiotics shown not to interact with these statins.

### Midazolam

Coadministering telithromycin with intravenous or oral midazolam resulted in two- and sixfold increases, respectively, in the midazolam AUC. A reduction in midazolam dose should be considered in patients taking telithromycin and requiring midazolam (i.e., peri-procedure). The patient's level of consciousness and airway status should be aggressively monitored while the patient is under the influence of midazolam.

### Warfarin

Telithromycin has been shown to elevate the International Normalized Ratio (INR) several days after starting therapy in a patient on chronic warfarin therapy. The INR increased form 3.1 before telithromycin was started to 11 after 5 days of telithromycin therapy. The INR returned to the therapeutic range 4 days after telithromycin was discontinued. Although the mechanism of the interaction is unknown, it is suspected that it is a result of the inhibition of the metabolism of the R-isomer, which is metabolized predominantly by CYP 1A2 and to a lesser extent CYP 3A4. The INR level should be measured in patients on warfarin who receive telithromycin in an effort to prevent bleeding complications *(126)*.

### Verapamil

A women receiving taking verapamil 180 mg daily for the treatment of hypertension experienced a sudden onset of shortness of breath, weakness, hypotension and brady-cardia after taking telithromycin for 2 days *(127)*. The patient required treatment with crystalloids, vasopressors, and transvenous pacing. Approximately 72 hours after dis-continuing telithromycin therapy that patient's heart rate and blood pressure returned to normal. It was suspected that the acute cardiac decompensation resulted from elevated verapamil secondary to the inhibition of its metabolism through the CYP 3A4 pathway by telethromycin. The cardiac status of susceptible patients should be monitored when telithromycin is added to a medication regimen containing verapamil.

### CYP3A4 Inducers

### Rifampin

Rifampin has been shown to reduce the $C_{max}$ and AUC of telithromycin by 79 and 86%, respectively when both agents were co-administered in repeated doses.

Co-administration with other 3A4 inducers phenytoin, carbamazepine, or phenobar-bital may result in subtherapeutic levels of telithromycin and therapeutic failure. Other classes of antibiotics should be considered in patients these agents.

### CYP 2D6 Substrates

### Metoprolol

There was a 38% increase in metoprolol $C_{max}$ and AUC when both agents were co-administered without any effect on metoprolol half-life. The increased metoprolol ex-posure in heart failure may have the potential to worsen heart failure. Other classes of antibiotics should be considered in patients these agents to avoid precipitating an epi-sode of acute decompensated heart failure.

### Digoxin

The co-administration of telithromycin and digoxin in healthy volunteers resulted in an increase in the peak and trough concentrations by 73 and 21%, respectively. Trough plasma digoxin concentrations ranged between 0.74#-#2.17 ng/mL without significant changes in ECG parameters and no signs of digoxin toxicity. Monitoring for digoxin side effects or digoxin levels should be considered when both agents are co-adminis-tered in patients.

### Theophylline

When theophylline was administered with repeated doses of theophylline, there was a 16 and 17% increase in theophylline $C_{max}$ and AUC, respectively.

### Sotalol

Telithromycin has been shown to decrease the $C_{max}$ and AUC of sotalol by 34 and 20%, respectively by decreasing the absorption of sotalol from the gastrointestinal tract.

## Oral Contraceptives

When telithromycin was coadministered with oral contraceptives containing ethinyl estradiol and levonorgestrel there was a 50% increase in the levonorgestrel AUC with no effect on ethinyl estradiol. Telithromycin did not interfere with the antiovulatory effects of oral contraceptives containing ethinyl estradiol and levonorgestrel.

---

### CASE STUDY 1

C.S. is a 76-year-old white female admitted to the hospital for periods of disorientation, confusion, hallucinations, and the inability to care for herself. On hospital day 2, the patient became tachypneic and tachycardiac. Anticoagulation with heparin and warfarin was initiated following a lung scan consistent with pulmonary embolism. On hospital day 4, TMP-SMX was started following a urine culture that was positive for *Escherichia coli*. Warfarin's hypoprothrombinemic effect was minimal after two 15-mg doses, with the PT 1.6 times the control value on hospital day 4. After administration of two doses of TMP-SMX and 10 mg warfarin on hospital day 4, the patient's PT/control value increased to 5.5 at 8 am the following morning. The PT remained consistently elevated over the next 5 days despite the fact that no further warfarin was administered. The last dose of TMP-SMX was administered on hospital day 7. The PT drawn on hospital day 7 was 6.1 times control. Later that afternoon, 10 mg of phytonadione was administered, and the patient's PT/control fell rapidly. The patient received 10 mg warfarin on hospital days 8 and 9. The PT again rose sharply but not to the same extent or for the same duration as it had when TMP-SMX was given simultaneously. The patient's condition eventually stabilized, and a maintenance dose of 2.5 mg every other day resulted in adequate anticoagulation. This case describes the rapid effect standard doses of TMP-SMX can have on warfarin metabolism.

---

### CASE STUDY 2

A 45-year-old male with a long history of probable schizoaffective disorder was admitted to the hospital after a suicide attempt. The most recent suicide attempt involved jumping out of a window, resulting in a T-6 spinal cord injury and paraplegia. While in the hospital, therapy was started with sertraline and risperidone and titrated to 200 mg daily and 1 mg twice daily, respectively. The patient's refractory depression necessitated the addition of 75 mg bupropion twice daily, 50 mg trazodone at bedtime, and 300 mg lithium carbonate twice daily. The patient developed a deep sacral decubitus ulcer requiring closure with a sacral flap and bilateral gluteal myocutaneous flaps. Postoperatively, the patient developed a fever and elevated white count. Serosanguinous drainage from his myocutaneous flap grew vancomycin-resistant *Enterococcus fecalis*. Linezolid 600 mg iv every 12 hours and 500 mg oral metronidazole every 6 hours were started. Lithium carbonate was stopped secondary to suspected toxicity. One week after stopping lithium and 10 days after starting linezolid, the patient complained of increasing tremor, nausea, and vomiting. At that time, the seratraline, bupropion, and trazodone were stopped. Twenty-four hours later, the patient became delirious, marked by acute confusion, visual hallucinations, and delusions. Temperature increased to 100.1°F, pulse was 101 beats/minute, respirations were 20/minute, and blood pressure was 100/71 mmHg. He exhibited coarse tremor and myoclonus. His pupils were dilated to 6 mm and minimally reactive. The patient was started on 8 mg cyproheptadine every 8 hours for 72 hours. Within 60 minutes of the first dose, the pupil size decreased to 4 mm. After 48 hours of treatment with cyproheptadine, the patient's altered mental status, tremor, gastrointestinal symptoms, myoclonus, pupil dilation, and fever resolved *(102)*. This case points out the rapid development of the serotonin syndrome when linezolid is added to a medication regimen taking a selective serotonin reuptake inhibitor.

## REFERENCES

1. Spika JS, Davis DJ, Martin SR, et al. Interaction between chloramphenicol and acetaminophen. Arch Dis Child 1986;61:1211–1124.
2. Kearns GL, Bocchini JA, Brown RD, et al. Absence of a pharmacokinetic interaction between chloramphenicol and acetaminophen in children. J Pediatr 1985;107:134–139.
3. Stein CM, Thornhill DP, Neill P, et al. Lack of effect of paracetamol on the pharmacokinetics of chloramphenicol. Br J Clin Pharmacol 1989;27:262–264.
4. Bloxham RA, Durbin GM, Johnson T, et al. Chloramphenicol and phenobarbitone Na drug interaction. Arch Dis Child 1979;54:76–77.
5. Powell DA, Nahata MC, Durrell DC, et al. Interactions among chloramphenicol, phenytoin, and phenobarbital in a pediatric patient. J Pediatr 1981;98:1001–1003.
6. Koup JR, Gibaldi M, McNamara P, et al. Interaction of chloramphenicol with phenytoin and phenobarbital. Clin Pharmacol Ther 1987;24:571–575.
7. Ballek RE, Reidenberg MM, Orr L. Inhibition of diphenylhydantoin metabolism by chloramphenicol. Lancet 1973;1:150.
8. Greenlaw CW. Chloramphenicol–phenytoin interaction. Drug Intell Clin Pharm 1979;13: 609–610.
9. Saltiel M, Stephens NM. Phenytoin–chloramphenicol interaction. Drug Intell Clin Pharm 1980;14:221.
10. Christensen LK, Skovsted L. Inhibition of metabolism by chloramphenicol. Lancet 1969; 2:1397–1399.
11. Brunova E, Slabochova Z, Platilova H, et al. Interaction of tolbutamide and chloramphenicol in diabetic patients. Int J Clin Pharmacol 1977;15:7–12.
12. Petitpierre B, Fabre J. Chlorpropamide and chloramphenicol. Lancet 1970;1:789.
13. Wallace JF, Smith RH, Garcia M, et al. Studies on the pathogenesis of meningitis. VI. Antagonism between penicillin and chloramphenicol in experimental pneumococcal meningitis. J Lab Clin Med 1967;70:408–418.
14. Jawetz E. The use of combinations of antimicrobial drugs. Annu Rev Pharmacol 1968;8: 151–170.
15. Deritis F, Giammanco G, Manzillo G. Chloramphenicol combined with ampicillin in treatment of typhoid. Br Med J 1972;4:17–18.
16. French GL, Ling TKW, Davies DP, et al. Antagonism of ceftazidime by chloramphenicol in vitro and in vivo during treatment of Gram negative meningitis. Br Med J 1985;291: 636–637.
17. Prober C. G. Effect of rifampin on chloramphenicol levels. N Engl J Med 1985;312:788–789.
18. Kelly HW, Couch RC, Davis RL, et al. Interaction of chloramphenicol and rifampin. J Pediatr 1988;112:817–820.
19. Koch-Weser J, Sellars EM. Drug interactions with coumarin anticoagulants (first of two parts). N Engl J Med 1971;285:487–498.

20. Koch-Weser J, Sellars EM. Drug interactions with coumarin anticoagulants (second of two parts). N Engl J Med 1971;285:547–558.

21. Finegold SM. Interaction of antimicrobial therapy and intestinal flora. Am J Clin Nutr 1970;23:1466–1471.

22. Klippel AP, Pitsinger B. Hypoprothrombinemia secondary to antibiotic therapy and manifested by massive gastrointestinal hemorrhage. Arch Surg 1968;96:266–268.

23. Bui LL, Huang DD. Possible interaction between cyclosporine and chloramphenicol. Ann Pharmacother 1999;33:252–253

24. Steinfort CL, McConachy KA. Cyclosporin–chloramphenicol drug interaction in a heart-lung transplant patient. Med J Aust 1994;161:455.

25. Schulman SL, Shaw LM, Jabs K, et al. Interaction between tacrolimus and chloramphenicol in a renal transplant recipient. Transplantation 1998;65:1397–1398.

26. Taber DJ, Dupuis RE, Hollar KD, et al. Drug–drug interaction between chloramphenicol and tacrolimus in a liver transplant recipient. Transplant Proc 2000;32:660–662.

27. Becker LD, Miller RD. Clindamycin enhances a nondepolarizing neuromuscular blockade. Anesthesiology 1976;45:84–87.

28. Best JA, Marashi AH, Pollan LD. Neuromuscular blockade after clindamycin administration: a case report. J Oral Maxillofac Surg 1999;57:600–603

29. al Ahdal O, Bevan DR. Clindamycin-induced neuromuscular blockade. Can J Anaesth 1995;42:614–617.

30. Sloan PA, Rasul M. Prolongation of rapacuronium neuromuscular blockade by clindamycin and magnesium. Anesth Analg 2002;94:123–124.

31. Rubbo JT, Sokoll MD, Gergis SD. Comparative neuromuscular effects of lincomycin and clindamycin. Anesth Analg 1977;56:329–332.

32. Wright JM, Collier B. Characterization of the neuromuscular block produced by clindamycin and lincomycin. Can J Physiol Pharmacol 1976;54:937–944.

33. Fiekers J, Henderson F, Marshall I, et al. Comparative effects of clindamycin and lincomycin on end-plate currents and quantal content at the neuromuscular junction. J Pharmacol Exp Ther 1983;227:308–315.

34. Atchinson W, Adgate L, Beaman C. Effects of antibiotics on the uptake of calcium into isolated nerve terminals. J Pharmacol Exp Ther 1988;245:394–401.

35. Butkus DE, de Torrente A, Terman DS. Renal failure following gentamicin in combination with clindamycin. Nephron 1976;17:307–313.

36. Spivey JM, Gal P. Vancomycin pharmacokinetic in neonates. Am J Dis Child 1986;140:859.

37. Huang KC, Heise A, Shrader AK, et al. Vancomycin enhances the neuromuscular blockade of vecuronium. Anesth Analg 1990;71:194–196.

38. Barg NL, Supena RB, Fekety R. Persistent staphylococcal bacteremia in an intravenous drug abuser. Antimicrob Agents Chemother 1986;29:209–211.

39. Angaran DM, Dias VC, Arom KV, et al. The comparative influence of prophylactic antibiotics on the prothrombin response to warfarin in the postoperative prosthetic cardiac valve patient. Ann Surg 1987;206:155–161.

40. Tilstone WJ, Gray JM, Nimmo-Smith RH, et al. Interaction between warfarin and sulphamethoxazole. Postgrad Med J 1977;53:388–390.

41. Kaufman JM, Fauver HE. Potentiation of warfarin by trimethoprim-sulfamethoxazole. Urology 1980;16:601–603.

42. Greenlaw CW. Drug interaction between co-trimoxazole and warfarin. Am J Hosp Pharm 1979;36:1155.

43. Errick JK, Keys PW. Co-trimoxazole and warfarin: case report of an interaction. Am J Hosp Pharm 1978;35:1399–1401.

44. O'Reilly RA, Motley CH. Racemic warfarin and trimethoprim-sulfamethoxazole interaction in humans. Ann Intern Med 1979;91:34–36.

45. O'Reilly RA. Stereoselective interaction of trimethoprim-sulfamethoxazole with the separated enantiomorphism of racemic warfarin in man. N Engl J Med 1980;302:33–35.

46. Jaffe JM, Colonize JL, Pouts RI, et al. Effect of altered urinary pH on tetracycline and doxycycline excretion in humans. J Pharmacokinet Bipolar 1973;1:267–282.

47. Jaffe JM, Pouts RL, Fled SL, et al. Influence of repetitive dosing and altered pH on doxycycline excretion in humans. J Pharm Sci 1974;63:1256–1260.

48. Chin TF, Latch JL. Drug diffusion and bioavailability: tetracycline metallic chelation. Am J Hosp Pharm 1975;32:625–529.

49. Ericsson CD, Feldman S, Pickering LK, et al. Influence of subsalicylate bismuth on absorption of doxycycline. JAMA 1982;247:2266–2267.

50. Albert KS, Welch RD, Descanted KA, et al. Decreased tetracycline bioavailability caused by a bismuth subsalicylate antidiarrheal mixture. J Pharm Sci 1979;68:586–588.

51. Friedman H, Greenbelt DJ, Leduc BW. Impaired absorption of tetracycline by colestipol is not reversed by orange juice. J Clin Pharmacol 1989;29:748–751.

52. Lindenbaum J, Round DG, Butler VP, et al. Inactivation of digoxin by the gut flora: reversal by antibiotic therapy. N Engl J Med 1981;305:789–794.

53. Penttilla O, Neuvonen PJ, Ahoy K, et al. Interaction between doxycycline and some ant epileptic drugs. Br Med J 1974;2:470–472.

54. Neuvonen PJ, Penttilla O, Lehtovaara R, et al. Effect of antiepileptic drugs on the elimination of various tetracycline derivatives. Eur J Clin Pharmacol 1975;9:147–154.

55. Neuvonen PJ, Penttila O. Interaction between doxycyline and barbiturates. Br Med J 1974;1:535–536.

56. Westfall LK, Mintzer DL, Wiser TH. Potentiation of warfarin by tetracycline. Am J Hosp Pharm 1980;37:1620–1625.

57. Caraco Y, Rubinow A. Enhanced anticoagulant effect of coumarin derivatives induced by doxycycline coadministration. Ann Pharmacother 1992;26:1084–1086.

58. McGennis AJ. Lithium carbonate and tetracycline interaction. Br Med J 1978;1:1183.

59. Fankhauser MP, Lindon JL, Connolly B, et al. Evaluation of lithium–tetracycline interaction. Clin Pharm 1988;7:314–317.

60. Steele M, Couturier J. A possible tetracycline–respiradone–sertraline interaction in an adolescent. Can J Clin Pharmacol 1999;6:15–17.

61. McCormack JP, Reid SE, Lawson LM. Theophylline toxicity induced by tetracycline. Clin Pharm 1990;9:546–549.

62. Kawai M, Honda A, Yoshida H, et al. Possible theophylline–minocycline interaction. Ann Pharmacother 1992;26:1300–1301.

63. Pfeifer HJ, Greenblatt DJ, Friedman P. Effects of three antibiotics on theophylline kinetics. Clin Pharmacol Ther 1979;26:36–40.

64. Mathis JW, Prince RA, Weinberger MM, et al. Effect of tetracycline hydrochloride on theophylline kinetics. Clin Pharm 1982;1:446–448.

65. Gotz VP, Ryerson GG. Evaluation of tetracycline on theophylline disposition in patients with chronic obstructive airways disease. Drug Intell Clin Pharm 1986;20:694–697.

66. Jonkman JHG, van der Boon WJV, Schoenmaker R, et al. No influence of doxycycline on theophylline pharmacokinetics. Ther Drug Monit 1985;7:92–94.

67. Bacon JF, Shenfield GM. Pregnancy attributable to interaction between tetracycline and oral contraceptives. Br Med J 1980;280:293.

68. DeSano EA, Hurley SC. Possible interactions of antihistamines and antibiotics with oral contraceptive effectiveness. Fertil Steril 1982;37:853–854.

69. Helms SE, Bredle DL, Zajic J, et al. Oral contraceptive failure rates and oral antibiotics. J Am Acad Dermatol 1997;36:705–710.

70. Neely JL, Abate M, Swinkler M, et al. The effect of doxycycline on serum levels of ethinyl estradiol, norethindrone, and endogenous progesterone. Obstet Gynecol 1991;77:416–420.

71. Murphy AA, Zacur HA, Charache P, et al. The effect of tetracycline on levels of oral contraceptives. Am J Obstet Gynecol 1991;164:28–33.
72. Tortajada-Ituren JJ, Ordovas-Baines JP, Llopis-Salvia P, et al. High-dose methotrexate–doxyxcycline interaction. Ann Pharmacother 1999;33:804–808.
73. Turck M. Successful psoriasis treatment then sudden "cytotoxicity." Hosp Pract 1984;19: 175–176.
74. Colmenero JD, Fernandez-Gallardo LC, Agundez JAG, et al. Possible implications of doxycycline–rifampin interaction for treatment of brucellosis. Antimicrob Agents Chemother 1994;38:2798–2802.
75. Churchill DN, Seely J. Nephrotoxicity associated with combined gentamicin-amphotericin B therapy. Nephron 1977;19:176–181.
76. Kroenfeld MA, Thomas SJ, Turndorf H. Recurrence of neuromuscular blockade after reversal of vecuronium in a patient receiving polymyxin/amikacin sternal irrigation. Anesthesiology 1986;65:93–94.
77. Warner WA, Sanders E. Neuromuscular blockade associated with gentamicin therapy. JAMA 1971;215:1153–1154.
78. Levanen J, Nordman R. Complete respiratory paralysis caused by a large dose of streptomycin and its treatment with calcium chloride. Ann Clin Res 1975;7:47–49.
79. Lippmann M, Yang E, Au E, et al. Neuromuscular blocking effects of tobramycin, gentamicin, and cefazolin. Anesth Analg 1982;61:767–770.
80. Dupuis JY, Martin R, Tetrault JP. Atracurium and vecuronium interaction with gentamicin and tobramycin. Can J Anaesth 1989;36:407–411.
81. Singh YN, Marshall IG, Harvey AL. Pre- and postjunctional blocking effects of aminoglycoside, polymyxin, tetracycline and lincosamide antibiotics. Br J Anaesth 1982;54:1295–1306.
82. Zarfarin Y, Koren G, Maresky D, et al. Possible indomethacin–aminoglycoside interaction in preterm infants. J Peds 1985;106:511–513.
83. Termeer A, Hoitsma AJ, Koene RAP. Severe nephrotoxicity caused by the combined use of gentamicin and cyclosporine in renal allograft recipients. Transplantation 1986;42: 220–221.
84. Christensen ML, Stewart CF, Crom WR. Evaluation of aminoglycoside disposition in patients previously treated with cisplatin. Ther Drug Monit 1989;11:631–636.
85. Gonzalez-Vitale JC, Hayes DM, Cvitkovic E, et al. Acute renal failure after *cis*-dichlorodiammineplatinum(II) and gentamicin-cephalothin therapies. Cancer Treat Rep 1978;62:693–698.
86. Salem PA, Jabboury KW, Khalil MF. Severe nephrotoxicity: a probable complication of *cis*-dichlorodiammineplatinum (II) and cephalothin-gentamicin therapy. Oncology 1982;39:31–32.
87. Kohn S, Fradis M, Podoshin L, et al. Ototoxicity resulting from combined administration of cisplatin and gentamicin. Laryngoscope 1997;107:407–408.
88. Dentino M, Luft F. C, Yum M. N, et al. Long-term effect of *cis*-diamminedichloride platinum (CDDP) on renal function and structure in man. Cancer 1978;41:1274–1281.
89. Lee EJ, Egorin MJ, Van Echo DA, et al. Phase I and pharmacokinetic trial of carboplatin in refractory adult leukemia. J Natl Cancer Inst 1988;80:131–135.
90. Bregman CL, Williams PD. Comparative nephrotoxicity of carboplatin and cisplatin in combination with tobramycin. Cancer Chemother Pharmacol 1986;18:117–123.
91. Kaka JS, Lyman C, Kilarski DJ. Tobramycin–furosemide interaction. Drug Intell Clin Pharm 1984;18:235–238.
92. Mathog RH, Klein WJ. Ototoxicity of ethacrynic acid and aminoglycoside antibiotics in uremia. N Engl J Med 1969;280:1223–1224.
93. Smith CR, Lietman PS. Effect of furosemide on aminoglycoside-induced nephrotoxicity and auditory toxicity in humans. Antimicrob Agents Chemother 1983;23:133–137.

94. Pillay VKG, Schwartz FD, Aimi K, et al. Transient and permanent deafness following treatment with ethacrynic acid in renal failure. Lancet 1969;1:77–79.

95. Meriweather WD, Mangi RJ, Serpick AA. Deafness following standard intravenous doses of ethacrynic acid. JAMA 1971;216:795–798.

96. Cimino MA, Rotstein C, Slaughter RL, et al. Relationship of serum antibiotic concentrations to nephrotoxicity in cancer patients receiving concurrent aminoglycoside and vancomycin therapy. Am J Med 1987;83:1091–1097.

97. Pauly DJ, Musa DM, Lestico MR, et al. Risk of nephrotoxicity with combination vancomycin-aminoglycoside antibiotic therapy. Pharmacotherapy 1990;10:378–382.

98. Mellor JA, Kingdom J, Cafferkey M, et al. Vancomycin toxicity: a prospective study. J Antimicrob Chemother 1985;15:773–780.

99. Ryback MJ, Albrecht LM, Boike SC, et al. Nephrotoxicity of vancomycin, alone and with an aminoglycoside. J Antimicrob Chemother 1990;25:679–687.

100. Wigen CL, Goetz MB. Serotonin syndrome and linezolid. Clin Infect Dis 2002;34: 1651–1652.

101. Hachem RY, Hicks K, Huen A, et al. Myelosuppression and serotonin syndrome associated with concurrent use of linezolid and selective serotonin reuptake inhibitors in bone marrow transplant recipients. Clin Infect Dis 2003;37:e8–e11.

102. Lavery S, Ravi H, McDaniel WW, et al. Linezolid and serotonin syndrome. Psychosomatics 2001;42:432–434.

103. Aga VM, Barklage NE, Jefferson JW. Linezolid, a monoamine oxidase inhibiting antibiotic, and antidepressants. J Clin Psychiatry 2003;64:609–611.

104. Hammerness P, Parada H, Abrams A. Linezolid:MAOI activity and potential drug interactions. Psychosomatics 2002;43:248–249

105. Hendershot PE, Antal EJ, Welshman IR. Linezolid: pharmacokinetic and pharmacodynamic evaluation of coadministration with pseudoephedrine HCl, phenylpropanolamine HCl, and dextromethorphan HBr. J Clin Pharmacol 2002;41:563–572.

106. Woodworth JR, Nyhart EH, Wolny JD, et al. Tobramycin and daptomycin disposition when co-administered to healthy volunteers. J Antimicrob Chemother 1994;33:655–659.

107. Synercid (quinupristin-dalfopristin) [package insert]. Bristol, TN: Monarch Pharmaceutical, 2003.

108. Stamatakis MK, Richards JG. Interaction between quinupristin/dalfopristin and cyclosporine. Ann Pharmacother 1997;31:576–578.

109. Lampasona V, Crass RE, Reines HD. Decreased serum tobramycin concentrations in patient with renal failure. Clin Pharm 1983;2:6–9.

110. Russo M. Penicillin-aminoglycoside inactivation: another possible mechanism of interaction. Am J Hosp Pharm 1980;37:702–704.

111. Chow MSS, Quintiliani R, Nightingale CH. In vivo inactivation of tobramycin by ticarcillin. JAMA 1982;247:658–659.

112. Kradjan WA, Burger R. In vivo inactivation of gentamicin by carbenicillin and ticarcillin. Arch Intern Med 1980;140:1668–1670.

113. Schentag JJ, Simons GW, Schultz RW, et al. Complexation vs hemodialysis to reduce elevated aminoglycoside serum concentrations. Pharmacotherapy 1984;4:374–380.

114. Uber WE, Brundage RR, White RL, et al. In vivo inactivation of tobramycin by piperacillin. Ann Pharmacother 1991;25:357–359.

115. Thompson MIB, Russo ME, Saxon BJ, et al. Gentamicin inactivation by piperacillin or carbenicillin in patients with end-stage renal disease. Antimicrob Agents Chemother 1982;21:268–273.

116. Ervin FR, Bullock WE, Nuttall CE. Inactivation of gentamicin by penicillins in patients with renal failure. Antimicrob Agents Chemother 1976;9:1004–1031.

117. Wallace SM, Chan LY. In vitro interaction of aminoglycosides with β-lactam penicillins. Antimicrob Agents Chemother 1985;28:274–281.

118. Henderson JL, Polk RE, Kline BJ. In vitro inactivation of gentamicin, tobramycin, and netilmicin by carbenicillin, azlocillin, or mezlocillin. Am J Hosp Pharm 1981;38: 1167–1170.

119. Pickering LK, Gearhart P. Effect of time and concentration upon interaction between gentamicin, tobramycin, netilmicin, or amikacin and carbenicillin or ticarcillin. Antimicrob Agents Chemother 1979;15:592–596.

120. Pickering LK, Rutherford I. Effect of concentration and time upon inactivation of tobramycin, gentamicin, netilmicin, and amikacin by azlocillin, carbenicillin, mecillinam, mezlocillin, and piperacillin. J Pharmacol Exp Ther 1981;217:345–349.

121. Hold HA, Broughall JM, McCarthy M, et al. Interactions between aminoglycoside antibiotics and carbenicillin or ticarcillin. Infection 1976;4:107–109.

122. Davies M, Morgan JR, Anand C. Interaction of carbenicillin and ticarcillin with gentamicin. Antimicrob Agents Chemother 1975;7:431–434.

123. Mclaughlin JE, Reeves DS. Clinical and laboratory evidence of inactivation of gentamicin by carbenicillin. Lancet 1971;1:261–264.

124. Rich DS. Recent information about inactivation of aminoglycosides by carbenicillin, and ticarcillin: clinical implications. Hosp Pharm 1983;18:41–43.

125. Prescribing Information. Kelek (telithromycin). Bridgewater, NJ: Aventis Pharmaceuticals, October 2004.

126. Kolilekas L, Anagnostopoulos GK, Lampaditis I, Eleftheriadis I. Potential interaction between telithromycin and warfarin. Ann Pharmacother 2004;38:1424–1427.

127. Reed M, Wall GC, Shah NP, Heun JM, Hicklin GA. Verapamil toxicity resulting from a probable interaction with telithromycin. Ann Pharmacother 2005;39:357–360.

# 12

# Drug–Food Interactions

**Kelly A. Harris, Kevin W. Garey, and Keith A. Rodvold**

## INTRODUCTION

Drug–food interactions can be a major source of patient inconvenience and nonadherence through disruptions in a patient's daily schedule. Unless advised to the contrary, patients often take drugs with meals as a suitable adherence reminder and to lessen gastrointestinal (GI) side effects. Lack of knowledge of potentially significant drug–food interactions can lead to poor clinical outcomes. This chapter describes mechanisms of drug–food interactions and US Food and Drug Administration (FDA) guidelines for drug–food interaction studies. Antimicrobial drug–food interactions based on drug classes and pharmacokinetics are described, as are the recommended dosing guidelines. In addition, anti-infectives and the disulfiramlike reaction and two case studies are included.

## MECHANISMS OF DRUG–FOOD INTERACTIONS

### Physiological Effects of Food

The majority of medications are absorbed in the small intestine, with very little absorption occurring directly from the stomach. However, changes in GI secretions and gastric pH can have an affect on subsequent absorption (1). GI secretions increase in response to food ingestion, which increases hydrochloric acid in the stomach, thus lowering stomach pH. This acidic environment will accelerate the dissolution and absorption of basic drugs but will cause increased degradation of acid-labile drugs (1).

The volume of a meal may also affect the subsequent absorption of the drug. Large fluid volumes tend to increase stomach-emptying rates, whereas large solid-food consumption tends to have the opposite effect (1). Delayed stomach emptying can increase the degradation of drugs that are unstable at low pH and increase absorption time. On the other hand, for drugs that take more time to dissolve, longer transit time may actually increase absorption by increasing the percentage of the drug in solution. Thus, the physiological effect of food may have variable affects on drug absorption, depending on the characteristics of each individual drug.

From: *Infectious Disease: Drug Interactions in Infectious Diseases, Second Edition*
Edited by: S. C. Piscitelli and K. A. Rodvold © Humana Press Inc., Totowa, NJ

*Food Composition*

The components of food may interact directly with medications in a number of ways. Examples include chelation of the drug by polyvalent metal ions or action as a mechanical barrier to inhibit the absorption of food across the mucosal surface of the intestines. The formulation of the drug will likely also affect the magnitude of drug–food interactions. Solutions and suspensions are generally less likely to be affected by foods because they pass rapidly through the stomach and become absorbed. Sustained-release formulations such as enteric-coated tablets are much more likely to be affected because the presence of food may delay absorption of the drug by several hours *(1)*.

*Effects of Food on Drug Absorption*

Drug–food interactions can be divided into three possible outcomes. Drug absorption may be increased, decreased, or not affected. Decreased absorption can be further subclassified into reduced vs delayed absorption. Reduced absorption is reflected by a decrease in the area under the concentration-time curve (AUC) of the drug. Delayed absorption is reflected by an increase in the time to reach maximum concentration $t_{max}$) of the drug. Alterations in the rate of drug absorption caused by the ingestion of food are generally not considered clinically significant as changes in the extent of drug absorption *(2)*.

*Effects of Food on Drug Metabolism*

A number of dietary factors are known to have potential for altering the metabolism of drugs *(3)*. Examples include dietary protein, cruciferous vegetables, and charcoal-broiled beef. In addition, malnutrition has been shown to alter the metabolism of certain drugs *(4)*. The effects of diet and nutrition have been described in a number of review articles *(3,4)*. Grapefruit juice has been demonstrated to increase the bioavailability of drugs known to be metabolized by cytochrome P450 (CYP) 3A4 enzymes *(5–7)*. It appears that grapefruit juice interactions are mediated by inhibition of gut wall metabolism, which results in reduced presystemic drug metabolism and therefore an increase in drug bioavailability, particularly for drugs with poor bioavailability. Although this field is still in its infancy, studies have shown an effect with grapefruit juice on protease inhibitors and macrolides, among others. The effect of grapefruit juice on P-glycoprotein-mediated drug transport is controversial *(8,9)*. A study reported that grapefruit juice, Seville orange juice, and apple juice were more potent inhibitors of the organic anion transporting polypeptides than of P-glycoprotein *(7)*. Although it appears that both drug-metabolizing enzymes and transporters determine drug disposition, further research in this field is necessary. A more complete review of transport proteins is provided in Chapter 3.

## DRUG–FOOD INTERACTION STUDIES

The Food-Effect Working Group of the Biopharmaceutics Coordinating Committee in the Center for Drug Evaluation and Research (CDER) at the FDA has published draft guidelines for food-effect bioavailability and bioequivalence studies for oral immediate-release or modified-release dosage forms. The guidance paper provides recommendations for study design, data analysis, and labeling, as well as specifying areas in which food-effect studies may not be important. These guidelines can be accessed at www.fda.gov. Using the FDA search engine on the Internet, limit the search to Center for Drug Evaluation and Research sites and type in "Food-effect working group" to access the document.

### Test Meal

The FDA guidance paper recommends that a food-effect study should be conducted under conditions expected to provide maximal effect with the presence of food in the GI tract. For this effect, they recommend a high-fat (50% of caloric value from the meal), high-calorie (approx 1000 cal) breakfast as the test meal. An example of such a meal would be two eggs fried in butter, two strips of bacon, two slices of toast with butter, 4 oz hash brown potatoes, with 8 oz whole milk. This would provide 150 protein calories, 250 carbohydrate calories, and 500–600 fat calories. Details of the meal should be provided in the protocol and final report.

### Study Design

A randomized, balanced, single-dose, two-treatment, two-period, two-sequence crossover study is recommended for food-effect studies. These studies are normally performed in healthy volunteers, with the formulation tested under fasted conditions in one treatment arm and immediately following the test meal in the other arm.

### Treatment Arms

Following an overnight fast of at least 10 hours, subjects should take the drug formulation with a full glass of water (180 mL or 6 fl oz). No food should be allowed for the following 4 hours, after which scheduled meals should be permitted. For fed subjects, following an overnight fast of at least 10 hours, subjects should be fed the test meal over not more than 30 minutes. The drug formulation should be given with a full glass of water no later than 5 minutes after finishing the test meal. As before, no other meals should be allowed for the following 4 hours, after which scheduled meals are permitted.

### Data and Statistical Analysis

A food effect will be concluded when the 90% confidence interval for the ratio of mean AUC or maximum concentration $C_{max}$ of fed vs fasted treatments falls outside 80 to 125% for AUC and 70 to 143% for $C_{max}$. Clinical relevance of the observed magnitude should be indicated by the sponsor of the study.

## ANTI-INFECTIVES AND DRUG–FOOD INTERACTION STUDIES

The following sections detail drug–food interaction studies of anti-infective agents by drug class. In the fluoroquinolones section, the effects of milk, yogurt, caffeine, and enteral feeds are also detailed. It is important to recognize that many of the earlier studies were completed prior to the FDA guidance paper. In addition, data have frequently been obtained in only one or two clinical studies, and observations made under these particular situations may not be relevant to the current clinical care of patients. However, more recently, well-controlled drug–food interaction studies have used the standardized test meals as recommended by the FDA.

A summary of selected studies reporting the effect of food on the $C_{max}$, $t_{max}$, and AUC of oral anti-infective agents is shown in Table 1 *(10–74)*.

## Table 1
## Effect of Food on the Pharmacokinetics of Oral Anti-Infectives

| | Ref. | Dosage form | Single or steady state | Status | n and gender | Oral dose (mg) | $C_{max}$ Fasting (µg/mL) | $C_{max}$ Fed (µg/mL) | AUC Fasting (µg·h/mL) | AUC Fed (µg·h/mL) | $t_{max}$ Fasting (h) | $t_{max}$ Fed (h) |
|---|---|---|---|---|---|---|---|---|---|---|---|---|
| *Penicillins* | | | | | | | | | | | | |
| Amoxicillin | 10 | Capsules | Single | Healthy | 16 M | 500 | 8.9 | 8.8 | 26.9/70 kg | 22.2/70 kg | 1.86 | 2.4 |
| Amoxicillin/clavulanate | 11 | Powder | Single | Healthy | 9 M, 9 F | 750 | 8.48 | 8.57 | 21.92 | 21.03 | NR | NR |
| Ampicillin | 10 | Capsules | Single | Healthy | 16 M | 500 | 5.4 | 4 | 17.4/70 kg | 12.0/70 kg | 1.49 | 2.48 |
| Bacampacillin | 12 | Tablets | Single | Healthy | 4 M, 2 F | 1600 | 12.188 | 6.138 | 29.912 | 22.043 | 0.923 | 1.667 |
| *Cephalosporins* | | | | | | | | | | | | |
| Cefadroxil | 13 | Capsules | Single | Healthy | 6 NR | 1000 | 32.1 | 32.7 | NR | NR | NR | NR |
| Cephalexin | 13 | Suspension | Single | Healthy | 6 NR | 1000 | 38.8 | 23.1 | 93 | 70 | 0.925 | 1.87 |
| Cefaclor | 14 | Tablets | Single | Healthy | 12 M | 250 | 8.7 | 4.3 | 8.6 | 7.6 | 0.6 | 1.3 |
| Cefprozil | 15 | Suspension | Single | Healthy | 12 M | 250 | 6.13 | 5.27 | 15 | 14.9 | 1.2 | 2 |
| Cefuroxime axetil | 16 | Suspension | Single | Healthy | 6 M, 6 F | 500 | 8 | 10.4 | 19 | 26.7 | 1.75 | 2 |
| Loracarbef | 17 | Capsules | Single | Healthy | 12 M | 400 | 19.21 | 13.64 | 33.04 | 35.38 | 1.125 | 2.35 |
| Cefixime | 18 | Tablets | Single | Healthy | 40 M | 100 | NR | NR | NR | NR | 2.6 | 3.2 |
| Cefditoren | 19 | Tablets | Single | Healthy | 8 M | 200 | 2.46 | 2.72 | 7.93 | 10.82 | 1.46 | 1.78 |
| Cefpodoxime | 20 | Suspension | Single | Healthy | 17 M | 200 | 2.62 | 3.02 | 13.5 | 16.3 | 2.75 | 3.22 |
| Ceftibuten | 21 | Capsules | Single | Healthy | 18 M | 200 | 9.85 | 6.6 | 42.07 | 33.7 | 1.6 | 3.8 |
| *Macrolides and combinations* | | | | | | | | | | | | |
| Erythromycin ethylsuccinate | 22 | Suspension | Single | Healthy | 12 M | 400 | 1.26 | 0.98 | 2.8441 | 2.3677 | 0.33 | 0.66 |
| Erythromycin stearate | 23 | Tablets | Single | Healthy | 4 M, 2 F | 500 | 3 | 1.4 | 13.2 | 5.2 | 2.7 | 2.3 |
| Erythromycin base | 24 | Tablets | Single | Healthy | 9 M, 6 F | 500 | 1.2 | 1 | 4.6 | 2.14 | 4 | 4.6 |
| Erythromycin estolate | 22 | Tablets | Single | Healthy | 25 M | 250 | 0.86 | 1.59 | 5.5706 | 8.8291 | 3 | 5 |
| Azithromycin | 25 | Suspension | Single | Healthy | 28 NR | 500 | 0.294 | 0.474 | 3.19 | 3.6 | NR | NR |
| Azithromycin | 25 | Tablets | Single | Healthy | 12 NR | 500 | 0.336 | 0.412 | 2.49 | 2.4 | NR | NR |

| | | | | | | | | | | | | |
|---|---|---|---|---|---|---|---|---|---|---|---|---|
| Azithromycin | 25 | Sachet | Single | Healthy | 12 NR | 1000 | 0.749 | 1.052 | 6.49 | 7.37 | NR | NR |
| Clarithromycin | 26 | Tablets | Single | Healthy | 26 M | 500 | 2.51 | 1.65 | 15.67 | 12.62 | 2 | 2.8 |
| Clarithromycin extended release | 27 | Tablets | SS | Healthy | 36 NR | 1000 | 2.33 | 3.91 | 35.9 | 49.2 | 5.5 | 5.6 |
| *Tetracyclines* | | | | | | | | | | | | |
| Tetracycline | 28 | Capsules | Single | Healthy | 4 M, 2 F | 500 | 4.5 | 2.7 | 55.7 | 31.7 | 3.8 | 4.7 |
| Doxycycline | 28 | Capsules | Single | Healthy | 4 M, 2 F | 200 | 5.1 | 4 | 85.3 | 78.6 | 3.2 | 5 |
| Minocycline | 29 | Capsules | Single | Healthy | 8 NR | 100 | 1.75 | 1.38 | 22.4 | 19.8 | 1.87 | 3.12 |
| *Quinolones* | | | | | | | | | | | | |
| Ciprofloxacin | 30 | Tablets | Single | Healthy | 12 M | 750 | 2.23 | 2.74 | 12.71 | 13.68 | 1.42 | 1.79 |
| Enoxacin | 31 | Tablets | Single | Healthy | 6 M, 2 F | 400 | 2.01 | 2.54 | 14.31 | 14.91 | 1 | 1 |
| Gatifloxacin | 32 | Tablets | Single | Healthy | 5 M, 7 F | 400 | 3.44 | 3.1 | 32.2 | 29.8 | 0.75 | 2 |
| Gatifloxacin | 33 | Tablets | Single | Healthy | 18 M | 400 | 3.5 | 3.2 | 32.8 | 30.5 | 2 | 2 |
| Gemifloxacin | 34 | Tablets | Single | Healthy | 13 M, 7 F | 320 | 1.21 | 1.07 | 7.57 | 7.38 | 1.5 | 2 |
| Levofloxacin | 35 | Tablets | Single | Healthy | 12 M, 12 F | 500 | 5.9 | 5.1 | 50.5 | 45.6 | 1 | 2 |
| Lomefloxacin | 36 | Tablets | Single | Healthy | 8 M, 4 F | 400 | 3.76 | 3.28 | 36.58 | 34.35 | 1.45 | 2.5 |
| Moxifloxacin | 37 | Tablets | Single | Healthy | 16 M | 400 | 2.8 | 2.5 | 38.5 | 37.7 | 1 | 2.5 |
| Ofloxacin | 38 | Tablets | Single | Healthy | 12 M | 200 | 2.24 | 1.56 | 13.18 | 11.26 | 0.83 | 1.85 |
| Sparfloxacin | 39 | Tablets | Single | Healthy | 10 M | 400 | 1.48 | 1.46 | 41.6 | 40.8 | 4.7 | 3.1 |
| *Miscellaneous anti-infective* | | | | | | | | | | | | |
| Trimethoprim | 40 | Suspension | Single | Healthy | 9 M, 3 F | 3 mg/kg | 2.35 | 1.84 | 37.1 | 28.9 | 2.68 | 2.76 |
| Albendazole | 41 | Capsules | Single | Healthy | 6 M | 10 mg/kg | 0.24 | 1.55 | 2.08 | 19.64 | 2.5 | 5.3 |
| Ivermectin | 42 | Tablets | Single | Healthy | 12 NR | 30 | 0.085 | 0.26 | 1.72 | 4.56 | 4.3 | 4.6 |
| Praziquantel | 43 | Tablets | Single | Healthy | 9 NR | 600 | 0.32 | 1.1 | 0.88 | 2.47 | 1.39 | 1.94 |
| Atovaquone | 44 | Suspension | SS | HIV positive | 21 M, 1 F | 750 | 12.4 | 15 | 238 | 301 | 6.5 | 8.9 |
| Linezolid | 45 | Tablets | Single | Healthy | 7 M, 5 F | 375 | 7.6 | 6.2 | 51.7 | 50 | 1.5 | 2.2 |
| Metronidazole | 46 | Capsules | Single | Healthy | 5 M, 5 F | 400 | 9.12 | 7.95 | 5587 | 5765 | 1.19 | 2.31 |
| *Antituberculosis agents* | | | | | | | | | | | | |
| Ethambutol | 47 | Tablets | Single | Healthy | 8 M, 6 F | 25 mg/kg | 4.55 | 3.83 | 29.8 | 27.5 | 2.48 | 3.21 |
| Isoniazid | 48 | Tablets | Single | Healthy | 8 M, 6 F | 300 | 5.53 | 2.73 | 20.16 | 17.72 | 1.02 | 1.93 |
| Pyrazinamide | 49 | Tablets | Single | Healthy | 8 M, 6 F | 30 mg/kg | 53.4 | 45.6 | 673 | 687 | 1.43 | 3.09 |
| Rifabutin | 50 | Capsules | Single | Healthy | 12 M | 150 | 0.1879 | 0.156 | 2.516 | 2.64 | 3 | 5.4 |
| Rifampin | 51 | Capsules | Single | Healthy | 8 M, 6 F | 600 | 10.93 | 7.27 | 57.15 | 55.2 | 2.305 | 4.43 |

*Continued on next page*

# Table 1 (Continued)
## Effect of Food on the Pharmacokinetics of Oral Anti-Infectives

| | Ref. | Dosage form | Single or steady state | Status | n and gender | Oral dose (mg) | $C_{max}$ Fasting (µg/mL) | $C_{max}$ Fed (µg/mL) | AUC Fasting (µg·h/mL) | AUC Fed (µg·h/mL) | $t_{max}$ Fasting (h) | $t_{max}$ Fed (h) |
|---|---|---|---|---|---|---|---|---|---|---|---|---|
| *Antifungals* | | | | | | | | | | | | |
| Griseofulvin | 52 | Microsize | Single | Healthy | 5 M, 1 F | 250 | NR | 0.6815 | NR | 14.14 | NR | 2.515 |
| Griseofulvin | 52 | Ultra-microsize | Single | Healthy | 5 M, 1 F | 250 | NR | 0.8043 | NR | 16.25 | NR | 2.44 |
| Itraconazole | 53 | solution | Single | Healthy | 30 M | 200 | 0.5457 | 0.3069 | 4.5199 | 3.1617 | 2.2 | 4.8 |
| Fluconazole | 54 | Tablets | Single | Healthy | 7 M, 5 F | 100 | 2.34 | 2.22 | 113 | 106 | 3.08 | 3.08 |
| Ketoconazole | 55 | Tablets | Single | Healthy | 8 M, 4 F | 200 | 4.37 | 4.42 | 15.25 | 20.47 | 1.21 | 2.33 |
| Voriconazole | 56 | Tablets | SS | Healthy | 12 M | 200 | 2.038 | 1.332 | 19.258 | 13.065 | 1.5 | 2.6 |
| *Nonnucleoside reverse transcriptase inhibitors* | | | | | | | | | | | | |
| Delavirdine | 57 | Tablets | SS | HIV positive | 11 M, 2 F | 400 | | 30 µM | 23 µM | NR | NR | NR |
| Efavirenz | 58 | Capsules | SS | Healthy | 5 NR | 1200 | NR | NR | 50% increase | NR | NR | NR |
| Nevirapine | 58 | Tablets | Single | Healthy | 12 M, 12 F | 200 | 2 | No change | NR | NR | NR | NR |
| *Nucleoside reverse transcriptase inhibitors* | | | | | | | | | | | | |
| Abacavir | 59 | Tablets | Single | HIV positive | 11 M, 7 F | 300 | 2.58 | 1.91 | 5.48 | 5.31 | 0.63 | 1.39 |
| Didanosine | 60 | Tablets | Single | HIV positive | 8 M | 375 | 2.789 | 1.291 | 3.902 | 2.083 | 0.5 | 0.5 |
| Didanosine enteric coated | 61 | Capsules | Single | Healthy | 20 NR | 400 | 1.204 | 0.653 | 3.196 | 2.599 | 2 | 3 |
| Lamivudine (as Combivir) | 62 | Tablets | Single | Healthy | 12 M, 12 F | 150 | 1.6203 | 1.3676 | 6.1376 | 6.0354 | 0.91 | 1.86 |
| Stavudine | 63 | Capsules | Single | HIV positive | 13 M, 4 F | 70 | 1.439 | 0.756 | 2.527 | 2.359 | 0.65 | 1.73 |
| Zalcitabine | 64 | Tablets | Single | HIV positive | 18 M, 2 F | 1500 | 0.0252 | 0.0155 | 0.072 | 0.062 | 0.8 | 1.6 |
| Zidovudine | 65 | Capsules | Single | HIV positive | 12 M, 6 F | 100 | 0.806 | 0.341 | 0.884 | 0.817 | 0.681 | 1.72 |
| *Protease inhibitors* | | | | | | | | | | | | |
| Amprenavir | 66 | Capsules | Single | Healthy | NR | 600 | | 46% decrease | | 23% decrease | | 2.5× increase |
| Fosamprenavir | 67 | Tablets | Single | Healthy | 40 M | 1200 | 4.58 | 3.93 | 20.2 | 17.6 | 1.25 | 2.5 |

388

| Drug | Ref | Formulation | Regimen | Subjects | n | Dose (mg) | | | | | | |
|---|---|---|---|---|---|---|---|---|---|---|---|---|
| Indinavir | 68 | Capsules | Single | Healthy | 11 M | 400 | 4.48 µM | 0.62 | 6.86 µM × h | 1.54 µM × h | 0.7 | 2 |
| Indinavir | 68 | Capsules | Single | Healthy | 11 M | 800 | 11.68 µM | 9.37 | 23.15 µM × h | 22.71 | 0.77 | 1.44 |
| Nelfinavir | 69 | Tablets | Single | Healthy | 6 NR | 800 | NR | NR | | 27–50% higher | NR | NR |
| Ritonavir | 58 | Capsules | Single | NR | 57 NR | 600 | NR | NR | 105.9 | 121.7 | NR | NR |
| Ritonavir | 58 | Solution | Single | NR | 18 NR | 600 | NR | 23% decrease | 120 | 129 | 2 | 4 |
| Saquinavir | 70 | Capsules | Single | Healthy | 8 NR | 600 | 0.003 | 0.051 | 0.024 | 0.161 | 2.4 | 3.8 |
| Saquinavir soft gel cap | 70 | Capsules | Single | Healthy | NR | 800 | NR | NR | 0.167 | 1.12 | NR | NR |
| *Non-HIV antivirals* | | | | | | | | | | | | |
| Famciclovir | 71 | Tablets | Single | Healthy | 12 M | 500 | 3.46 | 1.89 | 9.53 | 9.8 | 0.75 | 3 |
| Ganciclovir | 72 | Capsules | SS | HIV positive | 18 M, 2 F | 1000 | 0.85 | 0.96 | 4.7 | 5.6 | 1.8 | 3 |
| Rimantadine | 73 | Tablets | Single | Healthy | 11 M, 1 F | 100 | 0.109 | 0.115 | 4.14 | 4.07 | 4.3 | 3.4 |
| Valganciclovir | 74 | Tablets | SS | HIV positive | 37 M, 2 F | 875 | 5.33 | 6.07 | 19 | 24.8 | 1.5 | 1.5 |

SS, steady state; M, male; F, female; NR, not reported.

## PENICILLINS

The absorption of penicillin V and potassium penicillin are both decreased with the coadministration of food *(75)*. In a study performed in the late 1950s, six groups of 10 volunteers were given a standard meal served 60, 30, or 15 minutes before dosing, with the dose, or 1 or 2 hours after the dose of antibiotic. Blood concentrations of penicillin V or potassium penicillin were obtained at 0.5, 1, and 2 hours after dosing. Lower concentrations were observed with both drugs when given with food, although the effect was greater for potassium penicillin. In another study, healthy nurses were given 150-mg doses of penicillin V (K), potassium V (Ca), and potassium V (acid), with or without a standard meal *(1)*. Reported $C_{max}$ was markedly reduced with all formulations of penicillin V when given with a meal. However, in an earlier study, the absorption of penicillin V (acid) was unaffected by food, possibly because of its greater acid stability and its relatively slow dissolution *(1)*. Thus, penicillin V should be taken on an empty stomach; however, penicillin V (acid) can probably be safely taken with food if clinically indicated.

The AUC of penicillin G suspension decreased by approx 40% when given with milk or children's formula as compared to fasting and thus should be taken without food, if possible *(76)*.

Last, a study assessing the effect of food on nafcillin absorption also showed decreased and more erratic absorption when given with food *(77)*. Serum concentrations of nafcillin were below minimum inhibitory concentration values for common pathogens regardless of coadministration with food, and the authors did not recommend the use of oral nafcillin.

The AUC of ampicillin is decreased by approx 50% when given with food *(1)*. This effect was evident when volunteers were given ampicillin with a high-carbohydrate, -protein, or -fat meal; a standard breakfast; or a Sudanese diet *(10,78,79)*. Early research with amoxicillin demonstrated no effect on the absorption of amoxicillin when given with food *(80)*. In two follow-up studies, one showed decreased absorption when amoxicillin was given with food in 6 healthy volunteers, and another showed no effect in a crossover study of 16 healthy volunteers *(10,79)*. In both studies, the authors concluded that the effect was not clinically significant, and it was suggested that amoxicillin could be administered without regard to meals. Interestingly, the absorption of amoxicillin was decreased when given with 25 mL of water as compared to 250 mL. Thus, it is recommended that amoxicillin be taken with a full glass (250 mL) of water or other suitable liquid.

GI side effects appear to be reduced when the combination of amoxicillin and clavulanate potassium (Augmentin®) is administered with food *(11)*. In one study, after the administration of two 500-mg Augmentin tablets, no significant difference was seen in the AUC, peak concentration, or time to reach peak concentration for either amoxicillin or clavulanate when administered in the fed vs fasted state *(11)*. According to the manufacturer, Augmentin tablets, powder, and chewable tablets may be administered without regard to meals. There does not appear to be a difference in the pharmacokinetics of amoxicillin when administered in the fed vs fasted state. The absorption of clavulanate potassium is greater when Augmentin is administered at the start of a meal but reduced when it is given 30 and 150 minutes after the start of a high-fat breakfast *(1,81,82)*. The effect of food on the oral absorption of Augmentin-ES has not been evaluated *(83)*.

**Table 2**
**Penicillins**

| Generic | Brand | Company | Manufacturer recommendations |
|---|---|---|---|
| Amoxicillin | Amoxil capsules, powder, and chewable tablets | GlaxoSmithKline | Can be given without regard to meals |
| | Amoxil pediatric drops | GlaxoSmithKline | Can be given without regard to meals |
| Amoxicillin/ clavulanate | Augmentin powder, chewable tablets | GlaxoSmithKline | May be given without regard to meals; should be taken at the start of meals to minimize GI upset |
| | Augmentin tablets | GlaxoSmithKline | May be given without regard to meals; should be taken at the start of meals to minimize GI upset |
| | Augmentin ES-600 powder | GlaxoSmithKline | Should be taken at the start of meals to minimize GI upset |
| | Augmentin XR tablets | GlaxoSmithKline | Should be taken at the start of a meal to enhance absorption of amoxicillin and to minimize GI upset |
| Carbenicillin | Geocillin tablets | Pfizer | May be given without regard to meals; should be taken at the start of meals to minimize GI upset |
| Ampicillin | Omnipen capsules | Wyeth-Ayerst | Administer 0.5 hour before or 2 hours after meals for maximal absorption |
| | Omnipen for oral suspension | Wyeth-Ayerst | Administer 0.5 hour before or 2 hours after meals for maximal absorption |
| Penicillin V | Pen-Vee K for oral solution | Wyeth-Ayerst | May be given with meals; however, blood levels are slightly higher when given on an empty stomach |
| | Pen-Vee K tablets | Wyeth-Ayerst | May be given with meals; however, blood levels are slightly higher when given on an empty stomach |
| Bacampacillin | Spectrobid tablets | Pfizer | Can be given without regard to meals |

The pharmacokinetics of Augmentin XR®, an extended-release formulation, were evaluated in healthy volunteers when administered in the fasted state, at the start of a standardized meal, and 30 minutes after a high-fat meal. The absorption of amoxicillin is decreased in the fasted state. Clavulante potassium absorption is decreased after the administration of a high-fat meal. As a result, the manufacturer suggests that Augmentin XR is optimally administered at the start of a meal and should not be taken with a high-fat meal *(84)*. However, to minimize the potential for GI side effects, all amoxicillin-clavulanate potassium formulations should be given at the start of a meal. The manufacturers' dosing recommendations for penicillin antibiotics are shown in Table 2.

## CEPHALOSPORINS

### First-Generation Oral Cephalosporins

The administration of food with cephadrine delayed the $t_{max}$ but had minimal effects on the $C_{max}$ or the AUC *(85)*. Interestingly, the concomitant administration of cephalexin and food resulted in not only a delay in the $t_{max}$, but also a slower rate of drug clearance. This delay was minor, however, and not considered clinically significant (86,87). The rate and extent of absorption of cefadroxil, another first-generation cephalosporin, was not affected by the administration of a standard breakfast (13).

### Second-Generation Oral Cephalosporins

A number of studies have examined the effect of food on the absorption of cefaclor (15,88,89). The maximum achieved concentration of cefaclor pulvules is reduced by approx 50% and the $t_{max}$ is prolonged when given with food, whereas the AUC of the controlled-release formulation is enhanced with food (15,90). The AUC of cefaclor is also decreased by 10–20% when it is given concomitantly with food, but in clinical studies these results did not reach statistical significance (15,91). The administration of a standard breakfast did not affect the $C_{max}$ or the AUC for cefprozil but delayed the $t_{max}$ by approx 50 minutes (15,92). This delay in absorption was not statistically significant (15).

The absorption of cefuroxime axetil, an ester cephalosporin, is increased with food or milk (12,93,94). Administration with a standard breakfast caused an almost 100% increase in the $C_{max}$ and the AUC for cefuroxime. However, trough concentrations of cefuroxime were similar in both groups (12). Likewise, administration of cefuroxime with milk caused a 25–88% increase in the AUC and $C_{max}$ (93). Thus, it is recommended that cefuroxime axetil be taken ideally with food.

Loracarbef is a carbacephem antibiotic that is structurally similar to cefaclor (95). The effect of food on the pharmacokinetics of loracarbef capsules was evaluated in a crossover study of 12 healthy subjects. The ingestion of food delayed the $t_{max}$ and decreased the $C_{max}$ when compared to the fasting state. However, the AUC was similar between the fed and fasted states (17,96,97). The effect of food on the rate and extent of absorption of the oral suspension has not been studied to date.

### Extended-Spectrum Oral Cephalosporins

The food requirements with third-generation cephalosporins can be summarized by dividing this generation into the ester formulations and the nonester formulations. The bioavailability of the ester cephalosporins is enhanced by the presence of food (98). This effect is not caused by changes in the gastric pH but is probably secondary to increased contact time between the drug and the esterases of the intestinal mucosa secondary to delayed gastric emptying. The nonester cephalosporins, on the other hand, display a decrease in the AUC and $C_{max}$ when given with food.

The absorption of cefpodoxime proxetil, an ester cephalosporin, is higher when given with food (20,99). A four-way crossover study assessed a high- or low-fat and high- or low-protein meal vs a lead-in study assessing absorption under fasting conditions. In all cases, giving cefpodoxime with any meal increased the $C_{max}$ and the AUC by approx 22 and 34%, respectively (20). Absorption of cefixime, a nonester cephalosporin, is unaffected by food despite a slight delay in the time to reach peak concentration (100,101).

When cefdinir capsules were administered with a high-fat meal, the $C_{max}$ was reduced by 16%, and the AUC was reduced by 10%. However, the magnitude of these changes is not considered clinically significant, and cefdinir may be administered without regard to meals (102,103). The administration of cefdinir with 60 mg ferrous sulfate or a vitamin with 10 mg elemental iron reduced the extent of absorption by 80 and 31%, respectively. Another study evaluated the effect of a sustained-release ferrous sulfate preparation on the absorption of cefdinir *(104)*. The authors found that the AUC of cefdinir was significantly lower than when cefdinir was administered alone. The effect of foods fortified with elemental iron on the absorption of cefdinir has not been studied. The manufacturer recommends administering cefdinir at least 2 hours before or after iron supplements *(102)*.

Cefditoren is a prodrug ester cephalosporin. The $C_{max}$ and AUC values have been reported to increase when cefditoren is administered after a meal *(19)*. The estimated bioavailability of cefditoren, under fasting conditions, is approx 14%. When administered with a low-fat meal (693 cal), the bioavailability is increased to approx 16%. A moderate (648 cal) or high-fat meal (858 cal) resulted in a 70% increase in mean AUC and a 50% increase in mean $C_{max}$ compared with the fasted state. Thus, the manufacturer recommends taking cefditoren with food to enhance absorption *(105)*.

The administration of a standard meal (530 kcal) had no effect on the pharmacokinetics of ceftibuten except for a slight increase in the time to reach $C_{max}$ *(18,106)*. However, the administration of a high-fat breakfast contrasted these results by approx 20 and 33% decreases in the AUC and $C_{max}$, respectively *(21)*. However, the official labeling for ceftibuten recommends that the drug be taken 1 hour before or 2 hours after a meal. The manufacturers' dosing recommendations for cephalosporin antibiotics are shown in Table 3.

## MACROLIDES

### Erythromycin

A variety of dosage forms of erythromycin have been developed to improve stability and absorption of erythromycin when given with food. In general, two formulations were developed to improve the bioavailability of erythromycin *(1)*. The first was to develop erythromycin as an enteric-coated formulation, thus resisting acid degradation in the stomach. The second was to develop relatively acid-fast esters of erythromycin. The majority of these studies were performed in the 1950s and 1960s, making interpretation of results difficult because of the lack of standardization during this time period. However, for the most part, trends can be established for the various dosing forms of erythromycin.

Food decreases the total absorption of erythromycin base capsules and tablets *(1,107)*. This was improved by the development of erythromycin base coated tablets, which tended to improve the overall absorption of the erythromycin, and food tended simply to delay the time to peak absorption *(1,22,107)*. A small study did document decreased absorption with the coadministration of enteric-coated erythromycin with food *(1)*. The absorption of enteric-coated pellets of erythromycin base was delayed, but not reduced, when taken with a standard breakfast *(1)*.

The absorption of erythromycin stearate was reduced when given after meals in single- and multiple-dose studies *(1,23,108,109)*. However, the opposite effect was observed when erythromycin stearate was given before meals *(24)*. Significant increases in erythromycin concentrations occurred in healthy volunteers given erythromycin stearate-coated tablets immediately prior to a standard meal. This was hypoth-

**Table 3**
**Cephalosporins**

| Generic | Brand | Company | Manufacturer recommendations |
|---------|-------|---------|------------------------------|
| **First generation** | | | |
| • Cephradrine | Anspor capsules, oral suspension | GlaxoSmithKline | Can be given without regard to meals |
| | Velosef capsules, oral suspension | Bristol-Myers Squibb | Can be given without regard to meals |
| • Cefadroxil | Duricef capsules, suspension, tablets | Bristol-Myers Squibb | Can be given without regard to meals |
| • Cephalexin | Keflex oral suspension, capsules | Dista | Can be given without regard to meals |
| | Keftab tablets | Biovail, Eli Lilly | Absorption may be delayed by food, but the amount absorbed is not affected |
| **Second generation** | | | |
| • Cefaclor | Ceclor CD tablets | Dura | Should be administered with meals |
| | Ceclor pulvules, suspension | Lilly | Can be given without regard to meals |
| • Cefprozil | Cefzil for oral suspension | Bristol-Myers Squibb | Can be given without regard to meals |
| | Cefzil tablets | Bristol-Myers Squibb | Absorption may be delayed by food, but the amount absorbed is not affected |
| • Cefuroxime axetil | Ceftin for oral suspension | GlaxoSmithKline | Must be administered with food |
| | Ceftin tablets | GlaxoSmithKline | Can be given without regard to meals |
| • Loracarbef | Lorabid pulvules, oral suspension | Monarch | Should be taken at least 1 hour before or 2 hours after a meal |
| **Extended spectrum** | | | |
| • Cefixime | Suprax for oral suspension, tablets | Lederle labs | Can be given without regard to meals |
| • Cefdinir | Omnicef capsules, oral suspension | Abbott | Can be given without regard to meals |
| • Cefditoren | Spectracef tablets | TAP | Should be administered with meals |
| • Cefpodoxime | Vantin oral suspension | Pharmacia and Upjohn | Can be given without regard to meals |
| | Vantin tablets | Pharmacia and Upjohn | Should be administered with food |
| • Ceftibuten | Cedax capsules | Biovail | Absorption may be delayed by food, but the amount absorbed is not affected |
| | Cedax oral suspension | Biovail | Suspension must be administered at least 2 hours before or 1 hour after a meal |

esized to be caused by a rapid discharge of the dosage form from the stomach or the enteric coating of the formulation.

Erythromycin estolate, ethylcarbonate, and ethylsuccinate are esters of the erythromycin base and were developed for their improved absorption when coadministered with food. These esters are less water soluble and more resistant to acid degradation *(1)*. Consequently, studies have demonstrated no effect or increased absorption when these erythromycin esters are given with food *(22,110–112)*. Grapefruit juice has been reported to inhibit first-pass metabolism on CYP3A in the small intestine *(113)* and as a result can cause a significant increase in oral bioavailability of drugs that are CYP3A substrates *(114)*.

Although erythromycin is a potent inhibitor of CYP3A in the liver, less is known about its effect on CYP3A in the small intestine or if the metabolism of erythromycin is affected by inhibition of CYP3A in the small intestine. Therefore, six healthy male subjects were pretreated with 300 mL water or grapefruit juice 30 minutes before the single-dose administration of 400 mg erythromycin enteric-coated tablets in a crossover fashion to evaluate the effect of grapefruit juice on the pharmacokinetics of erythromycin *(114)*. The $C_{max}$ and AUC were significantly increased when erythromycin was administered with grapefruit juice compared with water. The $t_{max}$ and half-life values were not significantly different between the two phases. The authors concluded that the bioavailability of erythromycin was increased after the administration of grapefruit juice as a result of inhibition of CYP3A metabolism in the small intestine.

### Advanced-Generation Macrolides/Azalides

The bioavailability of clarithromycin is unaffected or increased in the presence of food *(26)*. In a study of healthy volunteers given a single dose of 500 mg clarithromycin, food increased the absorption of clarithromycin by 25%. The authors speculated that this would offer little clinical benefit and suggested that clarithromycin could be given without regard to food. The effect of grapefruit juice on the pharmacokinetics of clarithromycin and its active metabolite, 14-OH clarithromycin, has been evaluated in 12 healthy subjects *(115)*. After an overnight fast of at least 8 hours, subjects received a single 500-mg dose of clarithromycin with 240 mL of either water or freshly squeezed white grapefruit juice at times 0 and 2 hours after administration in a randomized, crossover fashion. Although administration of grapefruit juice significantly delayed the $t_{max}$ of both the parent and active metabolite, it did not affect the extent of absorption of clarithromycin *(115)*.

In contrast to the immediate-release formulation, the manufacturer recommends that clarithromycin extended-release tablets be taken with food *(116)*. Thirty-six healthy subjects were administered two 500-mg clarithromycin extended-release tablets once daily for 5 days in the fasting state and 30 minutes after starting a high-fat breakfast (1000 kcal) *(27)*. Although the absorption of 14-OH clarithromycin was not affected by food, absorption of the parent compound was 30% lower under fasting conditions.

Confusion has existed regarding the absorption of azithromycin with food. Early studies with azithromycin capsules demonstrated a 50% decrease in the overall absorption of azithromycin *(117)*. However, research with the currently marketed tablet, sachet, and suspension has shown little effect on the absorption when coadministered with a high-fat meal *(25)*. As well, an abstract also reported no interaction with food and an oral suspension of azithromycin when given to pediatric patients *(118)*.

Absorption of dirithromycin is decreased by up to 30% when taken on an empty stomach, and it should therefore be taken with a meal or within 1 hour of eating *(119,120)*. The manufacturers' dosing recommendations for macrolide and azalide antibiotics are shown in Table 4.

## TETRACYCLINES

In general, the tetracyclines are affected to various degrees by food, milk, and iron products. Tetracycline, the prototype antibiotic for this class, has amassed a substantial body of literature concerning its food and supplement interactions. Studies involving doxycycline and minocycline are plentiful as well, comparing their food, milk, and iron interactions with that of tetracycline. The reduced bioavailability of the tetracyclines is most likely because of chelation of the antibiotic with heavy metals such as iron and calcium and binding to macromolecules found in food *(1)*. Iron preparations and antacids containing calcium, magnesium, and aluminum cations form poorly soluble complexes that inhibit, to varying degrees, all of the tetracyclines *(121,122)*. It has been hypothesized that the tetracyclines with higher degrees of lipophilicity may display the least interaction with food or milk because of increased absorption and a decreased tendency to form complexes *(123)*. Of the three main tetracyclines, minocycline is most lipophilic, followed by doxycycline and then tetracycline *(121, 124)*.

The effect of food on the absorption of tetracycline was assessed in a number of healthy volunteer studies *(28,29,125–127)*. Test meals using high-carbohydrate, -fat, or -protein diets uniformly caused an approx 50% decrease in the absorption of tetracycline *(29,127,128)*. Likewise, the coadministration of tetracycline with 6 oz milk caused an even greater 65% decrease in tetracycline absorption, and 300 mg ferrous sulfate produced a 77% decrease in absorption *(29)*. Thus, it is always recommended that tetracycline be taken on an empty stomach with a full glass of water (1 hour before or 2 hours after food). Likewise, any patients who have failed tetracycline therapy should be questioned concerning how they administered the drug and whether the drug was coadministered with milk, multivitamins, or other supplements that might complex with the drug.

Doxycycline is less affected than tetracycline by coadministration with food or milk *(129)*. The coadministration of doxycycline with meals high in fat, carbohydrates, and protein or 6 oz homogenized milk produced approximately a 20% decrease in the overall absorption of the drug *(28)*. Another study reported a 30% decrease in AUC and a 24% decrease in the $C_{max}$ of doxycycline after it was administered with 300 mL milk compared to water *(130)*. The authors concluded that, similar to tetracycline, doxycycline should not be administered with milk. Minocycline also is minimally affected when given with food or milk, but coadministration with antacids or other divalent cations caused significantly decreased absorption and is contraindicated *(29,121,131)*.

A double-blind crossover study of seven volunteers given concomitantly with ferrous sulfate showed decreased doxycycline concentrations of 20–45% and a shortened half-life from 17 to 11 hours. The authors hypothesized that the half-life change was owing to enterohepatic recirculation of the drug leading to extended chelation with the

**Table 4**
**Macrolides/Azalides**

| Generic | Brand | Company | Manufacturer recommendations |
|---|---|---|---|
| Erythromycin ethylsuccinate | E.E.S. 200 and 400 liquid | Abbott | Can be given without regard to meals |
| | E.E.S. 400 filmtab tablets | Abbott | Can be given without regard to meals |
| | E.E.S. granules | Abbott | Can be given without regard to meals |
| | EryPed 200 and 400 granules | Abbott | Can be given without regard to meals |
| | EryPed drops and chewable tablets | Abbott | Can be given without regard to meals |
| Erythromycin delayed-release tablets | Ery-Tab tablets | Abbott | Well absorbed and may be given without regard to meals |
| Erythromycin stearate | Erythrocin stearate filmtab tablets | Abbott | Optimal serum levels of erythromycin are reached when taken in the fasting state or immediately before meals |
| Erythromycin base | Erythromycin base filmtab tablets | Abbott | Optimum blood levels are obtained when doses are given on an empty stomach |
| Enteric-coated pellets of ery-thromycin USP | Erythromycin delayed-release base capsules | Abbott | Optimum blood levels are obtained on a fasting stomach (administer at least 0.5 hours and preferably 2 hours before or after a meal) |
| Erythromycin estolate | Ilosone liquid, oral suspension | Dista | Plasma concentrations are comparable whether the estolate is taken in the fasting state or after food |
| | Ilosone pulvules, tablets | Dista | Plasma concentrations are comparable whether the estolate is taken in the fasting state or after food |
| Ethylsuccinate and sulfisoxazole | Pediazole suspension | Ross | Can be given without regard to meals |
| Troleandomycin | Tao capsules | Pfizer | Soluble and stable in the presence of gastric juice |
| Azithromycin | Zithromax capsules | Pfizer | Capsules should be given at least 1 hour before or 2 hours after a meal |
| | Zithromax for oral suspension | Pfizer | Give at least 1 hour before or 2 hours after a meal |
| | Zithromax tablets, sachet | Pfizer | Can be given without regard to meals |
| Clarithromycin | Biaxin filmtab tablets, granules | Abbott | Can be given without regard to meals |
| | Biaxin XL filmtab | Abbott | Should be taken with food |
| Dirithromycin | Dynabac tablets | Sanofi | Should be administered with food or within 1 hour of eating |

**Table 5**
**Decreased Absorption**
**of Tetracyclines With Food and Milk**

|            | Percentage decreased AUC | |
|------------|------|------|
| Antibiotic | Food | Milk |
| Tetracycline | 50 | 65 |
| Minocycline | 13 | 27 |
| Doxycycline | 20 | 20 |

iron salts remaining in the GI tract *(132)*. Although not as well documented, this interaction probably occurs to the same extent with tetracycline and minocycline as well because these drugs also undergo enterohepatic recirculation.

The inhibitory effects of various iron salts on the absorption of tetracycline was investigated in six healthy volunteers *(133)*. The iron salt types (each corresponding to 40 mg of elemental iron) all caused varying degrees of decreased absorption of tetracycline. Ferrous sulfate caused the most significant decrease in absorption (80–90%), followed by ferrous fumarate, ferrous succinate, ferrous gluconate (70–80%), ferrous tartrate (50%), and ferrous sodium edetate (30%).

Thus, it is recommended that minocycline and doxycline be given with food to decrease incidence of GI upset, but that the administration of all tetracyclines be spaced by at least 2 hours with antacids *(29,121,124)*. Because of the significant GI transit time of iron preparations, it is not advisable to prescribe tetracyclines for patients who are taking iron supplementation *(29)*. The interactions of tetracyclines with food, milk, and antacids is presented in Table 5, and the manufacturers' dosing recommendations for tetracycline antibiotics are shown in Table 6.

## FLUOROQUINOLONES

In general, food has little clinical effect on the pharmacokinetics of the quinolones. However, quinolones are affected by divalent and trivalent cations and thus are affected, to different extents, by calcium-containing foods, iron supplements, and antacids. As well, the effect of enteral feeds, which can contain significant amounts of di- and trivalent cations, on the pharmacokinetics of quinolones has been investigated in a number of published studies. Quinolones, to various extents, also inhibit the liver enzymes responsible for caffeine metabolism, creating another potential interaction.

Sparfloxacin is well absorbed after oral administration, with a bioavailability of greater than 80% *(134)*. Absorption of sparfloxacin is somewhat unusual in that it occurs via a passive and carrier-mediated process extending from the duodenum to the colon *(135)*. This corresponds to a longer $t_{max}$ and may increase the potential for interactions with foods that chelate fluoroquinolones. This has not been seen clinically, however, as food intake and high-fat meals do not affect the pharmacokinetics of sparfloxacin *(39)*.

Food (standard or high-fat meals) has minimal effects on the absorption of ciprofloxacin suspension, immediate-release tablets, or extended-release tablets

**Table 6**
**Tetracylines**

| Generic | Brand | Company | Manufacturer recommendations |
|---------|-------|---------|------------------------------|
| Tetracyclines | Achromycin V capsules | Lederly Labs | Give 1 hour before or 2 hours after meals |
| Demeclocycline | Declomycin tablets | Lederly Labs | Give 1 hour before or 2 hours after meals |
| Minocycline | Dynacin capsules | Medicis | Can be given without regard to meals |
| | Minocin oral suspension | Lederle Labs | Can be given without regard to meals |
| | Minocin pellet-filled capsules | Lederle Labs | Can be given without regard to meals |
| Doxycycline | Monodox capsules | Oclassen | May be given with food if GI upset occurs; administration with adequate amounts of fluid is recommended |
| Minocycline | Vectrin capsules | Warner Chilcott Professional Products | Can be given without regard to meals |
| Doxycycline | Vibra-tabs film coated | Pfizer | May be given with food if GI upset occurs; administration with adequate amounts of fluid is recommended |
| | Vibramycin calcium oral suspension | Pfizer | May be given with food if GI upset occurs; administration with adequate amounts of fluid is recommended |
| | Vibramycin monohydrate for oral suspension | Pfizer | May be given with food if GI upset occurs; administration with adequate amounts of fluid is recommended |

*(30,136–138)*. The effect of a fat- and calcium-rich breakfast on the pharmacokinetics of fleroxacin was studied in 20 healthy volunteers *(139)*. Administration with this breakfast reduced $C_{max}$ by approx 25%; however, no significant change was observed in the AUC. The clinical significance of the decreased $C_{max}$ was questionable, and the authors concluded that fleroxacin could be given without regard to meals. Food prolongs the $t_{max}$ of lomefloxacin by approx 1 hour but has no effect on the $C_{max}$ or AUC *(36)*. Likewise, food has minimal impact on enoxacin acid except for a somewhat lower $C_{max}$ and prolonged $t_{max}$.

Levofloxacin is well absorbed after oral administration, with a bioavailability of greater than 90% *(134)*. Administration with food decreases the $C_{max}$ by approx 14% and lengthens the $t_{max}$ by approx 1 hour. This is not considered clinically significant, and levofloxacin can be administered without regard to meals. Gatifloxacin has an absolute bioavailability of greater than 95% *(32,140)*. Concomitant administration of a high-fat or light breakfast had no effect on the absorption of gatifloxacin when com-

**Table 7**
**Quinolones**

| Generic | Brand | Company | Manufacturer recommendations |
|---|---|---|---|
| Ciprofloxacin | Cipro tablets | Bayer | Can be given without regard to meals |
| | Cipro XR tablets | Bayer | Can be given without regard to meals |
| Ofloxacin | Floxin tablets | Ortho-McNeil | Can be given without regard to meals |
| Levofloxacin | Levaquin tablets | Ortho-McNeil | Can be given without regard to meals |
| Lomefloxacin | Maxaquin tablets | Searle | Can be given without regard to meals |
| | Maxaquin tablets | Unimed | Can be given without regard to meals |
| Norfloxacin | Noroxin tablets | Merck | Administer 1 hour before or 2 hours after meals; patients should be well hydrated |
| | Noroxin tablets | Roberts | Administer 1 hour before or 2 hours after meals; patients should be well hydrated |
| Enoxacin | Penetrex tablets | Rhone-Poulen Rorer | Administer 1 hour before or 2 hours after meals |
| Sparfloxacin | Zagam tablets | Rhone-Poulenc Rorer | Can be given without regard to meals |
| Trovafloxacin | Trovan tablets | Pfizer | Can be given without regard to meals |
| Moxifloxacin | Avelox tablets | Bayer | Can be given without regard to meals |
| Gatifloxacin | Tequin tablets | Bristol-Myers Squibb | Can be given without regard to meals |
| Gemifloxacin | Factive tablets | Genesoft | Can be given without regard to meals |

pared to fasting conditions *(32,33,140,141)*. Similar to levofloxacin and gatifloxacin, moxifloxacin has excellent oral absorption, with an absolute bioavailability of approx 90% *(142)*. After the administration of a high-fat breakfast, the absorption of moxifloxacin is slightly delayed. The median $t_{max}$ values were 1.0 hour under fasting conditions and 2.5 hours in the fed state. The $C_{max}$ and AUC of moxifloxacin were decreased by approx 12 and 3%, respectively, after the administration of a high-fat meal. However, the magnitude of these effects is not considered clinically significant *(37)*. The absolute bioavailability of gemifloxacin is approx 71% and does not appear to be significantly altered by the administration of a high-fat meal *(34,143)*. The manufacturers' dosing recommendations for quinolone antibiotics are shown in Table 7.

### Quinolones and Milk or Yogurt

Coadministration with milk and yogurt significantly decreased the $C_{max}$ and AUC of ciprofloxacin in two healthy volunteer studies *(144,145)*. The effect of milk and yogurt on the absorption of norfloxacin was investigated in two other healthy volunteer trials *(146,147)*. The administration of milk caused more than a 50% decrease in the $C_{max}$ and AUC norfloxacin concentrations.

Coadministration with milk did not significantly decrease the $C_{max}$ and AUC of fleroxacin in 12 healthy volunteers *(144)*. Similarly, dairy products did not significantly affect the pharmacokinetics of enoxacin, lomefloxacin, moxifloxacin, or ofloxacin in other healthy volunteer studies *(31,147–149)*. Thus, it appears that patients should be counseled to avoid coadministration of milk with ciprofloxacin and norfloxacin and perhaps all the fluoroquinolones generally.

## Quinolones and Vitamin- or Mineral-Fortified Foods

Except for norfloxacin, the fluoroquinolones are labeled as able to be administered without regard to meals because of studies conducted with the standard FDA-mandated food-drug bioequivalency study meal of a high-fat, high-calorie, low-mineral breakfast *(150,151)*. The bioavailability of fluoroquinolones is reduced during the concomitant administration with multivalent cations (i.e., calcium, magnesium, iron, and aluminum). Thus, to minimize this drug interaction, it is recommended to administer the interacting agent at least 2–4 hours apart from the dosing of the fluoroquinolone *(152)*. There are an increasing number of food products available that have been fortified with essential vitamins and minerals. As a result, new drug–food interactions could exist that were not seen prior to the food products' fortification.

Most calcium-fortified food products have more calcium per serving than seen in the dietary calcium interaction studies conducted with milk or yogurt *(153)*. Several studies have evaluated the effect of calcium fortification on the bioavailability of fluoroquinolones using calcium-fortified orange juice *(151,153–155)*. In a randomized, three-way crossover study, 15 healthy subjects received a single dose of ciprofloxacin with 12 oz water, orange juice, and calcium-fortified orange juice. The $C_{max}$ and AUC decreased by 41 and 38%, respectively, when ciprofloxacin was administered with calcium-fortified orange juice compared to water. The authors concluded that administering ciprofloxacin with water was not bioequivalent to administering it with calcium-fortified orange juice *(153)*.

After administering a single 500-mg dose of levofloxacin to 16 healthy subjects, no significant difference in AUC was seen between the intake of either water or calcium-fortified orange juice. The $C_{max}$ was reduced by 18% and the $t_{max}$ increased by 58% when levofloxacin was coadministered with calcium-fortified orange juice compared to water. However, the degree of change in the $C_{max}$ and $t_{max}$ was about the same with both plain and calcium-fortified orange juices. The authors suggested that the interaction with levofloxacin and the orange juices seems less likely to be a chelation interaction like the one observed in the ciprofloxacin study *(153)*. Because levofloxacin is a P-glycoprotein substrate *(156)* and orange juice is a potential inhibitor of intestinal transport mechanisms *(7,157)*, one potential explanation includes inhibition of P-glycoprotein or organic anion transporting polypeptide in the GI tract by the orange juice in combination with minor chelation. No matter what the actual mechanism of the interaction, the $C_{max}$ of levofloxacin was significantly decreased with the administration of orange juice. The bioavailability of levofloxacin when taken with water alone, subject-measured portions of fortified orange juice and cereal, and subject-measured portions of fortified orange juice and cereal with milk was also studied *(155)*. Both phases of food intake were not considered bioequivalent to the water-alone phase in terms of the $C_{max}$.

When gatifloxacin was administered with fortified orange juice, the bioavailability was not bioequivalent to the administration with water according to FDA guidelines *(154)*. The AUC decreased by 12%, and volume of distribution and clearance increased by 13 and 15%, respectively, when administered with fortified orange juice. Although not statistically significant, the $C_{max}$ decreased by 13.5%, and the $t_{max}$ increased by 38% *(154)*.

Although a limited number of studies have evaluated the effect of foods fortified with vitamin or minerals on fluoroquinolone absorption, it may be prudent to instruct patients to avoid the concomitant administration of fluoroquinolones with fortified food products.

## Quinolones and Caffeine

Inhibition of CYP1A2 activity by certain quinolones results in prolonged half-life, increased AUC, and decreased clearance of caffeine (158). Coadministration of enoxacin and clinafloxacin caused more than 75% decrease in the clearance and 300% increase in the AUC of caffeine (159,160). Likewise, norfloxacin significantly altered the pharmacokinetics of caffeine, causing similar changes in the clearance and AUC (161). Ciprofloxacin caused approx 50% increase and decrease in the AUC and clearance of caffeine, respectively (162). In vitro tests with human liver microsomes assessed the inhibitory potency of various quinolone against CYP1A2. Enoxacin, ciprofloxacin, nalidixic acid, and norfloxacin were the strongest inhibitors of CYP1A2, followed by lomefloxacin and ofloxacin (158). Thus, caffeine should be avoided in patients with liver disorders, cardiac arrhythmias, or latent epilepsy or in intensive care units while individuals are undergoing treatment with quinolones known to interact with caffeine (163).

## Quinolones and Enteral Feeds

The effects of enteral feeds on the absorption of fluoroquinolones have produced controversial results. An enteral feeding product (Ensure®) reduced the relative oral bioavailability of ciprofloxacin by 28% in 13 healthy volunteers and decreased the $C_{max}$ and AUC (164). Another investigator showed no effect or increased ciprofloxacin absorption with concomitant enteral feeds (Pulmocare® or Osmolite®) through a nasogastric tube in six healthy volunteers (165). In another study, a jejunostomy tube, as opposed to a gastrostomy tube, produced a larger reduction in the bioavailability of ciprofloxacin (166).

The effect of gastric tube feeding on the bioavailability of gatifloxacin was evaluated in 16 critically ill patients (167). Both continuous and interrupted (held 2 hours before and after) tube feeding with Promote®, Jevity®, Glucerna®, Pulmocare®, or Impact® had no affect on gatifloxacin bioavailability; however, there was significant variability between patients.

Enteral feeds contain various cations that may affect the quinolones to different extents. Although not contraindicated, it is prudent to avoid the combination of enteral feeds and quinolones to ensure adequate absorption of the quinolones. It is recommended to hold enteral feeding for 2 hours before and after administration of quinolones (4 hours for sparfloxacin) (168).

## MISCELLANEOUS ANTIBIOTICS

### Nitrofurantoin

Food tends to enhance the absorption of nitrofurantoin (169–171). The increased dissolution time resulting from coadministration of food with nitrofurantoin has been hypothesized as the mechanism behind this increased absorption. Interestingly, food tends to have more of an effect on the urinary levels of nitrofurantoin than on the corresponding serum levels.

## Atovaquone

Food, especially fatty food, enhances the bioavailability of atovaquone two- to three-fold. Atovaquone has very poor bioavailability, and therapeutic concentrations may not be achieved when it is taken while fasting. Thus, it is recommended that atovaquone always be taken with a meal *(44,172)*.

## Metronidazole

The absorption of metronidazole is delayed but not reduced by the presence of food *(46)*. In a study of 10 healthy volunteers given a single dose of metronidazole with or without food, only slight interindividual variation in absorption was observed. Metronidazole has also been implicated with a disulfiramlike reaction when given with alcohol. A separate section of this chapter provides a full description of disulfiramlike reactions with anti-infectives.

## Antihelmintics

A fatty meal significantly enhances absorption of albendazole compared to the fasted state *(41,173,174)*. The mean $C_{max}$ was increased 6.5-fold and the AUC increased 9.5-fold in six healthy male subjects after the administration of a fatty meal *(41)*. Therefore, albendazole tablets are recommended to be administered with meals to enhance absorption.

Administration of ivermectin to healthy volunteers caused the absorption to be 2.5 times higher following a high-fat meal compared to the fasted state *(42)*. The manufacturer recommends that ivermectin be administered with water *(175)*.

Food has also been reported to increase the bioavailability of praziquantel *(43)*; therefore, it should be administered with meals *(176)*.

Compared to the fasting state, the administration of grapefruit juice enhanced the $C_{max}$ and AUC of albendazole 3.2-fold and 3.1-fold, respectively *(41)*. Praziquantel mean $C_{max}$ and AUC were also increased 1.62-fold and 1.9-fold, respectively, but with a large amount of interindividual variability *(177)*.

## Clindamycin

Food does not affect the absorption of clindamycin granules or capsules *(178,179)*.

## Linezolid

Linezolid is a novel oxazolidinone antibiotic that has activity against a variety of Gram-positive bacteria. The absolute bioavailability of linezolid is approx 100% *(45,180)*. When administered with a high-fat meal (850 cal), linezolid required a slightly longer time to reach peak plasma concentrations than when given under fasting conditions. $C_{max}$ was significantly lower following a high-fat meal compared to fasting. However, no difference was seen in mean AUC values under fasted and fed conditions. The effect of food on the bioavailability is considered minimal *(45)*. Linezolid is a weak, competitive (reversible) inhibitor of human monoamine oxidase A *(181)*. When linezolid is administered at a clinically approved dose (600 mg twice daily), dietary restriction of tyramine-containing foods is generally not necessary.

**Table 8**
**Miscellaneous Antibiotics**

| Generic | Brand | Company | Manufacturer recommendations |
| --- | --- | --- | --- |
| Sulfonamides and combinations | | | |
| • Trimethoprim and sulfamethoxazole | Bactrim DS tablets | Roche Laboratories | Not stated |
| | Bactrim pediatric suspension | Roche Laboratories | |
| | Bactrim tablets | Roche Laboratories | |
| • Ethylsuccinate and sulfisoxazole | Pediazole suspension | Ross | Can be given without regard to meals |
| • Trimethoprim and sulfamethoxazole | Septra DS tablets | GlaxoSmithKline | Not stated |
| | Septra grape suspension | GlaxoSmithKline | |
| | Septra suspension | GlaxoSmithKline | |
| | Septra tablets | GlaxoSmithKline | |
| Urinary anti-infectives and combinations | | | |
| • Nitrofurantoin | Furadantin oral suspension | Dura | Should be taken with food to improve absorption and tolerance |
| | Macrobid capsules | Proctor and Gamble | Should be taken with food to improve absorption and tolerance |
| | Macrodantin capsules | Proctor and Gamble | Should be taken with food to improve absorption and tolerance |
| • Fosfomycin | Monurol sachet | Forest | Can be given without regard to meals |
| • Nalidixic acid | NegGram caplets | Sanofi | Not stated |
| | NegGram suspension | Sanofi | Not stated |
| • Methenamine combination | Urised tablets | PolyMedica | Not stated |
| • Oxytetracycline | Urobiotic-250 capsules | Pfizer | To aid absorption of the drug, it should be given at least 1 hour before or 2 hours after eating |
| Antihelmintics | | | |
| • Albendazole | Albenza tablets | GlaxoSmithKline | Should be taken with food |
| • Ivermectin | Stromectol tablets | Merck | Should be taken with water |
| • Praziquantel | Biltricide tablets | Bayer | Should be taken with food |

*Continued on next page*

**Table 8 (*Continued*))**
**Miscellaneous Antibiotics**

| Generic | Brand | Company | Manufacturer recommendations |
|---|---|---|---|
| Other | | | |
| • Clindamycin | Cleocin HCL capsules | Pharmacia and Upjohn | To avoid the possibility of esophageal irritation, should be taken with a full glass of water |
| • Cycloserine | Seromycin capules | Dura | Not stated |
| • Vancomycin | Vancocin HCL, oral solution and pulvules | Lilly | Not stated |
| • Dapsone | Dapsone tablets USP J | acobus | Not stated |
| • Furazolidone | Furoxone liquid | Roberts | Can be given without regard to meals |
| | Furoxone tablets | Roberts | Can be given without regard to meals |
| • Atovaquone | Mepron suspension | GlaxoSmithKline | Administer with meals |
| • Atovaquone and proguanil | Malarone tablets, pediatric tablets | GlaxoSmithKline | Take with food or a milky drink |
| • Linezolid | Zyvoxx tablets, suspension | Pharmacia and Upjohn | Can be given without regard to meals |

However, patients should be advised to avoid consuming large amounts of foods with a high tyramine content (i.e., aged cheeses, fermented meats, sauerkraut, soy sauce, draught beers, and red wines) *(182)*.

The manufacturers' dosing recommendations for miscellaneous antibiotics are shown in Table 8.

## ANTIMYCOBACTERIALS

Peak concentrations and the relative bioavailability of isoniazid decreased by 70 and 40% with the addition of food, respectively, which suggests that isoniazid always be given on an empty stomach *(183)*. However, the manufacturer claims that isoniazid can be given with food if stomach upset occurs. A more recent study in 14 healthy volunteers investigated the effect of a high-fat breakfast on the absorption of isoniazid *(48)*. Relative to fasting, the high-fat meal reduced $C_{max}$ by 51%, doubled $t_{max}$, and reduced AUC by 12% *(48)*.

Because isoniazid is a weak monoamine oxidase inhibitor, several case reports have described adverse reactions in patients taking isoniazid who have ingested foods high in monoamines (e.g., tyramine) *(184)*. Flushing of the arms, face, and upper body were observed in patients after ingestion of cheese or red wine during isoniazid therapy *(185–187)*. Other possible symptoms include palpitatations, headache, and mild increases in systolic blood pressure. Isoniazid is also an inhibitor of histaminase, and at

**Table 9**
**Antimycobacterials**

| Generic | Brand | Company | Manufacturer recommendations |
|---------|-------|---------|------------------------------|
| Ethambutol | Myambutol tablets | Lederle Labs | Can be given without regard to meals |
| Rifabutin | Mycobutin capsules | Pharmacia and Upjohn | May be taken with meals if GI upset occurs |
| Aminosalicylic acid | Paser granules | Jacobus | Sprinkle on applesauce or yogurt or by swirling in the glass to suspend the granules in an acidic drink such as tomato or orange juice |
| Pyrazinamide | Pyrazinamide tablets | Lederle Labs | Not stated |
| Rifampin | Rifadin capsules | Hoechst Marion Roussell | Absorption reduced by 30% with food |
| Rifampin-isoniazid | Rifamate capsules | Hoechst Marion Roussell | Administer 1 hour before or 1 hour after meals |
| Cycloserine | Seromycin capules | Dura | Not stated |
| Ethionamide | Trecator-SC tablets | Wyeth-Ayerst | Administer at mealtimes to avoid GI upset |
| Isoniazid | Generic only | | Can be given without regard to food |

least 30 cases of adverse reactions after ingestion of fish with high histamine contents (e.g., tuna, mackerel, salmon, skipjack) have been reported in patients taking isoniazid *(184)*. Patients should be cautioned about the potential for adverse reactions with certain cheeses, red wine, and fish with high histamine content while taking isoniazid.

In a normal healthy volunteer study performed in the 1970s, the coadministration with food caused a 25% reduction in the $C_{max}$ and urinary excretion of rifampicin *(188)*. In a more recent analysis with 14 normal healthy volunteers, the addition of a high-fat meal reduced the $C_{max}$ of rifampin by 36% and the overall AUC by 6% *(51)*. An aluminum-magnesium antacid had no effect on the bioavailability of rifampin. Thus, rifampin should be taken on an empty stomach whenever possible but may be taken with food if stomach upset occurs.

The effect of a high-fat meal on the pharmacokinetics of rifabutin was studied in 12 healthy male volunteers *(50)*. Although a delay was seen in the $t_{max}$ (5.4 vs 3.0 hours), little effect was seen with the addition of food.

A standardized breakfast produced little to no effect on the mean AUC of ethambutol in 11 normal healthy volunteers *(189)*. A subsequent study in 14 male and female volunteers showed similar results with the coadministration of a high-fat meal with ethambutol *(47)*. However, the coadministration with an aluminum-magnesium antacid caused a 29% decrease in the $C_{max}$ and a 10% decrease in AUC. The authors of this article suggested that antacids should be avoided near the time of ethambutol dosing.

The effect of a high-fat meal on the pharmacokinetics of pyrazinamide was studied in 14 healthy volunteers *(49)*. A high-fat meal or an aluminum-magnesium antacid had minimal effect on the absorption of pyrazinamide. The manufacturers' dosing recommendations for antimycobacterial antibiotics are shown in Table 9.

## ANTIFUNGALS

### Azole Antifungals

A number of healthy volunteer studies have investigated the influence of food on the pharmacokinetics of ketoconazole, with conflicting results *(55,190–192)*.

A crossover study of 10 volunteers showed a 55–60% decrease in $C_{max}$ and AUC as well as a lengthened $t_{max}$ when 200 mg ketoconazole were given immediately after a low-fat breakfast *(55)*. Another study in 18 volunteers investigated the influence of a high-fat breakfast on the pharmacokinetics of ketoconazole over a wider dosing range (200–800 mg) *(190)*. This study determined that food did not reduce AUC or $C_{max}$ but did tend to lengthen $t_{max}$. At the 400- and 600-mg dosing regimens, there was a trend toward increased absorption that was not apparent at the 200- or 800-mg dosing regimens. Finally, a third study of 12 volunteers showed that a high-fat meal significantly prolonged $t_{max}$, and a high-carbohydrate meal significantly decreased $C_{max}$ *(191)*. There was a nonstatistically significant trend toward increased AUC values with the high-fat meal and decreased AUC values with the high-carbohydrate meals. The manufacturer recommends that ketoconazole be given with food, which appears reasonable given the conflicting results from pharmacokinetic studies.

The influence of a low-fat (1000-kJ) and a high-fat (3600-kJ) meal on the pharmacokinetics of 100 mg fluconazole and 100 mg itraconazole was investigated in 24 healthy volunteers *(54)*. The $C_{max}$, AUC, and $t_{max}$ of fluconazole were not significantly affected between test meals or compared to fasting. In contrast, the plasma AUC and $C_{max}$ of itraconazole were significantly increased with the two test meals vs fasting. The AUC of itraconazole when given on an empty stomach was approx 40% lower than when given with a high-fat meal. Similar results were seen when itraconazole was given to patients with superficial fungal infections *(193)*. The effect of food on a 200-mg oral solution of itraconazole was studied in 30 healthy male volunteers *(53)*. Unlike studies with itraconazole capsules, the $C_{max}$ and AUC decreased by 44 and 30%, respectively, when given with a high-fat meal. Thus, itraconazole capsules should be given with food; the oral solution should be given on an empty stomach.

The effect of cola beverages on the absorption of 100- and 200-mg doses of itraconazole has been assessed in two separate healthy volunteer studies *(194,195)*. Results from these studies showed that the addition of a cola product could increase the AUC and $C_{max}$ of itraconazole by approx 100%. Thus, the addition of an acidic beverage may be an option to increase absorption of itraconazole, especially in patients who are hypochlorhydric or who are taking gastric acid suppressants.

The effect of a high-fat breakfast on the pharmacokinetics of voriconazole was evaluated in 12 healthy male subjects *(56)*. At steady state (day 7), the bioavailability of voriconazole was reduced by approx 22% when taken with food compared to fasting. The rate of absorption was also significantly delayed by administering voriconazole with food. Therefore, voriconazole tablets should be taken at least 1 hour before or 1 hour after a meal.

### Griseofulvin

The effect of food on the pharmacokinetics of microsize and ultra-microsize griseofulvin was studied in nonfasting volunteers *(52)*. There were similar results between the two

**Table 10**
**Antifungals**

| Generic | Brand | Company | Manufacturer recommendations |
|---|---|---|---|
| Fluconazole | Diflucan tablets | Pfizer | Not stated |
| Ketoconazole | Nizoral tablets | Janssen | Administration with a meal may decrease absorption |
| Itraconazole | Sporanox capsules | Janssen | Should be taken with a full meal to ensure maximal absorption |
| Itraconazole | Sporanox oral solution | Janssen | If possible, do not take with food |
| Ultra-microsize crystals of griseofulvin | Fulvicin P/G tablets | Schering | Not stated |
|  | Fulvicin P/G 165 and 330 | Schering | Not stated |
| Griseofulvin microsize | Grifulvin V | Ortho | Better blood levels can probably be attained in most patients if the tablets are administered after a meal with a high-fat content |
| Ultramicrosize crystals of griseofulvin | Gris-PEG tablets | Allergan | Not stated |
| Terbinafine | Lamisil tablets | Novartis | An increase in the AUC of less than 20% is observed when administered with food |
| Voriconazole | Vfend tablets | Pfizer | Should be taken at least 1 hour before or 1 hour after a meal |

products when given with food. A study from the early 1960s showed that increased serum griseofulvin concentrations were higher when given with a high-fat meal, and thus it is recommended that griseofulvin be given with food (especially a high-fat meal) *(196)*.

The manufacturers' dosing recommendations for antifungal agents are shown in Table 10.

## HUMAN IMMUNODEFICIENCY VIRUS MEDICATIONS

### Nucleoside Reverse Transcriptase Inhibitors

Didanosine is variably absorbed after oral administration because of its poor solubility at low pH, with bioavailability ranging from 25 to 43% *(197,198)*. Acid-catalyzed hydrolysis results in significant degradation of the drug, which was slightly overcome by the buffered didanosine formulation *(199)*. Food alters the absolute bioavailability of didanosine by approx 50%, most likely because of increased hydrolysis at lower pH and delayed gastric emptying *(60)*. The effect of time of food administration on the bioavailability of didanosine using a chewable tablet formulation was studied in 10 human immunodeficiency virus (HIV)-positive patients. This study showed that the effect of food could be minimized if given 30–60 minutes before or 2 hours after a meal *(200)*. Based on these results, it is recommended that didanosine be administered 30 minutes to 1 hour before meals or at least 2 hours after a meal.

To eliminate the need for concurrent administration with antacids, an encapsulated enteric-coated bead formulation of didanosine was developed (Videx® EC). In healthy volunteers and in subjects infected with HIV, the AUC is equivalent for didanosine administered as the enteric-coated formulation relative to a buffered tablet formulation *(201)*.

The effect of food and timing of meals on the bioavailability of didanosine from encapsulated enteric-coated beads was evaluated in healthy subjects *(61)*. Concomitant administration with a high-fat (757 cal) or light meal (373 cal) decreased the rate of absorption. Regardless of the caloric content of the meal, the extent of the absorption of didanosine was reduced to a similar degree with a high-fat meal, light meal, yogurt, and applesauce. Administering the encapsulated enteric-coated beads 1.5, 2, or 3 hours before a meal resulted in similar absorption to that seen under fasting conditions. The overall reduction in AUC is approx 20 to 25% when didanosine is administered with food. Although this appears to be a moderate reduction, it is recommended to administer this formulation on an empty stomach *(202)*.

Zidovudine (ZDV) is fairly well absorbed after oral administration, with a bioavailability average of between 60 and 70% *(203)*. Several studies have examined the effect of certain types of food on ZDV absorption. Overall, food consumption (especially high-fat meals) tends to decrease the rate but not the extent of absorption of ZDV *(204,205)*. Another study investigated the pharmacokinetics of ZDV in 13 patients with acquired immunodeficiency syndrome (AIDS) who were either fasting or taking a standard breakfast. The mean AUC in the fed state was 24% lower than the fasted AUC and demonstrated more interpatient variability *(206)*. In a study by Shelton et al. *(65)*, a high-fat breakfast significantly reduced the $C_{max}$ of ZDV but did not significantly affect the extent of absorption (AUC). Previous studies sampled blood for ZDV concentrations for 4–6 hours postdose *(204,206)*. Shelton et al. *(65)* concluded that sample collection less than 10 hours may not have been adequate to determine the full effect of food on ZDV pharmacokinetics.

The administration of lamivudine with a standard breakfast (55% fat, 20% carbohydrates, 13% proteins) significantly increased $t_{max}$ and lowered $C_{max}$ but had no significant affect on the extent of absorption (AUC) *(207)*. Thus, lamivudine can be taken without regard to meals. Administration with meals, however, may decrease the likelihood of GI upset. Administration of a high-fat breakfast (1000 kcal) did not affect the extent of absorption of lamivudine or ZDV from the combined tablet, Combivir® *(62)*. Food slowed the rate of absorption, delaying the $t_{max}$ and decreasing the $C_{max}$ of lamivudine and ZDV, but these changes were not considered clinically significant.

Likewise, administration of zalcitabine with food tended to lengthen $t_{max}$ and decreased the AUC by approx 14% *(208)*. This is not considered clinically significant, and it is recommended that zalcitabine can be taken without regard to meals.

The absorption of stavudine is not affected by food, and therefore it can be taken without regard to meals *(209,210)*. As well, after single doses of abacavir taken with food, the $C_{max}$ was reduced by 35% and the AUC by 5% *(211)*. This was not considered clinically significant, and abacavir can be taken without regard to meals. Ethanol decreases the elimination of abacavir. Coadministration of ethanol and abacavir resulted in a 41% increase in abacavir AUC and a 26% increase in abacavir half-life *(58)*. The extent of absorption of Trizivir® tablets (abacavir, lamivudine, and ZDV) is not affected by the administration of a meal, and this formulation can be given with or without food *(212)*.

Emtricitabine systemic exposure (AUC) was not affected by the administration of a high-fat meal (1000 kcal), and the $C_{max}$ was reduced by 29% compared to the fasting state *(213)*. Following a high-fat meal (700–1000 kcal), the AUC of tenofovir increased by approx 40%, and the $C_{max}$ increased approx 14%. Administration with a light meal does not appear to significantly affect the pharmacokinetics of tenofovir *(214,215)*. Thus, emtricitabine and tenofovir can both be administered with or without food. When tenofovir is administered with didanosine, the $C_{max}$ and AUC of didanosine are significantly increased *(216,217)*. As a result, the manufacturers recommend reducing the didanosine dose when it is coadministered with tenofovir *(202,214,218)*. The exact mechanism of this interaction is unknown, but one hypothesis is that tenofovir inhibits an enzyme responsible for the degradation of didanosine *(219)*. Regardless of the mechanism, when tenofovir and didanosine enteric-coated capsules are coadministered, they should be taken under fasted conditions or with a light meal (less than 400 kcal). The didanosine buffered tablet formulation and tenofovir should be administered under fasting conditions *(214)*. Safety data on the combination of these two medications is limited.

### Nonnucleoside Reverse Transcriptase Inhibitors

A single-dose study of delavirdine showed an approx 30% reduction in AUC when delavirdine was given with food *(57)*. During steady-state dosing, delavirdine was not significantly affected by the presence of food, although the $t_{max}$ was delayed. Importantly, trough concentrations of the drug were similar in fasted vs nonfasted individuals *(57,220)*. Thus, delavirdine can be taken without regard to meals.

When efavirenz capsules were administered with a high-fat meal (894 kcal) or a reduced-fat/normal caloric meal (440 kcal), the AUC was increased by 22 and 17% and the $C_{max}$ was increased by 39 and 51%, respectively, when compared to fasting. Administration of a 600-mg efavirenz tablet with a high-fat meal (1000 kcal) caused a 28% increase in AUC and a 79% increase in $C_{max}$ relative to fasting conditions. To avoid an increase in the frequency of adverse events, it is recommended that efavirenz be administered on an empty stomach, preferably at bedtime *(221)*.

Absorption of nevirapine is not affected by food, and thus the drug can be taken without regard to meals *(210)*.

### Protease Inhibitors

Indinavir is known to be well absorbed after oral administration *(222)*, and the absolute bioavailability is approx 65% *(223)*. Eight healthy volunteers received indinavir with or without a high-fat meal consisting of eggs, toast, butter, bacon, whole milk, and hash browns *(68)*. The high-fat meal caused a reduction in the $C_{max}$ and AUC by 84 and 77%, respectively. A similar study in 12 healthy volunteers investigated the influence of various low-fat meals on the pharmacokinetics of indinavir. In this study, the meal consisted of toast, jelly, apple juice, coffee, skim milk, and sugar or cornflakes, sugar, and skim milk. These low-fat meals caused no significant reduction in the $C_{max}$ or AUC.

When indinavir is administered every 8 hours, it should be taken on an empty stomach (1 hour before or 2 hours after meals). Alternatively, administration with liquids such as skim milk, juice, coffee, tea, or a low-fat meal should not affect absorption. Indinavir should not be taken with or immediately after a heavy, high-fat meal (>2 g fat) *(210)*. Indinavir is metabolized by CYP3A4 enzymes in the liver and GI tract *(224)*. The addition of ritonavir, a known inhibitor of CYP3A4, at doses of 100–200 mg twice daily increases the AUC of indinivir by two- to threefold, respectively, and is not affected by the administration of food *(225)*. This pharmacokinetic interaction is advantageous because it eliminates the indinavir food restrictions and allows twice-daily dosing *(225)*. The manufacturer reports a decrease in the indinavir AUC by $26 \pm 18\%$ after a single 400-mg dose was administered to healthy volunteers with 8 oz single-strength grapefruit juice *(226)*.

Grapefruit juice and Seville orange juice have been used to evaluate the influence of intestinal CYP3A4 metabolism of CYP3A4 substrates *(227)*. Grapefruit juice seems to have the greatest effect on CYP3A4 substrates that undergo significant first-pass metabolism, particularly when bioavailability is less than 20% *(6)*. This is in contrast to two other studies in which the administration of grapefruit juice and Seville orange juice had no effect on the bioavailability of 800-mg doses of indinavir in HIV-infected patients and healthy volunteers *(227,228)*. Although double-strength grapefruit juice and Seville orange juice significantly delayed the $t_{max}$, no other significant differences in pharmacokinetic parameters were observed. These results are consistent with findings that, although indinavir undergoes extensive first-pass metabolism, intestinal metabolism accounts for less than 10% *(223)*. Grapefruit juice and Seville orange juice administration does not result in clinically significant changes in indinavir exposure *(227,228)*. To reduce the chance of nephrolithiasis, indinavir should be administered with plenty of liquids, thus increasing the solubility of the drug in urine *(68)*. Anecdotally, up to four large glasses of water or other liquid per day are recommended.

Saquinavir hard-gel capsule (Invirase®) has historically been poorly absorbed because of high first-pass metabolism and poor absorption, with an oral bioavailability of approx 4% *(229)*. Its bioavailability is improved with concomitant food consumption, particularly if given with high-fat meals. Administration of saquinavir with a high-fat meal can increase the bioavailability by approx 30% and increase the $C_{max}$ and AUC twofold *(229,230)*. Also, grapefruit juice increased the bioavailability and AUC by approximately twofold in eight healthy volunteers, which the authors attributed to inhibition of intestinal CYP3A4 *(231)*.

A saquinavir soft-gel capsule (Fortovase®) has also been approved for clinical use. This formulation, which utilizes the free base of saquinavir, as opposed to the mesylate salt, has improved the bioavailability by more than 300% *(232)*. As with the older formulation, the bioavailability of the newer formulation also improves with coadministration of food *(232)*. Thus, it is recommended that the older formulation of saquinavir be administered with a fatty snack; the newer, soft-gel formulation should be taken with food. When administered with a meal in ritonavir-boosted regimens, the plasma exposure with the hard-gel capsule formulation is similar to that observed with soft-gel capsules *(233,234)*. Because saquinavir is a substrate of CYP3A4 *(235)*, the effect of grapefruit juice on its bioavailability was evaluated. The administration of grapefruit juice to healthy volunteers increased the mean AUC of saquinavir hard-gel capsules by 50%, with large interindividual variability *(231)*.

**Table 11**
**HIV Antiretrovirals**

| Generic | Brand | Company | Manufacturer recommendations |
|---------|-------|---------|------------------------------|
| Nonnucleoside reverse transcriptase inhibitors | | | |
| • Delavirdine | Rescriptor tablets | Agouron | Can be given without regard to meals |
| • Nevirapine | Viramune tablets | Roxane | Can be given without regard to meals |
| • Efavirenz | Sustiva capsules, tablets | Bristol-Myers Squibb | Should be taken on an empty stomach, preferably at bedtime |
| Nucleoside reverse transcriptase inhibitors | | | |
| • Didanosine | Videx powder for oral solutions, buffered tablets | Bristol-Myers Squibb | Should be taken on an empty stomach, at least 30 minutes before or 2 hours after eating |
| | Videx EC capsules | Bristol-Myers Squibb | Should be taken on an empty stomach |
| • Zidovudine | Retrovir capsules, syrup | GlaxoSmithKline | May take with meals if GI upset occurs |
| | Retrovir tablets | GlaxoSmithKline | Not stated |
| • Lamivudine | Epivir oral solution, tablets | GlaxoSmithKline | Can be given without regard to meals |
| • Lamivudine/ Zidovudine | Combivir tablets | GlaxoSmithKline | Can be given without regard to meals |
| • Zalcitabine | Hivid tablets | Roche Laboratories | Can be given without regard to meals |
| • Stavudine | Zerit capsules, suspension | Bristol-Myers Squibb | Can be given without regard to meals |
| • Abacavir | Ziagen | GlaxoSmithKline | Can be given without regard to meals |
| • Abacavir/ lamivudine/ zidovudine | Trizivir tablets | GlaxoSmithKline | Can be given without regard to meals |
| • Emtricitabine | Emtriva capsules | Gilead | Can be given without regard to meals |
| • Tenofovir | Viread tablets | Gilead | Can be given without regard to meals |
| Protease inhibitors | | | |
| • Indinavir | Crixivan capsules | Merck | For optimal absorption, should be administered without food but with water 1 hour before or 2 hours after a meal |
| • Saquinavir | Invirase capsules | Roche | Take within 2 hours after a full meal |
| • Saquinavir soft gel cap | Fortovase capsules | Roche | Should be taken with a meal or up to 2 hours after a meal |
| • Ritonavir | Norvir capsules, oral solution | Abbott | Take with meals if possible |
| • Nelfinavir | Viracept tablets | Agouron | Should be taken with a meal |

*Continued on next page*

**Table 11** *(Continued)*
**HIV Antiretrovirals**

| Generic | Brand | Company | Manufacturer recommendations |
|---|---|---|---|
| • Amprenavir | Agenerase capsules | GlaxoSmithKline | Can be taken without regard to meals, but should not be taken with a high-fat meal |
| • Fosamprenavir | Lexiva tablets | GlaxoSmithKline | Can be taken without regard to meals |
| • Lopinavir/ ritonavir | Kaletra capsules | Abbott | Should be taken with food |
| • Atazanavir | Reyataz capsules | Bristol-Myers Squibb | Should be taken with food |

Nelfinavir appears to be well absorbed after oral administration, with a mean oral bioavailability ranging from 14 to 47% in various animal models *(232,236)*. Bioavailability in humans has not been studied, but increased drug concentrations were noted when the drug was taken concurrently with food. Nelfinavir AUC values in six fasted volunteers were 27 to 59% of those achieved in fed volunteers after administration of single 400- and 800-mg doses *(69)*. Thus, it is recommended that nelfinavir be administered with food.

Interestingly, administration of ritonavir with food appears to increase the absorption of the capsule while decreasing the absorption of the liquid formulation *(210)*. However, neither change is considered significant, and therefore it is recommended that ritonavir be given without regard to meals. However, it is most commonly administered with meals to improve GI tolerability.

The soft-gel capsule of amprenavir can be taken without regard to meals; however, it should not be taken with a high-fat meal *(237)*. To reduce the pill burden associated with amprenavir, a phosphate ester prodrug, fosamprenavir, has been approved. The administration of a high-fat meal had no influence on the AUC of fosamprenavir tablets compared to the fasting state. The $C_{max}$ was decreased by 12%. These changes are not considered clinically significant; fosamprenavir tablets can be taken without regard to meals *(67)*. In a randomized, crossover study of 12 healthy subjects, the coadministration of grapefruit juice did not significantly affect the pharmacokinetics of a single dose of amprenavir *(238)*.

The bioavailability of lopinavir/ritonavir capsules or liquid is increased with the administration of a meal moderate to high in fat *(239,240)*. There is also a clinically significant increase in the absorption of atazanavir when it is administered with food. After a single 400-mg dose, the AUC of atazanavir was increased by 35% with a light meal and by 70% with a high-fat meal *(241,242)*. The manufacturers' dosing recommendations for HIV antiretroviral antibiotics are shown in Table 11.

## NON-HUMAN IMMUNODEFICIENCY VIRUS ANTIVIRALS

The effect of a high-fat breakfast on the relative bioavailability of 1000 mg oral ganciclovir every 8 hours was assessed in 20 HIV-positive patients who were seroposi-

**Table 12**
**Non-HIV Antivirals**

| Generic | Brand | Company | Manufacturer recommendations |
|---------|-------|---------|------------------------------|
| Ganciclovir | Cytovene capsules | Roche | Administer with meals |
| Valgancicolovir | Valcyte tablets | Roche | Should be administered with food |
| Famciclovir | Famvir tablets | GlaxoSmithKline | Can be given without regard to meals |
| Valacyclovir | Valtrex caplets | Glaxo Wellcome | Can be given without regard to meals |
| Acyclovir | Zovirax capsules | Glaxo Wellcome | Can be given without regard to meals |
| | Zovirax sterile powder | Glaxo Wellcome | Can be given without regard to meals |
| | Zovirax suspension | Glaxo Wellcome | Can be given without regard to meals |
| | Zovirax tablets | Glaxo Wellcome | Can be given without regard to meals |
| Rimantadine | Flumadine syrup | Forest | Not stated |
| | Flumadine tablets | Forest | Not stated |
| Amantadine | Symmetrel capsules | Endo Labs | Not stated |
| | Symmetrel syrup | Endo Labs | Not stated |

tive for cytomegalovirus. $C_{max}$ and AUC were significantly increased, by 15 and 22%, respectively, with the presence of food, and it is recommended that ganciclovir be taken with food *(72)*. Because of the low bioavailability of ganciclovir, a prodrug has been developed, valganciclovir. The absolute bioavailability of oral valganciclovir is approx 10-fold higher than with oral ganciclovir *(243,244)*. Compared to the fasted state, the administration of valganciclovir with a standard breakfast increased the AUC by 23–57% depending on the dose administered *(74)*. Similar to oral ganciclovir, valganciclovir should be taken with food.

The effect of food was evaluated in two separate studies involving healthy volunteers given 250 or 500 mg famciclovir *(245,246)*. Administration with food decreased the $C_{max}$ by approx 53% and lengthened the $t_{max}$ by approx 2 hours. However, the AUC was unchanged in the fed-vs-fasting group, and the authors hypothesized that famciclovir could be given without regard to meals. Likewise, valacyclovir and the prototype, acyclovir, can be given without regard to meals *(247,248)*.

Amantadine and rimantadine can be taken without regard to meals *(73,249)*.

The manufacturers' dosing recommendations for non-HIV antiviral antibiotics are shown in Table 12.

## ANTI-INFECTIVES AND DISULFIRAMLIKE REACTIONS

The drug disulfiram (Antabuse®) is a therapeutic option in the treatment of alcoholism that acts to deter further ingestion of alcohol *(250)*. It works by inhibition of the enzyme aldehyde *(251,252)*. Disulfiram is a remarkably effective agent for inhibiting aldehyde dehydrogenase. Anecdotal reports have indicated local reactions in patients treated with disulfiram after using a beer-containing shampoo or contact lens solution

*(253,254)*. Indeed, a case report described a case of a women undergoing disulfiram therapy having a local vaginal reaction after engaging in sexual intercourse with her husband, who had ingested a large amount of alcohol *(255)*.

By the same mechanism, other compounds have been linked with causing a disulfiramlike reaction, and antibiotics are no exception. Cephalosporins, chloramphenicol, metronidazole, and other antibiotics have been associated with this reaction. In general, these reactions are rare and spontaneously occurring *(256)*. Although all patients should be counseled and warned of this potential interaction, it appears that patients who chronically consume large amounts of alcohol may be at higher risk of developing these reactions because of greater accumulation of acetaldehyde *(256)*. The likelihood of a reaction exists while the drug is still present in the body, and reactions have occurred with minimal amounts of alcohol up to a day after the last dose of an antibiotic *(257)*. Thus, generally it is recommended that patients abstain from alcohol during and for 2–3 days after therapy with any agents implicated in causing a disulfiramlike reaction.

### Signs and Symptoms

Patients experiencing a disulfiram reaction usually develop symptoms 5-10 minutes after consuming ethanol, and the reaction, assuming that no further alcohol is consumed, usually lasts from 30 minutes to several hours. In the majority of cases, symptoms are unpleasant but not life-threatening. However, a death has been reported that was attributed to a disulfiramlike reaction between alcohol and metronidazole *(258)*.

Reactions caused by the coingestion of alcohol and the drug disulfiram are manifested clinically by nausea, facial flushing, headache, tachycardia, and hypotension *(259,260)*. Disulfiramlike reactions caused by antibiotics present similarly *(261)*. Symptoms common to case reports describing a disulfiramlike reaction to antibiotics include tachycardia (up to 180 beats/minute), pronounced flushing of face and torso, and hypo- or hypertension. Headache, nausea, dizziness, and a feeling of enhanced intoxication are also common. Hypertension, as opposed to hypotension, which is normally seen with disulfiram reactions, is described in reactions with cephalosporins, especially moxalactam and cefoperazone, but this effect is not universal *(262,263)*. It has been hypothesized that this dichotomy is caused by inhibition of norepinephrine production by a metabolite of disulfiram, an effect that is not produced by cephalosporins *(264)*. However, this hypothesis is challenged by the fact that the hypotensive effect is also seen with other antialcohol drugs, such as cyanamide and coprine, which do not have an effect on norepinephrine.

### Metronidazole

Disulfiramlike reactions and a decreased desire to consume alcoholic beverages have been described with metronidazole *(265–267)*. In fact, it was suggested at one time that metronidazole may have a place in therapy as a preventative agent in the treatment of alcoholism *(268,269)*. However, studies using metronidazole in the treatment of alcoholism showed only minor beneficial effects, and metronidazole is not considered a therapeutic option in this area. Studies investigating the mechanism of the alcohol-metronidazole interaction published during the 1960s suggested that metronidazole noncompetitively inhibited liver alcohol dehydrogenase *(270)*. However, other studies in rats demonstrated that metronidazole did not act as an inhibitor for alcohol dehydrogenase. Authors have speculated that the disulfiramlike reaction with metronidazole might be mediated by the central nervous system *(271)*. Although rare, patients should still be informed about the possible disulfiramlike reaction when metronidazole is combined with alcohol.

### Cephalosporins

The majority of case reports and research involving disulfiramlike reactions and antimicrobials have focused on the cephalosporins and other β-lactams. Anecdotal reports have described a disulfiram reaction with cefmenoxime, cefotetan, cefoperazone, cefamandole, and moxalactam after the ingestion of an alcoholic beverage *(257,270,272–274)*. Other reactions have occurred in patients prescribed alcohol-containing medicinals and antibiotics. A case report described a hospitalized patient who was receiving moxalactam for presumed sepsis who had theophylline additionally prescribed for bronchospasm *(275)*. He received his dose of theophylline elixir (20% alcohol) and 30 minutes later became flushed and tremulous, hypotensive, and tachycardic. This reaction abated; however, the reaction reappeared when the patient was rechallenged with the theophylline elixir. His elixir was changed to tablets, and he continued to receive moxalactam without further incidents. Another case report described a similar incident in which the patient was receiving cefmenoxime and an alcohol-containing acetaminophen elixir *(257)*.

A number of studies in animal models and healthy volunteers have attempted to elucidate the mechanism and magnitude of disulfiramlike reactions with the cephalosporins *(259,261,276,277)*. In general, cephalosporins that have been implicated in causing a disulfiramlike reaction have in common a methyltetrazolethiol (MTT) side chain. Rats pretreated with β-lactams containing the MTT side chain experienced decreased alcohol elimination rates as well as increased acetaldehyde concentrations *(259,276)*. Those given β-lactams without the MTT side chain showed no such effect.

Volunteer trials have studied the potential of moxalactam, cefpirome, cefonicid, cefizoxime, and cefotetan to cause a disulfiramlike reaction when given with alcohol *(260,277–280)*. Patients given cefpirome or ceftizoxime, which do not contain a MTT side chain, and cefonicid, which contains methylsulfonic acid rather than a methyl group, displayed no signs or symptoms of a disulfiramlike reaction. No change in blood alcohol or aldehyde concentrations were observed in patients receiving cefpirome, ceftizoxime, or cefonicid. On the other hand, 5 of 8 and 2 of 10 volunteers given cefotetan or moxalactam, respectively, experienced a disulfiramlike reaction when combined with alcohol. Both these antibiotics contain the MTT side chain.

A hypothesis for the mechanism of this effect is that the MTT side chain becomes liberated from the rest of the cephalosporin molecule in vivo and is oxidized to a molecule that is structurally similar to disulfiram *(261)*. A study supporting this hypothesis demonstrated that the MTT side chain had no effect on the metabolizing capabilities of sheep liver cytoplasmic aldehyde dehydrogenase, but that a metabolite of the side chain was a potent inactivator *(261)*.

Thus, it appears that cephalosporins that contain the MTT side chain are at higher risk of precipitating a disulfiramlike reaction. Most case reports have involved patients receiving moxalactam, cefoperazone, and cefamondole; however, all cephalosporins with this side chain are likely to provide an increased risk *(281)*. All patients receiving these medications should be advised of the possibility of a disulfiramlike reaction. Chronic abusers of alcohol appear to be at the most risk of displaying a disulfiramlike reaction to these antibiotics, and an alternative agent may be prudent unless the patient can abstain from alcohol during therapy.

## Other Antibiotics

Isolated case reports have described disulfiramlike reactions with trimethoprim/ sulfamethoxazole, chloramphenicol, griseofulvin, or furazolidone when combined with alcohol *(256,282–284)*. Although most of these reports hypothesized that the reaction was secondary to an accumulation of acetaldehyde, the exact mechanism is unknown.

## Ritonavir Oral Solution

Ritonavir oral solution contains alcohol, and thus a potential interaction is possible when the solution is combined with disulfiram or anti-infectives associated with a disulfiramlike reaction *(285)*. It is advisable to avoid coadministration of disulfiram with ritonavir solution and to be aware of the potential interaction when ritonavir oral solution is coprescribed with metronidazole or cephalosporins containing the MTT side chain.

---

### CASE STUDY 1

K.R. is a 50-year-old male postal worker with a past medical history significant for hypertension and diabetes mellitus. He presents to his family physician with a 1-week history of a productive cough and decreased appetite. Chest X-ray and physical exam are consistent with community-acquired pneumonia. Sputum culture is positive for *Streptococcus pneumoniae*, which is sensitive to clarithromycin (among other agents). His physician prescribes Biaxin XL once daily for 2 weeks. After Day 3 of therapy, he returns to his physician's office without improvement in his symptoms. On speaking with the patient, his physician learns that he has not eaten a substantial amount of food for 2 days; he has primarily been drinking water. What is a likely cause of his therapeutic failure?

Although immediate-release clarithromycin can be taken without regard to meals, the extended-release formulation should be administered with food to enhance absorption *(26,116)*. Absorption of clarithromycin from the extended-release product was reduced by up to 30% when administered to healthy volunteers. Because this patient has not been eating, it is likely that he has been taking his Biaxin XL on an empty stomach, which may have reduced his exposure (AUC) of the medication to the causative organism(s).

---

### CASE STUDY 2

L.T. is a 34-year-old HIV-positive actor (CD4 = 39, undetectable viral load) currently prescribed 600 mg efavirenz at hour of sleep, 400 mg didanosine every morning, and 300 mg ZDV twice daily. His *Pneumocystis carinii* pneumonia prophylaxis of trimethoprim/sulfamethoxazole was changed to atovaquone secondary to development of a rash. He was counseled on the proper use of atovaquone and told to take it at the same time he takes his ZDV while continuing to take his didanosine 1 hour before breakfast on an empty stomach. Three months later,

L.T. was admitted to the hospital with PCP pneumonia. What is the likely reason for the failure of atovaquone?

Atovaquone has very poor bioavailability, and therapeutic concentrations may not be achieved when it is taken while fasting *(34)*. Food, especially fatty food, enhances the bioavailability of atovaquone three- to fourfold. On further questioning in the hospital, it was discovered that L.T. was taking his atovaquone with his evening dose of efavirenz and ZDV on an empty stomach, likely leading to subtherapeutic concentrations of atovaquone and clinical failure. Patients receiving atovaquone or other anti-infectives requiring food for optimal absorption should be specifically counseled concerning this interaction.

## REFERENCES

1. Welling PG. The influence of food on the absorption of antimicrobial agents. J Antimicrob Chemother 1982;9:7–27.
2. Yamreudeewong W, Henann NE, Fazio A, Lower DL, Cassidy TG. Drug–food interactions in clinical practice. J Fam Pract 1995;40:376–384.
3. Singh BN. Effects of food on clinical pharmacokinetics. Clin Pharmacokinet 1999;37: 213–255.
4. Krishnaswamy K. Drug metabolism and pharmacokinetics in malnourished children. Clin Pharmacokinet 1988;14:325–346.
5. Lown KS, Bailey DG, Fontana RJ, et al. Grapefruit juice increases felodipine oral availability in humans by decreasing intestinal CYP3A protein expression. J Clin Invest 1997; 99:2545–2553.
6. Bailey DG, Malcolm J, Arnold O, et al. Grapefruit-juice-drug interactions. Br J Clin Pharmacol 1998;46:101–110.
7. Dresser GK, Bailey DG, Leake BF, et al. Fruit juices inhibit organic anion transporting polypeptide-mediated drug uptake to decrease the oral availability of fexofenadine. Clin Pharmacol Ther 2002;71:120.
8. Takanaga H, Ohnishi A, Matsuo H, et al. Inhibition of vinblastine efflux mediated by P-glycoprotein by grapefruit juice components in caco-2 cells. Biol Pharm Bull 1998;21: 1062–1066.
9. Soldner A, Christians U, Susanto M, et al. Grapefruit juice activates P-glycoprotein-mediated drug transport. Pharm Res 1999;16:478–485.
10. Eshelman FN, Spyker DA. Pharmacokinetics of amoxicillin and ampicillin: crossover study of the effect of food. Antimicrob Agents Chemother 1978;14:539–543.
11. Staniforth DH, Lillystone RJ, Jackson D. Effect of food on the bioavailability and tolerance of clavulanic acid/amoxicillin combination. J Antimicrob Chemother 1982; 10:131–139.
12. Sommers DK, Van Wyk M, Moncrieff J, Schoeman HS. Influence of food and reduced gastric acidity on the bioavailability of bacampicillin and cefuroxime axetil. Br J Clin Pharmacol 1984;18:535–539.
13. Lode H, Stahlmann R, Koepp P. Comparative pharmacokinetics of cephalexin, cefaclor, cefadroxil, and CGP 9000.   Antimicrob Agents Chemother 1979;16:1–6.
14. Sourgens H, Derendorf H, Schifferer H. Pharmacokinetic profile of cefaclor. Int J Clin Pharmacol Ther 1997;35:374–380.
15. Barbhaiya RH, Shukla UA, Gleason CR, Shyu WC, Pittman KA. Comparison of the effects of food on the pharmacokinetics of cefprozil and cefaclor. Antimicrob Agents Chemother 1990;34:1210–1213.
16. Deppermann KM, Garbe C, Hasse K, Borner K, Keippe P, Lode H. Comparative pharmacokinetics of cefotiam hexetil, cefuroxime cefixime, cephalexin, and effect of H$_2$

blockers, standard breakfast and antacids on the bioavailability of cefuroxime hexetil. Twenty-ninth Interscience Conference on Antimicrobial Agents and Cemotherapy (ICAAC), September, 1989. Abstract 1223.

17. Roller S, Lode H, Stelzer I, Deppermann KM, Boeckh M, Koeppe P. Pharmacokinetics of loracarbef with acetylcysteine. Eur J Clin Microbiol Infect Dis 1992;11:851–855.
18. Nakashima M, Uematsu T, Takiguchi Y, Kanamaru M. Phase I study of cefixime, a new oral cephalosporin. J Clin Pharmacol 1987;27:425–431.
19. Li JT, Hou F, Lu H, et al. Phase I clinical trial of cefditoren pivoxil (ME 1207): pharmacokinetics in healthy volunteers. Drugs Exp Clin Res 1997;23:145–150.
20. Hughes GS, Heald DL, Barker KB, et al. The effects of gastric pH and food on the pharmacokinetics of a new oral cephalosporin, cefpodoxime proxetil. Clin Pharmacol Ther 1989;46:674–685.
21. Barr WH, Lin CC, Radwanski E, Lim J, Symchowicz S, Afrime M. The pharmacokinetics of ceftibuten in humans. Diagn Microbiol Infect Dis 1991;14:93–100.
22. Bechtol LD, Bessent CT, Perkal MB. The influence of food on the absorption of erythromycin esters and enteric-coated erythromycin in single-dose studies. Curr Ther Res 1979; 25:618–625.
23. Welling PG, Huang G, Hewitt PF, Lyons LL. Bioavailability of erythromycin stearate: influence of food and fluid volume. J Pharm Sci 1978;67:764–766.
24. Malmborg AS. Effect of food on absorption of erythromycin. A study of two derivatives, the stearate and the base. J Antimicrob Chemother 1979;5:591–599.
25. Foulds G, Luke DR, Teng R, Willavize SA, Friedman H, Curatolo WJ. The absence of an effect of food on the bioavailability of azithromycin administered as tablets, sachet, and suspension. J Antimicrob Chemother 1996;37(suppl C):37–44.
26. Chu S-Y, Park Y, Locke C, et al. Drug–food interaction potential of clarithromycin, a new macrolide antimicrobial. J Clin Pharmacol 1992;32:32–36.
27. Guay DR, Gustavson LE, Devcich KJ, et al. Pharmacokinetics and tolerability of extended-release clarithromycin. Clin Ther 2001;23:566–577.
28. Welling PG, Koch PA, Lau CC, Craig WA. Bioavailability of tetracycline and doxycycline in fasted and nonfasted subjects. Antimicrob Agents Chemother 1977;11:462–469.
29. Leyden JJ. Absorption of minocycline hydrochloride and tetracycline hydrochloride: effect of food, milk, and iron. J Am Acad Dermatol 1985;12(2 part 1):308–312.
30. Frost RW, Carlson JD, Dietz AJ Jr, Heyd A, Lettieri JT. Ciprofloxacin pharmacokinetics after a standard or high-fat/high- calcium breakfast. J Clin Pharmacol 1989;29:953–955.
31. Lehto PH, Kivisto KT. Effects of milk and food on the absorption of enoxacin. Br J Clin Pharmacol 1995;39:194–196.
32. Lacreta F, Kollia G, Duncan G, Behr D, Stoltz R, Grasela D. Effect of a high-fat meal in the bioavailability of gatifloxacin in healthy volunteers. 38th Interscience Conference on Antimicrobial Agents and Cemotherapy (ICAAC), September, San Diego, CA, September, 1998.
33. Mignot A, Guillaume M, Gohler K, et al. Oral bioavailability of gatifloxacin in healthy volunteers under fasting and fed conditions. Chemotherapy 2002;48:111–115.
34. Allen A, Bygate E, Clark D, et al. The effect of food on the bioavailability of oral gemifloxacin in healthy volunteers. Int J Antimicrob Agents 2000;16:45–50.
35. Lee LJ, Hafkin B, Lee ID, Hoh J, Dix R. Effects of food and sulcralfate on a single dose of 500 milligrams of levofloxacin in healthy subjects. Antimicrob Agents Chemother 1997;41:2196–2200.
36. Hooper WD, Dickinson RG, Eadie MJ. Effect of food on the absorption of lomefloxacin. Antimicrob Agents Chemother 1990;34:1797–1799.
37. Lettieri J, Vargas R, Agarwal V, et al. Effect of food on the pharmacokinetics of a single oral dose of moxifloxacin 400mg in healthy male volunteers. Clin Pharmacokinet 2001: 40(suppl 1):19–25.

38. Leroy A, Borsa F, Humbert G, et al. The pharmacokinetics of ofloxacin in healthy male volunteers. Eur J Clin Pharmacol 1987;31:629–630.
39. Shimada J, Nogita T, Ishibashi Y. Clinical pharmacokinetics of sparfloxacin. Clin Pharmacokinet 1993;25:358–369.
40. Hoppu K, Tuomisto J, Koskimies O, Simell O. Food and guar decrease absorption of trimethoprim. Eur J Clin Pharmacol 1987;32:427–429.
41. Nagy J, Schipper HG, Koopmans RP, et al. Effect of grapefruit juice or cimetidine coadministration on albendazole bioavailability. Am J Trop Med Hyg 2002;66:260–263.
42. Guzzo CA, Furtek CI, Porras AG, et al. Safety, tolerability, and pharmacokinetics of escalating high doses of ivermectin in healthy adult subjects. J Clin Pharmcol 2002;42: 1122–1133.
43. Castro N, Medina R, Sotelo J, et al. Bioavailability of praziquantel increases with concomitant administration of food. Antimicrob Agents Chemother 2000;44:2903–2904.
44. Mepron [package insert]. Research Triangle Park, NC: Glaxo Wellcome, 1998.
45. Welshman IR, Sisson TA, Jungbluth GL, et al. Linezolid absolute bioavailability and the effect of food on oral bioavailability. Biopharm Drug Dispos 2001;22:91–97.
46. Melander A, Kahlmeter G, Kamme C, Ursing B. Bioavailability of metronidazole in fasting and non-fasting healthy subjects and in patient's with Crohn's disease. Eur J Clin Pharmacol 1977;12:69–72.
47. Peloquin CA, Bulpitt AE, Jaresko GS, Jelliffe RW, Childs JM, Nix DE. Pharmacokinetics of ethambutol under fasting conditions with food and with antacids. Antimicrob Agents Chemother 1999;43:568–572.
48. Peloquin CA, Namdar R, Dodge AA, Nix DE. Pharmacokinetics of isoniazid under fasting conditions, with food and with antacids. Int J Tuberc Lung Dis 1999;3:703–710.
49. Peloquin CA, Bulpitt AE, Jaresko GS, Jelliffe RW, James GT, Nix DE. Pharmacokinetics of pyrazinamide under fasting conditions, with food, and with antacids. Pharmacotherapy 1998;18:1205–1211.
50. Narang PK, Lewis RC, Bianchine JR. Rifabutin absorption in humans: relative bioavailability and food effect. Clin Pharmacol Ther 1992;52:335–341.
51. Peloquin CA, Namdar R, Singleton MD, Nix DE. Pharmacokinetics of rifampin under fasting conditions, with food, and with antacids. Chest 1999;115:12–18
52. Bijanzadeh M, Mahmoudian M, Salehian P, et al. The bioavailability of griseofulvin from microsized and ultramicrosized tablets in non-fasting volunteers. Indian J Physiol Pharmacol 1990;34:157–161.
53. Barone JA, Moskovitz BL, Guarnieri J, et al. Food interaction and steady-state pharmacokinetics of intraconazole oral solution in healthy volunteers. Pharmacotherapy 1998;18: 295–301.
54. Zimmerman T, Yeates RA, Laufen H, et al. Influence of concomitant food intake on the oral absorption of two triazole antifungal agents, itraconazole and fluconazole. Eur J Clin Pharmacol 1994;46:147–150.
55. Lelawongs P, Barone JA, Colaizzi JL, et al. Effect of food and gastric acidity on absorption of orally administered ketoconazole. Clin Pharm 1988;7:228–235.
56. Purkins L, Wood N, Kleinermans D, et al. Effect of food on the pharmacokinetics of multiple-dose oral voriconazole. Br J Clin Pharmacol 2003;56:17–23.
57. Morse GD, Fischl MA, Cox SR, Thompson L, Della-Coletta AA, Freimuth WW. Effect of food on the steady-state pharmacokinetics of delavirdine mesylate in HIV[+] patients [abstract]. Program Abstracts, 35th Interscience Conference in Antimicrobial Agents and Chemotherapeutics (ICAAC), San Francisco, CA, September 17–20, 1995.
58. Hebel SK. Drugs Facts and Comparisons. St. Louis, MO: Facts and Comparisons, 2000.
59. Chittick GE, Gillotin C, McDowell JA, et al. Abacavir: absolute bioavailability, bioequivalence of three oral formulations, and effect of food. Pharmacotherapy 1999;19: 932–942.

60. Shuy WC, Knupp CA, Pittman KA, Dunkle L, Barbhaiya RH. Food-induced reduction in bioavailability of didanosine. Clin Pharmacol Ther 1991;50:503–507.

61. Damle BD, Yan JH, Behr D, et al. Effect of food on the oral bioavailability of didanosine from encapsulated enteric-coated beads. J Clin Pharmacol 2002;42:471–425.

62. Moore KH, Shaw S, Laurent AL, et al. Lamivudine/zidovudine as a combined formulation tablet: bioequivalence compared with lamivudine and zidovudine administered concurrently and the effect of food on absorption. J Clin Pharmacol 1999;39:593–605.

63. Kaul S, Christofalo B, Raymond RH, Stewart MB, Macleod CM. Effect of food on the bioavailability of stavudine in subjects with human immunodeficiency virus infection. Antimicrob Agents Chemother 1998;42:2295–2298.

64. Nazareno LA, Hotazo AA, Limjuco R, et al. The effect of food on pharmacokinetics of zalcitabine in HIV positive patients. Pharm Res 1995;12:1462–1465.

65. Shelton MJ, Portmore A, Blum MR, et al. Prolonged, but not diminished, zidovudine absorption induced by a high-fat breakfast. Pharmacotherapy 1994;14:671–677.

66. Nishiyama M, Koishi M, Fujioka M, et al. Phase I clinical trial with a novel protease inhibitor for HIV, KVX-478 in healthy male volunteers. Antiviral Res 1996;30:A35.

67. Falcoz C, Jenkins JM, Bye C, et al. Pharmacokinetics of GW433908, a prodrug of amprenavir, in healthy male volunteers. J Clin Pharamcol 2002;42:887–898.

68. Yeh KC, Deutsch PJ, Haddix H, et al. Single-dose pharmacokinetics of indinavir and the effect of food. Antimicrob Agents Chemother 1998;42:332–338.

69. Perry CM, Benfield P. Nelfinavir. Drugs 1997;54:81–87.

70. McEvoy GK. AHFS Drug Information. Bethesda, MD: American Society of Health System Pharmacists, 1999.

71. Pue MA, Benet LZ. Pharmacokinetics of famciclovir in man. Antiviral Chemistry Chemother 1993;4(suppl 1):47–55.

72. Lavelle J, Follansbee S, Trapnell CB, et al. Effect of food on the relative bioavailability of oral ganciclovir. J Clin Pharmacol 1996;36:238–241.

73. Wills RJ, Rodriguez LC, Choma N, Oakes M. Influence of a meal on the bioavailability of rimantadine HCL. J Clin Pharmacol 1987;27:821–823.

74. Brown F, Banken L, Saywell K, et al. Pharmacokinetics of valganciclovir and ganciclovir following multiple oral dosages of valganciclovir in HIV– and CMV-seropositive volunteers. Clin Pharmacokinet 1999;37:167–176.

75. Cronk GA, Wheatley WB, Fellers GF, Albright H. The relationship of food intake to the absorption of potassium alpha-phenoxyethyl penicillin and potassium phenoxymethyl penicillin from the gastrointestinal tract. Am J Med Sci 1960;240:219–225.

76. McCracken GH Jr, Ginsburg CM, Clahsen JC, Thomas ML. Pharmacologic evaluation of orally administered antibiotics in infants and children: effect of feeding on bioavailability. Pediatrics 1978;62:738–743.

77. Watanakunakorn C. Absorption of orally administered nafcillin in normal healthy volunteers. Antimicrob Agents Chemother 1977;11:1007–1009.

78. Ali HM, Farouk AM. The effect of Sudanese diet on the bioavailability of ampicillin. Int J Pharm 1980;6:301–306.

79. Welling PG, Huang H, Koch PA, Craig WA, Madsen PO. Bioavailability of ampicillin and amoxicillin in fasted and nonfasted subjects. J Pharm Sci 1977;66:549–552.

80. Neu HC. Antimicrobial activity and human pharmacology of amoxicillin. J Infect Dis 1974;129:S123–S131.

81. Augmentin tablets (amoxicillin/clavulanate potassium) [package insert]. Research Triangle Park, NC: GlaxoSmithKline, May 2002.

82. Augmentin suspension and chewable tablets (amoxicillin/clavulanate potassium) [package insert]. Research Triangle Park, NC: GlaxoSmithKline, January 2003.

83. Augmentin ES (amoxicillin/clavulanate potassium) [package insert]. Research Triangle Park, NC: GlaxoSmithKline, April 2003.

84. Augmentin XR (amoxicillin/clavulanate potassium) [package insert]. Research Triangle Park, NC: GlaxoSmithKline, November 2003.

85. Harvengt C, Schepper PD, Famy F, Hansen J. Cephradrine absorption and excretion in fasting and nonfasting volunteers. J Clin Pharmacol 1973;13:36–40.

86. Gower PE, Dash CH. Cephalexin: human studies of absorption and excretion of a new cephalosporin antibiotic. Br J Pharmacol 1969;37:738–747.

87. Tetzlaff TR, McCracken GH Jr, Thomas ML. Bioavailability of cephalexin in children: relationship to drug formulations and meals. J Pediatr 1978;92:292–294.

88. Glynne A, Goulbourn RA, Ryden R. A human pharmacology study of cefaclor. J Antimicrob Chemother 1978;4:343–348.

89. Sourgens H, Derendorf H, Schifferer H. Pharmacokinetic profile of cefaclor. Int J Clin Pharmacol Ther 1997;35:374–380.

90. Cefaclor [package insert]. Indianapolis, IN: Eli Lilly and Co., 1998.

91. Oguma T, Yamada H, Sawaki M, Narita N. Pharmacokinetic analysis of the effects of different foods on absorption of cefaclor. Antimicrob Agents Chemother 1991;35: 1729–1735.

92. Shukla UA, Pittman KA, Barbhaiya RH. Pharmacokinetic interactions of cefprozil with food, propantheline, metoclopramide, and probenecid in healthy volunteers. J Clin Pharmacol 1992;32:725–731.

93. Ginsburg CM, McCracken GH Jr, Petruska M, Olson K. Pharmacokinetics and bactericidal activity of cefuroxime axetil. Antimicrob Agents Chemother 1985;28:504–507.

94. Finn A, Straughn A, Meyer M, et al. Effect of dose and food on the bioavailability of cefuroxime axetil. Biopharm Drug Dispos 1987;8:519–526

95. Nelson JD, Shelton S, Kusmiesz H. Pharmacokinetics of LY163892 in infants and children. Antimicrob Agents Chemother 1988;32:1738–1739.

96. DeSante KA, Zeckel ML. Pharmacokinetic profile of loracarbef. Am J Med 1992;92 (suppl A):16S–19S.

97. Lorabid (loracarbef) [package insert]. Bristol, TN: Monarch Pharmaceuticals, September 2002.

98. Fassbender M, Lode H, Schaberg T, Borner K, Koeppe P. Pharmacokinetics of new oral cephalosporins, including a new carbacephem. Clin Infect Dis 1993;16:646–653.

99. Borin MT, Driver MR, Forbes KK. Effect of timing of food on absorption of cefpodoxime proxetil. J Clin Pharmacol 1995;35:505–509.

100. Nakashima M, Uematsu T, Takiguchi Y, et al. Phase I clinical studies of 7432-S, a new oral cephalosporin: safety and pharmacokinetics. J Clin Pharmacol 1988;28:246–252.

101. Faulkner RD, Bohaychuk W, Haynes JD, et al. The pharmacokinetics of cefixime in the fasted and fed state. Eur J Clin Pharmacol 1988;34:525–528.

102. Omnicef (cefdinir) [package insert]. North Chicago, IL: Abbott Laboratories, October 2001.

103. Guay DRP. Pharmacodynamics and pharmacokinetics of cefdinir, an oral extended spectrum cephalosporin. Pediatr Infect Dis J 2000;19:S141–S146.

104. Ueno K, Tanaka K, Tsujimura K, et al. Impairment of cefdinir absorption by iron ion. Clin Pharmacol Ther 1993;54:473–475.

105. Spectracef (cefditoren) [package insert]. Lake Forest, IL: TAP Pharmaceutical Products, 2001.

106. Kearns GL, Young RA. Ceftibuten pharmacokinetics and pharmacodynamics. Focus on paediatric use. Clin Pharmacokinet 1994;26:169–189.

107. Smith JW, Dyke RW, Griffith RS. Absorption following oral administration of erythromycin. JAMA 1953;151:805–810.

108. Hirsch HA, Finland M. Effect of food on the absorption of erythromycin propionate, erythromycin stearate and triacetyloleandomycin. Am J Med Sci 1959;237:693–708.

109. Clapper WE, Mostyn M, Meade GH. An evaluation of erythromycin stearate and propionyl erythromycin in normal and hospitalized subjects. Antibiotic Med Clin Ther 1960;7:91–96.

110. Hirsch HA, Finland M. Effect of food on absorption of a new form of erythromycin stearate and triacetyloleandomycin. Am J Med Sci 1959;239:198–202.

111. Thompson PJ, Burgess KR, Marlin GE. Influence of food on absorption of erythromycin ethylsuccinate. Antimicrob Agents Chemother 1980;18:829–831.

112. Coyne TC, Shum S, Chun ACH, Jeansonne L, Shirkey HC. Bioavailability of erythromycin ethylsuccinate in pediatric patients. J Clin Pharmacol 1978;18:192–202.

113. Ameer B, Weintraub RA. Drug Interactions with grapefruit juice. Clin Pharmacokinet 1997;33:103–121.

114. Kanazawa S, Ohkubo T, Sugawara K. The effects of grapefruit juice on the pharmacokinetics of erythromycin. Eur J Clin Pharmacol 2001;56:799–803.

115. Cheng KL, Nafziger AN, Peloquin CA, et al. Effect of grapefruit juice on clarithromycin pharmacokinetics. Antimicrob Agents Chemother 1998;42:927–929.

116. Biaxin XL (clarithromycin extended-release) [package insert]. North Chicago, IL: Abbott Laboratories, May 2003.

117. Hopkins S. Clinical toleration and safety of azithromycin. Am J Med 1991;91:40S–45S.

118. Thakker KM, Robarge L, Block S, Jefferson T, Broker R, Arrieta A. Pharmacokinetics of azithromycin oral suspension following 12 mg/kg/day (maximum 500 mg/day) for 5 days in fed pediatric patients. Thirty-eighth Interscience Conference on Antimicrobial Agents and Cemotherapy (ICAAC), San Diego, CA, September 24–27, 1998. Abstract A-59.

119. Sides GD, Cerimele BJ, Black HR, Busch U, DeSante KA. Pharmacokinetics of dirithromycin. J Antimicrob Chemother 1993;31(suppl C):65–75.

120. McConnell SA, Amsden GW. Review and comparison of advanced-generation macrolides clarithromycin and dirithromycin. Pharmacotherapy 1999;19:404–415.

121. Jonas M, Cunha BA. Minocycline. Ther Drug Monit 1982;4:137–145.

122. Mattila MJ, Neuvonen PJ, Gothoni G, Hackman R. Interference of iron preparations and milk with the absorption of tetracyclines. In: Baker SB, Neuhaus GA, eds. Toxicological Problems of Drug Combinations. Amsterdam, The Netherlands: Excerpta Medica, 1972, pp. 128–133.

123. von Wittenau MS. Some pharmacokinetic aspects of doxycycline metabolism in man. Chemother (Basel) 1968;13(suppl):41–50.

124. Cunha BA, Sibley CM, Ristuccia AM. Doxycycline. Ther Drug Monit 1982;4:125–135.

125. Kirby WMM, Roberts CE, Burdick RE. Comparison of two new tetracyclines with tetracycline and demethylchlortetracycline. Antimicrob Agents Chemother 1962;1961:286–292.

126. Poiger H, Schlatter C. Compensation of dietary induced reduction of tetracycline absorption by simultaneous administration of EDTA. Eur J Clin Pharmacol 1978;14:129–131.

127. Fabre J, Milek E, Kalfopoulos P, et al. The kinetics of tetracyclines in man. I. Digestive absorption and serum concentrations. Schweiz Med Wchr 1971;101:593–598.

128. Barr WH, Gerbracht LM, Letcher K, Plaut M, Strahl N. Assessment of the biologic availability of tetracycline products in man. Clin Pharmacol Ther 1971;13:97–108.

129. Rosenblatt JE, Barrett JE, Brodie JL, Kirby WMM. Comparison of in vitro activity and clinical pharmacology of doxycycline with other tetracyclines. Antimicrob Agents Chemother 1967;1966:134–141.

130. Meyer FP, Specht H, Quednow B, et al. Influence of milk on the bioavailability of doxycycline-new aspects. Infection 1989;17:245–246.

131. Allen JC. Minocycline. Ann Intern Med 1976;85:482–487.

132. Neuvonen PJ, Penttila O. Effect of oral ferrous sulphate on the half-life of doxycycline in man. Eur J Clin Pharmacol 1974;7:361–363.

133. Neuvonen PJ, Turakka H. Inhibitory effect of various iron salts on the absorption of tetracycline in man. Eur J Clin Pharmacol 1974;7:357–360.

134. Martin SJ, Meyer JM, Chuck SK, Jung R, Messick CR, Pendland SL. Levofloxacin and sparfloxacin: new quinolone antibiotics. Ann Pharmacother 1998;32:320–336.

135. Yamaguchi T, Yokogawa M, Sekine Y, Hashimoto M. Intestinal absorption characteristics of sparfloxacin. Xenobiotic Metab Disp 1991;6:53–59.

136. Heyd A, Shah A, Liu MC, Vaughan D, Heller AH. Oral bioavailability and efficacy of ciprofloxacin suspension for treatment of acute urinary tract infection. Thirty-eighth Interscience Conference on Antimicrobial Agents and Cemotherapy (ICAAC), San Diego, CA, September 24–27, 1998.

137. Shah A, Ming-Chung L, Vaughan D, et al. Oral bioequivalence of three ciprofloxacin formulations following single-dose administration: 500 mg tablet compared with 500 mg/10 mL or 500 mg/5 mL suspension and the effect of food on the absorption of ciprofloxacin oral suspension. J Antimicrob Chemother 1999;43(suppl A):49–54.

138. Cipro XR (ciprofloxacin extended-release) [package insert]. West Haven, CT: Bayer Pharmaceuticals Corp., 2003.

139. Bertino JS Jr, Nafziger AN, Wong M, Stragand L, Puleo C. Effect of a fat- and calcium-rich breakfast on pharmacokinetics of fleroxacin administered in single and multiple doses. Antimicrob Agents Chemother 1994;38:499–503.

140. Tequin (gatifloxacin) [package insert]. Princeton, NJ: Bristol-Meyers Squibb Co., October 2003.

141. Nakashima M, Uematsu T, Kosuge K, et al. Single- and multiple-dose pharmacokinetics of AM-1155, a new 6-fluoro-8-methoxy quinolone, in humans. Antimicrob Agents Chemother 1995;39:2635–2640.

142. Ballow C, Lettieri J, Agarwal V, et al. Absolute bioavailability of moxifloxacin. Clin Ther 1999;21:513–522.

143. Factive (gemifloxacin) [package insert]. Genesoft Pharmaceuticals, Seoul, Korea, 2003.

144. Hoogkamer JFW, Klenbloesem CH. The effect of milk consumption on the pharmacokinetics of fleroxacin and ciprofloxacin in healthy volunteers. Drugs 1995;49(suppl 2):346–348.

145. Neuvonen PJ, Kivisto KT, Lehto P. Interference of dairy products with the absorption of ciprofloxacin. Clin Pharmacol Ther 1991;50(5 Pt 1):498–502.

146. Minami R, Inotsume N, Nakano M, Sudo Y, Higashi A, Matsuda I. Effect of milk on absorption of norfloxacin in healthy volunteers. J Clin Pharmacol 1993;33:1238–1240.

147. Kivisto KT, Ojala-Karlsson P, Neuvonen PJ. Inhibition of norfloxacin absorption by dairy products. Antimicrob Agents Chemother 1992;36:489–491.

148. Stass H, Kubitza D. Study to assess the interaction between moxifloxacin and dairy products in healthy volunteers. Second European Congress of Chemotherapy and Seventh Biennial Conference of Antiinfective Agents and Chemotherapy, Hamburg, Germany, May 10–13, 1998.

149. Dudley MN, Marchbanks CR, Flor SC, Beals B. The effect of food or milk on the absorption kinetics of ofloxacin. Eur J Clin Pharmacol 1991;41:569–571.

150. Food and Drug Administration. Food-effect bioavailability and fed bioequivalence studies: study design, data analysis, and labeling. Draft guidance for industry. Bethesda, MD: US Department of Health and Human Services, Food and Drug Administration, Center for Drug Evaluation and Research, 2001.

151. Wallace AW, Victory JM, Amsden GW. Lack of bioequivalence when levofloxacin and calcium-fortified orange juice are coadministered to healthy volunteers. J Clin Pharmcol 2003;43:539–544.

152. Aminimanizani A, Beringer P, Jelliffe R. Comparative pharmacokinetics and pharmacodynamics of the newer fluoroquinolone antibacterials. Clin Pharmacokinet 2001;40:169–187.

153. Neuhofel AL, Wilton JH, Victory JM, et al. Lack of bioequivalence of ciprofloxacin when administered with calcium-fortified orange juice: a new twist on an old interaction. J Clin Pharmacol 2002;42:459–464.

154. Wallace AW, Victory JM, Amsden GW. Lack of bioequivalence of gatifloxacin when coadministered with calcium-fortified orange juice in healthy volunteers. J Clin Pharmacol 2003;43:92–96.

155. Amsden GW, Whitaker AM, Johnson PW. Lack of bioequivalence of levofloxacin when coadministered with a mineral-fortified breakfast of juice and cereal. J Clin Pharmacol 2003;43:990–995.

156. Yamaguchi H, Yano I, Saito H, et al. Pharmacokinetic role of P-glycoprotein in oral bioavailability and intestinal secretion of grepafloxacin in vivo. J Pharmacol Exp Ther 2002; 300:1063–1069.

157. Takanaga H, Ohnishi A, Yamada S, et al. Polymethoxylated flavones in orange juice are inhibitors of P-glycoprotein but not cytochrome P450 3A4. J Pharmacol Exp Ther 2000; 293:230–236.

158. Fuhr U, Anders EM, Mahr G, Sorgel F, Staib AH. Inhibitory potency of quinolone antibacterial agents against cytochrome P4501A2 activity in vivo and in vitro. Antimicrob Agents Chemother 1992;36:942–948.

159. Staib AH, Stille W, Dietlein G, et al. Interaction between quinolones and caffeine. Drugs 1987;34(suppl 1):170–174.

160. Randinitis JR, Koup G, Rausch G, Vassos AB. Effect of clinafloxacin administration on the single-dose pharmacokinetics of theophylline and caffeine. Thirty-eighth Interscience Conference on Antimicrobial Agents and Cemotherapy (ICAAC), San Diego, CA, September 24–27, 1998. Abstract A-19.

161. Carbo M, Segura J, De la Torre R, Badenas JM, Cami J. Effect of quinolones on caffeine disposition. Clin Pharmacol Ther 1989;45:234–240.

162. Healy DP, Polk RE, Kanawati L, Rock DT, Mooney ML. Interaction between oral ciprofloxacin and caffeine in normal volunteers. Antimicrob Agents Chemother 1989;33:474–478.

163. Staib AH, Harder S, Mieke S, Beer C, Stille W, Shah P. Gyrase-inhibitors impair caffeine elimination in man. Meth Find Exp Clin Pharmacol 1987;9:193–198.

164. Mueller BA, Brierton DG, Abel SR, Bowman L. Effect of enteral feeding with ensure on oral bioavailabilies of ofloxacin and ciprofloxacin. Antimicrob Agents Chemother 1994;38:2101–2105.

165. Yuk JH, Nightingale CH, Sweeney K, et al. Relative bioavailability in healthy volunteers of ciprofloxacin administered through a nasogastric tube with and without enteral feeding. Antimicrob Agents Chemother 1989;33:1118–1120.

166. Healy DP, Brodbeck MC, Clendening CE. Ciprofloxacin absorption is impaired in patients given enteral feedings orally and via gastrostomy and jejunostomy tubes. Antimicrob Agents Chemother 1996;41:6–10.

167. Kanji S, McKinnon PS, Barletta JF, et al. Bioavailability of gatifloxacin by gastric tube administration with and without concomitant enteral feeding in critically ill patients. Crit Care Med 2003;31:1347–1352.

168. Deppermann KM, Lode H. Fluoroquinolones: interaction profile during enteral absorption. Drugs 1993;45(suppl 3):65–72.

169. D'Arcy PF. Nitrofurantoin. Drug Intell Clin Pharm 1985;19:540–547.

170. Bates TR, Sequeira JA, Tembo AV. Effect of food on nitrofurantoin absorption. Clin Pharm Ther 1974;16:63–68.

171. Rosenberg HA, Bates TR. The influence of food on nitrofurantoin bioavailability. Clin Pharm Ther 1976;20:227–232.

172. Falloon, J, Sargent S, Piscitelli SC, et al. Atovaquone suspension in HIV-infected volunteers: pharmacokinetics, pharmacodynamics, and TMP-SMX interaction study. Pharmacotherapy 1999;19:1050–1056.

173. Albenza (albendazole) [package insert]. Research Triangle Park, NC: GlaxoSmithKline, September 2001.

174. Lange H, Eggers R, Bircher J. Increased systemic availability of albendazole when taken with a fatty meal. Eur J Clin Pharmacol 1988;34:315–317.

175. Stromectol (Ivermectin) [package insert]. Whitehouse Station, NJ: Merck and Co., October 2003.

176. Biltricide (praziquantel) [package insert]. West Haven, CT: Bayer Pharmaceuticals Corp., November 2003.

177. Castro N, Jung H, Medina R, et al. Interaction between grapefruit juice and praziquantel in humans. Antimicrob Agents Chemother 2002;46:1614–1616.

178. Cleocin [package insert]. Kalamazoo, MI: Pharmacia and Upjohn, 1998.

179. McGehee RF, Smith CB, Wilcox C, Finland M. Comparative studies of antibacterial activity in vitro and absorption and excretion of lincomycin and clinimycin. Am J Med Sci 1968;256:279–292.

180. Zyvox (linezolid) [package insert]. Kalamazoo, MI: Pharmacia and Upjohn Company, January 2002.

181. Martin JP, Herberg, JT, Slatter JG, et al. Although a novel microtier-plate assay demonstrates that linezolid (PNU-100766) is a weak, competitive (reversible) inhibitor of human monoamine oxidase (MAO A), no clinical evidence of MAO A inhibition in clinical trials has been observed. Paper presented at the 38th Interscience Conference on Antimicrobial Agents and Chemotherapy, San Diego, CA, September 1998.

182. Antal EJ, Hendershot PE, Batts DH, et al. Linezolid, a novel oxazolidinone antibiotic: assessment of monoamine oxidase inhibition using pressor response to oral tyramine. J Clin Pharmacol 2001;41:552–562.

183. Melander A, Danielson K, Hanson A, et al. Reduction of isoniazid bioavailability in normal men by concomitant intake of food. Acta Med Scand 1976;200:93–97.

184. Self TH, Chrisman CR, Baciewicz AM, et al. Isoniazid drug and food interactions. Am J Med Sci 1999;317:304–311.

185. Smith CK, Durack DT. Isoniazid and reaction to cheese. Ann Intern Med 1978;88:520–521.

186. Huser MJ, Baier H. Interactions of isoniazid with foods. Drug Intell Clin Pharm 1982;16: 617–618.

187. Baciewicz AM, Self TH. Isoniazid interactions. South Med J 1985;78:714–718.

188. Siegler DI, Bryant M, Burley DM, Citron KM, Standen SM. Effect of meals on rifampicin absorption. Lancet 1974;2:197–198.

189. Ameer B, Polk RE, Kline BJ, Grisafe JP. Effect of food on ethambutol absorption. Clin Pharm 1982;1:156–158.

190. Daneschmend TK, Warnock DW, Ene MD, et al. Influence of food on the pharmacokinetics of ketoconazole. Antimicrob Agent Chemother 1984;25:1–3.

191. Mannisto PT, Mantyla R, Nykanen S. Lamminsivu U, Ottoila P. Impairing effect of food on ketoconazole absorption. Antimicrob Agent Chemother 1982;21:730–733.

192. Brass C, Galgiani JN, Blaschke TF, et al. Disposition of ketoconazole, an oral antifungal in humans. Antimicrob Agents Chemother 1982;21:151–158.

193. Wishart JM. The influence of food on the pharmacokinetics of itraconazole in patients with superficial fungal infections. J Am Acad Dermatol 1987;17:220–223.

194. Lange D, Pavao JH, Klausner M. Effect of a cola beverage on the bioavailability of $H_2$ blockers. J Clin Pharmacol 1997;37:535–540.

195. Jaruratanasirikul S, Kleepkaew A. Influence of an acidic beverage (Coca-Cola) on the absorption of itraconazole. Eur J Clin Pharmacol 1997;52:235–237.

196. Crounse RG. Human pharmacology of griseofulvin: the effect of fat intake on gastrointestinal absorption. J Invest Dermatol 1961;37:529.

197. Hartman NR, Yarchoan R, Pluda JM, et al. Pharmacokinetics of 2',3'-dideoxy-adenosine and 2',3'-dideoxyinosine in patients with severe human immunodeficiency virus infection. Clin Pharmacol Ther 1990;47:647–654.

198. Knupp CA, Shyu WC, Dolin R, et al. Pharmacokinetics of didanosine in patients with acquired immunodeficiency syndrome-related complex. Clin Pharmacol Ther 1991;49: 523–535.

199. McGowan JJ, Tomaszewski JE, Cradock J, et al. Overview of the preclinical development of an antiretroviral drug, 2',3'-dideoxyinosine. Rev Infect Dis 1990;12(suppl 5):S513–S520.

200. Knupp CA, Milbrath R, Barbhaiya RH. Effect of time of food administration on the bioavailability of didanosine from a chewable tablet formulation. J Clin Pharmacol 1993; 33:568–573.

201. Damle BD, Kaul S, Behr D, et al. Bioequivalence of two formulations of didanosine, encapsulated enteric-coated beads and buffered tablet, in healthy volunteers and HIV-infected subjects. J Clin Pharmacol 2002;42:791–797.

202. Videx EC (didanosine) [package insert]. Princeton, NJ: Bristol-Meyers Squibb Co., February 2003.

203. Klecker RW Jr, Collins JM, Yarchoan R, et al. Plasma and cerebrospinal fluid pharmacokinetics of 3ɔ-azido-3ɔdeoxythymidine: a novel pyrimidine analog with potential application for the treatment of patients with AIDS and related diseases. Clin Pharmacol Ther 1987;41:407–412.

204. Unadkat JD, Collier AC, Crosby SS, Cummings D, Opheim KE, Corey L. Pharmacokinetics of oral zidovudine (azidothymidine) in patients with AIDS when administered with and without a high-fat meal. AIDS 1990;4:229–232.

205. Sahai J, Gallicano K, Garber G, et al. The effect of a protein meal on zidovudine pharmacokinetics in HIV-infected patients. Br J Clin Pharmacol 1992;33:657–660.

206. Lotterer E, Ruhnke M, Trautmann M, Beyer R, Bauer FE. Decreased and variable systemic availability of zidovudine in patients with AIDS if administered with a meal. Eur J Clin Pharmacol 1991;40:305–308.

207. Angel JB, Hussey EK, Mydlow PK, et al. Pharmacokinetics of (GR 109714X) 3TC administered with and without food to HIV-infected patients. Inf Conf AIDS 1992;8: B88. Abstract PoB 3008.

208. Shelton MJ, O'Donnell AM, Morse GD. Zalcitabine. Ann Pharmacother 1993;27:480–489.

209. Dudley MN, Graham KK, Kaul S, et al. Pharmacokinetics of stavudine in patients with AIDS or AIDS-related complex. J Infect Dis 1992;166:480–485.

210. Kaul S, Christofalo B, Raymond RH, Stewart MB, Macleod CM. Effect of food on the bioavailability of stavudine in subjects with human immunodeficiency virus infection. Antimicrob Agents Chemother 1998;42:2295–2298

211. Foster RH, Faulds D. Abacavir. Drugs 1998; 55:729–736.

212. Yuen GJ, Lou Y, Thompson NF, et al. Abacavir/lamivudine/zidovudine as a combined formulation tablet: bioequivalence compared with each component administered concurrently and the effect of food on absorption. J Clin Pharmacol 2001;41: 277–288.

213. Emtriva (emtricitabine) [package insert]. Gilead Sciences, Foster City, July 2003.

214. Viread (tenofovir disoproxil fumarate) [package insert]. Gilead Sciences, Foster City, October 2003.

215. Barditch-Crovo P, Deeks SG, Collier A, et al. Phase I/II trial of the pharmacokinetics, safety, and antiretroviral activity of tenofovir disoproxil fumarate in human immunodeficiency virus-infected adults. Antimicrob Agents Chemother 2001;45:2733–2739.

216. Kearney BP, Flaherty J, Wolf J, et al. Coadministration of tenofovir DF and didanosine: a pharmacokinetic and safety evaluation. Presented at the Eighth European Conference on Clinical Aspects and Treatment of HIV Infection, Athens, October 2001. Poster 172.

217. Kearney BP, Damle B, Plummer A, et al. Pharmacokinetic evaluation of tenofovir DF and enteric-coated didanosine. Fourteenth International AIDS Conference, Barcelona, Spain, July 2002. Abstract B10396.

218. Kearney BP, Isaacson E, Sayre J, et al. Didanosine and tenofovir DF drug-drug interaction: assessment of didanosine dose reduction. Presented at the Tenth Conference on Retroviruses and Opportunistic Infections, Boston, MA, February 2003. Poster 533.

219. Pecora Fulco P, Kirian MA. Effect of tenofovir on didanosine absorption in patients with HIV. Ann Pharmacother 2003;37:1325–1328.

220. Freimuth WW. Delavirdine mesylate, a potent non-nucleoside HIV-1 reverse transcriptase inhibitor. In: Mills J, Volberding PA, Corey L, eds. Antiviral Chemotherapy. Vol. 4. New York: Plenum, 1996, pp. 279–389.

221. Sustiva (efavirenz) [package insert]. Princeton, NJ: Bristol-Meyers Squibb Co., June 2003.

222. Moyle G, Gazzard B. Current knowledge and future prospects for the use of HIV protease inhibitors. Drugs 1996;51:701–712.

223. Williams GC, Sinko PJ. Oral absorption of the HIV protease inhibitors: a current update. Adv Drug Deliv Rev 1999;39:211–238.

224. Chiba M, Hensleigh M, Nishime JA, et al. Role of cytochrome P450 3A4 in human metabolism of MK-639, a potent human immunodeficiency virus protease inhibitor. Drug Metab Dispos 1996;24:307–314.

225. Saah AJ, Winchell GA, Nessly ML, et al. Pharmacokinetic profile and tolerability of indinavir-ritonavir combinations in healthy volunteers. Antimicrob Agents Chemother 2001;45:2710–2715.

226. Crixivan (indinavir sulfate) [package insert]. Whitehouse Station, NJ: Merck and Company, January 2003.

227. Penzak SR, Acosta EP, Turner M, et al. Effect of Seville orange juice and grapefruit juice on indinavir pharmacokinetics. J Clin Pharmacol 2002;42:1165–1170.

228. Shelton MJ, Wynn HE, Hewitt RG, et al. Effects of grapefruit juice on pharmacokinetic exposure to indinavir in HIV-positive subjects. J Clin Pharmacol 2001;41:435–442.

229. Noble S, Faulds D. Saquinavir: a review of its pharmacology and clinical potential in the management of HIV infection. Drugs 1996;52:93–112.

230. Muirhead GJ, Shaw T, Williams PEO, et al. Pharmacokinetics of the HIV-proteinase inhibitor, Ro 318959, after single and multiple oral doses in healthy volunteers. Br J Clin Pharmacol 1992;34:170P.

231. Kupferschmidt HH, Fattinger KE, Ha HR, Follath F, Krahenbuhl S. Grapefruit juice enhances the bioavailability of the HIV protease inhibitor saquinavir in man. Br J Clin Pharmacol 1998;45:355–359.

232. Beach JW. Chemotherapeutic agents for human immunodeficiency virus infection: mechanism of action, pharmacokinetics, metabolism, and adverse reactions. Clin Ther 1998: 20:2–25.

233. Kurowski M, Sternfeld T, Sawyer A, et al. Pharmacokinetic and tolerability profile of twice-daily saquinavir hard gelatin capsules and saquinavir soft gelatin capsules boosted with ritonavir in healthy volunteers. HIV Med 2003;4:94–100.

234. Cardiello PG, Monhaphol T, Mahanontharit A, et al. Pharmacokinetics of once-daily saquinavir hard-gelatin capsules and saquinavir soft-gelatin capsules boosted with ritonavir in HIV-1-infected subjects. J Acquir Immune Defic Syndr 2003;32:375–379.

235. Fitzsimmons ME, Collins JM. Selective biotransformation of the human immunodeficiency virus protease inhibitor saquinavir by human small-intestinal cytochrome P4503A4: potential contribution to high first-pass metabolism. Drug Metab Dispos 1997;25:256–266.

236. Shetty BV, Kosa MB, Khalil DA, Webber S. Preclinical pharmacokinetics and distribution to tissue of AG1343, an inhibitor of human immunodeficiency virus type 1 protease. Antimicrob Agents Chemother 1996;40:110–114.

237. Agenerase(amprenavir) [package insert]. Research Triangle Park, NC: GlaxoSmithKline, October 2002.

238. Demarles D, Gillotin C, Bonaventure-Paci S, et al. Single-dose pharmacokinetics of amprenavir coadministered with grapefruit juice. Antimicrob Agents Chemother 2002;46: 1589–1590.

239. Kaletra (lopinavir/ritonavir) [package insert]. North Chicago, IL: Abbott Laboratories, January 2003.

240. Gustavson L, Lam W, Bertz R, et al. Assessment of the bioequivalence and food effects for liquid and soft elastic capsule co-formulations of ABT-378/ritonavir (ABT-378/r) in

healthy subjects [poster]. Presented at the Fortieth Interscience Conference on Antimicrobial Agents and Chemotherapy, Toronto, Ontario, Canada, September 2000.

241. Reyataz (atazanavir sulfate) [package insert]. Princeton, NJ: Bristol-Meyers Squibb Co., June 2003.

242. O'Mara E, Mummaneni V, Randall D, et al. BMS-232632: A summary of multiple dose pharmacokinetic, food effect and drug interaction studies in healthy subjects. Presented at the Seventh Conference on Retroviruses and Opportunistic Infections. Available at Website: www.retroconference.org/2000/abstracts/504.htm.

243. Pescovitz MD, Rabkin J, Merion RM, et al. Valganciclovir results in improved oral absorption of ganciclovir in liver transplant recipients. Antimicrob Agents Chemother 2000;44:2811–2815.

244. Jung D, Dorr A. Single-dose pharmacokinetics of valganciclovir in HIV- and CMV-seropositive subjects. J Clin Pharmacol 1999;39:800–804.

245. Fowles SE, Fairless AJ, Pierce DM, et al. A further study of the effect of food on the bioavailability and pharmacokinetics of penciclovir after oral administration of famciclovir. Br J Clin Pharmacol 1991;32:657P.

246. Fowles SE, Pierce MC, Prince WT, et al. Effect of food on the bioavailability and pharmacokinetics of penciclovir, a novel antiherpes agent, following oral administration of the prodrug, famciclovir. Br J Clin Pharmacol 1990;29:620P–621P.

247. Acosta EP, Fletcher CV. Valacyclovir. Ann Pharmacother 1997;31:185–191.

248. Zovirax [package insert]. Research Triangle Park, NC: Glaxo Wellcome, 1998.

249. Aoki FY, Sitar DS. Clinical pharmacokinetics of amantadine hydrochloride. Clin Pharmacokinet (DG5), 1988;14:35–51.

250. Fuller RK, Roth HP. Disulfiram for the treatment of alcoholism: an evaluation in 128 men. Ann Intern Med 1979;90:901–904.

251. Kitson TM. The disulfiram-ethanol reaction. J Stud Alcohol 1977;38:96–113.

252. Jungnickel PW, Hunnicutt DM. Alcohol abuse. In: Young LY, Koda-Kimble MA, eds. Applied Therapeutics: The Clinical Use of Drugs. 6th Ed. Vancouver, WA: Applied Therapeutics, 1995, pp. 7–8.

253. Stoll K, King LE. Disulfiram-alcohol skin reaction to beer-containing shampoo. JAMA 1980;244:2045.

254. Refojo MF. Disulfiram-alcohol reaction caused by contact lens wetting solution. Contact Intraocul Lens Med J 1981;7:172.

255. Chick JD. Disulfiram reaction during sexual intercourse. Br J Psychiatry 1988;152:438.

256. Adams WL. Interactions between alcohol and other drugs. Int J Addict 1995;30:1903–1923.

257. Kannangara DW, Gallagher K, Lefrock JL. Disulfiram-like reactions with newer cephalosporins: cefmenoxime. Am J Med Sci 1984;287:45–47.

258. Cina SJ, Russell RA, Conrad SE. Sudden death due to metronidazole/ethanol interaction. Am J Forensic Med Pathol 1996;17:343–346.

259. Freundt KJ, Heiler C, Schreiner E. Ferrous sulfate combined with ascorbic acid does not significantly reduce acetaldehyde accumulation in the blood of alcoholized rats treated with disulfiram or betalactam antibiotics. Alcohol 1990;7:295–298.

260. Elenbaas RM, Ryan JL, Robinson WA, Singsank MJ, Harvey JM, Klaassen CD. On the disulfiram-like activity of moxalactam. Clin Pharmacol Ther 1982; 32:347–355.

261. Kitson TM. The effect of 5,5ɔ-dithiobis(1-methyltetrazole) on cytoplasmic aldehyde dehydrogenase and its implications for cephalosporin-alcohol reactions. Alcoholism: Clin Exp Res 1986;10:27–32.

262. McMahon FG. Disulfiram-like reaction to a cephalosporin. JAMA 1980;243:2397.

263. Neu HC, Prince AS. Interaction between moxalactam and alcohol. Lancet 1980;1:1422.

264. Kitson TM. The effect of cephalosporin antibiotics on alcohol metabolism: a review. Alcohol 1987;4:143–148.

265. Itil TM, Holden JM, Keskiner A, Shapiro D. Central effects of metronidazole. Psychiatr Res Rep Am Psychiatr Assoc. 1968 Mar;24:148–165.
266. Seixas FA. Alcohol and its drug interactions. Ann Intern Med 1975;83:86–92.
267. Campbell B, Taylor JAT, Haslett Wl. Anti-alcohol properties of metronidazole in rats. Proc Soc Exp Biol Med 1965;124:191–195.
268. Taylor JT. Metronidazole-a new agent for combined somatic and psychic therapy of alcoholism. Los Angeles Neurol Soc Bull 1964;29:158.
269. Penick SB, Carrier RN, Sheldon JB. Metronidazole in the treatment of alcoholism. Am J Psychiatry 1969;125:1063–1066.
270. Edwards JA, Price J. Metronidazole and human alcohol dehydrogenase. Nature 1967;214:190–191.
271. Kalant H, LeBlanc AE, Guttman M. Metabolic and pharmacologic interaction of ethanol and metronidazole in the rat. Can J Physiol Pharmacol 1972;50:476–484.
272. Foster TS, Raehl CL, Wilson HD. Disulfiram-like reaction associated with a parenteral cephalosporin. Am J Hosp Pharm 1980;7:858–859.
273. Umeda S, Arai T. Disulfiram-like reaction to moxalactam after celiac plexus alcohol block. Anesth Analg 1985;64:377.
274. Buening MK, Wold JS, Israel KS, et al. Disulfiram-like reaction to β-lactams [letter]. JAMA 1981;245:2027.
275. Brown KR, Guglielmo BJ, Pons VG, Jacobs RA. Theophylline elixir, moxalactam, and a disulfiram reaction. Ann Intern Med 1982;97:621–622.
276. Shimada J, Miyahara T, Otsubo S, Yoshimatsu N, Oguma T, Matsubara T. Effects of alcohol-metabolizing enzyme inhibitors and β-lactam antibiotics on ethanol elimination in rats. Jpn J Pharmacol 1987;45:533–544.
277. Kline SS, Mauro VF, Forney RB Jr, Freimer EH, Somani P. Cefotetan-induced disulfiram-type reactions and hypoprothrombinemia. Antimicrob Agents Chemother 1987;31:1328–1331.
278. Lassman HB, Hubbard JW, Chen BL, Puri SK. Lack of interaction between cefpirome and alcohol. J Antimicrob Chemother 1992;29(suppl 1):47–50.
279. McMahon FG, Ryan JR, Jain AK, LaCorte W, Ginzler F. Absence of disulfiram-type reactions to single and multiple doses of cefonicid: a placebo-controlled study. J Antimicrob Chemother 1987;20:913–918.
280. McMahon FG, Noveck RJ. Lack of disulfiram-like reactions with ceftizoxime. J Antimicrob Chemother 1982;10(suppl C):129–133.
281. Uri JV, Parks DB. Disulfiram-like reaction to certain cephalosporins. Ther Drug Monit 1983;5:219–224.
282. Heelon MW, White M. Disulfiram-cotrimoxazole reaction. Pharmacother 1998;18:869–870.
283. Azarnoff DL, Hurwitz A. Drug interactions. Pharmacol Physicians 1970;4:1–7.
284. Todd RG, ed. Extra Pharmacopoeia-Martindale. 25th Ed. London: Pharmaceutical Press, 1967, pp. 844–845.
285. Norvir Oral Solution [package insert]. Abbott Park, IL: Abbott Laboratories, 1998.

# 13
# Drug–Cytokine Interactions

## Curtis E. Haas and Jamie L. Nelsen

## INTRODUCTION

The term *drug–cytokine interaction* was proposed to describe the interactions between the mediators of the acute-phase response (APR) and drug metabolism *(1)*. This potential for drug–cytokine interactions has been appreciated in the laboratory since at least 1966 *(2)* and in clinical practice since the late 1970s *(3,4)*. The APR *(5)* to infection or injury, with its complex cascade of cytokines, endocrine hormones, free oxygen radicals, arachidonic acid metabolites, catecholamines, reactive oxygen species, and nitric oxide, can have multiple effects on the pharmacokinetic and pharmacodynamic properties of many drugs. Disturbances in drug disposition and action can be caused by many physiological changes, including alterations in protein binding, expansion of extracellular fluid volume, end-organ dysfunction (liver and kidney), changes in organ perfusion, hemodynamic compromise, hypoxia, and alterations in receptor availability or responsiveness *(6)*. A report put a novel twist on the drug–cytokine interaction definition. Brooks et al. *(7)* reported that the β-lactam antibiotic benzylpenicillin conjugated with interferon-γ and reduced the cytokine's immune responses.

Theoretically, all of these changes could fall under a broad description of drug–cytokine interactions. However, this chapter addresses the more commonly accepted, narrower focus of potentially important changes in hepatic drug metabolism *(8–10)* and limited data on changes in drug transporter activity *(11–13)* caused by cytokines, with an emphasis on the management of patients with infectious diseases.

Extensive research involving in vivo *(14–35)* and in vitro animal models *(36–50)*, and limited data from humans *(3,4,51–66)*, leave no doubt that the acute inflammatory response to infection and tissue injury can cause significant reductions in hepatic drug metabolism by the cytochrome P450 (CYP) system. Of the inflammatory mediators, the proinflammatory cytokines interleukin (IL)-1α and -1β, IL-6, and tumor necrosis factor (TNF)-α, and the interferons (IFN)-α, -β, and -γ appear to play the most important role in the downregulation of CYP gene expression and activity. The task for the clinician is determining the potential impact of this interaction on the individual patient, which may be influenced by the nature and extent of injury or infection, time since injury,

From: *Infectious Disease: Drug Interactions in Infectious Diseases, Second Edition*
Edited by: S. C. Piscitelli and K. A. Rodvold © Humana Press Inc., Totowa, NJ

therapeutic index and metabolic pathway of the drug in question, concomitant drug therapy, and the baseline physiological status of the patient. To date, the evidence defining the clinical importance of drug–cytokine interactions and useful predictors of the magnitude and time-course of the changes in drug metabolism remains very limited.

Traditional discussions of drug–cytokine interactions have focused primarily on the potential impact of the acute inflammatory response on hepatic drug metabolism *(8,10,67)*; however, with the evolving role of cytokine-based therapeutic agents in the treatment of cancer, viral infections, sepsis, and chronic inflammatory diseases, the importance of these interactions is expanding. The administration of exogenous cytokines has been associated with significant reductions in CYP enzyme activity or clinically important changes in hepatic drug clearance. These reports have included the administration of IFN preparations for chronic hepatitis B and C virus (HBV and HCV, respectively) *(68–71)*, IFN-α for metastatic cancer *(72)*, and infusions of IL-2 for renal cell carcinoma, human immunodeficency virus (HIV) infection, and hepatic metastases *(73–75)*. Although not yet reported, it is reasonable to suspect that anticytokine therapies currently approved for the treatment of chronic and refractory inflammatory conditions (e.g., severe rheumatoid arthritis and Crohn's disease) and acute inflammatory states may have the opposite effect of increasing the oxidative metabolism of some drugs.

There are several potential scenarios (Table 1) for how drug–cytokine interactions may result in clinically important changes in drug metabolism in patients presenting with or undergoing treatment for an infectious disease. Clinical presentations that could be associated with decreased drug metabolism may be infectious processes that affect concomitant drugs with a narrow therapeutic range (e.g., phenytoin) or may be noninfectious events (e.g., multiple trauma) that may affect the metabolism of concomitant anti-infective therapy (e.g., protease inhibitors). Proposed mechanisms and examples for these scenarios are presented in this chapter.

## CYTOKINES AND THE ACUTE-PHASE RESPONSE

For the purposes of this discussion, the definition of cytokines offered by Nicola *(76)* is used: "Cytokines are defined as secreted regulatory proteins that control the survival, growth, differentiation, and effector function of tissue cells. Cytokines encompass those families of regulators variously known as growth factors, colony-stimulating factors, interleukins, lymphokines, monokines, and interferons." Cytokines represent a broad array of proteins serving the role of signal transducers, from cells serving as biological sensors to responsive cells representing the means of affecting a biological response.

Cytokine expression is primarily a result of infection or injury indicating the presence of cellular "stress" and generally has a minimal role in homeostasis *(77)*. Cytokines mediate a complex, interacting, and often-confusing spectrum of biological responses, with considerable overlap of cytokine effects. Two key terms describing cytokine effects are pleiotropy and redundancy *(76)*. These properties of pleiotropy and redundancy appear to apply to drug–cytokine interactions as well *(8,10,32,35)*. There is considerable overlap in the effects of multiple cytokines on the gene expression and activity of an individual CYP enzyme, and individual cytokines appear to affect the activity of a broad spectrum of CYP enzymes.

**Table 1**

**Clinical Scenarios for Potential Drug–Cytokine Interactions in Infectious Diseases**

Decreased hepatic drug metabolism

- Acute inflammatory response: infections (viral, bacterial, fungal, and parasitic), trauma, major surgery
- Chronic viral infections: chronic active hepatitis, HIV
- Exogenous cytokine therapy: Interferons for hepatitis B and C

Increased hepatic drug metabolism

- Treatment/resolution of infectious diseases (acute or chronic)
- Recovery from trauma or tissue injury
- Anticytokine therapy for acute or chronic inflammatory conditions[a]

[a] Theoretical.

Tissue injury from a number of events, including infection, trauma, burns, and surgery, can precipitate the APR, leading to both local inflammation and a complex systemic response. Regardless of the triggering event, the first wave of the APR is mediated by the tissue macrophage or blood monocyte. Activated mononuclear cells release numerous inflammatory mediators, of which the IL-1 and TNF families are of greatest importance for the progression of the inflammatory response. This first wave of cytokines has both local and systemic effects. At the site of injury, IL-1 and TNF activate stromal cells, including fibroblasts and endothelial cells, to produce a second wave of cytokines that amplifies and propagates the inflammatory response. This second wave of cytokines includes potent chemotactic proteins (IL-8, monocyte chemoattractant protein, and other chemokines) that attract neutrophils and monocytes to the site of injury and the proinflammatory cytokines IL-6, TNF, and IL-1. Activated endothelial cells express surface integrin and adhesion molecules, which further encourage the migration of inflammatory cells to the site of injury. Other vascular effects include vasodilation and decreased endothelial adhesion, which contribute to vascular leak, local tissue edema, and systemic hemodynamic changes. These vascular effects are mediated by the release of low molecular weight substances such as reactive oxygen species, nitric oxide, and arachidonic acid metabolites. Platelet activation results in the release of other mediators, including platelet-activating factor, transforming growth factor-β, and serotonin *(5)*.

Systemic effects mediated by IL-1, IL-6, and TNF include fever and the generation of adrenocorticotropic hormone from the anterior pituitary with subsequent increases in circulating cortisol. The liver is thought to be the principal target of the systemic inflammatory mediators and is the organ responsible for regulating the availability of essential metabolites and functions needed for tissue defense, limitation of tissue destruction, removal of harmful substances, and support of tissue repair.

The regulation of the positive and negative acute-phase plasma proteins (APPs) is one of the hepatic responses to a systemic inflammatory response. The inflammatory mediators responsible for regulating APP gene expression in the hepatocyte fall into four major categories as defined by Baumann and Gauldie *(5)*: (1) IL-6-type cytokines (IL-6, IL-11, leukemia inhibitory factor, oncostatin m, and ciliary neurotrophic factor); (2) IL-1-type cytokines (IL-1α, IL-1β, TNF-α, and TNF-β); (3) glucocorticoids; and (4) growth factors (insulin, hepatocyte growth factor, fibroblast growth factor, and TGF-β). The two categories of cytokines appear to serve as the primary mediators of APP gene expression; the glucocorticoids and growth factors serve to modulate cytokine responses. Similar to the regulation of APP gene expression, data from an in vitro animal model suggested that many factors from these four major categories affect downregulation of CYP activity in an additive and time-dependent manner *(45)*. Although the physiological rationale is unclear, the downregulation of CYP activity in the liver appears to be as integral a part of the hepatic APR as the regulation of the APP response.

## THE CYTOCHROME P450 ENZYMES

The CYP enzymes are a large and diverse group of heme-containing enzymes located on the endoplasmic reticulum of cells present in many tissues of the body. These enzymes are responsible for the metabolism of many endogenous compounds (steroid hormones, biliary salts, fatty acids, etc.) and the detoxification of exogenous compounds (e.g., environmental pollutants, dietary contaminants, fungal and plant toxins, and xenobiotics). The highest concentrations of CYP enzymes are found in the liver and small intestines, with smaller amounts present in the kidneys, lung, and brain *(78)*.

A classification system for CYP nomenclature that groups CYP enzymes into families and subfamilies based on deoxyribonucleic acid (DNA) homology has been widely adapted *(79)*. The prefix CYP is used to designate all CYP enzymes, with families designated by an Arabic number (e.g., CYP3). All members of a CYP family have a greater than 40% identity in amino acid sequence. Subfamilies consist of enzymes with greater than 55% DNA homology and are designated by a capital letter (e.g., CYP2C and CYP2D are subfamilies of the CYP2 family). Last, an Arabic numeral (e.g., CYP3A4) designates individual enzymes. The gene associated with the individual enzyme is designated by italics (e.g., *CYP3A4*).

Although at least 14 mammalian CYP families and 26 subfamilies have been identified, a small number of CYP enzymes (1A2, 2A6, 2C8/9, 2C19, 2D6, and 3A4) account for more than 70% of the CYP content of the liver and are responsible for the metabolism of more than 90% of clinically important drugs in humans *(8,78)*. The content and activity of the major CYP enzymes is highly variable in humans and is regulated by a number of factors, including physiological, genetic, pathologic, and environmental factors *(78)*. CYP genes can be divided into two groups: those with expression that is mainly inducible and those with expression that is primarily constitutive. The CYP1 and CYP3 families are highly inducible, and their activity is greatly influenced by environmental factors known to induce or inhibit their gene expression, whereas the CYP2 family is constitutively expressed and more influenced by genetic factors. CYP2D6 and the CYP2C subfamilies are subject to genetic polymorphism with a bimodal distribution of extensive and poor metabolizers of enzyme substrates. The activities of these constitutively expressed CYPs are less influenced by epigenetic factors than the primarily inducible CYPs *(78,80)*.

Anti-infective agents that are substrates for the CYP enzymes, and therefore subject to pharmacokinetic alterations caused by drug–cytokine interactions, are very limited (Table 2) *(78,81,82)*. The majority of commonly used agents, including β-lactam antibiotics, aminoglycosides, fluoroquinolones, azole antifungals, and some antiviral drugs (e.g., acyclovir), are cleared predominantly by the kidney. Many of the agents metabo-

**Table 2**
**Anti-Infective Substrates for the CYP Enzymes**

| Protease inhibitors | Macrolides | Rifamycins | NNRTIs [a] | Miscellaneous |
|---|---|---|---|---|
| Amprenavir | Erythromycin | Rifabutin | Delaviridine | Caspofungin |
| Atazanavir | Clarithromycin | Rifampin | Efavirenz | Clindamycin |
| Fosamprenavir | | | Nevirapine | Dapsone |
| Indinavir | | | | Miconazole |
| Lopinavir/ritonavir | | | | Quinine |
| Nelfinavir | | | | |
| Ritonavir | | | | |
| Saquinavir | | | | |

[a] Nonnucleoside reverse transcriptase inhibitors.

lized by the CYP enzymes are also potent inhibitors (protease inhibitors, delaviridine, and macrolide antibiotics) or inducers (rifamycin derivatives and nevirapine) of these enzymes *(81)*, which serves to further confound the ability to predict the overall importance of drug–cytokine interactions in the setting of an acute inflammatory response. It is likely that the most important aspect of drug–cytokine interactions in the management of patients with infectious diseases is the effect of the acute or chronic infection, or its treatment, on the pharmacokinetics of concomitant therapies that may have narrow therapeutic indices.

## DRUG–CYTOKINE INTERACTION MECHANISMS

The use of in vivo experiments on animals and humans demonstrated that various inflammatory stimuli, including bacterial and viral infections, tissue injury by turpentine injection, and the administration of bacterial lipopolysaccharide (LPS), exogenous cytokines, and interferon-inducing agents, can significantly decrease the expression and activity of many CYP enzymes important in drug metabolism *(1,8–10)*. However, in vivo experiments do not permit the effects of individual inflammatory mediators on CYP activities and expressions to be studied because of the complex interplay of direct and indirect effects of any given stimulus on the synthesis and release of the inflammatory mediators of the APR. Several in vitro models using primary cultures of animal and human hepatocytes, as well as hepatoma cell lines, have been developed to explore the effects of specific cytokines. Although these in vitro models have provided considerable information concerning the effects of individual inflammatory mediators and the mechanisms underlying these effects, the models have several limitations that may decrease the ability to extrapolate the results to human hepatocyte function *in situ*.

Primary hepatocyte cultures demonstrate significant decay of CYP expression during the first 24–48 hours of growth *(42)*, requiring the manipulation of the culture environment to support the expression of CYP proteins. Some models show an initial decay followed by recovery of the expression of specific CYP proteins to stable levels at 4–5 days after initiation of growth *(40)*, indicating that the timing of experiments may have an important impact on the results. In addition, the inclusion of growth factors (e.g., growth hormone and insulin) and medium additives (e.g., bovine serum) may also affect the expression of CYP proteins. In summary, in vitro hepatocyte preparations cannot reproduce the stable expression of the full spectrum of hepatic P450s at levels consistent with the intact liver in vivo *(8)*.

Despite measures to remove contaminating cells, primary hepatocyte cultures do contain other cells, including Kupffer cells, fibroblasts, and endothelial cells *(39,48)*. Therefore, the addition of individual cytokines to these primary cultures may have both direct and indirect effects. The use of hepatoma cell lines, which are not contaminated by other cell types, avoids some of these indirect effects; however, hepatoma cells have different phenotypic expression than normal hepatocytes *(83)*. Hepatoma cultures also may not respond like hepatocytes to known inducers and inhibitors of CYP activity. In addition, hepatocytes are capable of synthesizing and releasing cytokines in response to inflammatory mediators, which may further confound any understanding of the effect of individual cytokines *(8)*.

Other limitations that may contribute to variability in the results from in vitro experiments include the use of heterologous vs homologous cytokines *(84)*, the use of variable concentrations of cytokines and incubation times *(39,85,86)*, and investigations involving induced vs constitutive expression or activity of the CYP proteins *(46)*.

A detailed discussion of the effects of individual cytokines on CYP activity is beyond the scope of this chapter, and the reader is referred to several reviews *(8–10)*. This literature indicates that the cytokines of greatest importance in drug–cytokine interactions appear to be IL-1 ($\alpha$ and $\beta$), IL-6, and TNF-$\alpha$, with the interferons ($\alpha$, $\beta$, and $\gamma$) having less effect. The growth factors (TGF-$\beta$1, TGF-$\alpha$, epidermal growth factor, and hepatocyte growth factor) may also have important effects on basal and induced expression of the CYP enzymes *(41,45,87)*.

Although the majority of investigations have focused on the effects of cytokines on oxidative hepatic drug metabolism by CYP enzymes, there is limited evidence that cytokines may also affect conjugative or Type II metabolic pathways. The addition of IL-1$\alpha$, TNF-$\alpha$, IL-6, IFN-$\gamma$, or a combination of IL-1$\alpha$, TNF-$\alpha$, and IFN-$\gamma$ all caused a significant decrease in uridine diphosphate (UDP) glucuronosyl transferase (UGT) activity in primary cultures of pig hepatocytes *(85)*. However, the same authors reported no effect of LPS administration on the glucuronidation of 1-naphthol using an in vivo pig model, despite significant negative effects on CYP enzyme activity and antipyrine clearance *(22)*.

The inconsistent effects on glucuronidation between in vitro and in vivo models may be because of the depletion of UDP glucuronic acid in vitro that is available at rather high concentrations in vivo *(85)*. Strasser and coworkers *(26)* evaluated the effects of inflammation on the expression of UGT1 and UGT2 isoforms using a turpentine-injected rat model and studied the influence of IL-1 and IL-6 on UGT expression in primary cultures of rat hepatocytes. The aseptic inflammatory response following turpentine injection resulted in a reduction of hepatic UGT2B3 and UGT1*1 messenger ribonucleic acid (mRNA) and a reduction in the glucuronidation of testosterone (a UGT2 substrate). The conjugation of *p*-nitrophenol, a UGT1 substrate, was unaffected by the inflammatory response, suggesting that some, but not all, UGT isoenzymes are downregulated during the acute inflammatory response. In vitro, IL-6 resulted in a dose-dependent suppression of UGT1*1 and UGT2B3 mRNA expression, consistent with the observation in vivo. IL-1 exposure did not affect expression of UGT1*1 or UGT2B3 in vitro *(26)*.

Contrary to effects on UGT expression, inflammation may induce *N*-acetyltransferase 2 gene expression. Using an in vivo rat model, Walter et al. *(88)* reported that the administration of streptolysin O, a toxin of streptococcal bacteria, or INF-γ inhibited microsomal drug oxidation but significantly increased the activity of procainamide *N*-acetyltransferase by 35 and 20%, respectively. These studies suggest that mediators of the inflammatory response have the potential to affect drug-metabolizing enzymes involved in conjugative metabolism, but considerably more research is needed to understand more completely the magnitude and direction of effect on the relevant systems.

Although several mechanisms by which cytokines decrease drug-metabolizing activity have been proposed, a decrease in gene expression, at the transcriptional or posttranscriptional level, appears to be the dominant mechanism *(8–10)*. Alternative or complementary mechanisms, which may affect CYP activity, include the induction of nitric oxide synthase *(89)*, xanthine oxidase (XO) *(37)*, and heme oxygenase (HO) *(90)* activities by cytokines.

### Regulation of Gene Transcription and Translation

Multiple in vitro and in vivo studies have shown that inflammatory stimuli *(13,17–19,28,30,31,33–35)* or the administration of proinflammatory cytokines *(12,25,29,31, 35,36,38,40,42,46,48,80,86,87,91–96)* cause a downregulation of various *CYP* mRNA with concomitant decreases in the corresponding CYP protein, supporting a regulation of gene transcription as a major mechanism in the decline of CYP activity. However, these studies do not provide direct evidence that the change in *CYP* mRNA content was caused by transcriptional regulation.

Wright and Morgan *(18)*, using a nuclear run-on assay, demonstrated that LPS or turpentine injection markedly decreased *CYP2C11* mRNA transcription, and that the magnitude of the effects was sufficient to explain the decreased mRNA content. However, turpentine injection in female rats caused a decrease in *CYP2C12* mRNA transcription that was of inadequate magnitude to explain the decline in *CYP2C12* mRNA, suggesting that posttranscriptional mechanisms were also important.

Delaporte and Renton *(21)* demonstrated that administration of the IFN-inducer polyinosinic acid-polycytidylic acid (pIC) to rats decreased the transcription rate of *CYP1A1* and *CYP1A2* genes using a nuclear run-on assay. When *de novo* transcription was inhibited by the addition of actinomycin D, IFN significantly augmented the rate of degradation of *CYP1A1* and *CYP1A2* mRNAs.

Cheng et al. *(32)* reported that the primary mechanism for downregulation of CYP following inflammatory stimuli was inhibition of transcription; however, increased rates of mRNA degradation must also contribute to explain the rapid achievement of the nadir CYP mRNA. These results support the involvement of both transcriptional and posttranscriptional events in cytokine-mediated downregulation of CYP mRNA expression.

The understanding of the molecular mechanisms involved in CYP gene regulation following acute injury or inflammation has increased over the past few years. The accumulating evidence suggests that individual cytokines may affect distinct regulatory mechanisms, and that the expression of individual CYP genes may be influenced by different and multiple regulatory pathways, which could explain the diverse response of the multiple CYP enzymes in various inflammatory models. The regulatory pathways are also likely to be species dependent, limiting the potential extrapolation from animal models to humans. An in-depth discussion of these molecular regulatory pathways is beyond the scope or intent of this chapter; however, a few examples are provided.

Tinel et al. *(97)* reported that the downregulation of CYP2C11 and CYP3A by IL-2 in cultured rat hepatocytes was related to induction of the proto-oncogene transcription factor c-*myc*. The addition of an antisense oligonucleotide to c-*myc* or inhibitors of c-*myc* transcription to the cultures blocked the IL-2-mediated suppression of CYP2C11 and CYP3A. Utilizing rat hepatocytes exposed to IL-1 or nuclear extracts of rat liver following in vivo LPS exposure, Iber and coworkers *(27)* demonstrated that the inflammatory cytokine-regulated transcription factor, nuclear factor-κB, bound to a low-affinity binding site, negative κB response element 1, in the promoter region of the *CYP2C11* gene. Mutations that inhibited binding of nuclear factor-κB at this site significantly decreased the ability of IL-1 and LPS to suppress *CYP2C11* transcription. These authors also demonstrated, however, that IL-6-mediated suppression of *CYP2C11* transcription was independent of negative κB response element 1 *(27)*, and the suppression of *CYP2C11* transcription by IL-1 and LPS may also be regulated by other mechanisms *(32)*, indicating that multiple and additive or redundant molecular mechanisms may contribute to decreased *CYP2C11* gene expression. The inflammatory response also appears to decrease hepatic nuclear factor (HNF-1α, HNF-3β, and HNF-4α)-mediated activation of the transcription of multiple rat CYP genes *(32,50)*.

Evidence indicates that IL-6 can downregulate in a dose-dependent manner the expression of the nuclear orphan receptors, constitutive androstane receptor (CAR) and pregnane X receptor (PXR), which are known to be important mediators of CYP2 and CYP3 induction following exposure to enzyme inducers *(13,98)*. IL-6 did not inhibit the transcriptional activity of CAR and PXR *(98)* but rather downregulated mRNA expression of the CAR and PXR genes *(13,98)*. IL-6 also decreased the expression of the retinoid X receptor, which is the obligatory heterodimeric partner of PXR and CAR necessary for high-affinity binding to DNA *(13)*. The depressive effects of systemic IL-1 administration on CYP2D activity and mRNA expression in rat hepatocytes is offset by the administration of rifampin, a potent transactivator of PXR *(25)*, providing indirect evidence that this may be an important mechanism. This evidence supports that the downregulation of the expression of members of the steroid/retinoid/thyroid hormone receptor superfamily of ligand-activated transcription factors (PXR, CAR, retinoid X receptor) play a role in attenuating CYP enzyme transcription; however, the mechanism responsible for this gene suppression by IL-6 is unknown.

Jover et al. *(99)* provided the most detailed study of the molecular mechanisms of IL-6-mediated downregulation of CYP3A4 utilizing a human hepatoma cell line, which they confirmed in primary human hepatocyte cultures. They demonstrated that IL-6 binding to the transmembrane gp130, the common receptor for IL-6-type cytokines, is essential to the subsequent downregulation of CYP3A4 by IL-6. They also demonstrated that CYP3A4 downregulation was independent of the JAK/STAT and SHP-2/Ras/MAPK signal transduction pathways, which are well-described pathways for the APR following IL-6 exposure. IL-6 caused induction of mRNA expression of the transcription factor CCAAT-enhancer binding protein β (C/EBPβ) gene and a translational induction of C/EBPβ-LIP (liver-enriched transcriptional inhibitory protein). C/EBPβ-LIP, devoid of the N-terminal activation domain, competes with the constitutively expressed

C/EBPβ liver-enriched transcriptional activating protein and C/EBPα, producing an inhibition of *CYP3A4* expression. These experiments demonstrated that an increased expression of C/EBPβ-LIP was the determining event in the downregulation of human CYP3A4. In another study, however, expression of C/EBPβ-LIP did not contribute to the early suppression of CYP transcription in the rat liver *(32)*. These studies demonstrated the complex molecular mechanisms that may be important in drug–cytokine interactions and that individual or multiple mechanisms may affect the cytokine and CYP gene combination under study.

## CYP Protein Synthesis or Degradation

Decreased CYP protein content and activity following exposure to cytokines could be explained by decreased protein synthesis (translational effect) or increased protein degradation, although there is considerably less evidence supporting these potential mechanisms. The treatment of female mice with endotoxin resulted in a rapid decline in hepatic *CYP2C12* mRNA and protein content. The decline in protein content could not be completely explained by pretranslational events, indicating that a posttranslational component must have contributed *(17)*. Calleja et al. *(46)* reported that IFN-γ significantly decreased constitutive and induced CYP3A6 enzyme content and activity without affecting the rate of mRNA transcription. This finding is consistent with a posttranscriptional mechanism such as enzyme degradation by XO induction *(37)* or reduction in mRNA translation.

The only study to evaluate the effects of a cytokine on CYP protein degradation directly did not support the enzyme degradation mechanism. Clark et al. *(100)* demonstrated that IL-6 inhibited phenobarbital-mediated induction of CYP2B1/2 activity in primary cultures of rat hepatocytes. To examine the possibility that IL-6 was affecting the degradation of CYP2B1/2, the effect of IL-6 on the loss of enzyme activity and content was measured in the presence of cycloheximide (a protein synthesis inhibitor). Cycloheximide led to loss of enzyme activity and content following phenobarbital-mediated induction, which was not further degraded by the addition of IL-6, supporting the conclusion that IL-6 did not promote the degradation of CYP2B1/2. *See* Induction of HO and Induction of XO sections for further discussion of cytokine effect on CYP protein degradation.

## CYP Enzyme Inhibition

Most studies that have measured CYP protein immunoreactivity and enzyme activity using "probe" compounds, which are specific for a given enzyme, have shown excellent correlation between the two *(16,20,22,23,36,39,43,44,48,87,93,100)*. This supports the argument that the loss of enzyme activity following cytokine exposure is caused by a loss of the corresponding immunoreactive protein; however, several exceptions *(43,44,46,89,30)* suggested that inhibition of enzyme catalysis may also be a contributing mechanism.

Khatsenko et al. *(89)* demonstrated that LPS exposure significantly decreased CYP2B1/2 activity in rats, which was correlated with nitric oxide synthase (NOS) induction, and was inhibited by the coadministration of an NOS inhibitor (L-NAME). In an in vitro experiment reported in the same publication, the authors demonstrated that the introduction of an NO-generating compound rapidly decreased CYP2B1/2 activity, consistent with direct inhibition of catalyzing activity *(see* the following section for more discussion of NOS induction).

Calleja and coworkers *(43)* evaluated the effects of IL-lβ, IL-2, and IFN-γ on the inducible expression of CYP1A1 and CYP1A2 activity and protein content in primary cultures of rabbit hepatocytes. IL-1β addition produced a more marked decrease in CYP1A1 activity compared to the decrease in protein content. Similarly, IL-1β had negligible effect on CYP1A2 protein content while producing a significant reduction in CYP1A2 activity. For the other cytokine/CYP combinations, changes in activity correlated with changes in immunoreactive protein content. These results suggest that IL-1β was capable of causing not only transcriptional effects, but also possibly a functional inhibition of catalytic activity. The same authors reported that IL-1β also decreased rifampin-induced CYP3A6 activity to a greater extent than the protein content, consistent with functional inhibition of enzyme activity *(46)*.

Paton and Renton *(44)* studied the effects of LPS and TNF-α on the downregulation of CYP1A1 activity and content using a unique coculture protocol utilizing murine hepatoma (Hepa 1) cells and murine-derived macrophage cells (IC-21). This methodology allowed the investigators to separate the direct and indirect effects of the inflammatory mediators. When TNF-α was added directly to the Hepa 1 cell cultures, CYP1A1 activity was decreased in a dose-dependent manner, but the cytokine had no effect on immunoreactive CYP1A1 protein content. These results support that TNF-α has posttranslational effects that inhibit CYP1A1 enzyme activity, but the protein is still recognized by the immunoassay.

The incubation of hepatocytes from turpentine-induced rabbits with serum from rabbits with an inflammatory reaction or serum from humans with a viral infection decreased CYP1A1 and CYP1A2 catalytic activity without a reduction in protein content. This decrease in catalytic activity was primarily mediated by IL-6 in rabbit serum and IL-6, IL-1β, and IFN-γ in human serum *(30)*.

### Induction of Nitric Oxide Synthase

Inflammatory mediators, particularly IL-1β, TNF-α, and LPS, are known to induce NOS with subsequent increases in cellular NO release by hepatocytes and other tissues *(89,92,101,102)*. Several in vitro studies have demonstrated that increased levels of NO, caused by either the induction of NOS by cytokines or the addition of NOS inducers, is correlated with a decrease in CYP activity and content, and that the inclusion of an NOS inhibitor reverses these effects *(89,103–105)*. However, the findings of other studies have not been consistent *(33,85,92)*. NO is proposed to have multiple potential effects on CYP-catalyzed metabolism, including both pretranscriptional and posttranscriptional mechanisms. NO may bind directly to the heme moiety of CYP enzymes, inhibiting their catalytic activity; it may accelerate the degradation of the protein by nitrosylation of heme or thiol groups on CYPs; or it may decrease transcription through nitrosylation of the thiol groups on nuclear transcriptional factors *(89)*.

Carlson and Billings *(104)* evaluated the effects of multiple cytokines on individual CYP protein content in primary rat hepatocyte cultures. The combination of IL-1β, TNF-α, and INF-γ depressed CYP1A2, CYP2C11, CYP2B1/2, and CYP3A2 content, with the greatest decrease seen for CYP2B1/2 (33 ± 9% of control). The addition of the NOS inhibitor (L-NMA) significantly prevented the cytokine-mediated decrease in the content of each CYP protein. When the hepatocyte cultures were treated with an NO donor (DETA/NONOate) in the absence of cytokines, there was a dose-dependent decrease in each of the CYP proteins, with the greatest decrease seen for CYP2B1/2 ($33 \pm 8\%$ of control). The treatment of cell cultures with individual cytokines caused increases in NO concentration and decreases in CYP content, which were also reversible by the inclusion of the NOS inhibitor. These data provide strong evidence that NO plays a role in the downregulation of CYP content following exposure to cytokines; however, the study did not evaluate any potential mechanism or measure enzyme activities.

In contrast to the findings in the previous paragraph, Sewer and Morgan *(92)* evaluated the effects of LPS, IL-1β, IL-6, TNF-α, and IFN-γ on the expression of *CYP2C11* mRNA in primary rat hepatocyte cultures. All of the cytokines except IFN-γ inhibited the expression of *CYP2C11* mRNA. IL-1β and LPS were potent inducers of NO release and iNOS mRNA expression; IL-6 and IFN-γ had no effect. The combination of IL-1β and LPS were additive on NO release but did not have additive effects on *CYP2C11* mRNA expression. In addition, the addition of L-NMA reduced NO release to control levels, but IL-1β and LPS downregulation of *CYP2C11* mRNA and protein expression were unaffected. The authors concluded that induction of NO release was not required for the cytokine-mediated downregulation of *CYP* gene expression.

The same group investigated the role of NO by comparing the effects of LPS administration to wild-type and *NOS2*-null mice. LPS significantly decreased phenobarbital-induced CYP2B enzymes by a pretranslantional mechanism in both wild-type and null mice. CYP2B protein was not rapidly suppressed. These results indicate that CYP2B expression was not dependent on NO production by NOS2 *(33)*. Monshouwer et al. *(85)* also reported that inhibition of NOS induction did not influence the effects of cytokines on decreasing CYP activity in primary pig hepatocyte cultures despite the complete suppression of NO release.

The differences in results concerning the role of NOS induction may be because of differences in culture conditions, duration of the studies, and cytokine/CYP combinations studied. For example, the results of Carlson and Billings *(104)* were short-term studies in which posttranslational effects would predominate, whereas the results of Sewer and Morgan *(92)* involved longer incubation times for which the responses are primarily transcriptional. This is consistent with the results reported by Paton and Renton *(44)*, in which decreases in CYP enzyme activity appeared to be at least partially caused by posttranslational effects and may have been mediated by the known effects of TNF on NOS induction. It is clear that NO may have an important effect on CYP activity but is not necessary for the inhibition of all CYP activity observed with inflammatory mediators. The effects of NO are likely to vary depending on the CYP of interest and the model of inflammation or infection under study *(8)*.

### Induction of HO

HO activity is increased in the liver of animals treated with inflammatory cytokines or infected with encephalomyocarditis virus *(15,90,103)*. This increase in HO activity appears to be primarily caused by increased transcription of HO mRNA *(90)*. Increased degradation of heme by HO could be associated with increased degradation of CYP protein. In rats, IL-1 and TNF were potent inducers of HO gene transcription; IL-6 was much less active, and IL-2 and IFN-γ had no effect.

In human hepatoma (HepG2) cell cultures, Fukuda and Sassa *(96)* demonstrated that IL-6 significantly suppressed the induced expression of *CYP1A1* mRNA using a nuclear run-off assay. They also demonstrated a rapid increase in the mRNA encoding for HO after treatment with IL-6. The addition of Sn-mesoporphyrin (a specific inhibitor of HO activity) partially reversed the IL-6-mediated suppression of *CYP1A1* gene transcription. These data suggest that induction of HO activity may be at least partially responsible for the downregulation of *CYP* gene transcription by IL-6. This and data from other studies *(105,106)* suggest that cytokine-mediated increases in heme catabolism may contribute to decreases in CYP activity but cannot account entirely for the changes observed.

### Induction of XO

The administration of IFNs and IFN inducers has been shown to increase the activity of XO in various tissues, including the liver, leading to the generation of superoxide radicals that may contribute to the degradation of CYP proteins. The administration of a free-radical scavenger, *N*-acetylcysteine, or an XO inhibitor, allopurinol, both attenuated downregulation of CYP activity by an IFN inducer, further supporting a role for XO in decreased CYP activity *(107,108)*. Moochhala and Renton *(37)* demonstrated a decrease in CYP3A and CYP1A1 activity in hamster livers by 36 and 38%, respectively, 24 h after administration of a synthetic IFN (IFN-α-Con₁). The activities of the D and O forms of XO were increased by 65 and 74%, respectively. In additional studies, the free-radical scavenger α-tocopherol and allopurinol prevented the loss of CYP activity mediated by the IFN inducer pIC. In chickens, in which XO cannot be formed, pIC had no effect on CYP content.

Although the above studies supported a role for XO in cytokine-mediated decreases in CYP activity, not all studies have supported this theory. Mannering and coworkers *(109)* demonstrated that the administration of IFN inducers or exogenous IFNs resulted in increases in XO activity and decreased levels of CYP protein. They also studied a cohort of mice administered tungsten in their drinking water, which decreased XO by approx 90% without changing CYP activity. The administration of the IFN inducer to the tungsten cohort resulted in a similar decrease in CYP activity as in the animals not receiving tungsten, suggesting that XO does not play an important role in IFN-mediated decreases in CYP activity. Cantoni et al. *(103)* showed a similar effect in a mouse model with administration of IL-2. Animals receiving tungsten in their drinking water had a preserved decrease in CYP content compared to controls but had XO activity equivalent to the basal state compared to a significantly increased XO activity in the control animals.

Clearly, the induction of XO activity is not necessary for CYP downregulation; however, because of the presence of redundant mechanisms, which may vary for different CYPs and cytokines, it is possible that XO may contribute to decreases in CYP activity *(8)*.

In conclusion, there are several potential mechanisms for the observed decrease in hepatic CYP content and activity associated with the APR. The interpretation and relevance of in vitro and in vivo animal models for predicting the response in the intact human are difficult because of the use of various experimental models, known species variability in CYP activity and response to inflammatory mediators, and the use of variable doses of inflammatory mediators. Although downregulation of CYP gene transcription is believed to be the predominant mechanism *(9,10)*, other mechanisms that contribute to decreased CYP synthesis, protein degradation, and inhibition of catalytic activity may play a role under certain conditions or at particular time-points in the inflammatory cascade.

## DRUG TRANSPORTERS

Preliminary evidence indicates that the inflammatory response may have important effects on drug transporters, which theoretically may contribute to pharmacokinetic or pharmacodynamic changes in patients following injury or infection. P-Glycoprotein (P-gp) is a cellular efflux pump that is widely distributed throughout the gut, liver, brain, and other tissues, including epithelial tissue-derived tumors. A diverse range of chemicals, including many clinically useful drugs, are substrates for P-gp, and changes in P-gp activity may have important effects on drug bioavailability, metabolism, elimination, and activity. P-gp is encoded by the multidrug resistance (*MDR*) gene family *(110)*.

A significant reduction in P-gp expression in the rat liver has been reported following turpentine- and endotoxin-induced inflammatory responses *(11)*. In rat hepatocyte cultures, both IL-1β and IL-6 resulted in significant reductions in P-gp protein content and efflux activity; however, only IL-6 resulted in a downregulation of *mdr-1a* and *mdr-1b* mRNA expression. This suggests that the reduction in P-gp may be caused by multiple mechanisms with IL-6 causing pretranslational effects; IL-1β may reduce translation or have posttranslational effects *(49)*.

Bertilsson et al. *(12)* utilized a vitamin $D_3$-induced Caco-2 cell line to evaluate the effects of proinflammatory cytokines (TNF-α, IL-1β, and IFN-γ) and LPS-induced macrophages on mRNA expression of *CYP3A4* and *MDR1* (coding for P-gp). CYP3A4 and P-gp share a significant overlap in their substrate specificities, and therefore relative changes in their activity may have clinical relevance. As expected, *CYP3A4* expression was significantly decreased by all cytokines and macrophage exposure with the exception of TNF-α and IFN-γ. The greatest suppression on *CYP3A4* mRNA expression was noted with the combinations of IL-6 and IFN-γ or of macrophages, IL-6, and IFN-γ. In contrast to what was reported with rat hepatocyte models, *MDR1* expression was induced by all of the cytokines and macrophage exposure with the exception of TNF-γ. Although this study did not evaluate the effects of these mediators on CYP3A4 and P-gp protein cellular content, downregulation of gene expression has the potential to result in significant alterations in drug bioavailability during acute inflammation if similar effects occur in vivo in the intestinal epithelium. Also, alterations in P-gp activity could have an important impact on tumor response in the presence of an acute or chronic inflammatory state.

Beigneux and coworkers *(13)* reported a significant decrease in expression of the $Na^+$-independent organic ion transporter protein 2 (*Oatp2*) gene in mice hepatocytes following LPS-induced inflammation.

These limited data suggest that mediators of the inflammatory response may affect the expression of several transporter protein systems, which may have important effects on drug response.

## CLINICAL DATA

Human clinical data investigating potential drug–cytokine interactions can be divided into four broad categories: (1) clinical observations or uncontrolled studies consistent with cytokine-mediated downregulation of CYP activity; (2) several studies evaluating the effects of influenza vaccination on drug metabolism; (3) controlled or quasi-experimental studies evaluating the impact of acute infectious diseases, acute inflammation, or inflammatory mediators (e.g., LPS),; and (4) studies involving the administration of recombinant human cytokines. The type of inflammatory response as well as the severity of the injury are likely to have an important impact on the nature and time-course of changes in CYP activity. Different inflammatory diseases will have different cytokine profiles, with the hepatocyte exposed to variable concentrations and temporal patterns of proinflammatory cytokines *(8)*. An acute viral infection will induce high concentrations of IFNs, and it appears the CYP downregulation during acute viral infections is mediated primarily by circulating IFNs *(16)*. With systemic inflammation, such as bacterial sepsis, the hepatocyte may be exposed to high concentrations of cytokines because of direct stimulation of local cytokine production by circulating LPS. In contrast, with localized, remote inflammation (e.g., surgery), the hepatocyte may be exposed to much lower concentrations of cytokines occurring at a later time-point, with circulating IL-6 serving more of an endocrine function *(8)*. All of these variables, combined with a high degree of variability in hepatic CYP activity and concomitant drugs that may alter CYP activity, make the prediction of the effect of any given injury or mediator very difficult.

### Clinical Observations

Table 3 summarizes the results of several clinical observations or uncontrolled studies that were consistent with downregulation of CYP activity associated with influenza infection, IL-2 administration, acute trauma, surgery, and critical illness. Chang et al. *(4)* reported prolongation of theophylline half-life during acute viral illnesses compared to 1 month after resolution of the infection in six children. Four children experiencing febrile illnesses without subsequent seroconversion did not have significant changes in theophylline half-life.

Vozeh et al. *(53)* reported changes in drug clearance in three critically ill patients receiving continuous-infusion theophylline; the changes paralleled changes in the patients' clinical condition. As clinical condition deteriorated, theophylline clearance decreased, and drug clearance increased as their clinical condition improved.

Shortly after these reports, an outbreak of influenza B in Washington State was associated with marked decreases in theophylline clearance associated with signs and symptoms of theophylline toxicity in 11 children receiving stable doses of theophylline. The most recent steady-state plasma theophylline concentrations prior to hospitalization were 8–15.8 µg/mL, which increased to a range of 22–48 µg/mL during the acute viral illness. The 6 patients who seroconverted to influenza B had the greatest decreases in theophylline clearance *(54)*.

Midazolam has been widely used in the critical care setting for sedation and anxiolysis, with a proposed benefit of a short-elimination half-life and subsequent predictable reversibility *(116)*. It is metabolized in the liver by CYP3A4 and has been used as an in vivo probe for assessing activity of this enzyme *(117)*. Soon after its introduc-

**Table 3**
**Clinical Observations or Uncontrolled Studies**

| Reference | Substrate drug | Provoking event | Effect |
|---|---|---|---|
| *4* | Theophylline | Influenza infection | ↑ $t_{1/2}$ |
| *53* | Theophylline | Critical illness | ↓ Cl |
| *5* | Theophylline | Influenza B infection | Toxicity |
| *111* | Midazolam | Critical illness | ↑ $t_{1/2}$ |
| *112* | Midazolam | Critical illness | ↑ $t_{1/2}$ |
| *55* | Midazolam | Critical illness | ↓ Cl |
| *113* | Midazolam | Critical illness | ↑ $t_{1/2}$ |
| *73* | Morphine | IL-2 infusion | Severe CNS toxicity |
| *57* | Cyclosporine | Allogeneic BM transplant | ↓ Cl |
| *59* | Carbamazepine | Temporal lobectomy | ↓ Cl |
| *114* | Phenytoin | Severe neurotrauma | ↓ $V_{max}$ |
| *115* | Methylprednisolone | Spinal cord injury | ↓ Cl |
| *65* | Omeprazole | Advanced cancer | ↓ CYP2C19 activity |
| *66* | Dextromethorphan | HIV positive (active disease) | ↓ CYP2D6 activity |
| *61* | ERMBT | Advanced cancer | ↓ CYP3A4 activity |
| *62* | Caffeine (CYP1A2) | Congestive heart failure | ↓ Cl |
| | Mephenytoin (CYP2C19) | | ↓ Cl |
| | Chlorzoxazone (CYP2E1) | | No Δ |
| | Dextromethorphan (CYP2D6) | | No Δ |

$t_{1/2}$, elimination half-life; Cl, total clearance; CNS, central nervous system; $V_{max}$, maximum rate of metabolism; BM, bone marrow; ERMBT, $^{14}$C-erythromycin breath test; , ↑, increased; ↓, decreased; no Δ, no significant change.

tion into critical care practice, it was reported that midazolam had a markedly prolonged effect and delayed time to awakening in this population *(55,111–113)*. Shelly and coworkers *(55)* reported two patients with decreased midazolam clearance during acute sepsis with no measurable plasma concentrations of the 1-OH metabolite. As the patients' condition improved, midazolam clearance improved markedly, and concentrations of the primary metabolite increased.

Chen et al. *(57)* evaluated the relationship between changes in serum IL-6 and TNF concentrations and the clearance of cyclosporine in six patients undergoing allogeneic bone marrow transplantation. Throughout the study period, cyclosporine was administered as a continuous intravenous infusion. Cyclosporine is a drug with low-to-intermediate extraction that is metabolized extensively by the liver via the isozymes of the CYP3A subfamily. Following bone marrow transplantation, there was a marked increase in dose-normalized cyclosporine blood concentrations, with peak values occurring 15.8 days after transplantation. The dose-normalized cyclosporine concentration increased 3.60- ± 0.68-fold compared to day 2. The increase in cyclosporine concentration occurred 4.83 ± 0.95 days after the peak in IL-6 concentrations, and the correlation between the two events suggested that the two parameters were interdependent. Concomitant measurement of two of the major metabolites of cyclosporine, AM1 and AM9, further support the hypothesis that the inflammatory response suppressed the CYP-mediated metabolism of cyclosporine.

Eleven patients undergoing temporal lobe resection experienced an average 30% increase in carbamazepine serum concentrations on postoperative day 3, which correlated with a significant increase in plasma IL-6 concentrations, which peaked on postoperative day 1 *(59)*. These two studies *(57,59)* involving patients with remote sites of inflammation support the hypothesis that the downregulation of CYP activity may be delayed, and that IL-6 may serve an endocrine function relaying this message to the liver.

Two reports suggested that severe neurotrauma may decrease drug metabolism in critically ill patients. McKindley et al. *(114)* reported changes in phenytoin metabolism over 10–14 days following severe head injury in nine patients. IL-6 plasma concentrations were inversely related to $V_{max't}$ and $V_{max\beta}$ for phenytoin. The lowest values for phenytoin metabolism occurred shortly after injury, when IL-6 plasma concentrations were highest.

The pharmacokinetics of high-dose, intravenous methylprednisolone (MP), administered to 11 men with acute spinal cord injury were compared to age-, gender-, and weight-matched, able-bodied historical controls. Total systemic clearance of MP was significantly lower in the patients with spinal cord injury compared to the historical controls (30.04 ± 12.03 vs 44.7 ± 4.90 L/hour, respectively). There was an inverse correlation between the neurological level of injury and the systemic clearance of MP *(115)*.

In contrast to studies evaluating the effect of acute illness on drug metabolism, recent studies have examined the relationship between the APR and drug metabolism in patients with chronic illness. In a study evaluating CYP2C19 genotype and phenotype in 16 patients with advanced cancer *(65)*, all of the patients possessed an extensive metabolizer genotype; however, 4 patients were phenotypically poor metabolizers. Compared to a reference population of healthy volunteers, the distribution of the omeprazole 2-hour hydroxylation index was significantly higher in the patients with advanced cancer, suggesting reduced metabolic activity in this cohort.

These findings are consistent with another study that evaluated hepatic CYP3A4 activity in 40 chemotherapy-naïve patients with advanced cancer by administering the $^{14}$C-erythromycin breath test (ERMBT) *(61)*. Patients were divided into two groups based on their serum C-reactive protein (CRP) concentration: control (≤ 10 μg/L) and APR (>10 μg/L). Patients in the APR group had an average 30% reduction in drug metabolism compared to the control group (*p* = 0.0062). CRP concentrations were significantly correlated with IL-6 concentrations and were associated with a poor performance status. Together, these observations indicate a potential for drug overexposure and toxicity in oncology patients, particularly those patients with evidence of chronic inflammation.

Frye et al. *(62)* evaluated the association between plasma cytokine concentrations and CYP enzyme activity in patients with chronic heart failure. They reported an inverse relationship between both TNF-α and IL-6 plasma concentrations and CYP2C19 activity. CYP1A2 activity was also negatively correlated with IL-6 plasma concentrations; however, elevated concentrations of neither TNF-α nor IL-6 had an appreciable correlation with CYP2D6 or CYP2E1 activity. The observed association among chronic illness, inflammation, and altered hepatic CYP activity *(61,62)* suggests a need to better define the factors affecting drug metabolism in chronic illness and the drug-metabolizing pathways most commonly affected and perhaps to reevaluate the efficacy and safety of drug regimens commonly used in these patients.

O'Neil et al. *(66)* examined the distribution of CYP2D6 phenotype, based on geno-type, potentially interacting drugs, and severity of illness, in 108 HIV-positive patients. When patients were stratified into acquired immunodeficiency syndrome (AIDS) and non-AIDS groups, there were no significant differences in the distribution of metabolic ratios of dextromethorphan, suggesting that chronic disease state did not affect CYP2D6 activity. However, when patients were stratified based on the presence or absence of an active illness at the time of phenotyping, significantly more patients with active disease were classified as "slow" extensive metabolizers, indicating a pos-sible relationship between acute illness and decreased CYP2D6 activity. In contrast to the above findings *(61,62,65)*, these data suggest that the severity of the chronic disease may have little effect on drug-metabolizing capacity.

Although these uncontrolled or observational studies do not prove any cause-and-effect relationship between the different inflammatory stimuli and changes in drug metabolism, the observations are consistent with the mechanisms and effects observed in the animal models. These reports provide some indication of the clinical importance of changes in drug metabolism that can be observed during various infectious or trau-matic inflammatory reactions.

### Influenza Vaccination Studies

Reports of decreased theophylline metabolism with influenza infection *(4,54)* and isolated case reports of decreased drug metabolism and toxicity following influenza vaccination prompted the performance of multiple trials evaluating the effects of influ-enza vaccination on drug metabolism *(118–127)*. These studies have shown inconsis-tent effects. Although some of the early studies showed significant reductions in drug metabolism *(118,119)*, the majority reported either small and transient changes or no overall effect on the pharmacokinetics or clinical effects of the drugs *(120–127)*. How-ever, it is notable that despite several studies reporting no significant changes in phar-macokinetics, individual patients in the study group did demonstrate what could be clinically important changes or drug toxicity.

Levine et al. *(122)* evaluated the effects of vaccination in 16 long-term-care resi-dents receiving chronic phenytoin therapy. Although there were no significant changes in mean phenytoin serum concentrations 7 and 14 days following vaccination, 4 patients experienced increases of 46 to 170% in their serum concentration. Fischer and coworkers *(120)* evaluated the effects of vaccination on theophylline serum concen-trations in 12 asthmatic patients receiving long-term theophylline therapy. Mean theo-phylline concentrations at 24 hours, 72 hours, 1 week, and 2 weeks after vaccination were unchanged; however, 1 patient required a dosage reduction at the first follow-up visit for a serum concentration of 24.5 µg/mL accompanied by signs of theophylline toxicity.

A study evaluating the effect of influenza vaccination on warfarin pharmacokinetics and pharmacodynamics reported no significant change in the half-lives of the warfarin enantiomers, but prothrombin time was increased to some degree in eight patients receiving long-term warfarin therapy. The authors suggested that the change in antico-agulant response might be caused by effects of the vaccine on procoagulant synthesis *(123)*. These findings were not consistent with two larger studies involving patients receiving chronic warfarin therapy *(121,124)*.

The relatively small and unimportant changes in drug metabolism observed in most patients following influenza vaccination are not surprising because the vaccine uncommonly causes systemic signs of inflammation, and IFN serum concentrations following vaccination have been low and transient or undetectable *(125–127)*. However, the results also support the conclusion that individual patients may experience clinically important changes in drug metabolism following influenza vaccination, and close monitoring of drugs with a low therapeutic index is warranted. This individual effect could be caused by a more pronounced inflammatory response following vaccination in isolated patients. The impact of other vaccinations on drug metabolism or CYP enzyme activity has not been studied.

### Infectious Diseases or Inflammatory Models

Table 4 summarizes the reports of acute infectious processes or in vivo models of inflammation on hepatic drug metabolism in humans. Elin et al. *(51)* compared antipyrine pharmacokinetics before and 6 h after injection of etiocholanolone (a steroidal pyrogen) or vehicle in a randomized, crossover study involving 33 healthy volunteers. Fourteen subjects developed fever following the pyrogen; 19 subjects remained afebrile. The febrile group experienced a statistically significant decrease in antipyrine clearance and a prolongation of half-life, and the afebrile group had no significant changes in antipyrine metabolism. The induction of fever and an APR by repeated doses of etiocholanolone have been shown to increase plasma concentrations of IL-1 in humans *(129)*, which may be responsible for the observed decrease in antipyrine metabolism. This steroid has been shown to directly inhibit CYP activity in the absence of hyperthermia, which may explain the above results *(130)*; however, this does not explain the difference between the febrile and afebrile subjects.

The intentional infection of five healthy subjects with *Plasmodium falciparum* was associated with a marked increase in steady-state plasma concentrations of quinine and with the development of signs and symptoms of cinochism in three subjects. The maximum plasma concentration $C_{max}$ before infection was 2.5–5 mg/L, compared to 4.2–12.8 mg/L during acute malaria, despite a quinine dosage reduction in three of the five subjects. The ratio of parent drug to metabolite also decreased during malaria, supporting the argument that the increased plasma concentrations were caused by inhibition of quinine metabolism *(3)*. Quinine is extensively metabolized by CYP3A4 in humans, suggesting that acute *P. falciparum* infections are associated with downregulation of CYP3A4 activity.

Akinyinka et al. *(131)* evaluated the metabolism of caffeine in 10 Nigerian patients with acute *P. falciparum* infections and 10 healthy controls. The caffeine:paraxanthine area under the plasma concentration–time curve (AUC) ratio (caffeine metabolic ratio), a measure of CYP1A2 enzyme activity, was significantly lower in the patients with acute malaria compared to the healthy volunteers ($0.48 \pm 0.13$ vs $0.34 \pm 0.16$; $p < 0.05$). These finding are similar to the changes observed for CYP3A4 activity during acute *P. falciparum* infections *(3)* and are consistent with a drug–cytokine interaction mechanism.

Soons et al. *(56)* conducted two pharmacokinetic studies involving 20 patients presenting with an acute, febrile infectious disease. Stereoselective pharmacokinetics of nitrendipine *(n = 10)* and the pharmacokinetics of racemic bisoprolol *(n = 10)* were

**Table 4**
**Effect of Infectious Diseases or Inflammatory Models**

| Reference | Substrate drug | Provoking event | Effect |
|---|---|---|---|
| *51* | Antipyrine | Etiocholanolone induced fever | Febrile group, ↓ Cl; afebrile group, no Δ |
| *3* | Quinine | Acute *P. falciparum* infection | ↑ Plasma concentrations |
| *56* | Nitrendipine | Acute febrile infectious disease | ↑ AUC and $C_{max}$ |
| | Bisoprolol | No Δ | |
| *58* | Antipyrine | Gram-negative LPS injection | ↓ Cl of all three probes |
| *60* | Hexobarbital | | |
| | Theophylline | | |
| *128* | Antipyrine | ZDV treatment of HIV | ↑ Cl |
| *131* | Caffeine MR | Acute *P. falciparum* infection | ↓ CYP1A2 activity |
| *63* | Antipyrine | Sepsis (pediatric) | ↓ Cl |
| *64* | ERMBT | Nonemergent surgery | ↓ CYP3A4 activity |

*See* Table 3 for definitions of abbreviations. AUC, area under the plasma concentration–time curve; $C_{max}$, maximum plasma concentration; ZDV, zidovudine; MR, metabolic ratio.

determined during the febrile illness and again 6 weeks later, following recovery from the illness. The AUC and $C_{max}$ of racemic nitrendipine increased 89 and 95%, respectively, during the infectious disease compared to the recovered state. The *R*- and *S*-enantiomers of nitrendipine increased similarly. In contrast to nitrendipine, none of the pharmacokinetic properties of bisoprolol were altered during the febrile illness. Nitrendipine is metabolized by CYP3A4, and bisoprolol is a substrate for CYP2D6, suggesting that acute infectious diseases may have a selective inhibition on the activity of individual CYP proteins.

Shedlofsky et al. evaluated the effects of Gram-negative endotoxin administration in healthy male *(58)* and female *(60)* volunteers on the clearance of three CYP probe drugs: antipyrine, hexobarbital, and theophylline. Subjects received two doses of intravenous endotoxin or saline on two consecutive mornings in a crossover design. Following endotoxin administration, the subjects demonstrated typical signs and symptoms of inflammation (fever, chills, nausea, headache, malaise, leukocytosis, and decreased albumin). The subjects also had transient elevations in IL-6 and TNF and marked and more persistent increases in serum CRP. Clearance of all three probe drugs was significantly decreased when administered 30 minutes after the second dose of endotoxin *(58,60)*, but only minor changes in clearance were seen when given after the first dose of endotoxin *(58)*. There did not appear to be any gender differences. These studies demonstrated relatively broad-spectrum downregulation of CYP-mediated drug metabolism following the administration of Gram-negative endotoxin to healthy volunteers, and that there is a lag in the time to inhibition of metabolism following induction of the inflammatory response.

A prospective, pediatric, case-control study by Carcillo et al. compared antipyrine metabolism in 51 septic patients enrolled within 24 hours of diagnosis, and 6 nonseptic, critically ill, posttransplant patients *(63)*. Septic patients had significantly reduced antipyrine metabolism compared to the control group, which was positively correlated with increasing IL-6 plasma concentrations, nitrite plus nitrate plasma concentrations, an indirect measure of NO synthesis, and the organ failure index score. Seventeen patients with persistent multiple organ failure were noted to have a 4- to 10-fold reduction in mixed CYP activity compared to patients without multiple organ failure or resolved multiple organ failure. Multivariate logistic regression analysis controlling for age, liver failure, transplantation status, and microbiological cause of sepsis revealed a small but significant association between reduced antipyrine metabolism and the development of respiratory and hematological failure.

The inference that decreased CYP activity may contribute to clinical outcome during sepsis is consistent with data from an animal model of sepsis reported by Crawford et al. *(34)*. Using the rat cecal ligation and puncture model of sepsis, the concomitant administration of 1-aminobenzotriazole, a potent broad-spectrum inhibitor of CYP enzymes, increased the 20-hour animal mortality rate from 0 to 100%. The clinical findings of Carcillo and coworkers *(63)* are consistent with the cytokine/NO/ONOO mechanism for reduced CYP activity *(104)* and support the idea that therapeutic drug regimens in septic patients with multiple organ failure need further evaluation to more clearly identify potentially serious drug–cytokine interactions and avoid related adverse events.

Elective surgery, as a form of programmed trauma, is an excellent model for studying the effects of acute injury on cytokine activation and regulation *(132,133)* and therefore provides a unique opportunity to study the effects of acute inflammation on CYP activity. Haas et al. *(64)* evaluated CYP3A4 activity using the ERMBT in 16 patients undergoing elective surgery for repair of an abdominal aortic aneurysm ($n = 5$), colon resection ($n = 6$), or peripheral vascular surgery with graft ($n = 5$). CYP3A4 activity and plasma cytokine concentrations (TNF-$\alpha$, IL-6, and IL-1$\beta$) were measured preoperatively and sequentially for 72 hours after the start of the surgical procedure. Patients undergoing aortic or colon surgery had a repeat ERMBT performed at hospital discharge. The ERMBT result, as a percentage of the preoperative result, declined significantly in all three groups, with the nadir observed 48–72 hours after surgery. CYP3A4 activity had returned to preoperative values by the time of hospital discharge in the aortic and colon surgery groups. The nadir ERMBT was significantly and negatively correlated with the peak IL-6 concentration. In a *post hoc* analysis, subjects with a peak IL-6 > 100 pg/mL had a significantly lower nadir ERMBT compared with subjects with a peak IL-6 of < 100 pg/mL regardless of the surgical procedure. The reduction in CYP3A4 activity from baseline in the patients undergoing aortic and colon surgery was comparable to the change in ERMBT results observed with well-known inhibitors of CYP3A4-mediated metabolism, including ketoconazole *(134,135)* and clarithromycin *(136)*. The results of this study are consistent with a significant drug–cytokine interaction and indicate that patients undergoing major surgery may be susceptible to clinically important changes in drug metabolism in the immediate postoperative period.

Only one study has been published that suggests that treatment of an infectious disease may be associated with an increase in hepatic drug metabolism. Brockmeyer et al. *(128)* studied the effect of zidovudine (ZDV) therapy on antipyrine clearance in HIV-infected patients. In the first study, they enrolled 10 patients with early HIV infection (Centers for Disease Control and Prevention/World Health Organization [CDC/WHO] A1) and 10 patients with a diagnosis of AIDS (CDC/WHO C3). Interferon plasma concentrations and antipyrine pharmacokinetics were evaluated in these two groups. The symptomatic AIDS patients had significantly higher IFN-$\alpha$ and IFN-$\gamma$ plasma con-

**Table 5**
**Effect of Exogenous Cytokines**

| Reference | Substrate drug/assay | Cytokine (indication) | Effect |
|---|---|---|---|
| 68 | Antipyrine | IFN-α (hepatitis B) | ↓ Cl |
| 69 | Theophylline | IFN-α (hepatitis B, volunteer) | ↓ Cl |
| 71 | In vitro CYP activity | IFN-α (hepatitis B) | ↓ Activity |
| 137 | Zidovudine | High-dose IFN-β (AIDS) | ↓ Cl |
| 70 | Theophylline | IFN-β (hepatitis C) | ↓ Cl |
| 72 | Theophylline | Low-dose IFN-α | No Δ (acute) |
|  | Antipyrine | (metastatic cancer) | ↓ Theo Cl (chronic) |
|  | Hexobarbital |  |  |
| 138 | Caffeine | IFN-α (hepatitis C) | No Δ |
|  | Urinary cortisol ratio |  |  |
| 139 | ERMBT | IFN-α (hepatitis C, volunteers) | ↓ CYP3A4 activity |
| 140 | Zidovudine | IL-2 (AIDS) | No Δ |
|  | Didanosine | IFN-α (AIDS) | No Δ |
| 74 | Indinavir | IL-2 (AIDS) | ↑ $C_{min}$, ↑ AUC |
| 75 | In vitro activity and CYP | IL-2 (metastatic cancer) | Low dose, no Δ |
|  |  |  | High-dose, ↓ activity and CYP |

*See* text and Tables 3 and 4 for definitions of abbreviations. $C_{min}$, minimum serum concentration.

centrations compared to the asymptomatic HIV-infected patients but no difference in IFN-β plasma concentrations. The symptomatic patients also had significantly longer antipyrine half-lives and decreased metabolic clearance but no difference in renal clearance of antipyrine.

The authors then studied 11 HIV-infected patients (CDC/WHO A1-2) and 11 patients with more advanced HIV infection (CDC/WHO B/C3). Plasma IFN concentrations and antipyrine pharmacokinetics were determined before and 1 day after a 14-day course of ZDV, 800 mg daily. Following ZDV therapy, plasma IFN-α and IFN-γ concentrations in the patients with more advanced disease decreased significantly, to concentrations similar to the patients with earlier-stage disease. In addition, antipyrine half-life decreased and clearance increased to values comparable to those in the patients with early-stage disease. ZDV therapy had no effects on IFN plasma concentrations or antipyrine pharmacokinetics in the patients with early disease *(128)*. These results suggest that decreased hepatic drug metabolism observed during chronic, symptomatic viral infections may improve significantly with antiviral treatment. This is similar to effects observed with the resolution of acute infectious diseases described by Soons et al. *(56)*.

## Exogenous Cytokine Administration

Table 5 summarizes the human trials investigating the effects of exogenous cytokines on hepatic drug metabolism. The effects of exogenous IFNs (α and β) on drug metabolism have been the most widely studied *(68–72,137–140)*. With few exceptions *(72,138)*, the IFNs have consistently decreased the metabolism of drugs and probe compounds that are metabolized by several different CYP enzymes (CYP1A and CYP3A subfamilies). The two studies that failed to show significant changes in hepatic drug metabolism were using low doses of IFN-α ($3 \times 10^6$ U three times per week), which were not associated with evidence of an APR *(72,138)*. Israel et al. *(72)* demonstrated that chronic administration of low-dose IFN-α was associated with a moderate decrease in theophylline metabolism, minimal effect on antipyrine clearance, and no effect on the metabolism of hexobarbital. Larger doses of IFN have been associated with more pronounced effects on theophylline and antipyrine clearance *(68–70)*. These data suggest that the effects of IFN on drug metabolism are dose dependent, and low doses associated with minimal inflammatory response have little to no effect on hepatic drug metabolism.

Piscitelli et al. *(140)* evaluated the effects of various doses of IFN-α ($1–15 \times 10^6$ U/day) on didanosine pharmacokinetics in 26 HIV-infected patients. IFN-α did not have any clinically significant effects on the apparent clearance of didanosine. Because didanosine is a nucleoside analog that is not metabolized by the CYP enzymes, this finding is not surprising. In contrast, IFN-β has been reported to decrease the clearance of another nucleoside analog, ZDV, significantly *(137)*. Eight patients, diagnosed with AIDS, initiated high-dose IFN-β therapy ($45 \times 10^6$ U/day by subcutaneous injection) after receiving 8 weeks of ZDV single-drug therapy. ZDV pharmacokinetic studies were conducted just prior to starting and after 3 and 15 days of combination therapy. Plasma concentrations of ZDV and its glucuronide metabolite were measured. The rate of metabolism of ZDV ($K_m$) declined from $1.43 \pm 0.94$/hour at baseline to $0.36 \pm 0.28$/hour on day 3 and $0.045 \pm 0.028$/hour on day 15. The elimination half-life of ZDV increased from $0.39 \pm 0.13$/hour on day 0 to $0.74 \pm 0.29$/hour on day 15. Plasma ZDV concentrations significantly increased over the 15-day study; the ratio of parent to metabolite decreased. These results are consistent with IFN-β having a negative effect on the metabolism of ZDV to its primary glucuronide metabolite.

High-dose infusions of IL-2 appear to have a potent inhibitory effect on CYP activity and content *(74,75)*. Elkahwaji et al. *(75)* administered variable doses of IL-2 ($3–12 \times 10^6$ U/m²/day) by continuous infusion from day 7 to day 3 prior to hepatic resection in patients with hepatic metastases. Effects of IL-2 on immunoreactive CYP content and enzyme activity consistent with CYP1A2 and CYP3A were compared to control patients not receiving IL-2. Patients receiving low doses of IL-2 ($3$ or $6 \times 10^6$ U/m²) showed little or no change in CYP content or activity compared to controls. Patients receiving high doses ($9$ or $12 \times 10^6$ U/m²) showed more marked changes in CYP content and activity. Total CYP was decreased by 32% and CYP1A2 activity and CYP3A activity by 63 and 50%, respectively. Immunoreactive CYP1A2, CYP2C, CYP2E1, and CYP3A4 were decreased to 37, 45, 60, and 39% of control values, respectively, although these differences did not reach significance because of a high degree of variability and small sample sizes. These results suggest that high-dose IL-2 can downregulate CYP protein content and catalytic activity from multiple CYP subfamilies, including CYP1A, CYP2s, and CYP3A.

Piscitelli and coworkers *(74)* evaluated the effects of variable doses of IL-2 on indinavir clearance, a protease inhibitor that is a substrate for CYP3A4. In the observation arm of this study involving eight patients, trough indinavir concentrations increased significantly, from $264 \pm 493$ ng/mL on day 1 of IL-2 therapy to $670 \pm 677$ ng/mL on day 5. Seven of eight patients had an increase in trough values. In a prospective pharmacokinetic study, eight of nine patients experienced an increase in their indinavir AUC, ranging from 27 to 215%. One patient had a 29% decrease in AUC for indinavir.

IL-2 therapy increased plasma IL-6 concentrations by approx 20-fold by day 5 of therapy, although there was no significant correlation between plasma IL-6 concentrations and changes in indinavir clearance.

In contrast to the effects observed with IL-1β *(137)*, IL-2 therapy was not associated with any marked alterations in ZDV pharmacokinetics *(140)*.

In conclusion, exogenous administration of cytokines (IFN and IL-2) is associated with clinically important decreases in hepatic drug metabolism in what appears to be a dose-dependent manner. The administration of higher doses of IFN or IL-2 in the management of infectious diseases (hepatitis or HIV infection) should be expected to inhibit the metabolism of drugs cleared predominantly by CYP1A, CYP2C, and CYP3A subfamilies, with low therapeutic index drugs of greatest clinical concern. The effect on drugs cleared by glucuronidation or other conjugative pathways requires further study.

## CASE STUDY 1

A.V. is a 66-year-old Caucasian male admitted to the intensive care unit with a diagnosis of severe community-acquired pneumonia. His past medical history is significant for congestive heart failure, hypertension, and chronic atrial fibrillation. His medications prior to admission were 25 mg carvedilol twice daily, 3 mg warfarin daily, 10 mg ramipril daily, 25 mg HCTZ daily, and 81 mg aspirin daily. Five days prior to admission, he presented to his primary care physician with upper respiratory infection symptoms, fever, myalgias, and malaise. A rapid diagnostic test for influenza B was positive, and he was prescribed 75 mg oseltamivir twice daily.

On admission, his temperature was 39.5°C, BP 90/40 mmHg, pulse 108 beats/min, 32 breaths/min respiratory rate. Arterial blood gas on room air was 7.31/46/58/22/87% (pH/pCO$_2$/pO$_2$/HCO$_3^-$/SaO$_2$). The white blood cell count was 12,300/μL. His chest radiograph revealed left middle and lower lobe infiltrates with consolidation at the left base. Because of worsening respiratory distress, the patient was intubated and placed on mechanical ventilation, carefully resuscitated with intravenous fluids, and started on 500 mg levofloxacin iv daily. His prior medications were held for now. Overnight the patient experienced multiple episodes of bright red blood per rectum. Physical exam revealed multiple ecchymotic areas on his upper and lower extremities. Laboratory exam revealed an international normalized ratio (INR) of 10.7. A.V. is seen regularly at the anticoagulation clinic, and his INR 2 weeks ago was 2.3. His aPTT was 43 seconds, platelet count was 234,000/μL, and fibrinogen was 225 mg/dL, so disseminated intravascular coagulation was not suspected. The resident discontinued the levofloxacin because of a suspected drug–drug interaction with warfarin and ordered 3 units of fresh frozen plasma and 10 mg vitamin K iv. A significant drug–drug interaction between levofloxacin and warfarin is unlikely, and the time-course is not consistent with this interaction. The most likely explanation for this serious adverse effect is decreased CYP2C9- and CYP3A4-mediated metabolism of warfarin secondary to persistently elevated plasma concentrations of proinflammatory cytokines and interferons over the course of his acute illness.

## CASE STUDY 2

H.G. is a 35-year-old Caucasian female diagnosed with HIV and hepatitis C (HCV), genotype 1a, infections. Three months ago, the patient started anti-retroviral treatment with Combivir® (300 mg ZDV/150 mg lamivudine) twice daily and 600 mg efavirenz daily at hour of sleep. At her last visit, an efavirenz plasma concentration was 3.5 $\mu M$/mL, and her HIV viral load and $CD4^+$ count were <50 copies/mL and 425 cells/cm$^3$, respectively. A liver biopsy revealed mild cirrhosis, reported as Grade 0, Stage 1. Treatment for HCV was started with 180 $\mu$g pegylated interferon-$\alpha$-2a once weekly and 600 mg ribavirin twice daily. Prior to initiating treatment, a baseline laboratory evaluation revealed an HCV viral load of 3 M copies/mL and liver transaminases within normal limits.

Two weeks after starting treatment for HCV, the patient came to the immuno-deficiency clinic complaining of fatigue, dizziness, myalgias, and "strange dreams." An efavirenz concentration was repeated and was significantly elevated at 9.8 $\mu M$/mL. The patient's adverse event may be attributed to the addition of pegylated interferon-$\alpha$-2a to antiretroviral therapy. Efavirenz is a substrate of CYP3A4 and CYP2B6, and downregulation of one or both of these pathways by exogenous interferon therapy could explain the elevated serum concentration of efavirenz 2 weeks after starting therapy. Efavirenz was held until symptoms resolved and a plasma concentration <4 $\mu M$/mL was obtained.

## CONCLUSIONS

The systemic inflammatory response with its resulting complex milieu of regulatory cytokines, hormones, catecholamines, and various other mediators can result in clini-cally significant decreases in drug metabolism for many commonly used drugs. Evi-dence also suggests that inflammatory mediators may have important effects on the expression and activity of drug transporters. Although data supporting the importance of these drug–cytokine interactions in the clinical use of drugs have increased, many more questions remain inadequately answered. Examples of questions to be addressed with future research include the following:

- What is the comparative impact of various inflammatory processes (bacterial infections, viral infections, blunt trauma, major surgery, burns, etc.) and injuries of different severity on hepatic drug metabolism? Are different families and subfamilies of CYP enzymes affected differently depending on the nature of the insult?
- Are there any readily available markers of the inflammatory process that will aid the bed-side clinician in predicting the importance of any potential drug–cytokine interaction?
- Are drug–cytokine interactions additive or synergistic with drug–drug interactions involv-ing enzyme inhibitors or antagonistic to drug–drug interactions involving enzyme inducers?
- What is the actual time-course of onset and resolution of drug–cytokine interactions, and do any clinical signs or laboratory markers reliably predict the evolution of the process?
- Do the mediators of the anti-inflammatory response (IL-1ra, IL-4, IL-10, IL-13, etc.) have the opposite effect of the proinflammatory cytokines? That is, will anti-inflammatory cyto-kines potentially induce hepatic CYP activity, causing a rebound in drug metabolism during the recovery from severe infections or trauma?

These and several other questions remain to be answered before there is a full under-standing of drug–cytokine interactions in humans. Until additional information is avail-able, it should be assumed that infection and injury that precipitate a systemic inflammatory response, or the administration of exogenous cytokines at an adequate dose to produce systemic inflammation, would potentially alter the pharmacokinetics of drugs that are cleared primarily by hepatic oxidative metabolism or possibly glucuronidation. This may warrant empiric dose reduction or intensified monitoring, depending on the pharmacodynamics or toxic potential of the drug, the ready availability of drug assays, or the urgency of patient need for the substrate drug.

## REFERENCES

1. Reiss WG, Piscitelli SC. Drug–cytokine interactions. Mechanisms and clinical implications. BioDrugs 1998;9:389–395.
2. Wooles WR, Borzelleca JF. Prolongation of barbiturate sleeping time in mice by stimulation of the reticuloendothelial system (RES). J Reticuloendothel Soc 1966;3:41–47.
3. Trenholme GM, Williams RL, Rieckmann KH, Firscher H, Carson PE. Quinine disposition during malaria and during induced fever. Clin Pharmacol Ther 1976;19: 459–467.
4. Chang KC, Bell TD, Lauer BA, Chai H. Altered theophylline pharmacokinetics during acute respiratory viral illness. Lancet 1978;1:1132–1133.
5. Baumann H, Gauldie J. The acute phase response. Immunol Today 1994;15:74–80.
6. Bodenham A, Shelly MP, Park GR. The altered pharmacokinetics and pharmacodynamics of drugs commonly used in critically ill patients. Clin Pharmacokinet 1988; 14:347–373.
7. Brooks BM, Flanagan BF, Thomas AL, Coleman JW. Penicillin conjugates to interferon-γ and reduces its activity: a novel drug–cytokine interaction. Biochem Biophys Res Commun 2001;288:1175–1181.
8. Morgan ET. Regulation of cytochromes P450 during inflammation and infection. Drug Metab Rev 1997;29:1129–1188.
9. Morgan ET. Regulation of cytochrome P450 by inflammatory mediators: why and how? Drug Metab Dispos 2001;29:207–212.
10. Renton KW. Alteration of drug biotransformation and elimination during infection and inflammation. Pharmacol Ther 2001;92:147–163.
11. Piquette-Miller M, Pak A, Kim H, Anari R, Shahzamiani A. Decreased expression and activity of PGP in rat liver during acute inflammation. Pharm Res 1998;15:706–711.
12. Bertilsson PM, Olsson P, Magnusson KE. Cytokines influence mRNA expression of cytochrome P450 3A4 and MDR1 in intestinal cells. J Pharm Sci 2001;90:638–646.
13. Beigneux AP, Moser AH, Shigenaga JK, Grunfeld C, Feingold KR. Reduction in cytochrome P-450 enzyme expression is associated with repression of CAR (constitutive androstane receptor) and PXR (pregnane X receptor) in mouse liver during the acute phase response. Biochem Res Commun 2002;293:145–149.
14. Renton KW, Mannering GJ. Depression of hepatic cytochrome P-450-dependent monoxygenase systems with administered interferon inducing agents. Biochem Biophys Res Commun 1976;2:343–348.
15. Renton KW. Depression of hepatic cytochrome P-450-dependent mixed function oxidases during infection with encephalomyocarditis virus. Biochem Pharmacol 1981;30: 2333–2336.
16. Singh G, Renton KW. Interferon-mediated depression of cytochrome P-450-dependent drug biotransformation. Mol Pharmacol 1981;20:681–684.
17. Morgan ET. Suppression of constitutive cytochrome P-450 gene expression in livers of rats undergoing an acute phase response to endotoxin. Mol Pharmacol 1989;36: 699–707.
18. Wright K, Morgan ET. Transcriptional and post-transcriptional suppression of P450IIC11 and P450IIC12 by inflammation. FEBS Lett 1990;271:59–61.

19. Morgan ET. Down-regulation of multiple cytochrome P450 gene products by inflammatory mediators in vivo. Independence from the hypothalamo-pituitary axis. Biochem Pharmacol 1993;45:415–419.

20. Monshouwer M, McLellan RA, Delaporte E, et al. Differential effect of pentoxifylline on lipopolysaccharide-induced downregulation of Cytochrome P450. Biochem Pharmacol 1996;52:1195–1200.

21. Delaporte E. Renton KW. Cytochrome P4501A1 and cytochrome P4501A2 are downregulated at both transcriptional and post-transcriptional levels by conditions resulting in interferon-$\alpha/\beta$ induction. Life Sciences 1996;60:787–796.

22. Monshouwer m. Witkamp RF, Nijmeijer SM, et al. A lipopolysaccharide-induced acute phase response in the pig is associated with a decrease in hepatic cytochrome P450-mediated drug metabolism. J Vet Pharmacol Ther 1996;19:382–388.

23. Nadai M, Sekido T, Matsuda I, et al. Time-dependent effects of *Klebsiella pneumoniae* endotoxin on hepatic drug-metabolizing enzyme activity in rats. J Pharm Pharmacol 1998; 50:871–879.

24. Warren GW, Poloyac SM, Gary DS, Mattson MP, Blouin RA. Hepatic cytochrome P-450 expression in tumor necrosis factor-$\alpha$ receptor (p55/p75) knockout mice after endotoxin administration. J Pharmacol Exp Ther 1999;288:945–950.

25. Kurokohchi K, Yoneyama H, Nishioka M, Ichikawa Y. Inhibitory effect of rifampicin on the depressive action of interleukin-1 on cytochrome P-450-linked monooxygenase system. Metabolism 2001;50:231–236.

26. Strasser SI, Mashford ML, Desmond PV. Regulation of uridine diphosphate glucuronosyltransferase during the acute-phase response. J Gastroenterol Hepatol 1998; 13:88–94.

27. Iber H, Chen Q, Cheng P, Morgan ET. Suppression of *CYP2C11* gene transcription by interleukin-1 mediated by NF-$\kappa$B binding at the transcription start site. Arch Biochem Biophys 2000;377:187–194.

28. Warren GW, Van Ess PJ, Watson AM, Mattson MP, Blouin RA. Cytochrome P450 and antioxidant activity in interleukin-6 knockout mice after induction of the acute-phase response. J Interferon Cytokine Res 2001;21:821–826.

29. Pan J, Xiang Q, Ball S. Use of a novel real-time quantitative reverse transcription-polymerase chain reaction method to study the effects of cytokines on cytochrome P450 mRNA expression in mouse liver. Drug Metab Dispos 2000;28:709–713.

30. Bleau AM, Levitchi MC, Maurice H, du Souich P. Cytochrome P450 inactivation by serum from humans with a viral infection and serum from rabbits with a turpentine-induced inflammation: the role of cytokines. Br J Pharmacol 2000;130:1777–1784.

31. Nicholson TE, Renton KW. Role of cytokines in the lipopolysaccharide-evoked depression of cytochrome P450 in the brain and liver. Biochem Pharmacol 2001;62:1709–1717.

32. Cheng PY, Wang M, Morgan ET. Rapid transcriptional suppression of rat cytochrome P450 genes by endotoxin treatment and its inhibition by curcumin. J Pharmacol Exp Ther 2003;307:1205–1212.

33. Li-Masters T, Morgan ET. Down-regulation of phenobarbital-induced cytochrome P4502B mRNAs and proteins by endotoxin in mice: independence from nitric oxide production by inducible nitric oxide synthase. Biochem Pharmacol 2002;64:1703–1711.

34. Crawford JH, Yang S, Zhou M, Simms H, Wang P. Down-regulation of hepatic CYP1A2 plays in important role in inflammatory responses in sepsis. Crit Care Med 2004;32:502–508.

35. Siewert E, Bort R, Kluge R, et al. Hepatic cytochrome P450 down-regulation during aseptic inflammation in the mouse is interleukin 6 dependent. Hepatology 2000;32: 49–55.

36. Williams JF. Bement WJ, Sinclair JF, Sinclair PR. Effect of interleukin 6 on phenobarbital induction of cytochrome P-450IIB in cultured rat hepatocytes. Biochem Biophys Res Commun 1991;178:1049–1055.

37. Moochhala SM, Renton KW. A role for xanthine oxidase in the loss of cytochrome P-450 evoked by interferon. Can J Physiol Pharmacol 1991;69:944–950.

38. Morgan ET, Thomas KB, Swanson R, et al. Selective suppression of cytochrome P-450 gene expression by interleukins 1 and 6 in rat liver. Biochim Biophys Acta 1994;1219: 475–483.

39. Clark MA, Hing HA. Gottschall PE, Williams JF. Differential effect of cytokines on the phenobarbital or 3-methylcholanthrene induction of P450 medicated monooxygenase activity in cultured rat hepatocytes. Biochem Pharmacol 1995;49:97–104.

40. Chen J, Strom A, Gustafsson J, Morgan ET. Suppression of the constitutive expression of cytochrome P-450 2C11 by cytokines and interferons in primary cultures of rat hepatocytes: comparison with induction of acute-phase genes and demonstration that CYP2C11 promoter sequences are involved in the suppressive response to interleukins 1 and 6. Mol Pharmacol 1995;47:940–947.

41. Ching KZ. Tenney KA, Chen J, Morgan ET. Suppression of constitutive cytochrome P450 gene expression by epidermal growth factor receptor ligands in cultured rat hepatocytes. Drug Metab Dispos 1996;24:542–546.

42. Tapner M, Liddle C, Goodwin H, George J, Farrell GC. Interferon gamma down-regulates cytochrome P450 3A genes in primary cultures of well-differentiated rat hepatocytes. Hepatology 1996;24:367–373.

43. Calleja C, Eeckhoutte C, Larrieu G, et al. Differential effects of interleukin-1β, interleukin-2, and interferon-γ on the inducible expression of CYP 1A1 and CYP 1A2 in cultured rabbit hepatocytes. Biochem Biophys Res Commun 1997;239:273–278.

44. Paton TE, Renton KW. Cytokine-mediated down-regulation of CYP1A1 in Hepa1 cells. Biochem Pharmacol 1998;55:1791–1796.

45. Iber H, Morgan ET. Regulation of hepatic cytochrome P450 2C11 by transforming growth factor-β, hepatocyte growth factor, and interleukin-11. Drug Metab Dispos 1998;26: 1042–1044.

46. Calleja C, Eeckhoutte C, Dacasto M, et al. Comparative effects of cytokines on constitutive and inducible expression of the gene encoding for the cytochrome P450 3A6 isoenzyme in cultured rabbit hepatocytes: Consequences on progesterone 6 β-hydroxylation. Biochem Pharmacol 1998;56:1279–1285.

47. Tinel M, Elkahwaji J, Robin MA, et al. Interleukin-2 overexpresses c-*myc* and down-regulates cytochrome p-450 in rat hepatocytes. J Pharmacol Exp Ther 1999;289: 649–655.

48. Milosevic N, Schawalder H, Maier P. Kupffer cell-mediated differential down-regulation of cytochrome P450 metabolism in rat hepatocytes. Eur J Pharmacol 1999;368:75–87.

49. Sukhai M, Yong A, Pak A, Piquette-Miller M. Decreased expression of P-glycoprotein in interleukin-1β and interleukin-6 treated rat hepatocytes. Inflamm Res 2001;50: 362–70.

50. Hakkola J, Hu Y, Ingelman-Sundberg M. Mechanisms of down-regulation of CYP2E1 expression by inflammatory cytokines in rat hepatoma cells. J Pharmacol Exp Ther 2003;304:1048–1055.

51. Elin RJ, Vesell ES, Wolff SM. Effects of etiocholanolone-induced fever on plasma antipyrine half-lives and metabolic clearance. Clin Pharmacol Ther 1975;17:447–457.

52. Lipton A, Hepner GW, White DS, Harvey HA. Decreased hepatic drug demethylation in patients receiving chemo-immunotherapy. Cancer 1978;41:1680–1684.

53. Vozeh S, Powell JR, Riegelman S, Costello JF, Sheiner LB, Hopewell PC. Changes in theophylline clearance during acute illness. JAMA 1978;240:1882–1884.

54. Kraemer MJ, Furukawa CT, Koup JR, Shapiro GS, Pierson WE, Bierman CW. Altered theophylline clearance during an influenza B outbreak. Pediatrics 1982;69:476–480.

55. Shelly MP, Mendel L, Park GR. Failure of critically ill patients to metabolize midazolam. Anaesthesia 1987;42:619–626.

56. Soons PA, Grib C, Breimer DD, Kirch W. Effects of acute febrile infectious diseases on the oral pharmacokinetics and effects of nitrendipine enantiomers and of bisoprolol. Clin Pharmacokinet 1992;23:238–248.

57. Chen YL, LeVraux V, Leneveu A, et al. Acute-phase response, interleukin-6, and alteration in cyclosporine pharmacokinetics. Clin Pharmacol Ther 1994;55:649–660.

58. Shedlofsky SI, Israel BC, McClain CJ, Hill DB, Blouin RA. Endotoxin administration to humans inhibits hepatic cytochrome P450-mediated drug metabolism. J Clin Invest 1994;94:2209–2214.

59. Gidal BE, Reiss WG, Liao IS, Pitterle ME. Changes in interleukin-6 concentrations following epilepsy surgery: potential influence on carbamazepine pharmacokinetics [letter]. Ann Pharmacother 1996;30:545–546.

60. Shedlofsky SI, Israel BC, Tosheva R, Blouin RA. Endotoxin depresses hepatic cytochrome P450-mediated drug metabolism in women. Br J Clin Pharmacol 1997;43: 627–632.

61. Rivory LP, Slaviero KA, Clarke SJ. Hepatic cytochrome P450 3A drug metabolism is reduced in cancer patients who have an acute-phase response. Br J Cancer 2002;87: 277–280.

62. Frye RF, Schneider VM, Frye CS, et al. Plasma levels of TNF-$\alpha$ and IL-6 are inversely related to cytochrome P450-dependent drug metabolism in patients with congestive heart failure. J Card Fail 2002;8:315–319.

63. Carcillo JA, Doughty L, Kofos D, et al. Cytochrome P450 mediated drug metabolism is reduced in children with sepsis-induced multiple organ failure. Int Care Med 2003;29: 980–984.

64. Haas CE, Kaufman DC, Jones CE, et al. Cytochrome P450 3A4 activity after surgical stress. Crit Care Med 2003;31:1338–1346.

65. Williams ML, Bhargava P, Cherrouk I, et al. A discordance of the cytochrome P450 2C19 genotype and phenotype in patients with advanced cancer. Br J Clin Pharmacol 2000;49:485–488.

66. O'Neil WM, Gilfix BM, Markoglou N, et al. Genotype and phenotype of cytochrome P450 2D6 in human immunodeficiency virus-positive patients and patients with acquired immunodeficiency syndrome. Eur J Clin Pharmacol 2000;56:231–240.

67. Farrell GC. Drug metabolism in extrahepatic diseases. Pharmacol Ther 1987;35:375–404.

68. Williams SJ, Farrell GC. Inhibition of antipyrine metabolism by interferon. Br J Clin Pharmacol 1986;22:610–612.

69. Williams SJ, Baird-Lambert JA, Farrell GC. Inhibition of theophylline metabolism by interferon. Lancet 1987;2:939–941.

70. Okuno H, Takasu M, Kano H, et al. Depression of drug-metabolizing activity in the human liver by interferon-$\beta$. Hepatology 1993;17:65–69.

71. Okuno H, Kitao Y, Takasu M, et al. Depression of drug metabolizing activity in the human liver by interferon-$\alpha$. Eur J Clin Pharmacol 1990;39:365–367.

72. Israel BC, Blouin RA, McIntyre W, Shedlofsky SI. Effects of interferon-$\alpha$ monotherapy on hepatic drug metabolism in cancer patients. Br J Clin Pharmacol 1993;36:229–235.

73. Bortulossi R, Fabiani F, Savron F, et al. Acute morphine intoxication during high-dose recombinant interleukin-2 treatment for metastatic renal cell cancer. Eur J Cancer 1994;30A:1905–1907.

74. Piscitelli SC, Vogel S, Figg WD, et al. Alteration in indinavir clearance during interleukin-2 infusions in patients infected with the human immunodeficiency virus. Pharmacotherapy 1998;18:1212–1216.

75. Elkahwaji J, Robin MA, Berson A, et al. Decrease in hepatic cytochrome P450 after interleukin-2 immunotherapy. Biochem Pharmacol 1999;57:951–954.

76. Nicola NA. An introduction to the cytokines. In: Nicola NA, ed. Guidebook to the Cytokines and Their Receptors. Oxford, England: Oxford University Press, 1994, pp. 1–7.

77. Dinarello CA. Proinflammatory cytokines. Chest 2000;118:503–508.
78. Slaughter RL, Edwards DJ. Recent advances: the cytochrome P450 enzymes. Ann Pharmacother 1995;29:619–624.
79. Nebert DW, Adesnick M, Coon MJ, et al. The P450 gene superfamily: recommended nomenclature. DNA 1987;6:1–11.
80. Muntane-Relat J, Ourlin JC, Domergue J, Maurel P. Differential effects of cytokines on the inducible expression of CYP1A1, CYP1A2, and CYP3A4 in human hepatocytes in primary culture. Hepatology 1995;22:1143–1153.
81. Piscitelli SC, Flexner C, Minor JR, Polis MA, Masur H. Drug interactions in patients infected with human immunodeficiency virus. Clin Infect Dis 1996;23:685–693.
82. Rendic S, DiCarol FJ. Human cytochrome P450 enzymes: a status report summarizing their reactions, substrates, inducers and inhibitors. Drug Metab Rev 1997;29:413–580.
83. Jover R, Bort R, Gomez- Lechon J, Castell JV. Re-expression of C/EBPα induces CYP2B6, CYP2C9 and CYP2D6 genes in HepG2 cells. FEBS Lett 1998;431:227–230.
84. Craig PI, Williams SJ, Cantrill E, Farrell GC. Rat but not human interferon suppresses hepatic oxidative metabolism in rats. Gastroenterology 1989;97:999–1004.
85. Monshouwer M, Witkamp RF, Nijmeijer SM, Van Amsterdam JG, Van Miert A. Suppression of cytochrome P450- and UDP glucuronosyl transferase-dependent enzyme activities by proinflammatory cytokines and possible role of nitric oxide in primary cultures of pig hepatocytes. Toxicol Appl Pharmacol 1996;137:237–244.
86. Abdel-Razzak Z, Loyer P, Fautrel A, et al. Cytokines down-regulate expression of major cytochrome P-450 enzymes in adult human hepatocytes in primary culture. Mol Pharmacol 1993;44:707–715.
87. Abdel-Razzak Z, Corcos L, Fautrel A, Campio JP, Guillouzo A. Transforming growth factor-β1 down-regulates basal and polycyclic aromatic hydrocarbon-induced cytochromes P-450 1A1 and 1A2 in adult human hepatocytes in primary culture. Mol Pharmacol 1994;46:1100–1110.
88. Walter R, Siegmund W, Scheuch E. Effects of interferon-γ and streptolysin O on hepatic procainamide N-acetyltransferase and various microsomal cytochrome P450-dependent monooxygenases in rats. Immunopharmacol Immunotoxicol 1996;18:571–586.
89. Khatsenko OG, Gross SS, Rifkind AB, Vane JR. Nitric oxide is a mediator of the decrease in cytochrome P450-dependent metabolism caused by immunostimulants. Proc Natl Acad Sci USA 1993;90:11,147–11,151.
90. Rizzardini M, Terao M, Falciani F, Cantoni L. Cytokine induction of haem oxygenase mRNA in mouse liver. Interleukin 1 transcriptionally activates the haem oxygenase gene. Biochem J 1993;290:343–347.
91. Trautwein C, Ramadori G, Gerken G, et al. Regulation of cytochrome P450 IID by acute phase mediators in C3H/HeJ mice. Biochem Biophys Res Commun 1992;182:617–623.
92. Sewer MB, Morgan ET. Nitric oxide-independent suppression of P450 2CII expression by interleukin-1β and endotoxin in primary rat hepatocytes. Biochem Pharmacol 1997;54:729–737.
93. Sindhu RK, Sakai H, Okamoto T, Kikkawa Y. Differential effect of interleukin-1α on rat hepatic cytochrome P450 monooxygenases. Toxicology 1996;114:37–46.
94. Craig PI, Mehta I, Murray M, et al. Interferon down regulates the male-specific cytochrome P450IIIA2 in rat liver. Mol Pharmacol 1990;38:313–318.
95. Fukuda Y, Ishida N, Noguchi T, Kappas A, Sassa S. Interleukin-6 down regulates the expression of transcripts encoding cytochrome P450 IA1, IA2 and IIIA3 in human hepatoma cells. Biochem Biophys Res Commun 1992;184:960–965.
96. Fukuda Y, Sassa S. Suppression of cytochrome P450IAl by interleukin-6 in human HepG2 hepatoma cells. Biochem Pharmacol 1994;47:1187–1195.
97. Tinel M, Elkahwaji J, Robin M, et al. Interleukin-2 overexpresses c-*myc* and down-regulates cytochrome P-450 in rat hepatocytes. J Pharmacol Exp Therap 1999;289:649–55.

98. Pascussi JM, Gerbal-Chaloin S, Pichard-Garcia L, et al. Interleukin-6 negatively regulates the expression of pregnane X receptor and constitutively activated receptor in primary human hepatocytes. Biochem Biophys Res Commun 2000;274:707–713.

99. Jover R, Bort R, Gomez-Lechon J, Castell JV. Down-regulation of human CYP3A4 by the inflammatory signal interleukin-6: molecular mechanism and transcription factors involved. FASEB J September 5, 2002;10.1096/fj.02-0195fje.

100. Clark MA, Williams JF, Gottschall PE, Wecker L. Effects of phenobarbital and interleukin-6 on cytochrome P4502B1 and 2B2 in cultured rat hepatocytes. Biochem Pharmacol 1996;51:701–706.

101. Beasley D, Eldridge M. Interleukin-1 β and tumor necrosis factor-α synergistically induce NO synthase in rat vascular smooth muscles cells. Am J Physiol 1994;266:R1197–R1203.

102. Geller DA, Freeswick PD, Nguyen D, et al. Differential induction of nitric oxide synthase in hepatocytes during endotoxemia and the acute-phase response. Arch Surg 1994; 129:165–171.

103. Cantoni L, Carelli M, Ghezzi P, et al. Mechanisms of interleukin-2-induced depression of hepatic cytochrome P-450 in mice. Eur J Pharmacol 1995;292:257–263.

104. Carlson TJ, Billings RE. Role of nitric oxide in the cytokine-mediated regulation of cytochrome P-450. Mol Pharmacol. 1996;49:796–801.

105. el Azhary R, Renton KW, Mannering GJ. Effect of interferon inducing agents (polyriboinosinic acid-polyribocytidylic acid and tilorone) on the heme turnover of hepatic cytochrome P-450. Mol Pharmacol 1980;17:395–399.

106. Singh G, Renton KW. Inhibition of the synthesis of hepatic cytochrome P-450 by the interferon-inducing agent poly rI-rC. Can J Physiol Pharmacol 1984;62:379–383.

107. Ghezzi P, Bianchi M, Gianera L, et al. Role of reactive oxygen intermediates in the interferon-mediated depression of hepatic drug metabolism and protective effect of N-acetylcysteine in mice. Cancer Res 1985;45:3444–3447.

108. Ghezzi P, Bianchi M, Mantovani A, Spreafico F, Salmona M. Enhanced xanthine oxidase activity in mice treated with interferon and interferon inducers. Biochem Biophys Res Commun 1984;119:144–149.

109. Mannering GJ, DeLoria LB, Abbott V. Role of xanthine oxidase in the interferon-mediated depression of the hepatic cytochrome P-450 system in mice. Cancer Res 1988;48: 2107–2112.

110. Fardel O, Lecurer V, Guillouzo A. The P-glycoprotein multidrug transporter. Gen Pharmacol 1996;27:1283–1291.

111. Byatt CM, Lewis LD, Dawling S, Cochrane GM. Accumulation of midazolam after repeated dosage in patients receiving mechanical ventilation in an intensive care unit. Br Med J 1984;289:799–800.

112. Byrne AJ, Yeoman PM, Mace P. Accumulation of midazolam in patients receiving mechanical ventilation [letter]. Br Med J 1984;289:1309.

113. Shafer A, Doze VA, White PF. Pharmacokinetic variability of midazolam infusions in critically ill patients. Crit Care Med 1990;18:1039–1041.

114. McKindley DS, Boucher BA, Hess MM, et al. Effect of acute phase response on phenytoin metabolism in neurotrauma patients. J Clin Pharmacol 1997;37:129–139.

115. Segal JL, Malt by BF, Langdorf MI, et al. Methylprednisolone disposition kinetics in patients with acute spinal cord injury. Pharmacotherapy 1998;18:16–22.

116. Allonen H, Ziegler G, Klotz U. Midazolam kinetics. Clin Pharmacol Ther 1981;30: 653–661.

117. Thummel KE, Shen DD, Podoll TD, et al. Use of midazolam as a human cytochrome P450 3A probe: I. *In vitro-in vivo* correlations in liver transplant patients. J Pharmacol Exp Ther 1994;271:549–556.

118. Renton KW, Gray JD, Hall RI. Decreased elimination of theophylline after influenza vaccination. CMAJ 1980;123:288–290.

119. Kramer P, McClain CJ. Depression of aminopyrine metabolism by influenza vaccination. N Engl J Med 1981;305:1262–1264.

120. Fischer RG, Booth BH, Mitchell DQ, Kibbe AH. Influence of trivalent influenza vaccine on serum theophylline levels. CMA J 1982;126:1312–1313.

121. Patriarca PA, Kendal AP, Stricof RL, et al. Influenza vaccination and warfarin or theophylline toxicity in nursing-home residents [letter]. N Engl J Med 1983;308:1601–1602.

122. Levine M, Jones MW, Gribble M. Increased serum phenytoin concentration following influenza vaccination. Clin Pharm 1984;3:505–509.

123. Kramer P, Tsuru M, Cook CE, McClain CJ, Holtzman JL. Effect of influenza vaccine on warfarin anticoagulation. Clin Pharmacol Ther 1984;35:416–418.

124. Lipsky BA, Pecoraro RE, Roben NJ, deBlaquiere P, Delaney CJ. Influenza vaccination and warfarin anticoagulation. Ann Intern Med 1984;100:835–837.

125. Grabowski N, May JJ, Pratt DS, Richtsmeier WJ, Bertino JS. The effect of split virus influenza vaccination on theophylline pharmacokinetics. Am Rev Respir Dis 1985;131:934–938.

126. Meredith CG, Christian CD, Johnson RF, et al. Effects of influenza virus vaccine on hepatic drug metabolism. Clin Pharmacol Ther 1985;37:396–401.

127. Hannan SE, May JJ, Pratt DS, Richtsmeier WJ, Bertino JS. The effect of whole virus influenza vaccination on theophylline pharmacokinetics. Am Rev Respir Dis 1988;137:903–906.

128. Brockmeyer NH, Barthel B, Mertins L, Goos M. Effect of zidovudine therapy in patients with HIV infection on endogenous interferon plasma levels and the hepatic cytochrome P450 enzyme system. Chemotherapy 1998;44:174–180.

129. Watters JM, Bessey PQ, Dinarello CA, Wolff SM, Wilmore DW. The induction of interleukin-1 in humans and its metabolic effects. Surgery 1985;98:298–305.

130. Anari MR, Renton KW. Modulatory effect of hyperthermia on hepatic microsomal cytochrome P450 in mice. Biochem Pharmacol 1993;46:307–10.

131. Akinyinka OO, Sowunmi A, Honeywell R, Renwick AG. The effects of acute falciparum malaria on the disposition of caffeine and the comparison of saliva and plasma-derived pharmacokinetic parameters in adult Nigerians. Eur J Clin Pharmacol 2000;56:159–165.

132. Van Deuren M, Twickler TB, de Waal Malfety MC, et al. Elective orthopedic surgery, a model for study of cytokine activation and regulation. Cytokine 1998;10:897–903.

133. DiPadova F, Pozzi C, Tondre MJ, et al. Selective and early increase of IL-1 inhibitors, IL-6 and cortisol after elective surgery. Clin Exp Immunol 1991;85:137–142.

134. Jamis-Dow CA, Pearl ML, Watkins PB, et al. Predicting drug interactions in vivo from experiments in vitro: human studies with paclitaxel and ketoconazole. Am J Clin Oncol 1997;20:592–599.

135. Polk RE, Crouch MA, Israel DS, et al. Pharmacokinetic interaction between ketoconazole and amprenavir after single doses in healthy men. Pharmacotherapy 1999;19:1378–1384.

136. Brophy DF, Israel DS, Pastor A, et al. Pharmacokinetic interaction between amprenavir and clarithromycin in healthy male volunteers. Antimicrob Agents Chemother 2000;44:978–984.

137. Nokta M, Loh JP, Douidar SM, Ahmed AE, Pollard RE. Metabolic interaction of recombinant interferon-β and zidovudine in AIDS patients. J Interferon Res 1991;11:159–164.

138. Pageaux GP, LeBricquir Y, Berthou F, et al. Effects of interferon-α on cytochrome P-450 isoforms 1A2 and 3A activities in patients with chronic hepatitis C. Eur J Gastro Hepatol 1998;10:491–495.

139. Craig PI, Tapner M, Farrell GC. Interferon suppresses erythromycin metabolism in rats and human subjects. Hepatology 1993;17:230–235.

140. Piscitelli SC, Amantea MA, Vogel S, et al. Effects of cytokines on antiviral pharmacokinetics: an alternative approach to assessment of drug interactions using bioequivalence guidelines. Antimicrob Agents Chemother 1996;40:161–165.

# 14

# Circumventing Drug Interactions

## Douglas N. Fish

## INTRODUCTION

There are numerous opportunities for drug interactions involving antimicrobial agents. The potential for drug interactions encountered in clinical practice continues to grow as the number of different antimicrobial classes expands, the number of specific agents within these drug classes increases, and antimicrobial drug regimens become more complex (e.g., treatment of mycobacterial infection and human immunodeficiency virus [HIV] disease). In addition, antimicrobials are commonly used in certain patient populations (e.g., critically ill, elderly, or HIV-infected patients) for whom many drugs of various classes are used, and the potential for drug interactions therefore increases as a function of the number and types of drugs present. Many interactions are of minimal clinical importance and often ignored. However, other interactions are associated with substantial risk of adverse pharmacokinetic or pharmacodynamic interactions, resulting in decreased therapeutic efficacy, increased incidence of drug toxicities, or potential for increased antimicrobial resistance. Thus, the ability to prevent or minimize adverse drug interactions is of vital importance in optimizing the appropriate and effective use of antimicrobials and enhancing patient outcome.

The objective of this chapter is to review strategies for avoiding or minimizing adverse drug interactions. It must be emphasized, however, that the key to avoiding drug interactions is for practitioners to possess a thorough understanding of the drugs they are most often prescribing or otherwise encountering in their practices. There is no substitute for adequate knowledge regarding potential interactions and familiarity with literature addressing the clinical importance of these interactions. Because objective studies of many potential interactions either have not been performed or have produced inconsistent recommendations, familiarity with the pharmacokinetic and pharmacodynamic characteristics of the particular agents may also assist clinicians in predicting the likelihood of possible interactions. Only after practitioners possess a thorough knowledge of the specific agents can strategies for circumventing drug interactions be effectively employed.

One additional point must be emphasized when considering strategies to circumvent drug interaction. It will often be extremely challenging to use only agents with no pos-

From: *Infectious Disease: Drug Interactions in Infectious Diseases, Second Edition*
Edited by: S. C. Piscitelli and K. A. Rodvold © Humana Press Inc., Totowa, NJ

sibility of drug interactions. One such difficult situation is the management of patients with advanced HIV disease, for which patients are often receiving multiple antimicrobial and non-antimicrobial agents for treatment of the HIV infection as well as treatment or prevention of associated opportunistic infections. In such cases, the relative risks of drug use must be weighed vs the relative benefits to be gained. Risk-vs-benefit considerations regarding the use of potentially interacting drugs should be carefully contemplated when initiating or continuing any agent. Often, the relative risks and benefits to the patient will be clear based on the indication for antimicrobial use, other underlying disease states, and existing data regarding the probable significance of the drug interaction in question. In many other cases, however, the decision regarding relative risks and benefits will be quite subjective and based primarily on the clinical expertise and previous clinical experience of the practitioner. Again, the key to making such decisions is for practitioners to possess a thorough understanding of the drugs they are using and to exercise common sense when making management decisions.

The most effective way to avoid significant drug interactions is obviously to completely avoid the use of drugs that are likely to be involved in such interactions in a specific patient. This requires that drugs be prospectively evaluated for potentially significant interactions as they are initially selected for use and prior to actual administration to the patient. Because it is often the case that drug therapy has already been initiated prior to the practitioner becoming involved in management of the patient, it is also important to be able to evaluate preexisting drug regimens for potentially important interactions before they become clinically significant. In either scenario, the goal is to *prospectively* evaluate the potential for interactions to make appropriate decisions regarding drug management rather than reacting to an adverse interaction after it has already occurred.

Finally, it must be noted that most literature, indeed, including this chapter, usually considers drug interactions from the perspective of creating potential for doing the patient harm. However, it would certainly be inaccurate to characterize all drug interactions as negative. Situations also exist in which drug interactions are advantageous for improving pharmacokinetic profiles and enhancing the potential therapeutic efficacy of antimicrobial agents.

A classic example of a beneficial drug interaction is the concomitant use of probenecid with penicillin G or amoxicillin in the treatment of syphilis. By decreasing the renal tubular secretion of the penicillins, probenecid helps maintain these drugs at treponemicidal concentrations over longer periods of time than would otherwise be possible given their short elimination half-lives *(1)*. Another common example is the use of "boosted" protease inhibitor regimens such as the concomitant use of ritonavir and saquinavir, in which inhibition of cytochrome P450 (CYP) 3A4 by ritonavir results in decreased saquinavir metabolism, significantly increased saquinavir exposure, and enhanced therapeutic efficacy of this protease inhibitor combination *(2)*.

A thorough knowledge of the pharmacology and pharmacokinetics of antimicrobial agents and potentially interacting drugs may allow creative clinicians to utilize drug interactions to achieve beneficial therapeutic results rather than putting patients at risk for negative outcomes. Although this chapter focuses on circumventing negative interactions, the potential for beneficial drug interactions must also be recognized and may often be equally as clinically significant as negative interactions.

**Table 1**
**Strategies for Avoiding Adverse Drug Interactions When Selecting Agents for Use**

- Obtain detailed patient medication histories prior to selecting antimicrobial therapy
- Do not add a drug with interaction potential if not necessary
- If possible, delay initiation of potentially interacting drugs until after antimicrobial treatment course is completed
- Consider concomitant disease states, particularly organ dysfunction
- Select drug classes and specific agents with the least potential for known interactions
- When possible, avoid agents associated with serious adverse effects or toxicities
- Avoid concurrent administration of agents with overlapping adverse effect profiles
- Use the smallest effective drug doses
- Do not overestimate the ability of patients to adhere to recommended dosing schedules

## STRATEGIES FOR AVOIDING DRUG INTERACTIONS WHEN SELECTING AGENTS FOR USE

As previously stated, the most effective way to avoid significant drug interactions is to completely avoid the use of drugs that are likely to be involved in such interactions in a specific patient. In addition to choosing antimicrobial agents for use in patients already receiving other drugs, practitioners are frequently choosing agents for treatment of noninfectious problems in patients already receiving antimicrobials for some indication. In either case, there are a number of considerations that should be taken into account to minimize the potential for, or clinical significance of, drug interactions involving antimicrobials; these are listed in Table 1. Many of these considerations are relatively straightforward and dictated by common sense and clinical experience as much as by any drug-specific data.

### Obtain Detailed Patient Medication Histories Prior to Selecting Antimicrobial Therapy

Clinicians must be fully aware of medications used by a patient before potential drug–drug interactions can be considered and appropriate antimicrobial agents selected. Detailed medication histories, including both prescription and nonprescription medications, should therefore be carefully obtained from all patients. Although most therapeutically significant drug–drug interactions involve prescription medications, a number of common over-the-counter drugs have also been demonstrated to cause potentially significant drug–drug interactions with various classes of antimicrobials. Such nonprescription medications include antacids, histamine$_2$-receptor antagonists, and multivitamin preparations that include zinc or iron *(2–9)*. Information regarding drug–drug interactions involving herbal preparations and natural products is currently scarce. However, certain compounds, such as St. John's wort *(10)*, are known to have the potential to cause significant interactions, and additional such products are likely to be identified in the future.

Medication histories must therefore be thorough, and clinicians should remember to ask patients regarding both prescription and nonprescription drugs as well as use of natural products. Such detailed medication histories are important for inpatients and outpatients alike.

### *Do Not Add a Drug With Interaction Potential If Not Necessary*

Although this point appears to be self-evident, it is not unusual for patients to be initiated on drug therapy for poorly understood or poorly justified indications. An attempt must always be made to differentiate between necessary and unnecessary concomitant medications. If a drug is not clearly indicated, it should not be used if potentially significant drug interactions exist.

### *If Possible, Delay Initiation of Other Drugs With Interaction Potential*

Occasionally, patients receiving antimicrobials for treatment of an acute infection will also need to begin additional drug therapy for some other indication. Because the antimicrobial is administered for some brief and well-defined duration of therapy, it is often possible to delay initiation of another potentially interacting agent until the course of antimicrobial therapy has been completed. This may occur not only in hospitalized patients who are prepared for discharge but also in ambulatory settings as well.

Examples of such situations may include initiation of benzodiazepine therapy in patients receiving CYP inhibitors such as macrolides or azole antifungals; initiation of carbamazepine for headache or neuropathic disorders in patients receiving agents such as macrolides or azole antifungals; or initiation of theophylline for chronic management of uncontrolled chronic obstructive pulmonary disease in patients receiving certain fluoroquinolones for treatment of an acute exacerbation of bronchitis. When such situations arise, it is often possible to delay initiation of other potentially interacting drugs until after the course of antimicrobial therapy has been completed without placing patients at undue risk or inconvenience.

### *Consider Concomitant Disease States, Particularly Organ Dysfunction*

Practitioners must be aware of concomitant disease states or conditions that may affect the safe use of antimicrobials. Conditions associated with decreased renal or hepatic function may have important effects on the potential for adverse drug interactions, including both pharmacokinetic and pharmacodynamic interactions. Use of agents such as aminoglycosides, amphotericin B, or foscarnet in patients with underlying renal dysfunction increases the risk of antimicrobial-induced nephrotoxicity and would increase the potential for pharmacokinetic alterations of other concomitantly administered agents that are renally eliminated [2,3,11,12]. Patients with significant liver disease or other conditions associated with hypoalbuminemia may be predisposed to interactions involving decreased binding of drugs to albumin-binding sites.

Pharmacodynamic interactions may also be of special concern in patients with organ dysfunction, particularly those interactions associated with overlapping adverse effect profiles of concomitantly administered drugs. Pharmacokinetic alterations in drug metabolism or elimination caused by organ dysfunction may lead to increased concentrations of concurrently administered drugs and thus perhaps predispose patients to pharmacodynamic interactions that would otherwise be relatively minor. Important examples of such interactions include use of ganciclovir and trimethoprim/ sulfamethoxazole in patients with renal insufficiency (increased potential for bone marrow suppression) [11] or combined use of nucleoside reverse transcriptase inhibitors, which is associated with peripheral neuropathy in patients with hepatic or renal disease [2].

Although many of the potential drug interactions in the examples above would be present in patients with normal organ function as well, the risk of significant interactions is often increased in patients with preexisting diseases. The risk of adverse drug interactions in patients with organ dysfunction may often be reduced by modification of dosage regimens to allow for pharmacokinetic alterations; however, data regarding appropriate dosage modifications are sometimes unavailable *(13)*. Alternatively, antimicrobials should be selected based on known pharmacokinetic and pharmacodynamic properties to minimize the potential impact of preexisting diseases on adverse drug interactions.

### Select Drugs With the Least Potential for Known or Predictable Interactions

Once the need for treatment has been established, preexisting patient factors have been evaluated, and other concomitant medications have been considered, agents with the least known or theoretical potential for significant drug interactions should be selected. Again, this particular strategy seems rather obvious. However, several specific aspects are worth reiterating.

Antimicrobial agents are often selected first on the basis of the desired antimicrobial class to be used, after which a specific agent within the class is selected based on differences in antimicrobial spectrum, pharmacokinetics, adverse effect profiles, cost, compliance issues, formulary considerations, and so on. Practitioners must initially consider whether certain classes of antimicrobials should be avoided in a particular patient (e.g., fluoroquinolones in a patient on chronic antacid therapy for gastroesophageal reflux disease or sulfonamides in a patient receiving warfarin for chronic atrial fibrillation).

After the decision to use a certain class of antimicrobials has been made, the practitioner should then consider whether there are any differences between specific agents within the class in terms of potentially significant drug interactions. If a macrolide-type drug is to be used, azithromycin may be a better choice than erythromycin or clarithromycin based on concurrent medications or other risk factors for significant drug interactions *(14,15)*. Specific fluoroquinolones also differ from each other in their potential for CYP-mediated drug interactions; thus, levofloxacin or gatifloxacin may be better choices than ciprofloxacin in patients receiving drugs such as theophylline or warfarin *(4,16–19)*. Because not all agents within the same antimicrobial class necessarily share the same potential for significant interactions, appropriate selection of a specific agent within a class must include considerations of differences in pharmacokinetics, degree of CYP inhibition or induction, and so on.

Differences in in vitro activity among specific agents within an antimicrobial class should also be considered when evaluating the potential for significant drug interactions. For example, in the treatment of *Staphylococcus aureus* infection, inadvertent coadministration of calcium carbonate and the resultant 50% decrease in absorption of fluoroquinolones may be less clinically significant for moxifloxacin than for ciprofloxacin because of moxifloxacin's significantly greater in vitro staphylococcal activity and lower minimum inhibitory concentrations (MICs) for staphylococci *(20)*.

In summary, differences among antimicrobial classes as well as among specific agents within each class must be considered when selecting drugs to avoid or minimize the potential for significant drug interaction.

## *When Possible, Avoid Drugs Associated*
## *With Serious Adverse Effects or Toxicities*

General principles of appropriate drug selection dictate that agents with serious adverse effect potential should be avoided when possible. From the perspective of avoiding or minimizing drug interactions, practitioners should remember that neither the occurrence nor the magnitude of drug interactions is always known or accurately predicted. Therefore, antimicrobials with potential for causing toxicities should be avoided when possible to minimize the potential severity of unpredictable drug interactions and resulting increased drug exposure should they occur.

## *Avoid Concurrent Administration of Drugs*
## *With Overlapping Adverse Effect Profiles*

When prospectively designing or modifying drug regimens, attention should be given to avoiding the use of agents with overlapping adverse effect profiles. Well-documented examples of important pharmacodynamic interactions include increased incidence of neutropenia with concurrent administration of zidovudine and ganciclovir, trimethoprim/sulfamethoxazole, sulfadiazine, or interferon-$\alpha$ *(21–23)*. As noted, patients with acute illnesses or organ system dysfunction may be more predisposed to the occurrence of certain additive or synergistic toxicities. Adverse pharmacodynamic interactions are often unpredictable and are best avoided or minimized by not providing opportunities for such interactions to occur.

## *Use the Smallest Effective Drug Doses*

Many drugs, antimicrobials as well as non-antimicrobials, are associated with dose- and concentration-dependent toxicities. The severity and clinical significance of drug interactions, particularly pharmacokinetic interactions associated with decreased metabolism and increased concentrations of the affected drugs, are often closely related to the relative increase in drug concentrations above normally observed ranges. One strategy to minimize the significance of potential drug interactions is therefore to reduce this relative increase in drug concentrations and thus avoid the concentration-related toxicities that result. This can be accomplished by using the smallest effective doses and lowest effective concentrations for drugs that may potentially be involved in drug interactions.

The occurrence and magnitude of drug interactions are not always predictable, and some potential drug interactions may not be readily avoidable because of the nature of the disease states involved and necessity for use of other concomitant medications. However, using the smallest possible doses may minimize the severity of the interactions should they occur.

## *Do Not Overestimate the Ability of Patients*
## *to Adhere to Recommended Dosing Schedules*

Many well-recognized pharmacokinetic drug interactions are related to decreased absorption of medications because of chelation or pH-dependent mechanisms in the gastrointestinal tract. Studies have clearly demonstrated that spacing the administration of medications at least 1–2 hours apart minimizes many of these significant absorption-related drug interactions; examples include decreased bioavailability of fluoroquinolones caused by antacids, sucralfate, and didanosine; decreased bioavailability of ketoconazole and itraconazole caused by antacids, didanosine, and gastric acid-suppressive agents; and decreased bioavailability of indinavir caused by didanosine *(24–34)*.

Although it is possible to minimize these interactions by proper spacing of medications, practitioners should not rely on the abilities of patients to adhere properly to very detailed and specific administration schedules. This is particularly true when the antimicrobials are used for the treatment of moderate-to-severe infections or those infections caused by difficult pathogens such as *Pseudomonas aeruginosa* or fungi; in these situations, patient nonadherence may result in therapeutic failure or development of antimicrobial resistance.

Proper spacing of medications in the treatment of HIV-infected patients may also be problematic because of the sheer number of drugs involved and the association of both nonadherence and low serum concentrations of antiretroviral agents with viral response to therapy *(35–40)*; the use of newer medications that require only once- or twice-daily administration has eased this difficulty to some extent but not overcome it. Concomitant administration of medications shown to result in significant drug interactions should be avoided whenever possible, despite the fact that such interactions can perhaps be prevented by manipulation of administration techniques or schedules.

## STRATEGIES FOR EVALUATING PREEXISTING DRUG REGIMENS FOR POTENTIAL DRUG INTERACTIONS

As previously stated, the most effective way to avoid significant drug interactions is to completely avoid the use of drugs that are likely to be involved in such interactions in a specific patient. However, practitioners often become involved in the management of patients after the selection and initiation of drug therapy has already occurred. It is therefore vital that practitioners are also able to evaluate these preexisting drug regimens prospectively for potentially important interactions before they become clinically significant (e.g., before the patient starts exhibiting signs or symptoms of toxicities).

Comprehensive knowledge of the pharmacokinetics and pharmacodynamics of antimicrobial agents, as well as knowledge of significant drug interactions associated with each, is the most reliable method of detecting and managing drug interactions. However, as the number of antimicrobial agents continues to increase and the number of documented or presumed drug interactions continues to expand, it becomes ever more difficult for practitioners to keep personal knowledge bases comprehensive and complete. Practitioners must therefore develop methods for quickly evaluating multidrug regimens for potential drug interactions. To do this, there are a number of considerations that should be taken into account to recognize the potential for significant drug interactions involving antimicrobials. Again, many of these considerations are relatively straightforward and dictated by common sense and clinical experience as much as by drug-specific data.

As previously discussed, a number of nonprescription drugs and natural products are capable of causing clinically significant drug interactions. Clinicians must be careful to consider such nonprescription drug use as well as prescription medications when evaluating preexisting drug regimens.

**Table 2**
**Clues That Should Prompt Careful Evaluation**
**of Preexisting Drug Regimens for Potential Drug Interactions**

- Drugs with well-documented drug interaction potential
- Drugs with known, relatively narrow therapeutic ranges
- Drugs with well-described pharmacodynamic determinants of efficacy or toxicity
- Drugs associated with serious adverse effects or toxicities
- Presence of extensive medication profiles in patients who cannot be easily monitored for drug efficacy and toxicity

The following section presents a number of drug and patient characteristics that, when observed, should alert practitioners to closely scrutinize the complete drug regimen for potentially significant interactions. These clues signaling the need for careful evaluation of regimens are listed in Table 2. One very basic rule that should be remembered when evaluating drug regimens for interactions is this: Any drug in the regimen that is unnecessary or of questionable benefit should be discontinued. Drugs that the patient does not take will not interact with any other drug.

### Drugs With Well-Documented Drug Interaction Potential

The presence of antimicrobials such as erythromycin, clarithromycin, tetracyclines, fluoroquinolones, metronidazole, sulfonamides, azole-type antifungals (particularly itraconazole and voriconazole), rifamycins, nucleoside or nonnucleoside reverse transcriptase inhibitors, and protease inhibitors should immediately alert practitioners to the need to evaluate the complete drug regimen for potentially significant drug interactions. These agents have been well documented to be involved in a number of pharmacokinetic or pharmacodynamic drug interactions that have resulted in therapeutic failure because of lack of efficacy or drug toxicities of these or concomitantly administered drugs. The presence of certain non-antimicrobials should also immediately prompt practitioners to evaluate regimens thoroughly for potential drug interactions with antimicrobials; these include drugs such as warfarin, digoxin, theophylline, phenytoin, carbamazepine, phenobarbital, antiarrhythmic agents, immunosuppressant agents (e.g., cyclosporine, mycophenolate, sirolimus), antacids, sucralfate, and tricyclic antidepressants. Drug interactions involving the aforementioned antimicrobial and non-antimicrobial agents have been reasonably well characterized and should be readily recognizable to experienced practitioners in nearly every area of clinical practice.

### Drugs With Known, Relatively Narrow Therapeutic Ranges

Drugs such as warfarin, digoxin, theophylline, phenytoin, carbamazepine, and cyclosporine are known to possess relatively narrow therapeutic ranges that are associated with efficacy or toxicity. These agents are also well known to be involved in adverse interactions with antimicrobial agents. The presence of these types of drugs should therefore prompt practitioners to examine the complete drug regimen carefully for potentially significant interactions. Fortunately, most of these agents are capable of being monitored by measured plasma drug concentrations or laboratory measures of pharmacological effect (e.g., warfarin), and suspected interactions may be rapidly evaluated.

However, the effects of these drugs on concomitant antimicrobial therapy may not be as easily assessed; the first sign of adverse drug interactions involving antimicrobials is often therapeutic failure in the treatment of the infection.

## Drugs With Well-Described Pharmacodynamic Determinants of Efficacy or Toxicity

The pharmacodynamic determinants of therapeutic efficacy or toxicity have not yet been well described for many antimicrobials. For agents such as the penicillins and cephalosporins, pharmacodynamic properties (e.g., time during which concentrations are above the MIC) have been well associated with bactericidal effects and therapeutic efficacy *(41)*; however, these drugs are relatively free of clinically significant interactions, and failure to achieve optimal plasma concentrations is usually attributed to underdosing or high MICs of difficult pathogens rather than to adverse drug interactions.

There are certain antimicrobials for which the pharmacodynamics have been reasonably well described and that are subject to clinically significant drug interactions. The bactericidal efficacy of the fluoroquinolones, for example, is related to achieving favorable peak plasma concentration-to-MIC ratios ($C_{max}$ :MIC ratio) or ratios of the favorable area under the plasma concentration–time curve (AUC) to MIC (AUC:MIC ratio) *(41–44)*. Therapeutic efficacy of the protease inhibitors has been related to the minimum plasma concentration $C_{min}$ of the drugs in plasma; risk of selecting resistant strains of HIV has also been related to low protease inhibitor $C_{min}$ during therapy *(36,45–47)*. Both the fluoroquinolones and the protease inhibitors have been associated with a multitude of drug interactions that have the potential for adversely affecting plasma concentrations and thus adversely affecting pharmacodynamic determinants of efficacy; practitioners should be alert to the possibilities of potential drug interactions when these agents are part of multidrug regimens.

## Drugs Associated With Severe Toxicities

Antimicrobials such as amphotericin B, ganciclovir, foscarnet, high-dose trimethoprim/sulfamethoxazole, pentamidine, and zidovudine are frequently associated with severe toxicities and should prompt careful review of drug regimens for potential interactions. Non-antimicrobials such as warfarin, digoxin, carbamazepine, antiarrhythmic agents, cyclosporine and other immunosuppressants, and chemotherapeutic agents are also associated with severe toxicities as a result of drug interactions, and regimens that include such agents should be carefully evaluated. The presence of overlapping adverse effect profiles and potential for additive or synergistic toxicities should also always be carefully evaluated.

## Presence of Extensive Medication Profiles in Patients Who Cannot Be Easily Monitored

Particularly in the outpatient setting, the presence of extensive drug regimens should serve as a signal that the practitioner must carefully assess the regimen for potential drug interactions. Many patients are seen as outpatients and returned home with minimal or no follow-up after additions or modifications to their drug regimens have occurred. Individuals treated as inpatients may also be discharged from the hospital shortly after changes to their medication regimens have been made and before potential interactions can be fully assessed. Without the ability to provide careful follow-up and monitoring for drug interactions, any interactions that occur may lead to severe toxicities, premature discontinuation of medication because of adverse effects, or unsuccessfully treated disease states that may reappear in the future with more severe and previously preventable complications. The inability to ensure adequate follow-up necessitates a thorough evaluation of medication regimens for possible interactions before the patient leaves the clinic.

## OTHER CONSIDERATIONS FOR CIRCUMVENTING OR MINIMIZING DRUG INTERACTIONS

Unfortunately, the majority of antimicrobials and non-antimicrobials alike are not routinely monitored by plasma concentration determinations, and there are no readily available laboratory measures of pharmacological effect (e.g., international normalized ratio for warfarin). Practitioners must thus be alert to the possibility of drug interactions that are not easily observed until the patient's disease state fails to improve or evidence of toxicities develops. This is particularly true in the treatment of infectious diseases; the first sign that an adverse drug interaction has occurred may be when the pathogen develops resistance to agents to which it was previously susceptible, or when a patient with HIV infection returns to the clinic with a significantly decreased CD4+ lymphocyte count and evidence of significant disease progression. Good clinical skills and conscientious patient monitoring and follow-up are usually the best tools for detecting and minimizing drug interactions as they occur.

In this regard, as previously discussed, patients treated in acute care or other inpatient settings may be at less risk for significant drug interactions than those treated as outpatients. Patients treated in inpatient settings have more closely supervised medical care, often have extensive and frequent laboratory testing performed, and are often under the watchful eye of a number of various health care professionals during their hospital stay. As a result, drug interactions occurring in this setting are often detected at an earlier point in time before serious complications have occurred and are able to be managed more effectively. Conversely, patients treated in various outpatient settings often go for long periods of time between follow-up visits and are at higher risk for more severe complications caused by any drug interactions that may occur. As a result, patients for whom follow-up is sporadic or scheduled at relatively long intervals must have their medications carefully scrutinized for any potentially significant interactions before they are released under their own supervision.

It should also be particularly noted that many patients treated as outpatients may be receiving drug prescriptions from more than one health care provider and may have their prescriptions filled at more than one pharmacy. As a result, drugs with potentially significant interactions may unknowingly be simultaneously prescribed by separate practitioners; these potential drug interactions may then go undetected because of the unavailability of complete medication profiles. Patients evaluated in the outpatient setting should be specifically asked whether they are seen by more than one health care provider and whether their prescriptions are filled at more than one pharmacy. Patients should be encouraged to use only one pharmacy for all prescriptions to avoid this potentially dangerous situation.

Finally, the importance of good patient education and counseling cannot be too strongly emphasized. Patients whose medical care is not closely supervised and moni-

**Table 3**
**Useful Drug Interaction Resources for Clinicians**

Drug Topics Red Book 2004. Montvale, NJ: Medical Economics Company, 2004
  (drug–food, drug–alcohol, and drug–tobacco interactions)

Hansten PD, Horn JR. Drug Interactions: Analysis and Management.. St. Louis, MO:
  Facts and Comparisons, 2004 (quarterly)

Pronsky ZM. Food–Medication Interactions. 13th ed. Birchrunville, PA:
  Food-Medication Interactions, 2003

Stockley IH. Drug Interactions. 5th ed. London, England: Pharmaceutial Press, 1999

Tatro DS. Drug Interaction Facts. St. Louis, MO: Facts and Comparisons, 2004 (quarterly)

Tatro DS. Drug Interaction Facts: Herbal Supplements and Food. St. Louis, MO:
  Facts and Comparisons, 2004 (quarterly)

Zucchero FJ, Hogan MJ, Sommer CD. Evaluations of Drug Interactions (EDI).
  Vol. 1. St. Louis, MO: First Databank, 2001 (bimonthly)

Zucchero FJ, Hogan MJ, Sommer CD. Evaluations of Drug Interactions (EDI).
  Vol. 2. St. Louis, MO: First Databank, 2001 (bimonthly)

Computer databases and Internet resources
  • Micromedex Drugdex® System, Drug-REAX® System, and AltMed-REAX™
    for the Professional, and Drug Interaction Tool for the Hand-Held PDA. Englewood, CO:
    Micromedex
  • http://www.medscape.com
  • www.drkoop.com/drugstore/pharmacy/interactions-entry.asp
  • http://www.hiv-druginteractions.org
  • http://www.aidsinfo.nih.gov/guidelines
  • http://www.hivatis.org
  • http://www.foodmedinteractions.com

tored on a regular basis require more complete education regarding the purpose of their medications, any special instructions for drug administration or scheduling of doses, and signs and symptoms that may be early indicators of significant drug interactions. The last should consist of appropriate education regarding the expected time-course of improvement of their diseases state (including resolution of infections) and signs of potential drug toxicity. Patients should be given sufficient information to appropriately evaluate for both obvious treatment failure and any possibly drug-related toxicities, which may be indicative of potential drug interactions.

## RESOURCES FOR CLINICIANS

A number of excellent resources are available to assist the clinician in identifying and managing potential drug interactions (Table 3). These references include general drug interaction compendia as well as resources dedicated to specific types of interactions (e.g., drug–food interactions). Several references for information regarding interactions with natural products and alternative medicines are also now available. In addition to printed literature and textbooks of various types, several Internet Web sites are also available or currently under development. The clinician must bear in mind that these reference sources may lag behind new drug development and often do not include recently approved agents. These references also often include only those interactions that have been specifically studied and for which documenting literature is available.

Thus, interactions that are likely to occur based on agents possessing pharmacological properties similar to other drugs known to cause interactions (e.g., CYP-mediated interactions) but have yet to be proven are not always be included. Although these resources are not always current or comprehensive, they are nevertheless useful in supplementing the practitioner's personal knowledge base and aiding in the assessment of the potential clinical significance of interactions.

## SUMMARY

Given the number of antimicrobials available for use, the complexity of treating certain types of infections, and the number of various medications used in certain patient populations, the potential for clinically significant drug interactions is very high. Many interactions are of minimal clinical importance and often ignored; other interactions are associated with substantial risk of adverse pharmacokinetic or pharmacodynamic interactions, resulting in decreased therapeutic efficacy, increased incidence of drug toxicities, or potential for increased antimicrobial resistance. Thus, the ability to prevent or minimize adverse drug interactions is of vital importance in optimizing the appropriate and effective use of antimicrobials and enhancing patient outcome.

The key to avoiding or minimizing the significance of drug interactions is for practitioners to possess a thorough understanding of the drugs they are most often using. There is no effective substitute for adequate knowledge regarding potential interactions and familiarity with the literature addressing the actual clinical importance of these interactions. In the absence of specific data, familiarity with the pharmacokinetic and pharmacodynamic characteristics of the particular agents may assist clinicians in predicting the likelihood of possible interactions. Only after practitioners possess a thorough knowledge of the specific agents can strategies for circumventing drug interactions be effectively employed.

Risk-vs-benefit considerations regarding the use of potentially interacting drugs should be contemplated when initiating or continuing any agent. Appropriate management decisions are again based on a thorough understanding of the drugs used and the exercise of some degree of common sense.

A number of strategies can be employed, and characteristics of patients or drugs should be examined, which will facilitate the avoidance or minimization of significant drug interactions. Drugs should be prospectively evaluated for potential interactions as they are initially selected for use and prior to actual administration to the patient. A number of "red flags" also exist that should prompt the evaluation of preexisting drug regimens for potentially important interactions. In either scenario, the goal is to evaluate the potential for interactions *prospectively* to make appropriate decisions regarding drug management before problems resulting from drug interactions actually arise.

### CASE STUDY 1

S.D. is a 39-year-old male who was diagnosed with HIV infection in 2001. His illness has been complicated by failure of multiple antiretroviral regimens, severe hypersensitivity reaction to abacavir, cryptococcal meningitis, and disseminated *Mycobacterium avium* complex infection that has been slow to respond to medical management and multiple surgical resections. At the last clinic visit, his CD4 lymphocyte count was 80 cells/mm$^3$, and his HIV viral load was 89,300 RNA copies/mL; all antiretroviral agents were stopped at that time pending the results of viral phenotyping for drug susceptibility. He is now seen in clinic 2 weeks later and is to be started on a susceptibility-guided antiretroviral drug regimen consisting of 300 mg tenofovir once daily, 300 mg lamivudine once daily, 100 mg ritonavir once daily, 300 mg atazanavir once daily, and 600 mg efavirenz once daily at night. His other current medications are 160/800 mg trimethoprim/sulfamethoxazole once daily, 500 mg clarithromycin twice daily, 1200 mg ethambutol once daily, 150 mg rifabutin every other day, and 200 mg fluconazole every other day.

This case illustrates the complexities of management of HIV infection and provides an example of a drug regimen containing numerous potential drug interactions involving multiple classes of drugs. This case also provides examples of taking advantage of certain drug interactions to counteract other potentially harmful interactions and produce overall favorable pharmacokinetic and therapeutic effects. Considering interactions between the various antiretroviral agents, tenofovir has been shown to decrease the atazanavir AUC by approx 25% and $C_{min}$ by approx 40% *(46,48)*. These changes are enough to result in potentially subtherapeutic concentrations of atazanavir. Conversely, however, ritonavir may increase the atazanavir AUC by more than 300% and the $C_{min}$ by 1000% *(49,50)*. This "boosting" of atazanavir by ritonavir-induced inhibition of CYP3A4 enzymes is more than sufficient to overcome the effects of concomitant tenofovir use and allows atazanavir to be used in safe and convenient low, once-daily doses. The AUC of tenofovir may be increased approx 25% by atazanavir, but this interaction is not felt to be significant *(46)*. Ritonavir's CYP3A4 inhibition also increases the AUC of efavirenz by approx 20% *(46)*; the inhibition of CYP2C9 or CYP2C19 pathways by efavirenz likewise results in a 20% increase in the AUC of ritonavir *(50,51)*.

This patient is also receiving multiple medications for treatment or prevention of opportunistic infections, and several potential drug interactions involving these drugs are present. Ritonavir increases the plasma AUC of rifabutin approximately fourfold and can result in increased rifabutin-induced toxicities *(52)*; reduction of the rifabutin dose is therefore recommended *(53)*. Although rifabutin is an inducer of CYP3A4, the interaction with ritonavir is not sufficient to require an increase in ritonavir dosage *(53)*. Similar to ritonavir, atazanavir also increases the AUC of rifabutin by approx 250% *(46,48)*; however, efavirenz decreases rifabutin's AUC by approx 35% *(46,50,51,54)*. Mixed effects may also be seen on the plasma concentrations of clarithromycin as a result of interactions with antiretrovirals. The AUC of clarithromycin is increased approx 75% by ritonavir and 95% by atazanavir; concomitant use of efavirenz results in a 40% decreased clarithromycin AUC *(46,55)*. Rifabutin can also substantially decrease concentrations of clarithromycin *(56)*. The overall effects on clarithromycin pharmacokinetics as a result of these interactions probably do not necessitate changes in clarithromycin dosing in patients with normal renal function *(55)*. Finally, fluconazole can inhibit CYP3A4 and increase the AUC of rifabutin by up to 75% *(57)*. This potential interaction must also be considered along with those caused by the antiretroviral drugs that affect the pharmacokinetics of rifabutin.

These numerous potential interactions involving both increased or decreased concentrations of multiple drugs must all be carefully evaluated by clinicians involved in the management of such patients. Although the use of fewer drugs with decreased potential for significant drug interactions would have been desirable, the choice of drugs in this patient was dictated by clinical circumstances and allowed little flexibility in the design of the total drug regimen. The drugs in S.D.'s regimen appear to be dosed appropriately in consideration of the types and magnitudes of the various interactions. However, close monitoring of S.D. for response to therapy and clinically important toxicities will obviously be required.

## CASE STUDY 2

T. R. is a 44-year-old female with a past medical history significant for severe gastroesophageal reflux disease (GERD) and recurrent urinary tract infection (UTI). Her current medications include 40 mg omeprazole orally twice daily, multivitamin with iron orally once daily, and 1–2 tablespoons aluminum hydroxide/magnesium hydroxide antacid every 2 hours as needed for breakthrough acid reflux symptoms. She was last treated for a UTI 5 weeks ago and received a 10-day course of amoxicillin/clavulanate at that time.

She is now seen in the internal medicine clinic complaining of cough, fever, fatigue, and anorexia. Physical examination reveals a temperature of 38.8°C, heart rate of 95 beats/minute, and respiratory rate of 26 breaths/minute; blood pressure is within normal limits. A chest radiograph performed in the clinic reveals a middle right lobe infiltrate, and the diagnosis of community-acquired pneumonia is made based on clinical and radiographic findings. She is judged to be moderately ill and is to be treated as an outpatient. What antimicrobial regimen should be selected for treatment of T. R.'s pneumonia?

Current guidelines for treatment of community-acquired pneumonia recommend that macrolides and doxycycline are the preferred agents in patients without significant comorbidities who are to be treated as outpatients (58,59). However, T. R.'s recent course of antibiotic therapy may put her at increased risk of infection with drug-resistant strains of *Streptococcus pneumoniae*. A treatment regimen consisting of the combination of a β-lactam (amoxicillin or amoxicillin/clavulanate) plus a macrolide or monotherapy with a fluoroquinolone may therefore be preferred (59). The lack of any significant drug interactions between β-lactams or macrolides and her other current medications would make this regimen an attractive choice for treatment of her pneumonia. The fact that she received amoxicillin/clavulanate for her most recent UTI, however, may perhaps make a fluoroquinolone the clinically preferred therapy for her respiratory tract infection.

Fluoroquinolones such as levofloxacin, gatifloxacin, and moxifloxacin would be potentially appropriate choices in this patient because of favorable activity against respiratory tract pathogens, including strains resistant to β-lactams, and proven clinical efficacy in the treatment of community-acquired pneumonia. These fluoroquinolones have been shown not to have any significant drug interactions when administered concurrently with acid-suppressive agents such as histamine$_2$-receptor antagonists and proton pump inhibitors *(4,27,28,60–65)*. The concomitant use of omeprazole and a fluoroquinolone should therefore not be of concern in this patient. However, divalent cation-containing antacids have been shown to decrease the bioavailability of fluoroquinolones by as much as 70 to 90% *(4,27,60–63,65,66)*. T. R.'s use of antacids for relief of breakthrough GERD symptoms therefore has the potential to cause a significant interaction with any fluoroquinolone regimen, and concomitant use of these drugs would be contraindicated.

Two potential options would still allow the use of fluoroquinolones for the treatment of T. R.'s infection: either discontinue as-needed use of antacids for the duration of antibiotic therapy or time the administration of the antacids so that they are not administered within 2 hours before or 4–6 hours after taking the fluoroquinolone *(4,60,63,66)*. Whether one of these options would be appropriate for T. R. would depend on her frequency of antacid use and her perceived ability to adhere to a carefully timed administration schedule for her medications. If the severity of her GERD and frequency of breakthrough symptoms is such that antacid use cannot be temporarily discontinued for the duration of antibiotic therapy, careful timing of drug administration becomes the necessary option. However, if T. R. is not able to adhere to the required drug administration schedule, then fluoroquinolone therapy may not be an appropriate option for T. R. despite the clinical reasons for selecting a fluoroquinolone for treatment of her pneumonia. The decision of whether to use a fluoroquinolone or return to a β-lactam-based regimen is a decision that must be made by the clinician in concert with T. R.

Multivitamins with iron also pose a problem for the use of fluoroquinolones in T. R. Similar to antacids, ferrous sulfate- and iron-containing multivitamins have been demonstrated to decrease fluoroquinolone bioavailability by as much as 70% as a result of the formation of chelation complexes *(4,61–63,67–69)*. Should a fluoroquinolone be used by T. R., the best strategy to avoid an undesirable drug interaction would be to discontinue multivitamin use for the duration of antibiotic therapy.

Although a fluoroquinolone is perhaps the preferred antibiotic for this patient's pneumonia based on current recommendations, T. R.'s use of antacids for severe GERD poses some difficulty because of the significant clinical consequences of the potential drug interaction. Again, the decision whether to use a fluoroquinolone as would normally be recommended or alternatively to use a regimen of β-lactam plus macrolide is a decision that must be made after consideration of clinical risks and benefits as well as T. R.'s ability to adhere to potentially necessary changes in her antacid use.

## REFERENCES

1. Fantry LE, Tramont EC. *Treponema pallidum.* In: Yu V, Merigan T, Barriere SL, eds. Antimicrobial Chemotherapy and Vaccines. Baltimore, MD: Williams and Wilkins, 1998, pp. 462–471.
2. Piscitelli SC, Gallicano KD. Interactions among drugs for HIV and opportunistic infections. N Engl J Med 2001;344:984–996.
3. Albengres E, Le Louet H, Tillement JP. Systemic antifungal agents. Drug interactions of clinical significance. Drug Safety 1998;18:83–97.

4. Fish DN. Fluoroquinolone adverse effects and drug interactions. Pharmacotherapy 2001; 21(suppl):253S–272S.

5. Sommers DK, Van Wyk M, Moncrieff J. Influence of food and reduced gastric acidity on the bioavailability of bacampicillin and cefuroxime axetil. Br J Clin Pharmacol 1984;18: 535–539.

6. Saathoff N, Lode H, Neider K, et al. Pharmacokinetics of cefpodoxime proxetil and interactions with an antacid and an $H_2$ receptor antagonist. Antimicrob Agents Chemother 1992;36:796–800.

7. Satterwhite JH, Cerimele BJ, Coleman DL. Pharmacokinetics of cefaclor AF: effects of age, antacids and $H_2$-receptor antagonists. Postgrad Med J 1992;68:S3–S9.

8. Peloquin CA, Bulpitt AE, Jaresko GS, Jelliffe RW, Childs JM, Nix DE. Pharmacokinetics of ethambutol under fasting conditions, with food, and with antacids. Antimicrob Agents Chemother 1999;43:568–572.

9. Chin TF, Lach JL. Drug diffusion and bioavailability: tetracycline metal chelation. Am J Hosp Pharm 1975;32:625–629.

10. Piscitelli SC, Burstein AH, Chaitt D, et al. Indinavir concentrations and St. John's wort. Lancet 2000;355:547–548.

11. Tseng AL, Foisy MM. Management of drug interactions in patients with HIV. Ann Pharmacother 1997;31:1040–1058.

12. Lee BL, Safrin S. Interactions and toxicities of drugs used in patients with AIDS. Clin Infect Dis 1992;14:773–779.

13. Hilts AE, Fish DN. Dosing of antiretroviral agents in patients with organ dysfunction. Am J Health-Syst Pharm 1998;55:2528–2533.

14. Periti P, Mazzei T, Mini E, Novelli A. Pharmacokinetic drug interactions of macrolides. Clin Pharmacokinet 1992;23:106–131.

15. Rodvold KA, Piscitelli SC. New oral macrolide and fluoroquinolone antibiotics: an overview of pharmacokinetics, interactions, and safety. Clin Infect Dis 1993;17(suppl 1): S192–S199.

16. Okimoto N, Niki Y, Soejima R. Effect of levofloxacin on serum concentration of theophylline. Chemotherapy 1992;40(suppl 3):68–74.

17. Gisclon LG, Curtin CR, Fowler CL, et al. Absence of a pharmacokinetic interaction between intravenous theophylline and orally administered levofloxacin. J Clin Pharmacol 1997;37:744–750.

18. Stass H, Kubitza D. Profile of moxifloxacin drug interactions. Clin Infect Dis 2001;32 (suppl 1):S47–S50.

19. Liao S, Palmer M, Fowler C, Nayak RK. Absence of an effect of levofloxacin on warfarin pharmacokinetics and anticoagulation in male volunteers. J Clin Pharmacol 1996;36: 1072–1077.

20. Blondeau JM. A review of the comparative in-vitro activity of 12 antimicrobial agents, with a focus on five new "respiratory quinolones." J Antimicrob Chemother 1999;43 (suppl B):1–12.

21. Causey D. Concomitant ganciclovir and zidovudine treatment for cytomegalovirus retinitis in patients with HIV infection: an approach to treatment. J Acquir Immune Defic Syndr 1991;4(suppl 1):S16–S21.

22. Hochster H, Dieterich D, Bozzette S, et al. Toxicity of combined ganciclovir and zidovudine for cytomegalovirus disease associated with AIDS: an AIDS clinical trials group study. Ann Intern Med 1990;113:111–117.

23. Burger DM, Meenhorst PL, Koks CHW, Beijnen JH. Drug interactions with zidovudine. AIDS 1993;7:445–460.

24. Lomaestro BM, Baillie GR. Effect of staggered dose of calcium on the bioavailability of ciprofloxacin. Antimicrob Agents Chemother 1991;35:1004–1007.

25. Flor S, Guay DRP, Opsahl JA, et al. Effects of magnesium-aluminum hydroxide and calcium carbonate antacids on bioavailability of ofloxacin. Antimicrob Agents Chemother 1990;34:2436–2438.
26. Knupp CA, Barbhaiya RH. A multiple-dose pharmacokinetic interaction study between didanosine (Videx®) and ciprofloxacin (Cipro®) in male subjects seropositive for HIV but asymptomatic. Biopharm Drug Dispos 1997;18:65–77.
27. Nix DE, Watson WA, Lener ME, et al. Effects of aluminum and magnesium antacids and ranitidine on the absorption of ciprofloxacin. Clin Pharmacol Ther 1989;46:700–705.
28. Grasela TH Jr, Schentag JJ, Sedman AT, et al. Inhibition of enoxacin absorption by antacids or ranitidine. Antimicrob Agents Chemother 1989;33:615–617.
29. Van Slooten AD, Nix DE, Wilton JH, Love JH, Spivey JM, Goldstein HR. Combined use of ciprofloxacin and sucralfate. DICP Ann Pharmacother 1991;25:578–582.
30. Lee L-J, Hafkin B, Lee I-D, Hoh J, Dix R. Effects of food and sucralfate on a single oral dose of 500 mg of levofloxacin in healthy subjects. Antimicrob Agents Chemother 1997;41:2196–2200.
31. Sahai J, Gallicano K, Oliveras L, Khaliq S, Hawley-Foss N, Garber G. Cations in the didanosine tablet reduce ciprofloxacin bioavailability. Clin Pharmacol Ther 1993;53:292–297.
32. Piscitelli SC, Goss TF, Wilton JH, D'Andrea DT, Goldstein H, Schentag JJ. Effects of ranitidine and sucralfate on ketoconazole bioavailability. Antimicrob Agents Chemother 1991;35:1765–1771.
33. Blum RA, D'Andrea DT, Florentino BM, et al. Increased gastric pH and the bioavailability of fluconazole and ketoconazole. Ann Intern Med 1991;114:755–757.
34. Crixivan (indinavir sulfate) capsules product monograph. Whitehouse Station, NJ: Merck and Co., 2003.
35. Preston SL, Postelnick M, Purdy BD, Petrolati J, Aasi H, Stein DS. Drug interactions in HIV-positive patients initiated on protease inhibitor therapy [letter]. AIDS 1998;12:228–230.
36. Erice A, Balfour HH Jr. Resistance of human immunodeficiency virus type 1 to antiretroviral agents: a review. Clin Infect Dis 1994;18:149–156.
37. Singh N, Squier C, Sivek C, et al. Determinants of compliance with antiretroviral therapy in patients with human immunodeficiency virus: prospective assessment with implications for enhancing compliance. AIDS Care 1996;8:261–269.
38. Chesney MA. Factors affecting adherence to antiretroviral therapy. Clin Infect Dis 2000;30(suppl 2):S171–S176.
39. Nieuwkerk PT, Sprangers MA, Burger DM, et al. ATHENA Project. Limited patient adherence to highly active antiretroviral therapy for HIV-1 infection in an observational cohort study. Arch Intern Med 2001;161:1962–1968.
40. Samet EH, Libman H, Steger KA, et al. Compliance with zidovudine therapy in patients infected with human immunodeficiency virus, type 1: a cross-sectional study in a municipal hospital clinic. Am J Med 1992;92:495–502.
41. Craig WA. Pharmacokinetic/pharmacodynamic parameters: rationale for antibacterial dosing of mice and men. Clin Infect Dis 1998;26:1–12.
42. Maderas-Kelly KJ, Ostergaard BE, Hovde LB, Rotschafer JC. Twenty-four-hour area under the concentration-time curve/MIC ratio as a generic predictor or fluoroquinolone antimicrobial effect by using three strains of *Pseudomonas aeruginosa* and an in vitro pharmacodynamic model. Antimicrob Agents Chemother 1996;40:627–632.
43. Preston SL, Drusano GL, Berman AL, et al. Pharmacodynamics of levofloxacin. A new paradigm for early clinical trials. JAMA 1998;279:125–129.
44. Forrest A, Nix DE, Ballow CH, Goss TF, Birmingham MC, Schentag JJ. Pharmacodynamics of intravenous ciprofloxacin in severely ill patients. Antimicrob Agents Chemother 1993;37:1073–1081.

45. D'Aquila RT, Johnson VA, Wells SL, et al. Zidovudine resistance and HIV-1 disease progression during antiretroviral therapy. Ann Intern Med 1995;122:401–408.

46. US Department of Health and Human Services. Guidelines for the Use of Antiretroviral Agents in HIV-1 Infected Adults and Adolescents. November 10, 2003. Available at: http://aidsinfo.nih.gov/guidelines. Accessed: March 18, 2005.

47. Acosta EP, Henry K, Baken L, Page LM, Fletcher CV. Indinavir concentrations and antiviral effect. Pharmacotherapy 1999;19:708–712.

48. BMS Virology. Reyataz™ (atazanavir) product monograph. Princeton, NJ: Bristol-Myers Squibb, 2003.

49. Agarwala S, Russo R, Mummaneni V, Randall D, Geraldes M, O'Mara E. Steady-state pharmacokinetic interaction study of atazanavir with ritonavir in healthy subjects. American Society for Microbiology: Programs and Abstracts of the 42nd Interscience Conference on Antimicrobial Agents and Chemotherapy, San Diego, CA, September 27–30, 2002. Abstract H-1716.

50. Guidelines for the Use of Antiretroviral Agents in HIV-1-Infected Adults and Adolescents. Revised October 29, 2004. Available at: http://AIDSinfo.nih.gov/guidelines. Accessed: March 18, 2005.

51. Fiske W, Benedek IH, Joseph JL, et al. Pharmacokinetics of efavirenz (EFV) and ritonavir (RIT) after multiple oral doses in healthy volunteers [abstract]. Proceedings of the 12th World AIDS Conference, Geneva, Switzerland, June, 1998.

52. Cato A III, Cavanaugh J, Shi H, Hsu A, Leonard J, Granneman R. The effect of multiple doses of ritonavir on the pharmacokinetics of rifabutin. Clin Pharmacol Ther 1998;63:414–421.

53. Centers for Disease Control and Prevention. Updated guidelines for the use of rifabutin or rifampin for the treatment and prevention of tuberculosis among HIV-infected patients taking protease inhibitors or nonnucleoside reverse transcriptase inhibitors. MMWR Morb Mortal Wkly Rep 2000;49:185–189.

54. Hollender E, Stambaugh J, Ashkin D, et al. The concomitant use of rifabutin and efavirenz in HIV/TB coinfected patients. Proceedings of the 10th Conference on Retroviruses and Opportunistic Infections, Boston, MA, February, 2003. Abstract 785.

55. Ouellet D, Hsu A, Granneman GR, et al. Pharmacokinetic interaction between ritonavir and clarithromycin. Clin Pharmacol Ther 1998;64:355–362.

56. Hafner R, Bethel J, Power M, et al. Tolerance and pharmacokinetic interactions of rifabutin and clarithromycin in human immunodeficiency virus-infected volunteers. Antimicrob Agents Chemother 1998;42:631–639.

57. Trapnell CB, Narang PK, Li R, Lavelle JP. Increased plasma rifabutin levels with concomitant fluconazole therapy in HIV-infected patients. Ann Intern Med 1996;124:573–576.

58. Niederman MS, Mandell LA, Anzueto A, et al. Guidelines for the management of adults with community-acquired pneumonia. Diagnosis, assessment of severity, antimicrobial therapy, and prevention. Am J Respir Crit Care Med 2001;163:1730–1754.

59. Mandell LA, Bartlett JG, Dowell SF, File TM Jr, Musher DM, Whitney C. Update of practice guidelines for the management of community-acquired pneumonia in immunocompetent adults. Infectious Diseases Society of America. Clin Infect Dis 2003;37:1405–1433.

60. Balfour JAB, Wiseman LR. Moxifloxacin. Drugs 1999;57:363–373.

61. Shiba K, Kuaajima H, Momo K. The effects of aluminum hydroxide, cimetidine, ferrous sulfate, green tea, and milk on the pharmacokinetics of gatifloxacin in healthy humans [abstract]. Proceedings of the 21st International Congress of Chemotherapy, Birmingham, UK, July, 1999.

62. Tequin® (gatifloxacin) product monograph. Princeton, NJ: Bristol-Myers Squibb Co., October 2003.

63. Shiba K, Sakai O, Shimada J, Okazaki O, Aoki H, Hakusui H. Effects of antacids, ferrous sulfate, and ranitidine on absorption of DR-3355 in humans. Antimicrob Agents Chemother 1992;36:2270–2274.

64. Stuht H, Lode H, Koeppe P, Rost KL, Schaberg T. Interaction study of lomefloxacin and ciprofloxacin with omeprazole and comparative pharmacokinetics. Antimicrob Agents Chemother 1995;39:1045–1059.

65. Teng R, Dogolo LC, Willavize SA, Friedman HL, Vincent J. Effect of Maalox and omeprazole on the bioavailability of trovafloxacin. J Antimicrob Chemother 1997;39 (suppl B):93–97.

66. Lober S, Ziege S, Rau M, et al. Pharmacokinetics of gatifloxacin and interaction with an antacid containing aluminum and magnesium hydroxide. Antimicrob Agents Chemother 1999;43:1067–1071.

67. Polk RE, Healy DP, Sahai J, Drwal L, Racht E. Effect of ferrous sulfate and multivitamins with zinc on absorption of ciprofloxacin in normal volunteers. Antimicrob Agents Chemother 1989;33:1841–1844.

68. Kanemitsu K, Hori S, Yanagawa A, Shimada J. Effect of ferrous sulfate on the absorption of sparfloxacin in healthy volunteers and rats. Drugs 1995;49(suppl 2):352–356.

69. Lacreta FP, Kaul S, Kollia GD, Duncan G, Randall DM, Grasela DM. Pharmacokinetics (PK) and safety of gatifloxacin in combination with ferrous sulfate or calcium carbonate in healthy volunteers. American Society for Microbiology: Programs and Abstracts of the 39th Interscience Conference on Antimicrobial Agents and Chemotherapy, San Francisco, CA, September, 1999. Abstract 198.

# 15

# Design and Data Analysis
# of Drug Interaction Studies

## David E. Nix and Keith Gallicano

## STUDY RATIONALE

Drug interaction studies should be considered for drugs that are likely to be administered concomitantly to large numbers of patients. The drugs may be indicated for the same disease process, and their use in combination is considered therapeutically rational. Alternatively, the drugs may have different indications, but the two disease processes occur frequently in the same population. Drugs involved in interactions are divided into precipitant drugs (drugs that cause a change in the pharmacokinetics or pharmacodynamics of another drug) and the object drug (drug affected by the precipitant drug). A drug can act as a precipitant drug and an object drug at the same time when two drugs affect each other during concomitant administration.

To study large numbers of potential interactions routinely for all drugs is not feasible or desirable. Consequently, screening methods are required to identify drugs that are likely to interact. A chemist who is knowledgeable about drug interactions affecting gastrointestinal absorption may be able to identify potential interactions involving chelation, physical binding, or other incompatibility. Metabolism of object drugs may be studied using in vitro cytochrome P450 (CYP) enzyme preparations to identify enzymes involved in the metabolism (1,2). Databases are available of drugs that inhibit or induce various CYP subtypes. Once metabolism is determined to be a major elimination pathway and the responsible enzyme subtypes are known, these databases can be used to identify potentially interacting drugs (3). Preliminary interaction studies of substrates with metabolic inhibitors and inducers can be performed using the same in vitro enzyme preparations as those used to determine metabolic pathways of substrates (2,4). Similar methods have been adapted to investigate drug interactions involving intestinal metabolism and drug transport (5–7).

Interactions involving protein-binding displacement are not usually clinically significant. However, protein-binding interactions should be examined for drugs that (1) exhibit high binding to plasma proteins (>95%); (2) have a narrow therapeutic index; (3) occupy most of the available plasma protein-binding sites at clinically relevant concentrations; and (4) have a small volume of distribution (<10 L/70 kg),

From: *Infectious Disease: Drug Interactions in Infectious Diseases, Second Edition*
Edited by: S. C. Piscitelli and K. A. Rodvold © Humana Press Inc., Totowa, NJ

are restrictively cleared by the major organ of elimination (e.g., low hepatic clearance) or are nonrestrictively cleared (e.g., high renal clearance), and are administered parenterally *(8,9)*. Preliminary protein-binding studies can be carried out in vitro, recognizing that metabolites may contribute to protein displacement interactions. Interactions involving renal clearance changes may be expected for drugs that rely heavily on renal excretion for their elimination. For these drugs, the presence of significant tubular secretion or reabsorption suggests possible interactions. Pharmacodynamic interactions should be suspected for drugs that have similar pharmacological or toxicological effects.

## STUDY DESIGN: GENERAL ISSUES

Current regulatory guidances provide some insight into designs for in vivo drug interaction studies *(10,11)*. These guidances recommend three designs: (1) randomized crossover, (2) one-sequence crossover, or (3) parallel. A position paper by the Pharmaceutical Research and Manufacturers of America Drug Metabolism and Clinical Pharmacology Technical Working Groups has defined a minimal best practice for in vitro and in vivo pharmacokinetic drug–drug interaction studies targeted to drug development, with the goal of harmonizing approaches by regulatory agencies and industry sponsors *(12)*.

Drug interaction studies involve the measurement of pharmacokinetics or a specific pharmacodynamic effect in the presence and absence of a precipitant drug. Such studies typically employ a within-subject design in which individuals receive both treatments in either fixed or random order. A fixed-order design denotes a longitudinal or one-sequence crossover study in which the treatments are administered sequentially over two or more time periods, and all participants are grouped into a single sequence. Longitudinal studies are often conducted in patients who are receiving long-term therapy of the object drug or taking drugs with long elimination half-lives (>72 hours). A two-period, longitudinal study involves the administration of the object drug alone followed by measurement of the pharmacokinetics or effect parameter(s) over time in Period 1. A washout period may or may not be necessary. Then, the object and suspected precipitant drugs are concomitantly administered simultaneously or at different times in Period 2. Measurements of the pharmacokinetics or effect parameters are performed following administration of the combination treatment. In the longitudinal design, potential period effects are merged with the treatment effects. If a 30% change in the clearance of the object drug is observed, the change may have been caused by the precipitant drug or some other intercurrent event. Perhaps the food intake differed between the two periods (treatment phases), or a portion of the subjects acquired a mild viral infection between the two periods. If females are included as subjects, the number of subjects in the luteal phase of the menstrual cycle may differ between the two periods.

The study must be designed with full knowledge of the pharmacokinetics of both drugs. If the study involves single doses of the object drug, then adequate washout of the first dose must be allowed before starting the second treatment phase. For the control treatment, measuring serum concentrations or effect for at least 4–5 half-lives is important. If reduced clearance is expected with the interaction, the sampling time may need to be extended following concomitant treatment. If the study involves multiple-dose administration of the object drug, then the serum concentrations should reach steady state during both periods, particularly if the object drug has time-dependent pharmacokinetics, before assessing the pharmacokinetic or effect parameter(s).

The major advantage of a two-period, longitudinal design is that the potential for carryover effect from prior administration of the precipitant drug is avoided. A switchback design in which the object drug is replicated at least once after the precipitant drug is discontinued is useful to determine the effects of starting and stopping a metabolic inhibitor or inducer on the baseline characteristics of the object drug. Such a design was used to establish the rebound-to-baseline pharmacokinetic parameters of steady-state zidovudine at 14 days after rifampin was discontinued in Period 2 *(13)*.

Administration of the treatments in random order signifies a crossover study. A crossover design consists of a set of *S* sequences that describes the order in which all or some of the *T* treatments are to be given to the subjects in *P* periods and are designated as *T, P, S* designs, in which *T, P,* and *S* are greater than 1 *(14)*. The order of the treatments is randomized to the defined sequences, and the subjects are randomly assigned to one of the sequences. Designs that have a single (fixed) sequence are sometimes referred to as "crossover-like" but should be considered as a longitudinal study rather than a crossover study because single sequences cannot be randomized.

There are two main types of crossover designs: nonreplicated and replicated. Nonreplicated designs have the same number of treatments as periods, and the number of sequences increases as the factorial of *T* (i.e., when $T = 3$, $S = 6$). Replicate designs have more periods than treatments, such that at least one treatment is replicated within a subject. Optimum designs are those that are balanced with equal numbers in each sequence and balanced for carryover effects and variance for the given number of treatments. A design that has each treatment followed by a different treatment the same number of times is balanced for carryover. In a variance-balanced design, each treatment appears the same number of times in each period. The presence of a carryover effect is important to assess in drug interaction studies, and enough subjects in each sequence are needed to allow testing of this effect.

The simplest nonreplicated crossover design is the 2, 2, 2 design. This design is the most frequently used crossover design in drug interaction studies. Suppose Treatment A involves giving the object drug alone, and Treatment B involves giving the object drug with the precipitant drug. Subjects would receive the two treatments in one of two sequences, AB or BA, in which Treatment A or B would be given during the first period and then switched to the other treatment during the second period. Carryover effects may be introduced for subjects receiving Treatment B (Sequence BA) in the first period if drug exposures of the object drug are increased by the precipitant drug. An adequate washout period must be planned between the two periods to prevent differential carryover in the two sequences. This may sometimes be difficult if the duration of an "adequate" washout period is not known *a priori*. Carryover and sequence effects, however, are confounded in the 2, 2, 2 design, and studies in which the two treatments are replicated must be conducted for optimal evaluation of carryover effects.

When nonreplicated studies involve more than two periods, the number of sequences should be carefully planned rather than testing all possible sequences. Usually, a subset of sequences is chosen that defines a variance-balanced design. In a three-period, crossover pharmacokinetic study with Treatments A, B, and C, the six possible sequences

ABC, ACB, BAC, BCA, CAB, and CBA must be included to maintain a carryover-balanced design. If carryover is a concern when the object and precipitant drugs are given together in Treatments B and C, then a large sample size may be required to ensure an adequate number of subjects per sequence to test the carryover effect. A three-period crossover design in which two drugs are given alone and together during the three phases is often used to investigate bidirectional drug interactions. A four-period crossover study would have 4! or 24 possible sequences. However, only four sequences, ABCD, BDAC, CADB, and DCBA, are necessary for a variance- and crossover-balanced study.

There is considerable interest in replicate crossover designs for bioequivalence studies in which the test and reference treatments are administered each on two separate occasions. This allows for assessment of intraindividual variability in systemic exposure and estimation of carryover effects. The analysis of replicate designs considers that some individuals may differ from the mean response and allows for the determination of "individual bioequivalence." Optimal designs for carryover estimation of the two treatments are AA, BB, AB, and BA for two-period designs; ABB and BAA for three-period designs; and AABB, BBAA, ABBA, and BAAB for four-period designs (14–17). Switchback designs, either ABA and BAB or ABAB and BABA, are preferred to estimate the intraindividual variability (14). Similar designs may be employed for drug interaction studies because they increase the confidence that a drug interaction detected is a true interaction and not an expression of intraindividual variability.

Replicate measurements may also be obtained in more traditional study designs. As an example, the object drug may be administered as a multiple-dose regimen, and measurements can be made during more than 1 day or dosing interval before changeover to the next treatment. This was done in a randomized crossover study to investigate the interaction between cimetidine and theophylline (18). Theophylline was administered at a subject-specific dose (concentration controlled) for 23 days. Subjects received Treatment 1 (cimetidine or placebo) on days 5–11, cimetidine/placebo washout on days 12–16, and Treatment 2 (cimetidine or placebo) on days 17–23. Cimetidine and placebo treatments were assigned by a randomized crossover allocation. The pharmacokinetics of theophylline was assessed on the first, fourth, and seventh days of each treatment period. In the analysis, the data from the fourth and seventh days were treated as replicate measurements of the effect at steady state. Because theophylline exhibits large intersubject variability in clearance, doses were adjusted in a run-in phase to provide similar mean steady-state concentrations before evaluating the interaction. This example also shows how concentration control can be incorporated into the design of a drug interaction study.

Randomization codes can be generated for crossover studies using a variety of methods. One suggested method involves equally dividing the subjects into two to four blocks. For example, a study planned for 16 subjects could be divided into four blocks of 4 subjects each or two blocks of 8 subjects each. The number of subjects per block and total sample size should be a multiple of the number of sequences planned. A list of sequences needed (as described earlier in this section) is made, and the list is repeated to provide one sequence entry (row) for each subject based on the planned sample size. Random numbers are then assigned to each entry along with the block label (1, 2, etc.). At this point, there will be three columns: block, sequence, and random number. The entries (rows) are sorted *within each block* in either ascending or descending order, keeping the random numbers and sequence labels together. Finally, subject numbers are added in sequential order (e.g., 01, 02, 03, etc.) in a new column. This procedure will produce a random code that assigns each subject number to a particular treatment sequence. The subject numbers are assigned to individual subjects in the order that they were screened or accepted into the study.

A parallel design may be used for evaluating drug interactions. However, such designs are less desirable, usually because the drug variability is greater between individuals than within individuals. A simple parallel design study consists of two groups of subjects/patients, one group that is receiving the object drug and one that is receiving the object drug concomitantly with the suspected precipitant drug. Most studies of this type are performed in patient populations who are receiving the drug or drugs therapeutically. There may be problems with comparability of the two patient groups in terms of pharmacokinetics of the object drug regardless of the precipitant drug. The two groups may or may not be randomly selected. If random assignment is not used, additional issues of bias must be considered. When studies of this type are necessary, the use of population modeling is recommended for evaluating the presence or absence of the interaction. An example of using population modeling to evaluate a drug interaction involved imipramine and alprazolam *(19)*. The parallel design may be advantageous for drugs with long elimination half-lives in studies in which a long washout period is impractical for a crossover design.

A placebo-controlled, parallel-group study can be conducted when possible inherent group differences in a parallel design or time-dependent effects in a single-sequence longitudinal design are a concern. Subjects in each group receive treatment on more than one occasion, and treatment effects are adjusted for baseline values in the first period of each treatment group. Alternatively, the mean treatment differences are estimated within each group, and then these differences are compared between treatment groups. A placebo-controlled, parallel-group design was used to show no clinically significant effect of indinavir on the pharmacokinetics of voriconazole *(20)* and to demonstrate that ritonavir inhibited the metabolism of rifabutin *(21)*.

Drug interactions may be very complex. The mechanism of potential interaction is important to hypothesize from in vitro studies, previous clinical and preclinical studies, and experience with other related drugs. Such knowledge is essential to planning a good drug interaction study. Most studies are designed to evaluate the effect of a precipitant drug on an object drug. The precipitant drug may cause some physical or physiological effect that alters the pharmacokinetics or pharmacodynamics of the object drug. Several questions need to be posed about the precipitant drug in relation to developing the study methods. What are the doses and administration schedules that are relevant to clinical practice? Is the interaction concentration dependent within the range of clinically achievable concentrations? Does the interaction take time to develop (e.g., P450 induction)? What is the primary goal of the study (e.g., to find the maximum potential interaction)? In limited circumstances, one may be interested in whether the pharmacokinetics or pharmacodynamics of both drugs are affected by concomitant administration.

Multiple dosing of the precipitant drug is often desirable. The object drug may be administered as a single- or multiple-dose regimen designed to achieve steady state. A single dose may be appropriate when inhibition of elimination is suspected and safety concerns are substantial. In such cases, unpredictable accumulation would be avoided. One exception occurs when an object drug undergoes extensive first-pass metabolism, and the precipitant drug inhibits this metabolism. Much greater systemic bioavailability may result even with single-dose administration.

Concerns about multiple-dose studies are exemplified by a study of voriconazole effects on cyclosporine pharmacokinetics. This study included renal transplant patients receiving treatment with cyclosporine, which was continued throughout the study. Subjects received voriconazole or placebo for 7.5 days (Period 1), underwent a washout period of at least 4 days, then received the alternate treatment (voriconazole or placebo) for 7.5 days. Although 14 subjects were entered, only 7 completed the study, and all 7 were withdrawn during the voriconazole treatment. Voriconazole resulted in a mean 1.7-fold increase in cyclosporine exposure *(22)*.

Although a multiple-dose regimen of the object drug may simulate clinical use and provide greater applicability, safety would favor a single-dose study in healthy subjects first. The addition of procedures to limit exposure to high concentrations during the interaction phase for a follow-up multiple-dose study needs to be considered. For example, the study could employ a dose reduction during the combination treatment. More extensive knowledge of the potential study outcomes, frequent and careful clinical monitoring, and perhaps real-time drug concentration monitoring may be necessary when the object drug is administered in a multiple-dose regimen.

Drug interaction studies are most commonly performed in healthy volunteers. Healthy subjects are easier to recruit, the investigators can better control concomitant medications and activities, and study participation may be safer compared to patients with target illnesses. There is no compelling reason why performing a pharmacokinetic interaction study in healthy volunteers is less desirable than performing the study in a target population likely to receive both drugs unless disease effects in the target population influence the magnitude of interaction differently or safety considerations prevent the use of healthy volunteers. The elderly are often cited as a group more susceptible to drug interactions. This is true because elderly patients in general receive more drugs, and interactions only occur when two or more drugs are given concurrently *(23)*. In addition, geriatric patients may eliminate drugs more slowly and therefore achieve higher concentrations than young counterparts. Administering a dose regimen to healthy volunteers that provides serum concentrations and systemic exposure (area under the serum concentration–time curve, AUC) similar to those expected in elderly patients may control the latter factor. The same is true for patients with organ failure, who have reduced drug clearance. However, dose adjustments used for these patients in clinical practice should also be considered.

Interaction studies that involve pharmacodynamic assessments may or may not be best performed in the target population, depending on the nature of the pharmacodynamic effect. Suppose an object drug reduces wheezing and acute bronchospasm and increases forced expiratory volume in 1 second in patients with asthma. Administration of a precipitant drug in combination with the object drug leads to worsening of symptoms and lowering the 1-second forced expiratory volume in asthma patients. However, these effects are not seen in patients without asthma. Such an interaction would need to be studied in the target population.

One report of an interaction between a laxative polymer and digoxin found a pharmacokinetic interaction consistent with a 30% decrease in digoxin absorption. The concluding statement was "there was no consequence of this interaction on heart rate and atrial ventricular conduction." The study was conducted in healthy volunteers and digoxin administration was not associated with changes in atrial ventricular conduction with or without the laxative administration. Although a small decrease in heart rate was noted following digoxin dosing, the laxative did not alter the observed change *(24)*. This study demonstrated the importance of using relevant pharmacodynamic parameters and the importance of the study population. The pharmacodynamic parameter should be a validated surrogate marker and be sensitive to changes in response. Had the study been conduced in patients with atrial fibrillation, changes may have been more apparent. Discussions of specific issues relating to pharmacodynamic drug interactions are beyond the scope of this chapter because the endpoint parameters depend on the pharmacology of the specific drug class and the characteristics of the parameter itself.

## PHARMACOKINETIC INTERACTION STUDIES

### Absorption

Drug interactions may involve absorption or other aspects of drug delivery. This chapter does not address pharmaceutical or physicochemical interactions that occur in vitro or ex vivo, such as incompatibility in intravenous admixtures or interactions that occur within intravenous administration tubes. Drug interactions commonly occur with drugs that are administered orally. Most of these interactions involve the effect of a precipitant drug on gastric pH or physical interactions between the two drugs. If an acidic environment in the stomach is required for optimal dissolution, reduced absorption in the presence of drugs that increase gastric pH may occur. The interaction between acid suppressants (e.g., cimetidine or omeprazole) and ketoconazole or itraconazole are classic examples of this type of interaction *(25,26)*. Interaction studies should be performed for drugs that have greatly reduced solubility at neutral pH compared to pH less than 3.0. One must be careful to provide sufficient doses of the acid suppressant to increase gastric pH to above 6.0 during the absorption period *(27)*. Continuous monitoring of gastric pH is recommended to ensure that the target pH is attained.

Many drugs bind or complex with other drugs, thereby preventing gastrointestinal absorption. Examples of this type of interaction include those between tetracycline and calcium carbonate, ciprofloxacin and aluminum antacids or iron products, and norfloxacin and sucralfate *(28–30)*. These interactions occur when both drugs are present in the stomach and upper gastrointestinal tract at the same time. Maximum interaction usually occurs when the precipitant drug is administered slightly before or at the same time as the object drug *(29)*. Although not well studied, differences in gastric pH, gastric emptying time, and transintestinal secretion of drug may influence the extent of these interactions.

### Distribution

Drug distribution may be affected by drug interactions. However, many studies conclude differences in volume of distribution that represent artifact rather than true differences. Changes in volume of distribution should be examined using intravenous dosing whenever possible. When oral administration is used, apparent changes in volume of distribution may represent changes in bioavailability. Comparisons should be made using steady-state volume of distribution $V_{ss}$ only. Frequently $V_{area}$ (also designated as $V_z$) is used for comparisons. However, this parameter is greatly affected by changes in the terminal elimination rate constant for pharmacokinetic models more complex than models involving monoexponential decay.

Steady-state volume of distribution may also be affected by experimental problems. Suppose a drug is well described using a three-compartment model when administered alone. The same drug is given after 10 days of rifampin treatment, and the clearance is greatly enhanced. Drug concentrations are substantially lower following rifampin treatment, and the profile is best described using a two-compartment model. Presumably, the third exponential phase would remain present, but the concentrations may be undetectable with the assay used. $V_{ss}$ is equal to mean residence time (AUMC/AUC) multiplied by systemic clearance (Cl) for an intravenous bolus dose, where AUMC is the area under the first moment of the plasma concentration–time curve. Although AUC would be decreased and Cl increased as a result of the interaction, these parameters would be affected minimally by missing the third exponential phase. However, the third exponential phase contributes a large portion of the total AUMC for the control treatment. Excluding this phase following rifampin treatment will cause an apparent decrease in the $V_{ss}$. Thus, problems fitting the control and interaction phases to the same model with equal reliability could result in apparent changes in $V_{ss}$ when no true change occurred. Similar problems would occur with noncompartmental analysis, but the problem would not be as apparent.

Examples of drug interactions affecting distribution include the interaction between ceftriaxone and drugs that increase free fatty acid concentrations (e.g., heparin). Free fatty acids displace ceftriaxone from protein binding (31). This interaction is generally not clinically significant because the increased free fraction (microbiologically active drug) results in no change in average steady-state unbound concentrations in plasma even though renal clearance is increased. In general, for orally administered drugs that are highly protein bound, protein displacement interactions may be clinically relevant when the object drug has a narrow therapeutic range, a small volume of distribution (<10 L/70 kg), and long elimination half-life (8,9).

Another potentially significant situation involves parenterally administered drugs that exhibit a high extraction ratio. Here, nearly all of the drug that passes through the organ is removed or metabolized, including both bound and unbound drug. Displacement from protein binding will have no effect on the total clearance of the drug. However, the increased free fraction of drug may result in greater pharmacodynamic activity while the precipitant drug is present. For the interaction to be significant, the object drug must have a narrow therapeutic index so that the increase in free drug concentration will have toxicological significance. Overall, protein-binding displacement interactions are rarely clinically significant.

### Renal Excretion

Changes in renal excretion of drugs can be subdivided into filtration, secretion, and reabsorption. Glomerular filtration of drugs is limited by protein binding, and only unbound drug is filtered. Drug interactions involving displacement of an object drug from serum protein will result in transiently higher unbound serum concentrations and lead to increased renal clearance for object drugs that have a low renal extraction ratio. The clinical significance of protein-binding displacement is somewhat limited by the compensatory increase in renal clearance. Lower total serum concentrations from increased clearance may compensate for the increased free fraction.

Tubular secretion involves active transport of drugs from the serum to the tubular lumen. Separate transport systems are present for acids and bases, but these transport systems have a very low degree of specificity. Precipitant drugs may inhibit tubular secretion, resulting in reduced renal clearance. Drugs that are extensively eliminated in the urine and have significant tubular secretion (renal clearance of free drug greater than 150% of glomerular filtration or high renal extraction ratio) are good candidates for studying this interaction mechanism. The normal glomerular filtration rate (GFR) is about 120 mL/minute, and the renal blood flow is approx 1100 mL/minute for a 70-kg adult. A drug can have a renal clearance approaching renal blood flow rate, as is observed with para-aminohippuric acid owing to its extensive tubular secretion. The partitioning of a drug into red blood cells and the ability to diffuse out of red blood cells may also influence tubular secretion.

Probenecid is an example of a drug that inhibits tubular secretion by competing for the transport system. Probenecid may be administered with certain β-lactam drugs to prolong their elimination rate. The β-lactam agents most affected by this interaction have a high ratio of renal clearance to GFR and rely on the kidney as their major clearance organ. Before penicillin resistance was prevalent, a combination of probenecid and high-dose amoxicillin was used to provide single-dose treatment for uncomplicated gonorrhea *(32)*.

To assess drug interactions involving renal excretion, collection of both urine and plasma (or serum) is required. A measure of the GFR before or during the study is helpful to explore the mechanism of interaction. GFR can be determined by radiolabeled $^{99m}$Tc-diethylenetriamine pentaacetic acid clearance, $^{125}$I-iothalamate clearance, inulin clearance, or creatinine clearance (with concurrent cimetidine treatment) *(33–35)*. Measurement of creatinine clearance also serves as a rough measure of GFR. However, overestimation of GFR is expected owing to a small component of tubular secretion. The tubular secretion of creatinine is sometimes quite large. As cimetidine inhibits the tubular secretion of creatinine, concurrent treatment during urine collection can improve the estimate of GFR *(35)*. Estimates of GFR from serum creatinine have been improved using a new prediction equation *(36)*.

Competitive inhibition of tubular secretion is typically concentration dependent and is influenced by the concentration of the precipitant and object drugs. Concentration-dependent renal clearance of the object drug is established by collecting urine in intervals less than or equal to one half-life duration. Blood samples collected at the beginning and end of each urine collection interval are a minimum requirement, but more blood samples taken during the collection interval will provide a better estimate of plasma AUC. The renal clearance is calculated for each interval and would be expected to increase as drug concentrations (plasma AUC) decline. A precipitant drug may have only minor effect on the renal clearance when concentrations of the object drug are high because saturation may already be present. However, the precipitant drug should prevent the increase in renal clearance seen at low concentrations of the object drug. The precipitant drug must be present in sufficient concentrations through-out the observation period to observe inhibition. Thus, continuous infusion or fre-quent dosing of the precipitant drug may be required unless the half-life of the precipitant drug is long. An interaction study also may be planned using dosing regi-mens likely to be used in clinical practice. However, information about the mecha-nism of interaction may be lost. An assumption usually made in pharmacokinetics is that clearance of the object drug is stable during each assessment period. If there are large differences in peak and trough drug concentrations of the precipitant drug over the period in which the pharmacokinetics of the object drug is assessed, this assump-tion may be violated because the degree of inhibition depends on inhibitor concentra-tion. Information about the mechanism of interaction may also be lost if urine is collected in only one interval to obtain the average renal clearance.

Tubular reabsorption is usually a passive process by which drug present in the tubu-lar lumen (high concentration) diffuses back into the capillary lumen and returns to circulation. The drug must be un-ionized to diffuse across the tubular membrane. Inter-actions occur from altered pH in the tubular lumen or from physical interaction between the precipitant and object drug within the tubular lumen. An independent measure of tubular secretion, filtration, and reabsorption is not possible in the clinical setting. Instead, only the overall renal clearance is measured, and the intrinsic clearance is compared to GFR to classify the elimination as net tubular reabsorption, filtration, or net tubular secretion.

### Metabolism

CYP enzymes metabolize many anti-infective drugs with pharmacokinetics that are affected by drugs that inhibit or induce these enzymes. Several anti-infective agents act as inhibitors (ritonavir, ciprofloxacin, etc.) or inducers (rifampin, rifabutin, etc.) of CYP enzymes. Goals for a metabolism interaction study are important to set. The goal may be to determine if a clinically significant interaction is likely between two drugs or to determine more broadly if a drug serves as a precipitant drug involving a particular enzyme system. The precipitant drug should be administered in a clinically relevant, multiple-dose regimen for sufficient duration to achieve steady-state pharmacokinetic conditions. Longer durations of treatment may be required for time-dependent interac-tions. For example, maximum induction with rifampin takes 10–13 days (37). When no prior knowledge is available, multiple dosing for at least 1 week is usually sufficient. A longitudinal design in which the object drug is studied alone, then following treatment with the precipitant drug is preferred in the absence of prior knowledge about the inter-action offset time. If the offset time is of interest, the object drug may be studied again at various times after the precipitant drug is stopped.

More than 50% of drugs that undergo metabolism are metabolized primarily by CYP3A enzymes. These enzymes are induced by rifampin, rifabutin, phenytoin, car-bamazepine, and barbiturates and are present in the gastrointestinal tract, liver, and other organs. CYP3A4 enzymes are responsible for first-pass metabolism of many drugs, and their inhibition may lead to pronounced increases in systemic bioavailability of orally administered object drugs. Precipitant drugs may induce or inhibit CYP3A4. Candidate object drugs are those that rely on metabolism by CYP3A4 enzymes for a substantial portion of their clearance. Midazolam is an excellent marker of CYP3A4 activity because its elimination depends almost entirely on hydroxylation by the CYP3A subfamily of enzymes to form 1-hydroxy midazolam *(38,39)*.

Drugs that affect CYP3A activity in the gastrointestinal tract or liver may affect the apparent clearance of oral midazolam. *N*-Demethylation of erythromycin is also catabolized by CYP3A, and this metabolism occurs mostly in the liver. The intravenous administration of [$^{14}$C-*N*-methyl]-erythromycin and measurement of $^{14}CO_2$ in breath provides a convenient marker of CYP3A4 activity in the liver (not gastrointestinal tract) *(40–42)*, even though potential limitations of the test have been identified *(43)*. Cortisol is metabolized to 6β-hydroxycortisol by CYP3A4 isozymes. The measurement of urinary 6β-hydroxycortisol/cortisol ratio remains fairly stable without circadian differences. Agents that affect CYP3A4 enzyme activity usually cause changes in the 6β-hydroxycortisol/cortisol ratio *(41,42)*. All of these markers are useful tools to identify induction or inhibition of CYP3A4, even though changes in clearance may not directly correlate among the different markers.

Other common metabolic enzyme pathways involve CYP1A2 and the polymorphic CYP2D6 and CYP2C19 isozymes. Probe drugs are caffeine and theophylline for CYP1A2 *(44,45)*, debrisoquin and dextromethorphan for CYP2D6 *(46)*, and omeprazole and mephenytoin for CYP2C19 activity *(47)*. For caffeine and theophylline, changes in systemic clearance are usually evaluated. The measurement of paraxanthine/caffeine ratio in saliva at 6 hours after caffeine intake also correlates with CYP1A2 activity *(48)*. CYP2D6 activity can be assessed by measuring changes in the dextromethorphan/dextrophan ratio in urine *(46)*. CYP2C19 activity can be evaluated from the urinary *S*-mephenytoin/*R*-mephenytoin ratio after administration of racemic mephenytoin *(49)*.

Markers of CYP isozyme activity are useful to evaluate whether a potential precipitant drug effects metabolism. There is also need to evaluate whether a drug serves as an object drug resulting in toxicity, loss of therapeutic activity, or reduced effectiveness. Agents that are known to inhibit CYP1A2 (cimetidine, enoxacin), CYP3A4 (itraconazole, ketoconazole), CYP2D6 (quinidine, cimetidine), and CYP2C19 (omeprazole, fluconazole) are well known *(50–54)*. However, not all of these drugs have specific effects on only one isozyme. Rifampin, rifabutin, carbamazepine, and phenytoin are inducers of CYP3A4 and other enzymes *(50,51)*. Lists of enzyme inhibitors and enzyme substrates can be found in several publications *(50,52,53)*. Many of the listed drugs are not specific for one enzyme subgroup.

If feasible, active or toxic metabolites in plasma and urine should be measured because the magnitude and direction of metabolite pharmacokinetic changes are often unpredictable. Multiple metabolic enzymes and pathways can confound predictions. The AUC of metabolite may be altered even if the metabolite is not the directly affected pathway. Alterations in metabolite pharmacokinetics do not always translate to measurable effects on AUC of parent drug. Detectable changes in AUC of the parent drug may not be apparent if a minor metabolic pathway is affected or if compensatory changes in hepatic and renal clearance occur. Thus, there is a danger in concluding "no interaction" from data involving only the parent drug. Metabolic parameters such as the metabolic AUC ratio and the urinary recovery ratio of metabolite to parent drug can give useful information on mechanisms of interaction, particularly if the metabolite is eliminated exclusively by renal excretion.

## Other Elimination Pathways

Some drugs are eliminated by fecal excretion and are excreted in bile or by transintestinal secretion. Enterohepatic recycling occurs when drugs are eliminated in bile as conjugates. Deconjugation occurs in the small intestine, thereby allowing for reabsorption of the parent drug. A precipitant drug that interferes with deconjugation will prevent enterohepatic recycling (reabsorption) and increase the apparent clearance. Potential examples of this interaction type involve antibacterial drugs and oral contraceptives *(55)*. Precipitant drugs that physically trap or bind another drug within the gastrointestinal lumen may also enhance the clearance of the object drug. Examples of this interaction include iron salts or aluminum hydroxide with doxycycline *(56,57)* and aluminum hydroxide with temafloxacin *(58)*.

## PHARMACOSTATISTICAL TECHNIQUES

Advances have been made in the past decade to facilitate detection and evaluation of drug interactions. The intent of this section is to focus on the recommended approaches for presenting and analyzing pharmacostatistical drug interaction data. In this section, the terms *test* and *reference* treatments refer to the administration of the object and precipitant drugs in combination (test) and administration of the object drug alone (reference).

There are many approaches, both parametric and nonparametric, to analyzing comparative data from drug interaction studies. The recommended strategy by regulatory agencies in the United States *(10)* and Europe *(59,60)*, editors of clinical pharmacology journals *(61,62)*, and others *(63,64)* is to adapt the confidence interval approach used in average bioequivalence studies *(14,65)*. The purpose of a bioequivalence or comparative bioavailability study is to demonstrate that the shape and magnitude of blood or plasma concentration–time profiles produced by the drug formulations under study are sufficiently alike that therapeutic equivalence can be assumed. In drug interaction studies, the aim is usually to show that an interaction is not clinically meaningful by the similarity of concentration–time profiles or other pharmacokinetic characteristics. In traditional analysis, the null hypothesis stipulates that parameters for the object drug are equivalent for the test and reference treatment. When a significant difference is found, the null hypothesis would be rejected, and a difference would be concluded. A small, clinically unimportant difference may be statistically significant at the 5% level of significance ($\alpha = 0.05$).

The lack of significance does not necessarily imply no interaction. In such cases, the statistical power, or probability of detecting a specified difference, must be considered. The specified difference should be a change that would be considered clinically important given the available pharmacodynamic and toxicological information. A large, clinically important difference between treatments may not be statistically significant if sample size is small and within- and between-individual pharmacokinetic variability is large. Therefore, classical statistical approaches that attempt to confirm an interaction by rejecting the null hypothesis of no difference are inappropriate because the consumer risk is not controlled.

An alternative approach is required that adequately defines the risk to the consumer. Because a drug–drug interaction consists of different drug treatments, one should test the null hypothesis of nonequivalence by demonstrating equivalence or lack of pharmacokinetic interaction, as first proposed by Steinijans et al. *(66).* In this manner, the risk to the patient of a clinically relevant interaction can be defined within established limits.

Two important assessment criteria must be defined before invoking the equivalence approach: (1) the range of clinically acceptable variation in pharmacokinetic response of the affected drug and (2) the risk to the consumer of incorrectly concluding a "lack of pharmacokinetic interaction." The range of clinically acceptable variation defines the equivalence range (clinical no-effect boundary). The range can be determined from population (group) average dose or concentration–response relationships, pharmacokinetic and pharmacodynamic models, and other available information for the object drug *(10).* The consumer risk is the Type I or "$\alpha$ error" in statistics and is usually set at 5%.

The equivalence method is based on the two one-sided *t*-test procedures of rejecting the interval hypotheses that the test/reference ratio is less than the lower equivalence limit and greater than the upper equivalence limit. At the 5% level of consumer risk, this procedure is operationally identical to the method of declaring equivalence (or lack of interaction) if the shortest 90% confidence interval for the ratio is entirely within the prespecified equivalence range. More generally, the $100 \times (1 - 2\alpha)\%$ confidence limits around the ratio (test/reference) of the means or medians of the test and reference treatments constrain the consumer risk to $100 \times (\alpha)\%$ as well as indicate the precision of a negative outcome. In bioequivalence studies, the accepted equivalence range is ±20%, which corresponds to a lower limit of 80% and an upper limit of 120% for original data or 125% for logarithmic transformed data. A range of ±20% seems reasonable to assess product quality, but for drug interactions these limits may be wider or narrower depending on the patient population and the therapeutic index and pharmacokinetic variability of the object drug. For example, a range of clinically acceptable variation of 30% for changes in zidovudine AUC was suggested *(67),* whereas a range variation of 50% for changes in indinavir AUC was proposed *(68).* No dose adjustment is required if the confidence interval falls within the no-effect boundary, and the boundary does not have to be symmetrical around the mean difference on the original or logarithmic scales *(10,69).* Equivalence limits of the form ($\theta$, 1/$\theta$) have been proposed for data on both the original and logarithmic scales *(70).*

Statistical inferences are made on either absolute (Test – Reference) or relative (Test/Reference) differences in the arithmetic means, geometric means (from logarithmic transformed data), harmonic means (from reciprocal transformed data), or medians of pharmacokinetic variables. Parametric analysis of variance (ANOVA) models appropriate for the study design are used to test differences in means, and nonparametric methods such as the Wilcoxon rank sum test or Wilcoxon signed rank test are used to test differences in medians. If the study design is unbalanced from an unequal number of subjects in each sequence (crossover) or from missing data, then assessments are based on least-squares means. Because clinicians prefer to think in terms of relative rather than absolute changes, pharmacokinetic differences are usually expressed as a ratio.

Confidence limits around these mean differences (mean ratios) for within-subject comparisons in crossover studies and between-group comparisons in parallel studies are constructed from the residual mean-square error (MSE) term in ANOVA. The

ANOVA provides exact confidence limits for relative differences of geometric means if the distribution of variables is truly lognormal. Only approximate limits for relative differences of arithmetic means are possible because ANOVA ignores variability in the reference mean unless Fieller's theorem is applied *(71)*. Nonparametric approximate 90% confidence limits can be calculated for two-period, two-sequence crossover studies *(72)*. One should be cautious in concluding no interaction when approximate confidence limits generated from parametric or nonparametric techniques are within but near the equivalence limits. Also, inferences on mean data may not reflect how certain individuals in the study population respond to the interaction. A particular strata of individuals may show an apparent interaction even though the overall mean data indicate no pharmacokinetic interaction.

### Logarithmic Transformation of Pharmacokinetic Variables

All pharmacokinetic variables, except those such as $t_{max}$ that depend on discreet sampling times, are logarithmically transformed before ANOVA *(14,66,73)*. Harmonic means have been proposed for inferences on half-life *(74)*. Transformation converts a multiplicative model to an additive model, which is the basis of ANOVA [ln(Test/Reference) = ln(Test) − ln(Reference)]. Decisions on $t_{max}$ are best handled by nonparametric analysis. Most pharmacokinetic data have positively skewed distributions created by the truncation of these quantities at zero and have variances that depend on the mean. Transformation reduces the skewness and brings the distribution of data closer to normal. However, the main reason for transforming the data is to stabilize or make equal the within-subject (crossover study) or between-group (parallel study) variance and not to normalize the between-subject parameters *(73)*. Another advantage of transformation is that it is the best way to handle ratios for relative or proportional differences, and calculation of the associated confidence limits is straightforward.

For most studies, the outcome will not change regardless of whether the original or log scale is used. There are two instances when conclusions can be opposite in a within-subject design *(73)*. If certain subjects with larger-than-average responses show larger-than-expected absolute differences, variability is increased on the original scale, whereas larger-than-expected absolute differences for smaller-than-average responses are expanded on the log scale. If this occurs, for example, when fast and slow metabolizers are studied together, then the within-subject variability and the relative mean changes can be different on the two scales.

### Crossover Design and Analysis of Variance

The ANOVA for a crossover design includes the effects of sequence, subject within sequence, treatment, period, and, except for the 2, 2, 2 design, carryover. All effects except the sequence effect are tested by the MSE term. The sequence effect is tested against the subject-within-sequence effect. Any subgroup comparison of fixed effects (e.g., males and females) is tested with the subject mean-square term.

The sequence effect measures the differences between the groups of subjects defined by their sequence. In statistical parlance, this effect is known as the treatment-by-period interaction, which is a measure of the differential effect of the treatment (Test − Reference) in each of the periods. In the 2, 2, 2 design, the sequence effect is caused by three confounded sources: (1) a difference between subjects in the two sequences (i.e., group effects), (2) an unequal carryover of one treatment into the next period compared to the other treatment, and (3) a treatment-by-period interaction.

The period effect measures the differences between study periods. This effect is known as the treatment-by-sequence interaction, which is a measure of the differential effect of the treatment in each of the sequences. The period effect can be caused by equal carryover in each sequence from period to period, bias in analytical data if samples in each period were analyzed in different batches, differences in the study environment or procedures, and changes with time in stage of disease.

The period-by-sequence interaction represents the direct treatment effect if no differential carryover effects are present. The estimate of treatment differences will not be biased if a period effect is present.

The MSE term is a measure of the intrasubject variability and is usually converted to a coefficient of variation $CV_W$ to estimate the consistency of the magnitude of interaction among the subjects *(75)*. The $CV_W$ is estimated as $100\% \times (e^{MSE} - 1)^{1/2}$ for logarithmic transformed data and as $100\% \times (MSE)^{1/2}/Y$ for original data, where $Y$ is either the least-squares mean of the reference treatment or the grand mean of the two least-squares treatment means under comparison.

The goal of any within-subjects design is to minimize the $CV_W$. The interaction is considered highly variable for a particular pharmacokinetic parameter if the $CV_W$ is >25%. The $CV_W$ is a very informative parameter but is rarely reported in the literature. Values for a number of drugs orally administered in crossover bioequivalence studies have been tabulated by Steinijans et al. *(76)*. The $CV_W$ is important to know because the width of the confidence interval around the difference of treatment means, the calculation of *post hoc* power to detect these differences, and an estimation of sample sizes for planning future interaction studies is directly related to this value.

There are a number of sources of variation in $CV_W$: the true intrasubject pharmacokinetic variation exhibited by a single person, analytical variability (measurement errors), within-batch variation in manufacture of the drug formulation, nonadherence to the medications, and the random subject-by-treatment interaction. This last source is caused by random variability of treatments within subjects or within identifiable subgroups of the population studied. Each individual may behave differently to the test treatment, or subjects in subgroups may show similar variation within subgroups but different responses to the test treatment among subgroups. An example could be smokers responding differently from nonsmokers to one of the treatments. On the log scale, the random subject-by-treatment interaction is minimized if all subjects show the same relative change in the same direction.

## Sample Size and Post Hoc Power Calculations

The sample size of the study needs to be planned with consideration of the purpose of the study. If the purpose of the study is to evaluate a potential drug interaction that is suspected based on preliminary data, the sample size can be somewhat conservative. However, if the goal is to demonstrate the lack of interaction for an individual drug when a member of the same drug class exhibits the interaction (class labeling), then the sample size should be larger.

Estimations of sample size for a within-subject drug interaction study require a knowledge of $CV_w$ for the interaction. These values may be greater than those reported for drugs in bioequivalence studies *(76)* because not all subjects will respond to the precipitant drug to the same degree. Tables of sample sizes for 2, 2, 2 crossover designs to attain a power of 80 or 90% at the 5% nominal level for a given $CV_w$ and expected relative difference in treatment medians or means are published for the multiplicative (logarithmic) model with equivalence ranges of 0.7–1.43 *(77)*, 0.8–1.25 *(70,78)*, and 0.9–1.11 *(77)*. Similar tables are published for the additive (original) model *(79)* and for parallel designs *(70,80)*. The minor influence of the between-subject coefficient of variability on sample size estimates for the 2, 2, 2 crossover design is demonstrated in ref. *70*.

*Post hoc* power calculations are useful for negative studies to estimate differences that can be detected with a certain power (usually 80% at the 5% significance level) or to estimate the power of the study to detect a specified difference (usually 20% of reference at the 5% significance level). These calculations require an estimation of the standard error of the difference in mean or medians. General equations for point hypothesis testing for original and logarithmic data using a central *t*-distribution are provided in refs. *71* and *81*. General equations for interval hypothesis testing using a noncentral *t*-distribution for crossover and parallel designs are given in refs. *70* and *71*.

## PHARMACOKINETIC METRICS AND CHARACTERISTICS

The major assumptions in bioequivalence are that the Cl of the drug under investigation is constant over the course of the study, and that AUC is a pure characteristic of extent of bioavailability *F*. In drug interactions, both clearance and bioavailability can change after oral administration. Therefore, changes in AUC can result from alterations in either parameter. Schall et al. *(82)* proposed the terminal elimination half-life $t_{1/2,z}$ and the ratio of $AUC/t_{1/2,z}$ as characteristics for Cl and *F*, respectively, in drug–drug interaction studies. Assuming a constant volume of distribution, an increase in Cl will decrease $t_{1/2,z}$, and an increase in the ratio of $AUC/t_{1/2,z}$ suggests an increase in *F*. In single-dose bioequivalence studies, both AUC from time of dosing to the time of last measurable sample $t_z$ ($AUC_{0-tz}$) and $AUC_{0-tz}$ extrapolated to infinity ($AUC_{0-\infty}$) are used as metrics to characterize *F* because $t_{1/2,z}$ is assumed to be unaffected by changes in only *F*. However, if $t_{1/2z}$ changes from drug interactions, then only $AUC_{0-\infty}$ should be used to characterize drug exposure because changes in $AUC_{0-tz}$ and $AUC_{0-\infty}$ may not be proportional.

Because AUC is a composite characteristic of Cl and *F* and peak drug concentrations ($C_{max}$) reflect both rate and extent of absorption assuming a constant volume of distribution, there are recommendations that these metrics be expressed in terms of drug exposure *(83)*. AUC is the ideal metric for total systemic drug exposure, and $C_{max}$ is a measure of peak systemic exposure. The term *drug exposure* conveys more clinical relevance than the term *rate and extent of drug absorption* because drug safety and effectiveness are concerns in drug interaction studies.

## PRESENTATION AND INTERPRETATION
## OF DRUG INTERACTION DATA

There are generally three ways to present comparative pharmacokinetic data for changes in the test treatment relative to the reference treatment: (1) a test/reference ratio expressed as a percentage; (2) an $x$-fold change, where $x$ is the test/reference ratio; or (3) a percentage change [(Test/Reference ratio – 1) × 100%]. For example, an AUC ratio of 200% indicates a twofold increase and a 100% increase in AUC. Often, $x$-fold changes are confused with percentage change, and the reader needs to be aware of which method of calculation was used.

Current thinking favors expressing the results in terms of a test/reference geometric mean ratio and the corresponding 90% confidence limits for AUC and $C_{max}$ parameters. A search for formal clinical drug interaction studies of anti-infective medications over the period 2001–2003 (assessed January 6, 2004, via Medline) found 23 published studies. Only five (22%) of these studies provided 90% confidence limits and used bioequivalence testing. It is important not to confuse reporting of 95% confidence limits with 90% confidence limits. The former bounds will be wider and may lead to different conclusions in equivalence testing. Reporting the 95% confidence limits is another way of reporting a test of significance at the 5% level of significance. For example, AUC of bosentan increased 2.1-fold (95% confidence interval 1.5–2.7) after concomitant administration with ketoconazole *(84)*. The 95% confidence interval would be examined to determine if it includes the value 1.0, and if not, as in this case, a statistically significant interaction at the 5% level of significance ($p < 0.05$) would be concluded.

The no-effect boundary or acceptable range needs to be established *a priori*. If a drug interaction is concluded, the clinical significance of the interaction and recommendations on how to mange the interaction need to be formulated. The Food and Drug Administration guidance for metabolic interaction studies allows three approaches for developing a no-effect boundary. The first approach is to describe the range of the selected exposure parameters over a range of doses that are normally used. The sponsor should include information on dose or concentration–response studies or pharmacokinetic/pharmacodynamic models to support the recommendation. If the exposure parameters remain within this range in the presence of a potential precipitant drug, the sponsor could conclude that no interaction is expected. The second approach requires a replicate study design and addresses the question of switchability. This approach involves assessment of individual bioequivalence rather than average bioequivalence. Studies employing this second approach for a drug interaction study have not been published. The third approach defaults to bioequivalence criteria when the 90% confidence interval for geometric mean exposure parameter ratio (Test/Reference) falls within 80 to 125% *(10)*. This last approach is most commonly used.

The use of bioequivalence criteria should eliminate a substantial portion of studies that statistically conclude a drug interaction when only small, clinically insignificant differences occur. As an example, digoxin steady-state AUC was 25.5 ng·hour/mL after digoxin alone and 23.9 ng·hour/mL after digoxin plus zaleplon (a hypnotic agent). From a test of significance (ANOVA, $p = 0.018$), a drug interaction would have been concluded. The geometric mean ratio (Test/Reference) was 93%, with a 90% confidence interval of 89 to 98%, and this would more appropriately lead to a no-effect conclusion *(85)*. Potential problems with the bioequivalence approach include too small sample size and high variability. If the sample size is too small, confidence intervals tend to be wide, and this could result in a 90% confidence interval that falls outside the no-effect boundary despite a mean ratio near 100%. Too large of a sample size with the bioequivalence approach does not cause adverse consequences other than excessive study costs. For tests of significance, too small of a sample size will lead to low power and inability to detect an important drug interaction, and too large of a study population may cause detection of small, clinically insignificant changes.

Not only does the no-effect boundary need to be established *a priori*, use of unconventional ranges needs to be justified. In a study evaluating the effect of montelukast on digoxin, several problems are apparent. The authors used a no-effect boundary of 70–143% without appropriate justification. Digoxin exhibits a narrow therapeutic index and relatively low variability in exposure parameters in a healthy population. The mean digoxin $AUC_{0-\infty}$ was 43.2 ng·hour/mL for digoxin alone and 39.2 ng·hour/mL for digoxin plus montelukast. Although the 90% confidence interval for $AUC_{0-\infty}$ was 70–118%, the authors concluded that montelukast has no effect on the pharmacokinetics of digoxin *(86)*. The use of this expanded no-effect boundary for a drug with a narrow therapeutic index is concerning. Moreover, the 90% confidence interval is too wide to fit within the range of 80–125%. The study involved a small sample size ($n = 10$) and did not address power.

In another study, which evaluated the effects of proton pump inhibitors on theophylline, the no-effect boundary was expanded to 70–143% for steady-state $C_{max}$ but not for steady-state AUC *(87)*. There is no pharmacokinetic basis to suspect a change in rate of absorption of theophylline from acid suppression, and the reason for the expanded boundary was not addressed. Because the observed 90% confidence limit for steady-state $C_{max}$ fell within the range of 80–125%, conclusions remain appropriate. In some cases involving drugs (e.g., ethionamide) with moderate-to-high variability in exposure parameters, it may be difficult to obtain 90% confidence intervals that fall within the usual no-effect boundaries, requiring the use of large sample sizes or expanded boundaries *(88)*.

An example of a study that used an expanded no-effect boundary and provided justification involved interactions between didanosine and indinavir, ketoconazole, and ciprofloxacin *(89)*. A no-effect boundary of 75–133% was used. The authors cited a study in which the AUC of indinavir was increased 29% with clarithromycin administration, and the interaction was concluded to be not clinically significant. For ciprofloxacin, the authors cited the package insert and a publication and considered that a 48% increase in ciprofloxacin AUC in elderly subjects did not result in a recommendation for reducing the dose. For ketoconazole, the authors cited a study that reported a 59% increase in ketoconazole AUC when administered with food compared to fasting and considered that the labeling did not contain a recommendation for administering ketoconazole with food *(89)*. In another study, in which ketoconazole significantly increased the exposure of desloratadine, the interaction was concluded to be not clinically relevant as no changes in electrocardiogram parameters were observed *(90)*. Although such observation does not totally rule out clinical significance in special populations, the value of concomitant pharmacodynamic assessment is apparent.

Another potential area of misinterpretation is when the doses or dosing intervals of the drug under investigation are different in the test and reference arms of the study. This may occur if the purpose is to obtain equivalent drug exposures over a specified time period in the absence and presence of an interacting drug. The magnitude of pharmacokinetic effect can appear smaller or larger if the control dose is larger or smaller.

For example, 800 mg indinavir every 8 hours was estimated to give about the same AUC over 24 hours as 400 mg indinavir every 12 hours in the presence of 400 mg ritonavir every 12 hours *(91)*. From single-dose indinavir data, the magnitude of the interaction was actually about a fivefold increase in AUC if 400 mg indinavir was used as the reference *(91)*. Depending on the purpose of the study, the analysis should be based on dose-normalized or dose-independent parameters (e.g., clearance or AUC/ dose) for drugs that display linear pharmacokinetics, and the reporting should reflect the actual differences in these parameters to avoid misinterpretation.

Many issues remain to be resolved concerning optimal design of drug interaction studies. Traditional issues such as defining the research hypothesis (question of interest); determining the appropriate study population (healthy volunteers or patients); determining the study design (crossover, longitudinal, or parallel; washout requirements; etc.); deciding between single dose or steady state; and deciding which pharmacokinetic or pharmacodynamic endpoints to evaluate, should depend on knowledge of the drugs involved, preliminary data on the potential interaction, and general knowledge of pharmacokinetics and drug interactions. Defining whether a drug interaction exists is now considered an equivalence problem in which endpoints are compared between the object drug given with and without the precipitant drug. The acceptable clinical no-effect boundary associated with equivalence must be somewhat flexible depending on the therapeutic index of the object drug and variability of the endpoints. The use of replicate designs improves the ability to examine carryover, reduces the required sample size, and allows determination of intrasubject variability in the interaction. However, studies involving replicate treatments are more expensive, and the analysis is more complex. Although replicate designs are used for bioequivalence studies and are widely discussed, such designs are not uniformly accepted as a promising new standard in drug interaction studies.

## REFERENCES

1. Ekins S. Past, present, and future applications of precision–cut liver slices for in vitro xenobiotic metabolism. Drug Metabol Rev 1996;28:591–623.
2. Decker CJ, Laitinen LM, Bridson GW, Raybuck SA, Tung RD, Chaturvedi PR. Metabolism of amprenavir in liver microsomes: role of CYP3A4 inhibition for drug interactions. J Pharm Sci 1998;87:803–807.
3. Bonnabry P, Sievering J, Leemann T, Dayer P. Quantitative drug interactions prediction system (Q–DIPS): a computer-based prediction and management support system for drug metabolism interactions. Eur J Clin Pharmacol 1999;55:341–347.
4. Rodrigues AD, Wong SL. Application of human liver microsomes in metabolism-based drug–drug interactions: in vitro–in vivo correlations and the Abbott Laboratories experience. Adv Pharmacol 1997;43:65–101.
5. Koudriakova T, Iatsimirskaia E, Utkin I, et al. Metabolism of the human immunodeficiency virus protease inhibitors indinavir and ritonavir by human intestinal microsomes and expressed cytochrome P4503A4/3A5: mechanism-based inactivation of cytochrome P4503A by ritonavir. Drug Metab Dispos 1998;26:552–561.
6. Hochman JH, Yamazaki M, Ohe T, Lin JH. Evaluation of drug interactions with P-glycoprotein in drug discovery: in vitro assessment of the potential for drug–drug interactions with P-glycoprotein. Curr Drug Metab 2002;3:257–273.
7. Benet LZ, Cummins CL, Wu CY. Transporter-enzyme interactions: implications for predicting drug–drug interactions from in vitro data. Curr Drug Metab 2003;4:393–398.

8. Rolan PE. Plasma protein binding displacement interactions–why are they still regarded as clinically important? Br J Clin Pharmacol 1994;37:125–128.

9. Sansom LN, Evans AM. What is the true clinical significance of plasma protein binding displacement interactions? Drug Safety 1995;12:227–233.

10. Guidance for Industry. In vivo drug metabolism/drug interaction studies—study design, data analysis, and recommendations for dosing and labeling. November 1999. US Department of Health and Human Services, Food and Drug Administration. Center for Drug Evaluation and Research, Center for Biologics Evaluation and Research.

11. Therapeutic Products Programme Guidance Document. Drug–drug interactions: studies in vitro and in vivo. September 21, 2000. Therapeutic Products Directorate, Health Canada.

12. Bjornsson TD, Callaghan JT, Einolf HJ, et al. The conduct of in vitro and in vivo drug–drug interaction studies: a Pharmaceutical Research and Manufacturers of America (PhRMA) perspective. Drug Metab Dispos 2003;31:815–832.

13. Gallicano KD, Sahai J, Shukla VK, et al. Induction of zidovudine glucuronidation and amination pathways by rifampicin in HIV-infected patients. Br J Clin Pharmacol 1999;48: 168–179.

14. Ormsby E. Statistical methods in bioequivalence. In: Jackson AJ, ed. Generics and Bioequivalence. Boca Raton, FL: CRC Press, 1994, pp. 1–27.

15. Fleiss JL. A critique of recent research on the two-treatment crossover design. Controlled Clin Trials 1989;10:237–243.

16. Vuorinen J. A practical approach for the assessment of bioequivalence under selected higher-order cross-over design. Statist Med 1997;16:2229–2243.

17. Chow SC, Liu JP. On assessment of bioequivalence under a higher-order crossover design. J Biopharm Stat 1992;2:239–256.

18. Nix DE, Di Cicco RA, Miller AK, et al. The effect of low-dose cimetidine (200 mg twice daily) on the pharmacokinetics of theophylline. J. Clin Pharmacol 1999;39:855–865.

19. Grasela TH Jr, Antal EJ, Ereshefsky L, Wells BG, Evans RL, Smith RB. An evaluation of population pharmacokinetics in therapeutic trials. Part II. Detection of a drug–drug interaction. Clin Pharmacol Ther 1987;42:433–441.

20. Purkins L, Wood N, Kleinermans D, Love ER. No clinically significant pharmacokinetic interactions between voriconazole and indinavir in healthy volunteers. Br J Clin Pharmacol 2003;56:62–68.

21. Cato A, Cavanaugh J, Shi H, Hsu A, Leonard J, Granneman R. The effect of multiple doses of ritonavir on the pharmacokinetics of rifabutin. Clin Pharmacol Ther 1998;63: 414–421.

22. Romero AJ, Pogamp PL, Nilsson LG, Wood N. Effect of voriconazole on the pharmacokinetics of cyclosporine in renal transplant patients. Clin Pharmacol Ther 2002;71: 226–234.

23. Cadieux RJ. Drug interactions in the elderly. How multiple drug use increases risk exponentially. Postgrad Med 1989;86:179–186.

24. Ragueneau I, Poirier JM, Radembino N, Sao AB, Funck-Brentano C, Jaillon P. Pharmacokinetic and pharmacodynamic drug interactions between digoxin and macrogol 4000, a laxative polymer, in healthy volunteers. Br J Clin Pharmacol 1999;48:453–456.

25. Piscitelli SC, Goss TF, Wilton JH, D'Andrea DT, Goldstein H, Schentag JJ. Effects of ranitidine and sucralfate on ketoconazole bioavailability. Antimicrob Agents Chemother 1991;35:1765–1771.

26. Blum RA, D'Andrea DT, Florentino BM, et al. Increased gastric pH and the bioavailability of fluconazole and ketoconazole. Ann Intern Med 1991;114:755–757.

27. Lebsack ME, Nix D, Ryerson B, et al. Effect of gastric acidity on enoxacin absorption. Clin Pharmacol Ther 1992;52:252–256.

28. Lehto P, Kivisto KT, Neuvonen PJ. The effect of ferrous sulphate on the absorption of norfloxacin, ciprofloxacin and ofloxacin. Br J Clin Pharmacol 1994;37:82–85.

29. Nix DE, Watson WA, Lener ME, et al. Effects of aluminum and magnesium antacids and ranitidine on the absorption of ciprofloxacin. Clin Pharmacol Ther 1989;46:700–705.

30. Parpia SH, Nix DE, Hejmanowski LG, Goldstein HR, Wilton JH, Schentag JJ. Sucralfate reduces the gastrointestinal absorption of norfloxacin. Antimicrob Agents Chemother 1989;33:99–102.

31. Jungbluth GL, Pasko MT, Beam TR, Jusko WJ. Ceftriaxone disposition in open-heart surgery patients. Antimicrob Agents Chemother 1989;33:850–856.

32. Megran DW, Lefebvre K, Willetts V, Bowie WR. Single–dose oral cefixime vs amoxicillin plus probenecid for the treatment of uncomplicated gonorrhea in men. Antimicrob Agents Chemother 1990;34:355–357.

33. Gaspari F, Perico N, Remuzzi G. Measurement of glomerular filtration rate. Kidney Int 1997;63(suppl):S151–S154.

34. Brochner-Mortensen J. Current status on assessment and measurement of glomerular filtration rate. Clin Physiol 1985;5:1–17.

35. Hellerstein S, Berenbom M, Alon US, Warady BA. Creatinine clearance following cimetidine for estimation of glomerular filtration rate. Pediatr Nephrol 1998;12:49–54.

36. Levey AS, Bosch JP, Breyer-Lewis J, Greene T, Rogers N, Roth D. A more accurate method to estimate glomerular filtration rate from serum creatinine: a new prediction equation. Ann Intern Med 1999;130:461–470.

37. Baciewicz AM, Self TH. Rifampin drug interactions. Arch Intern Med 1984;144:1667–1671.

38. Wandel C, Bocker R, Bohrer H, Browne A, Rugheimer E, Martin E. Midazolam is metabolized by at least three different cytochrome P450 enzymes. Br J Anaesth 1994;73: 658–661.

39. Thummel KE, Shen DD, Podoll TD, et al. Use of midazolam as a human cytochrome P450 3A probe: II. Characterization of inter- and intraindividual hepatic CYP3A variability after liver transplantation. J Pharmacol Exper Ther 1994;271:557–566.

40. Lown KS, Thummel KE, Benedict PE, et al. The erythromycin breath test predicts the clearance of midazolam. Clin Pharmacol Ther 1995;57:16–24.

41. Watkins PB, Turgeon DK, Saenger P, et al. Comparison of urinary 6-β-cortisol and the erythromycin breath test as measures of hepatic P450IIIA (CYP3A) activity. Clin Pharmacol Ther 1992;52:265–273.

42. Hunt, CM, Watkins, PB, Saenger P, et al. Heterogeneity of CYP3A isoforms metabolizing erythromycin and cortisol. Clin Pharmacol Ther 1992;51:18–23.

43. Chiou WL, Jeong HY, Wu TC, Ma C. Use of the erthromycin breath test for in vivo assessments of cytochrome P4503A activity. Clin Pharmacol Ther 2001;70:305–310.

44. Sarkar MA, Jackson BJ. Theophylline N-demethylations as probes for P4501A1 and P4501A2. Drug Metab Dispos 1994;22:827–834.

45. Ziebell J, Shaw-Stiffel T. Update on the use of metabolic probes to quantify liver function: caffeine vs lidocaine. Digest Dis 1995;13:239–250.

46. Anthony LB, Boeve TJ, Hande KR. Cytochrome P-450IID6 phenotyping in cancer patients: debrisoquin and dextromethorphan as probes. Cancer Chemother Pharmacol 1995;36:125–128.

47. Flockhart DA. Drug interactions and the cytochrome P450 system. The role of cytochrome P450 2C19. Clin Pharmacokin 1995;29(suppl 1):45–52.

48. Fuhr U, Rost KL, Engelhardt R, et al. Evaluation of caffeine as a test drug for CYP1A2, NAT2 and CYP2E1 phenotyping in man by in vivo vs in vitro correlations. Pharmacogenetics 1996;6:159–176.

49. Brockmoller J, Rost KL, Gross D, Schenkel A, Roots I. Phenotyping of CYP2C19 with enantiospecific HPLC–quantification of *R*- and *S*-mephenytoin and comparison with the intron4/exon5 G→A-splice site mutation. Pharmacogenetics 1995;5:80–88.

50. Tanaka E. Clinically important pharmacokinetic drug–drug interactions: role of cytochrome P450 enzymes. J Clin Pharm Ther 1998;23:403–416.

51. Lomaestro BM, Piatek MA. Update on drug interactions with azole antifungal agents. Ann Pharmacother 1998;32:915–928.
52. Caraco Y. Genetic determinants of drug responsiveness and drug interactions. Ther Drug Monitor 1998;20:517–524.
53. Shannon M. Drug–drug interactions and the cytochrome P450 system: an update. Pediatr Emerg Care 1997;13:350–353.
54. Guengerich FP. Role of cytochrome P450 enzymes in drug–drug interactions. Adv Pharmacol 1997;43:7–35.
55. Zachariasen RD. Loss of oral contraceptive efficacy by concurrent antibiotic administration. Women Health 1994;22:17–26.
56. Nguyen VX, Nix DE, Gillikin S, Schentag JJ. Effect of oral antacid administration on the pharmacokinetics of intravenous doxycycline. Antimicrob Agents Chemother 1989;33: 434–436.
57. Neuvonen PJ, Penttila O. Effect of oral ferrous sulphate on the half–life of doxycycline in man. Eur J Clin Pharmacol 1974;7:361–363.
58. Sorgel F, Granneman GR, Mahr G, Kujath P, Fabian W, Nickel P. Hepatobiliary elimination of temafloxacin. Clin Pharmacokin 1992;22(suppl 1):33–42.
59. Note for Guidance on the Investigation of Drug Interactions. December 1997. Committee for Proprietary Medicinal Products (CPMP), the European Agency for the Evaluation of Medicinal Products Human Medicines Evaluation Unit.
60. Müller HJ, Gundert-Remy U. The regulatory view on drug-drug interactions. Int J Clin Pharmacol Ther 1994;32:269–273.
61. Hitzenberger G, Steinijans VW. To reject or not to reject recent experience with bioequivalence papers. Int J Clin Pharmacol Ther 1994;32:161–164.
62. Waller PC, Jackson PR, Tucker GT, Ramsay LE. Clinical pharmacology with confidence. Br J Clin Pharmacol 1994;37:309–310.
63. Fuhr U, Weiss M, Kroemer HK, et al. Systematic screening for pharmacokinetic interactions during drug development. Int J Clin Pharmacol Ther 1996;34:139–151.
64. Kuhlmann J. Drug interaction studies during drug development: which, when, how? Int J Clin Pharmacol Ther 1994;32:305–311.
65. Pidgen AW. Statistical aspects of bioequivalence—a review. Xenobiotica 1992;22:881–893.
66. Steinijans VW, Hartmanns M, Huber R, Radtke HW. Lack of pharmacokinetic interaction as an equivalence problem. Int J Clin Pharmacol Ther Toxicol 1991;29:323–328.
67. Gallicano KD, Sahai J, Swick L, Seguin I, Pakuts A, Cameron DW. Effect of rifabutin on the pharmacokinetics of zidovudine in patients infected with human immunodeficiency virus. Clin Infect Dis 1995;21:1008–1011.
68. De Wit S, Debier M, De Smet M, et al. Effect of fluconazole on indinavir pharmacokinetics in human immunodeficiency virus-infected patients. Antimicrob Agents Chemother 1998;42:223–227.
69. Huang S-M, Lesko LJ, Williams RL. Assessment of the quality and quantity of drug–drug interaction studies in recent NDA submissions: study design and data analysis issues. J Clin Pharmacol 1999;39:1006–1014.
70. Hauschke D, Kieser M, Diletti E, Burke M. Sample size determination for proving equivalence based on the ratio of two means for normally distributed data. Statist Med 1999; 18:93–105.
71. Chow S-C, Liu J-P, eds. Design and Analysis of Bioavailability and Bioequivalence Studies. 2nd Ed. New York, NY: Marcel Dekker, 2000.
72. Wijnand HP. Some nonparametric confidence intervals are non-informative, notably in bioequivalence studies. Clin Research Reg Affairs 1996;13:65–75.
73. Midha KK, Ormsby ED, Hubbard JW, et al. Logarithmic transformation in bioequivalence: application with two formulations of perphenazine. J Pharm Sci 1993;82:138–144.

74. Roe DJ, Karol MD. Averaging pharmacokinetic parameter estimates from experimental studies: statistical theory and application. J Pharmaceut Sci 1997;86:621–624.

75. Hauschke D, Steinijans VW, Diletti E, et al. Presentation of the intrasubject coefficient of variation for sample size planning in bioequivalence studies. Int J Clin Pharmacol Ther 1994;32:376–378.

76. Steinijans VW, Sauter R, Hauschke D, et al. Reference tables for the intrasubject coefficient of variation in bioequivalence studies. Int J Clin Pharmacol Ther 1995;33:427–430.

77. Diletti E, Hauschke D, Steinijans VW. Sample size determination: extended tables for the multiplicative model and bioequivalence ranges of 0.9 to 1.11 and 0.7 to 1.43. Int J Clin Pharmacol Ther Tox 1992;8:287–290.

78. Hauschke D, Steinijans VW, Diletti E, Burke M. Sample size determination for bioequivalence assessment using a multiplicative model. J Pharmacokin Biopharm 1992; 20:557–561.

79. Lui, J-P, Chow S-C. Sample size determination for the two one-sided tests procedure in bioequivalence. J Pharmacokin Biopharm 1992;20:101–104.

80. Chow SC, Wang H. On sample size calculation in bioequivalence studies. J Pharmacokin Pharmacodyn 2001;28:155–169.

81. Gallicano K, Sahai J, Zaror-Behrens G, Pakuts A. Effect of antacids in didanosine tablet on bioavailability of isoniazid. Antimicrob Agents Chemother 1994;38:894–897.

82. Schall R, Hundt HKL, Luus HG. Pharmacokinetic characteristics for extent of absorption and clearance in drug/drug interaction studies. Int J Clin Pharmacol Ther 1994;32: 633–637.

83. Tozer TN, Bois FY, Hauck WW, Chen M-L, Williams RL. Absorption rate vs exposure: which is more useful for bioequivalence testing? Pharm Res 1996;13:453–456.

84. van Giersbergen PL, Halabi A, Dingemanse J. Single and multiple dose pharmacokinetics of bosentan and its interaction with ketoconazole. Br J Clin Pharmacol 2002;53: 589–595.

85. Sanchez GarcRa P, Paty I, Leister CA, et al. Effect of zaleplon on digoxin pharmacokinetics and pharmacodynamics. Am J Health-Syst Pharm 2000;57:2267–2270.

86. Depré M, Van Hecken A, Verbesselt R, et al. Effect of multiple doses of montelukast, a CysLT1 receptor antagonist, on digoxin pharmacokinetics in healthy volunteers. J Clin Pharmacol 1999;39:941–944.

87. Dilger K, Zheng Z, Klotz U. Lack of drug interaction between omeprazole, lansoprazole, pantoprazole and theophylline. Br J Clin Pharmacol 1999;48:438–444.

88. Auclair B, Nix DE, Adam RD, James GT, Peloquin CA. Pharmacokinetics of ethionamide administered under fasting conditions or with orange juice, food, or antacids. Antimicrob Agents Chemother 2001;45:810–814.

89. Damle BD, Mammaneni V, Kaul S, Knupp C. Lack of effect of simultaneously administered didanosine encapsulated enteric bead formulation (Videx EC) on oral absorption of indinavir, ketoconazole, or ciprofloxacin. Antimicrob Agents Chemother 2002; 46:385–391.

90. Banfield C, Herron J, Keung A, Padhi D, Affrime M. Desloratadine has no clinically relevant electrocardiographic or pharmacodynamic interactions with ketoconazole. Clin Pharmacokinetics 2002;41(suppl 1):37–44.

91. Hsu A, Granneman GR, Cao G, et al. Pharmacokinetic interaction between ritonavir and indinavir in healthy volunteers. Antimicrob Agents Chemother 1998;42:2784–2791.

# Index